D0392522

GENDER AND PTSD

Gender and PTSD

Edited by

RACHEL KIMERLING
PAIGE OUIMETTE
JESSICA WOLFE

THE GUILFORD PRESS
New York   London

Library of Congress Cataloging-in-Publication Data

Gender and PTSD / edited by Rachel Kimerling, Paige Ouimette, Jessica Wolfe.
    p. cm.
Includes bibliographical references and index.
  ISBN 1-57230-783-8
  1. Post-traumatic stress disorder. 2. Women—Mental health. I. Kimerling, Rachel. II. Ouimette, Paige. III. Wolfe, Jessica, 1950–
  RC552.P67 G46 2002
  616.85′21—dc21

                          2002008924

About the Editors

Rachel Kimerling, PhD, is a psychologist at the VA Palo Alto Healthcare System and the Clinical Laboratory and Education Division of the National Center for PTSD. She is also Assistant Professor at the Pacific Graduate School of Psychology in Palo Alto, California. She was formerly Assistant Adjunct Professor in the Department of Psychiatry at the University of California, San Francisco, where she conducted PTSD research at San Francisco General Hospital. Dr. Kimerling is interested in the detection, prevention, and treatment of PTSD in health care settings.

Paige Ouimette, PhD, is Associate Professor of Psychology at Washington State University (WSU). Prior to WSU, she was a Research Associate at the Center for Health Care Evaluation at the VA Palo Alto Healthcare System and Consulting Assistant Professor of Psychiatry and Behavioral Sciences at Stanford University School of Medicine. Her research addresses PTSD and comorbid conditions in clinical settings. Dr. Ouimette maintains a clinical practice in Pullman, Washington.

Jessica Wolfe, PhD, MPH, is Clinical Instructor in Psychiatry, Harvard Medical School, and Associate Professor of Psychiatry, Boston University School of Medicine. She founded the Women's Health Sciences Division of the VA's National Center for PTSD and cofounded the Boston University School of Medicine Center for Excellence in Women's Health.

Contributors

Sudie E. Back, MA, Center for Drug and Alcohol Programs, Department of Psychiatry and Behavioral Sciences, Medical University of South Carolina, Charleston, South Carolina

Mary C. Blehar, PhD, Women's Mental Health Program, National Institute of Mental Health, Bethesda, Maryland

Kathleen T. Brady, PhD, Center for Drug and Alcohol Programs, Department of Psychiatry and Behavioral Sciences, Medical University of South Carolina, Charleston, South Carolina

Pamela J. Brown, PhD, Private Practice and Department of Psychiatry and Human Behavior, Brown University, Providence, Rhode Island

Todd C. Buckley, PhD, Psychology Service, VA Boston Healthcare System/Boston University School of Medicine, Boston, Massachusetts

Christina A. Byrne, PhD, Department of Psychology, Western Washington University, Bellingham, Washington

Dana Cason, PhD, Columbia, South Carolina

Marylene Cloitre, PhD, Anxiety and Traumatic Stress Program, Payne Whitney Clinic, and Department of Psychiatry, Weill Medical College of Cornell University, New York Presbyterian Hospital, New York, New York

Gretchen Clum, PhD, Department of Psychology, University of Missouri–St. Louis, St. Louis, Missouri

Karen Cusack, PhD, Trauma Initiative, South Carolina Department of Mental Health, Charleston, South Carolina

Bruce Cuthbert, PhD, Adult Psychopathology and Prevention Research Branch, Division of Mental Disorders, Behavioral Research and AIDS, National Institute of Mental Health, Bethesda, Maryland

Michael de Arellano, PhD, National Crime Victims Research and Treatment Center, Department of Psychiatry and Behavioral Sciences, Medical University of South Carolina, Charleston, South Carolina

Anne P. DePrince, PhD, Department of Psychology, University of Denver, Denver, Colorado

Ruth R. DeRosa, PhD, North Shore University Hospital, Manhasset, New York, and Family Therapy Institute of Suffolk, Smithtown, New York

Sherry Falsetti, PhD, National Crime Victims Research and Treatment Center, Department of Psychiatry and Behavioral Sciences, Medical University of South Carolina, Charleston, South Carolina

Edna B. Foa, PhD, Center for the Treatment and Study of Anxiety, University of Pennsylvania School of Medicine, Philadelphia, Pennsylvania

Jennifer J. Freyd, PhD, Department of Psychology, University of Oregon, Eugene, Oregon

Matthew J. Friedman, MD, National Center for PTSD, VA Medical and Regional Office Center, White River Junction, Vermont, and Departments of Psychiatry and Pharmacology, Dartmouth Medical School, Hanover, New Hampshire

Jennifer D. Foster, MA, Department of Psychology, Georgia State University, Atlanta, Georgia

Kim L. Gratz, MS, Department of Psychology, University of Massachusetts, Boston, Massachusetts

Anouk Grubaugh, MA, Center for Trauma Recovery, University of Missouri–St. Louis, St. Louis, Missouri

Charity Hammond, BA, National Center for PTSD, Women's Health Sciences Division, VA Boston Healthcare System, Boston, Massachusetts; present address: Department of Psychology, University of Georgia, Athens, Georgia

Matthew Jakupcak, MS, Department of Psychology, University of Massachusetts, Boston, Massachusetts

Terence M. Keane, PhD, Psychology Service, VA Boston Healthcare System/Boston University School of Medicine, Boston, Massachusetts

Rachel Kimerling, PhD, VA Palo Alto Healthcare System, National Center for PTSD, and Pacific Graduate School of Psychology, Palo Alto, California

Daniel W. King, PhD, National Center for PTSD and Boston University School of Medicine, Boston, Massachusetts

Lynda A. King, PhD, National Center for PTSD and Boston University School of Medicine, Boston, Massachusetts

Karestan C. Koenen, PhD, Psychiatric Epidemiology Program, School of Public Health, Columbia University, New York, New York

Elizabeth D. Krause, MA, Department of Psychology: Social and Health Sciences, Duke University, Durham, North Carolina

Kathryn M. Magruder, PhD, Department of Psychiatry and Behavioral Sciences, Medical University of South Carolina, Charleston, South Carolina

Joy McQuery, MD, Department of Psychiatry, Cambridge Hospital, Cambridge, Massachusetts

Tamara L. Newton, PhD, Department of Psychological and Brain Sciences, University of Louisville, Louisville, Kentucky

Fran H. Norris, PhD, Department of Psychology, Georgia State University, Atlanta, Georgia

Holly K. Orcutt, PhD, Department of Psychology, Northern Illinois University, DeKalb, Illinois

Susan M. Orsillo, PhD, National Center for PTSD, Women's Health Sciences Division, VA Boston Healthcare System/Boston University, Boston, Massachusetts

Paige Ouimette, PhD, Department of Psychology, Washington State University, Pullman, Washington

Jessica M. Peirce, PhD, Department of Psychiatry, Johns Hopkins University School of Medicine, Baltimore, Maryland

Sheela Raja, PhD, Hines VA Medical Center and Psychology Service, Department of Veterans Affairs, Edward Hines Jr. Hospital, Hines, Illinois

Ann M. Rasmusson, MD, VA National Center for PTSD, West Haven, Connecticut, and Department of Psychiatry, Yale University School of Medicine, New Haven, Connecticut

Patricia Resick, PhD, Center for Trauma Recovery, University of Missouri–St. Louis, St. Louis, Missouri

David S. Riggs, PhD, Center for the Treatment and Study of Anxiety, University of Pennsylvania School of Medicine, Philadelphia, Pennsylvania

Susan Roth, PhD, Department of Psychology: Social and Health Sciences, Duke University, Durham, North Carolina

Paula P. Schnurr, PhD, National Center for PTSD, VA Medical and Regional Office Center, White River Junction, Vermont, and Department of Psychiatry, Dartmouth Medical School, Hanover, New Hampshire

Sherry H. Stewart, PhD, Departments of Psychology, Psychiatry, and Community Health and Epidemiology, Dalhousie University, Halifax, Nova Scotia, Canada

David F. Tolin, PhD, Anxiety Disorders Center, The Institute of Living, Hartford, Connecticut

Deborah L. Weisshaar, MA, Department of Psychology, Georgia State University, Atlanta, Georgia

Preface

Current conceptualizations of posttraumatic stress disorder (PTSD) arose from two major groups of clinical observations. Terms such as "war neurosis" and "shellshock" were derived to describe the stress reactions observed among veterans of combat, while the constellation of symptoms known as "rape trauma syndrome" developed from mental health and advocacy work with survivors of sexual assault. Because most combat veterans have been male, and sexual assault survivors presenting in treatment settings have been predominantly female, these early conceptualizations of what we now call PTSD resulted with inherently gendered concepts. In other words, the construct of PTSD has been shaped by judgments regarding gender from the very beginning, though gender has been implicit, rather than explicit, in the way the construct has been shaped.

To say that gender is important to the construct of PTSD makes sense. Biological differences between men and women may moderate the impact of trauma exposure and the expression of PTSD symptoms. Gender is also a major factor in the type of trauma exposure experienced by the individual, the social relationships that mediate the impact of exposure, and the systems of meaning into which the traumatic event is encoded. To tease apart the specific effects of sex and gender in the prevalence, etiology, assessment, diagnosis, and treatment of PTSD may be impossible. However, awareness and consideration of gender issues in research and service delivery can only enhance our understanding of this disorder and our abilities to help traumatized individuals. This book is intended for this purpose. It is a foundation for understanding a gender-based analysis of the PTSD literature and the resulting implications for treatment and research.

The chapters presented here are not merely intended to catalogue sex-based differences observed between men and women with PTSD. Instead, this volume seeks to examine existing research on PTSD through a gender-based perspective. This distinction is substantive: to document the way in which trauma-exposed men and women are different and the ways in which they are the same would serve only a descriptive purpose, and be of little value to our efforts to prevent and treat PTSD. Such a narrow focus excludes the complex and powerful influences of social, cultural, and economic contexts on behavior. Ultimately we must work toward explanatory models that can account for the social, cultural, and economic processes that create a context in which men and women are exposed to different forms of traumatic stress, experience different social responses following exposure, and see different outcomes. Therefore, we conceptualize gender differences as an interaction between biologically based sex differences and the individual's social context. This framework accounts for intragender diversity as well as differences between genders by assuming that gender differences are context-dependent. That is, the extent to which men and women differ may be more pronounced in some situations and among some populations than others. The factors that describe these gender differences are important cues to the social, cultural, or psychological structures that create different experiences for men and women in society and in mental health treatment. Identification of these factors as they relate to PTSD will bolster our ability to provide effective services by helping us to tailor assessment, diagnosis, and treatment to the realities of the patients we serve.

One of the most notable gender issues in PTSD is its epidemiology: the disorder is found among women at approximately twice the rate as in men. We therefore begin this book with an investigation of the epidemiology of PTSD. The extent to which these gender differences in prevalence rates vary across age, ethnicity, and culture, and occur in more and less developed nations, will yield inferences regarding important factors that influence the relationship between gender and PTSD. The remaining chapters in Part I investigate etiological factors that might explain these gender differences. Chapter 2 explores biologically based sex differences in relation to the neurobiology of PTSD. This chapter addresses an essential question—are there sex-based differences in neurobiological stress-response pathways that would contribute to a vulnerability for PTSD?—including the complex issues of the menstrual cycle and women's reproductive status. Since early research in social psychology established empirical support for the Schachter–Singer theory of emotion, we have known that social factors can mediate the effect of biologically based sensations on behavior and emotion by means of cognitive processing. Chapter 3 explores the ways in which the cognitive processing of traumatic events might further help to explain gender-based differential vulnerabilities to PTSD. Chapter 4 explores similar issues with an emphasis on interpersonal trauma and the ways in which socially defined familial roles and gender roles have an impact on close relationships and the cognitive processing of traumatic events that occur within these relationships.

A necessary adjunct to an investigation of gender issues relevant to the etiology of PTSD is an examination of the diagnostic category itself, and how we decide which individuals do or do not meet criteria. This line of inquiry is consistent with a longstanding concern among health professionals who treat a variety of health and mental health disorders—namely, that treatment for women may be based on a male model, or that some conditions are manifested differently in women and men. Certain clinical characteristics associated with trauma exposure are significantly more common in women than men. For example, since the publication of Judith Herman's influential book *Trauma and Recovery*, clinicians and researchers have grappled with the difficulties in applying the PTSD construct to individuals who experience prolonged and chronic exposure to trauma or present with an onset of symptoms in childhood. As a result, we are posed with difficult questions: Does the PTSD construct fit women less well than men, or are women more likely to meet criteria for another syndrome following trauma, an elaborated or complex PTSD? Chapter 5 addresses these difficult questions in the differential diagnosis of PTSD. The remaining two chapters in Part II focus on issues of gender in the assessment of PTSD. Comprehensive assessment of PTSD can involve a structured diagnostic interview, psychometric evaluation, or psychobiological evaluation. Chapter 6 reviews diagnostic interviews and psychometric instruments that assess exposure to trauma and PTSD. The authors explore the generalizability of measures with limited psychometric data from women and minorities, and the utility of measures developed specifically for either males or females. Chapter 7 analyzes gender differences in psychophysiology studies of PTSD in an effort to sharpen assessment paradigms and the interpretation of these data with men and women.

Part III addresses men's and women's distinctive comorbid symptoms and degree of comorbid pathology. Chapters explore psychiatric comorbidity with PTSD, the complex gender differences in the comorbidity between PTSD and substance use disorders, and medical comorbidity with PTSD. Comorbid conditions such as these increase an individual's risk for functional impairment and treatment failure. Gender differences in comorbid conditions may have multiple determinants. For example, Chapter 5 notes that when PTSD is overlooked in women patients, these women are likely to be diagnosed with multiple Axis I disorders instead. These data suggest a possible diagnostic bias whereby symptoms resulting from trauma exposure that are more common among women than men, or expressed differently in women than men, are less likely to be conceptualized as hallmark symptoms of traumatic stress and labeled as comorbid diagnoses. Such a bias would overpathologize women exposed to trauma with excess diagnoses of Axis I and Axis II disorders. One way to read these chapters on comorbidity, then, is as informing the "goodness of fit" for our current construct of PTSD in women. However, significant portions of the literature in each of these chapters suggest that some gender differences, such as those in rates of major depression or medical morbidity, where we expect a higher prevalence among women than men, are attenuated by trauma exposure. In these cases, the authors' discussions of data that find genders more similar than different still yield important information regarding gender issues in PTSD. Finally, Chapter 9, on substance use disorders (SUDs), describes the importance of incorporating gender into case formulations for trauma patients even when comorbid symptoms are similar. In this population, the etiology of PTSD-SUD comorbidity differs for men and women, and these differences hold important treatment implications. This section highlights the context-dependent nature of gender differences and the importance that awareness of clinical characteristics associated with gender can play in diagnosis and treatment.

The issue of gender is relatively unexplored with respect to the treatment of PTSD. The authors in Part IV review PTSD treatment to determine our effectiveness in treating both men and women. Given that gender issues have an impact on so many aspects of traumatic stress, their relevance to the treatment of PTSD is important to explore. Chapter 11 explores the efficacy and effectiveness of PTSD treatment. The treatment outcome literature suggests that different types of treatment are indicated for women and for men. Furthermore, the effect sizes found in this treatment literature suggest that our most efficacious treatments may be those developed for women. The pharmacotherapy literature, reviewed in Chapter 12, suggests that women may evidence a more robust response to certain types of drug treatment than men, although premenopausal women may differ from postmenopausal women. Because genders differ in the types of trauma exposure, in the meaning ascribed to traumatic events, and potentially in treatment outcomes, two chapters in this section explore whether the content and process of psychotherapy are different for men and women. Chapter 13 explores themes in individual psychotherapy in an analysis of qualitative treatment data, and Chapter 14 reviews indications for couple and family therapy.

As noted in each of the literature reviews in this book, there is a dearth of data in many areas of the trauma literature that directly compare women and men. Precisely because of the inherent gendered nature of PTSD, appropriate research designs for sex-based comparisons are particularly difficult to achieve. As a result, more research is needed before we can make comprehensive and definitive statements about assessment, treatment, and service delivery. Such research would make a critical contribution to improving the gender sensitivity of our efforts to prevent and treat PTSD.

In Part V we focus on efforts to galvanize further work in this area. The book therefore concludes with two important chapters regarding future directions in research and policy. Chapter 15 reviews research methods for investigating gender differences, and Chapter 16 completes the volume with a discussion of the relevance of gender issues in PTSD for health policy and suggestions for future research.

This book is only the beginning of efforts to achieve an awareness of gender in PTSD research and clinical activities. The chapters provide important, data-based information on the diagnosis, assessment, and treatment of PTSD. As much as each chapter illuminates important gender issues and clinical implications, each chapter also highlights how much remains to be learned about gender and PTSD. Difficult and complex questions arise regarding the research methods, clinical techniques, and policies that can be used to address gender issues in PTSD. Addressing these unanswered questions is a formidable, but essential, task. However, it is important to recognize that considerable knowledge has been amassed in the field of traumatic stress. When revisited, this knowledge base can be tremendously useful to clinicians, researchers, and administrators who want to use an awareness of gender issues to improve the effectiveness of their work with trauma-exposed populations.

RACHEL KIMERLING

Acknowledgments

Each of these chapters represents a remarkable effort from the authors, and the results represent an important and novel lens through which to understand the PTSD literature. We extend heartfelt thanks and admiration to each of the contributors. In addition, we thank the many other individuals who were essential to the preparation of this book. The impetus for this undertaking was born from the ideas and enthusiasm of John Wilson. Advice from Terence Keane, Mary Koss, and Rudolf Moos was much appreciated and helped shape the conceptualization of this book. Constance Dahlenberg, Cheryl Hankin, Mardi Horowitz, Laura Mayorga, Rudolf Moos, and Judith Stewart shared their expertise as reviewers for these chapters. Rachel Kimerling thanks Alessandra Rellini and Shannon Mullen, who were indispensable in kindly offering their editorial assistance. Paige Ouimette thanks Rudolf Moos for support and guidance while working on this book at the Center for Health Care Evaluation at the Veterans Affairs Palo Alto Health Care System in Menlo Park. Last, our personal thanks and recognition to Terence Keane and Matthew Friedman of the Department of Veterans Affairs National Center for PTSD, pioneers and continuous supporters of all work in this increasingly important field.

RACHEL KIMERLING
PAIGE OUIMETTE
JESSICA WOLFE

Contents

Part I | Etiology

1 | The Epidemiology of Sex Differences in PTSD across Developmental, Societal, and Research Contexts

FRAN H. NORRIS
JENNIFER D. FOSTER
DEBORAH L. WEISSHAAR

In this chapter, we review the epidemiological evidence regarding sex differences in posttraumatic stress disorder (PTSD). Our primary goal is to determine how consistent or inconsistent these differences are across developmental (youth vs. adults vs. older adults), societal ("Western"/developed vs. non-Western/developing), and research contexts (general population vs. disaster-stricken vs. violence-torn). Because of our focus on gender differences, we included a study in our review only if the investigators sampled both sexes and compared male and female exposure or vulnerability to trauma. We also limited our review to studies that have examined the distribution or impact of trauma in community-dwelling samples. Issues and findings regarding clinical, service-seeking, military, or professional (e.g., firefighters) samples may be very different. Despite this limitation, our review is reasonably comprehensive because three different types of community samples (or research contexts) are considered. Each may have different implications for gender effects. Whereas the first context, general population research, provides normative (and typically lifetime) data, the latter two contexts represent situations in which levels of trauma are unusually and presently high. In the case of disasters, the onset of the trauma is sudden and acute, but in the case of political or community violence, the onset is less well defined and the course is more chronic. The boundary between these last two contexts is not always clear, but the distinction generally works for our purposes.

Within each research context, we first review evidence regarding sex differences in exposure and then in effects. In each section, we begin with studies of adult populations in "Western" or developed countries; often, these studies compose the bulk of the literature and have shaped mainstream thought. We then review studies of youth and older adults in those same countries, followed by studies conducted in non-Western or developing countries. Assignment of areas of the world to the dichotomy of Western/developed versus non-Western/developing countries was not without ambiguity. We placed research conducted in the United States (including Puerto Rico), Canada, western Europe, Australia, and New Zealand in the former category, and studies conducted in Latin America, eastern Europe, Asia, and the Middle East (except for Israel) in the latter. We recognize that our comparative conclusions sometimes stand on shaky empirical ground. First, in most studies of trauma, developmental stage and cohort are hopelessly confounded. This confound could be especially important for interpreting the influence of age on gender effects, because the last three decades have witnessed considerable social change with regard to gender roles, at least in the United States and similar countries. Second, there are still relatively few studies from non-Western or developing countries in the published literature, especially given our reliance on English language journals. The studies we describe are illustrative, not exhaustive.

Because of our attention both to context and to distinctions between exposure and effects, this chapter is more detailed, complex, and longer than it would otherwise have been. So we should perhaps begin by explaining why we believed these distinctions might be important to consider in our review. Epidemiological studies usually have a descriptive rather than an explanatory purpose. With only a few exceptions, specific studies describe differences between men and women but do not, and really cannot, say much about the reasons for these differences. Current conceptualizations pertaining to gender and PTSD run the gamut from biological to psychological to social to cultural. Each is as capable as the next of explaining the most general observation that women typically show higher rates of PTSD than men. However, these perspectives may be able to differentially explain patterns of findings that vary (or do not) across developmental, cultural, or research contexts. For example, if the sexes differ to about the same degree regardless of participants' culture, conclusions regarding the relative etiological importance of biological versus cultural mechanisms should be different from conclusions that would be reached if the sexes differ only in certain cultural contexts.

Similarly, we thought it would be useful to distinguish sex differences in objective exposure from those in subjective experience and in symptom outcomes. This sequence corresponds to the criteria for PTSD outlined in the fourth edition of the *Diagnostic and Statistical Manual of Mental Disorders* (DSM-IV; American Psychiatric Association, 1994). The distinction between event (A1) and subjective experience of the event (A2) is new in DSM-IV, and still relatively few published studies have considered its diagnostic implications. Of most relevance here is the question of when in this sequence sex differences arise. Identifying this point could have implications for both theory development and intervention efforts. For example, one might draw very different etiological conclusions if sex-linked risk for PTSD can be explained by sex differences in the frequency or nature of trauma exposure than if it occurs later in the process. This is a critical issue, because epidemiological studies of the general population show that men and women do tend to experience different types of trauma. Only a few studies have been large enough to test for differences in conditional risk (i.e., risk given exposure) with type of trauma held constant. This is another reason to include studies of communities in which the trauma is shared. Studies of disaster, war, and community violence tell us little about the overall frequency or impact of trauma in the population but are better able to hold timing and type of stress constant. Thus, for example, if women are more at risk for PTSD than men only or primarily because of their greater risk for sexual violence, sex differences should be minimal in disaster studies in which this is not a factor.

We conclude this chapter by considering implications of the observed patterns for theory, research, and intervention. However, we offer our conclusions as "food for thought" rather than as the final word on such matters. More importantly, we hoped to identify gaps in the research base and to inspire others to sharpen their own conceptualizations of gender effects and, in so doing, to begin to make theory-based, a priori predictions about when sex differences should be observed and when they should not. Most importantly, our goal is to describe the accumulated database with sufficient objectivity and detail, so that it is useful to researchers regardless of their own theoretical bent. In this regard, our intent is to let the facts speak for themselves.

SEX DIFFERENCES IN THE GENERAL POPULATION

Methodology

In the last decade, an explosion of interest in the epidemiology of trauma has resulted in dramatic progress in knowledge of the distribution and impact of traumatic events in the population. We need to attend, at least briefly, to the methodological changes that have occurred along the way. Epidemiological studies of the general population usually rely on structured diagnostic inventories designed for use by lay interviewers. Despite the recency of the research on PTSD, we are clearly in our third generation of these measures, perhaps even our fourth. First-generation measures, perhaps unavoidably, were flawed. The PTSD module included in the Diagnostic Interview Schedule (DIS) for DSM-III assessed symptoms of posttraumatic stress and then probed for the causal event. The Epidemiologic Catchment Area Survey, which used this module, yielded unreliably low estimates of PTSD and little data about trauma itself (Davidson, Hughes, Blazer, & George, 1991; Helzer, Robins, & McEvoy, 1987). The second generation of measures, primarily DIS for DSM-III-R, began with a single-item screen providing examples of unusually stressful events that sometimes happen to people. Respondents were asked whether these or similar events had ever happened to them and, if so, were asked about criterion symptoms that followed the worst and up to three of the events. Studies that used these measures (e.g., Breslau, Davis, Andreski, & Peterson, 1991) appear to have yielded quite reliable estimates of the prevalence of PTSD but to have underestimated the prevalence of potentially traumatic events and overestimated the conditional risk for PTSD associated with particular events. Third-generation measures replaced single-item screens with more detailed event inventories. Studies using these measures, most notably the National Comorbidity Survey (NCS; Kessler, Sonnega, Bromet, Hughes, & Nelson, 1995), yielded overall prevalence estimates of PTSD that were quite similar to those provided by second-generation measures. However, they yielded higher rates of trauma exposure and, accordingly, lower rates of conditional risk (PTSD rates given exposure). Because symptom questions are anchored to the worst event, estimates of conditional risk remain biased. The Detroit Area Survey of Trauma (Breslau et al., 1998) may have inaugurated a fourth generation of measures. This study employed an expanded version of the PTSD module from the Composite International Diagnostic Interview (CIDI 2.1; World Health Organization, 1993) that corrects for the reporting of multiple traumas associated with the same occasion and provides estimates of PTSD for both the worst event and a randomly selected event, thereby providing unbiased estimates of conditional risk. This module is very long and complex, but as computerized interviewing becomes more common, it may become the standard for epidemiological assessment in the field.

Interpretation of the database emerging over time is further complicated by changes in the diagnostic criteria for PTSD. The changes from DSM-III to DSM-III-R were relatively minor, but the changes from DSM-III-R to DSM-IV were significant from an epidemiological perspective. With DSM-IV, the conceptualization of the qualifying event shifted from one that is beyond the realm of normal experience to one that is experienced with helplessness, terror, or horror (the A2 criterion). Furthermore, a new criterion (F) was added, which states that the event must cause significant distress or functional impairment. Prevalence rates made on the basis of DSM-IV criteria are expected to be lower than those based on DSM-III-R criteria (Breslau, 1998).

We now summarize results from various epidemiological studies. For estimating sex differences in exposure to trauma and conditional risk for PTSD associated with particular events, we rely most heavily on studies that have used third- or fourth-generation measures (i.e., event inventories rather than single-item screens). For estimating sex differences in the overall prevalence of PTSD, results from second-generation measures are included as well. Although we do not include studies that used first-generation measures, we acknowledge their pioneering contributions to the field by identifying the complex issues surrounding the measurement of trauma and PTSD.

Exposure: Sex Differences in Prevalence and Types of Trauma

Studies of Adults in Western/Developed Societies

The NCS (Kessler et al., 1995) provided our only estimates to date based on a nationwide probability sample of adult residents of the United States. Over 2,800 men and 3,000 women, ages 15–54, were interviewed in their homes and asked about 12 specific types of trauma, such as life-threatening accident, sexual assault, sexual molestation, witnessing, fire/disaster, combat, or physical assault. Previous studies had prompted a new understanding of trauma as frequent rather than rare (e.g., 69% in Norris, 1992; 69% in Resnick, Kilpatrick, Dansky, Saunders, & Best, 1993), but this study made the point unequivocally: 61% of men and 51% of women (a significant difference) reported at least one traumatic event during their lives. More women than men reported sexual molestation, sexual assault, and child abuse, but more men than women reported fire/disaster, life-threatening accident, physical assault, combat, being threatened with a weapon, and being held captive. Using an expanded inventory of qualifying events, Breslau et al. (1998) found an even higher lifetime prevalence of exposure (90%) in the Detroit Area Survey of Trauma, in which approximately 2,200 adults ages 18–45 were randomly selected and interviewed by telephone. Men reported an average of 5.3 distinct traumatic events, and women 4.3, a significant difference. More women than men reported rape and sexual assault, but more men than women reported being threatened with a weapon, being shot or stabbed, or being badly beaten up. More men than women experienced other forms of injury or shock, such as accidents or fires, as well. Men and women differed little in their reports of secondary trauma experienced because of traumatic events in the lives of others or the unexpected death of a loved one. Similarly, Stein, Walker, Hazen, and Forde's (1997) telephone survey of 1,000 randomly selected Canadian adults yielded prevalence rates for lifetime exposure of 74% of women and 81% of men, with more men (55%) than women (46%) experiencing multiple events. Comparable results emerged in an ethnically diverse sample of 1,500 randomly selected residents of New Zealand, ages 18–90, interviewed by phone (Flett, Kazantzis, Long, MacDonald, & Millar, 2000). Overall, 49% of women and 55% of men had experienced at least one event. Women were more likely than men to report sexual assault (both in adulthood and childhood), domestic violence, and sudden death of a loved one, and men were more likely than women to report motor vehicle accidents, other serious accidents, physical assault, and robbery.

Other studies, although less representative, have nonetheless replicated the finding that men are more exposed to trauma than women. Norris (1992) studied 1,000 adults ages 18–90, selected purposively rather than randomly across sex (50% female), age (33% each young, middle-aged, and older adults), race (50% black or African American), and city (25% each from four cities in the southeast United States). She found overall lifetime prevalence rates for exposure of 74% of men and 65% of women; these rates did not include Hurricane Hugo, which had struck two of the studied cities the year before the data were collected. In contrast to the lifetime rates, past-year rates did not differ between men (19.5%) and women (22.4%), suggesting that the differential risk associated with males accumulates over time or occurs earlier in life. (We later return to this point.) Consistent with other studies, over the course of their lives, more men than women had experienced physical assault, motor vehicle crashes, and combat, whereas more women than men had experienced sexual assault or molestation. Men and women were equally likely to have been robbed or bereaved, or to have experienced a fire or other disaster. Breslau, Davis, and Andreski (1995) studied the occurrence of events over a 3-year period in a prospective study of almost 1,000 randomly selected young adult members of a health maintenance organization (HMO) in the Detroit metropolitan area. The difference between men and women in exposure rates for the 3-year period did not reach, but approached, statistical significance, with men scoring higher, suggesting, as did Norris's results, that either the differential risk associated with males accumulates gradually or lessens with age. Vrana and Lauterbach (1994) studied 440 undergraduates selected from a introductory psychology subject pool. These students averaged 20 years of age, with a range from 17 to 49 years. Despite being young, 84% of the sample had experienced at least one of the listed events and, again, men averaged more events than women. More men than women reported accidents, life threats, fire, witnessing, and combat. More women than men reported rape and sexual abuse. Finally, in a study of nearly 1,000 Israeli students, averaging 24 years of age, Amir and Sol (1999) found an overall prevalence rate of 67%, with men again averaging more events than women, especially from exposure to military trauma. Women were more likely to experience sexual assault than men and equally as likely to have experienced the sudden death of a loved one or a terrorist attack.

Studies of Youth in Western/Developed Societies

As expected, fewer studies have examined prevalence of trauma in adolescent samples, and the list narrows further when we restrict inclusion to third-generation measures. Boney-McCoy and Finkelhor (1995) conducted an important study of interpersonal violence in a national random telephone sample of 1,042 boys and 958 girls ages 10–16. Completed incidents were reported by 26% of the girls and 44% of the boys. When attempted victimizations are added, these rates increase to 33% and 47%, respectively. Consistent with the adult literature, more boys than girls had experienced physical assaults, and more girls than boys had experienced sexual assaults. Roughly 15 months later, these same young people were reinterviewed (Boney-McCoy & Finkelhor, 1996). Over the interim, 20% of the girls and 22% of the boys had experienced one of the studied events. Once again, it appears that the difference between males and females in exposure to trauma is less evident when the reporting period is short. Similarly, Kilpatrick and Saunders (1999) assessed prevalence of victimization in a random telephone sample of 4,023 adolescents ages 12–17. Boys had significantly higher lifetime prevalence rates of physical assault and witnessing violence (21%, 44% among boys; 13%, 35% among girls), girls had significantly higher rates of sexual assault (13% among girls; 3% for boys), and boys and girls had equal rates of exposure to physically abusive punishment (8.5% for boys; 10.2% for girls). Singer, Anglin, Song, and Lunghofer (1995) likewise found boys to be more exposed to violence than girls in their sample of 3,735 youth ages 14–19 from six public schools in three cities. Exceptions were victimization at home and sexual assault and abuse.

Perkonigg and Wittchen (1999) presented the only study we identified that examined traumatic events other than violence (e.g., serious accidents, sudden deaths of loved ones) in a sample that included a high proportion of adolescents. These investigators interviewed over 3,000 persons ages 14–24 in metropolitan Munich, Germany. They used the CIDI and DSM-IV criteria. Before Criterion A2 was taken into account, the prevalence of exposure was 25% for males and 18% for females. More males than females reported physical attacks, serious accidents, and witnessing; more females than males reported sexual assault and sexual abuse as a child. As noted earlier in this chapter, few studies have yet published data on Criterion A2, but this study was an exception. A2 is the new DSM-IV criterion stating that the event must have been experienced subjectively as involving terror, horror, or helplessness. Of respondents meeting Criterion A1 (objective event), 74% of males and 87% of females met the A2 criterion (subjective trauma). Thus, when based on A2 as well as A1 criteria, exposure prevalence rates differed less: For males, these rates were 19% overall, 16% among those ages 14–17, and 20% among those ages 18–24; and for females, the rates were 15% overall, 11% among those ages 14–17, and 17% among those ages 18–24.

Studies of Older Adults in Western/Developed Societies

Older people have often been excluded from general population studies of adult mental health. The upper age limit was 55 for the NCS, and 45 for the Detroit Area Survey. Given the evidence that exposure to trauma peaks for individuals between the ages of 16 and 20 (Breslau et al., 1998), the exclusion of older adults is often justified. Their exclusion nonetheless leaves gaps in our knowledge, because older people constitute a significant, and growing, portion of the population. Norris (1992) and Flett et al. (2000) both included older adults in their samples and found that past-year exposure decreases sharply with age. We identified no study that examined whether sex differences in exposure change over the adult life course, but it is reasonable to think they might. In a reanalysis of Norris's data (see Figure 1.1), male sex was associated with greater past-year exposure only among adults less than 26 years of age (37% vs. 26%). From about age 30 onward, men's exposure was no higher than women's. After age 55, the 1-year exposure rates for both sexes were approximately 15%. In noting that, in *relative* terms, this rate is low, we should pause to note that in *absolute* terms, it is not.

Studies of Non-Western/Developing Societies

Few data on trauma exposure in general populations have emerged from developing or non-Western countries. Together with our colleagues, Art Murphy and Julia Perilla, we have been conducting an epidemiological study of trauma in Mexico (e.g., Norris, Murphy, Baker, & Perilla, 2000). For U.S. researchers, Mexico offers exceptional opportunities to examine the influences of context and culture on trauma and PTSD. Though its economy is developing, Mexico remains a much poorer country than the United States. Moreover, despite the heterogeneity within each society, these two neighboring countries have strikingly different cultural heritages. The United States has been characterized (Hofstede, 1980) as among the world's most individualistic and change-oriented, moderately egalitarian societies. Of special interest here, it also has been characterized as moderately low in masculinity (i.e., the value placed on traditional gender roles). In contrast, Mexico has been characterized (Hofstede, 1980) as being collectivist, avoiding change and uncertainty, and high on power, distance, and masculinity. Yet the country is easily accessible and sufficiently modern to accommodate collaborative research.

We interviewed 1,289 Mexicans in their own homes between February 1999 and January 2000. Participants were randomly selected from Guadalajara, a large city in central Mexico, and Oaxaca, a small city in southern Mexico. The sample is approximately two-thirds female and averages 37 years of age (range 18–92). We used the CIDI (Version 2.1) PTSD module

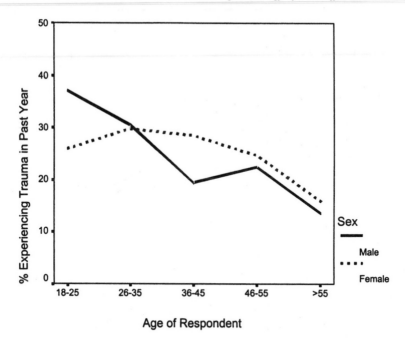

FIGURE 1.1. Past-year exposure to potentially traumatic events by sex and age in a sample of 1,000 adults from the southeastern United States.

for DSM-IV. In this sample, 83% of men and 74% of women had experienced at least one potentially traumatic event at some point in their lives, 27% of men and 22% of women in the past year. Men were disproportionately exposed to combat, life-threatening accidents, witnessing someone killed or injured, physical assault, and threats with weapons. Women were disproportionately exposed to sexual assault and sexual molestation. There were no sex differences in the lifetime prevalence of fire, disaster, or traumatic bereavement. These results generally replicate findings from comparable studies conducted in the United States, with two exceptions. First, the overall sex difference is detectable even over a 1-year interval, and second, men retain their elevated risk until approximately age 50 (see Figure 1.2).

Because the Mexico trauma study used DSM-IV criteria, we assessed Criterion A2 (subjective experience) as well as A1 (objective event). The relative risks for men and women reversed at this point. Of those reporting an event, 52% of men and 72% of women experienced terror, and 60% of men and 71% of women experienced helplessness. Thus comparable percentages, 60% of men and 61% of women, met Criterion A2. This pattern of effects in illustrated in Figure 1.3.

Although the study was conducted in the United States, results from

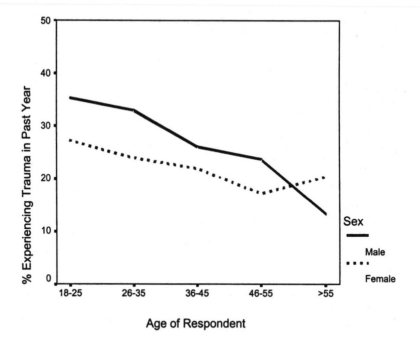

FIGURE 1.2. Past-year exposure to potentially traumatic events by sex and age in a sample of 1,289 adults from Guadalajara and Oaxaca, Mexico.

the Chinese American Psychiatric Epidemiology Study (CAPES) are useful for considering whether findings from the previously mentioned studies generalize to a non-Western context. These findings are not yet published but were made available to us by David Takeuchi, Principal Investigator, NIMH Grant No. 47460, and his associate, Lisa Tracey. This study had a total of 1,747 participants, of whom 50% were female and 95% were immigrants. As assessed by the CIDI for DSM-III-R, 32% of the women and 42% of the men experienced one or more traumatic events, a significant difference. These rates are quite intriguing in that they are notably lower than those found in other U.S. studies. Nonetheless, the pattern of men reporting more events than women still held.

Summary of Sex Differences in Trauma Exposure

The most general conclusion to be drawn from these data is that men are exposed to Criterion A events more frequently than women. This disproportionate exposure of men held in studies of adults from the United States (Breslau et al., 1998; Kessler et al., 1995; Norris, 1992), Canada (Stein et al., 1997), New Zealand (Flett et al., 2000), and Mexico (Norris et al.,

2000). It held in studies of college students from the United States (Vrana & Lauterbach, 1994) and Israel (Amir & Sol, 1999), and in studies of youth from the United States (Boney-McCoy & Finkelhor, 1996; Kilpatrick & Saunders, 1999) and Germany (Perkonigg & Wittchen, 1999). With regard to objective exposure (Criterion A1), the largest gap in the literature concerned older adults. Reanalyses of available data from samples in the United States and Mexico suggested that the sex difference in exposure decreases with age and is absent by late life. However, this appears to be the only qualification to the fact of greater male exposure to criterion events.

Because men are almost universally more exposed, whereas (as we detail later) women are typically more distressed, is it safe to rule out exposure as the source of the sex difference in PTSD? Unfortunately for lovers of parsimony, it is not this simple. First of all, screening instruments, such as those found in the DIS and the CIDI, undoubtedly identify some "false positives" (i.e., events that, for whatever reason, are not actually experienced as involving terror, horror, or helpless); that is, they are not actually *traumatic*. In two studies (youth in Germany; adults in Mexico) that examined Criterion A2, males and females differed little or did not differ in their prevalence of the subjective experience of *trauma*. Second, and perhaps

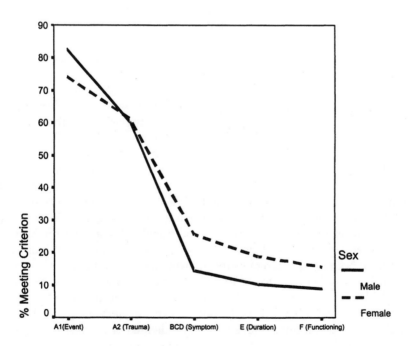

FIGURE 1.3. Percentages of men and women meeting criteria for PTSD in the Mexican sample.

more importantly, almost all of the studies summarized here found significant differences between men and women, or boys and girls, in the nature or types of events they experienced. When such data were reported, there was no exception to the rule that females are exposed to sexual violence far more often than males. To the extent that sexual violence is associated with a higher conditional risk for PTSD than physical violence or other forms of trauma (e.g., life-threatening accidents, sudden deaths of loved ones), the importance of exposure as the source of the sex difference cannot be ruled out.

Effects: Sex Differences in Risk and Conditional Risk for Lifetime and Current PTSD

Studies of Adults in Western/Developed Societies

The first published epidemiological study to report statistically significant sex differences in the prevalence of PTSD was conducted by Breslau et al. (1991). They interviewed 1,000 randomly selected members of an HMO, ages 21–30, in Detroit, Michigan, using the Revised DIS for DSM-III-R. The study yielded lifetime prevalence rates of 11.3% in women, 6% in men, and 9.2% overall that were very similar to those later found in the NCS, a nationwide study of adults ages 15–54 (Kessler et al., 1995). Those rates were 10.4% in women, 5.0% in men, and 7.8% overall. Thus, women appear to be approximately twice as likely as men to meet all PTSD criteria. Gender differences were even stronger in NCS rates of conditional risk; 20.4% of exposed women and 8.2% of exposed men developed PTSD. Among both men and women, the event with the highest conditional risk was rape. For all "most upsetting traumas" other than rape or neglect, a higher proportion of women than men met diagnostic criteria.

On the basis of DSM-IV criteria, the Detroit Area Survey of Trauma (Breslau et al., 1998) found the conditional probability of lifetime PTSD to be 13% in women and 6.2% in men, when estimated on the basis of a randomly selected event, compared to 17.7% in women and 9.5% in men, when estimated on the basis of the respondent's worst event. These results confirm suspicions that estimates of conditional risk made on the basis of most upsetting events are biased, yet the excess vulnerability of women is evident in both cases and retains the approximate 2:1 ratio observed in earlier studies. Breslau et al. found that this greater risk associated with female sex held even in a regression analysis that controlled for other sociodemographic factors and type of trauma. The risk of developing PTSD related to the index trauma increased if the individual had a history of previous trauma, but the sex difference remained comparable with previous exposure controlled (Breslau, Chilcoat, Kessler, & Davis, 1999).

Women also show greater chronicity of symptoms than do men. This is an important facet to examine, because PTSD fails to remit in more than one-third of individuals who develop it, even after many years (Kessler et al., 1995). The Detroit Area Survey of Trauma (Breslau et al., 1998) showed that the median time from onset to remission was 4 years for women compared to only 1 year for men. Using data from the first wave of the earlier Detroit HMO study of young adults, Breslau and Davis (1992) likewise found that women were overrepresented among lifetime PTSD cases of more than 1-year duration. Given exposure, 22% of women compared to 6% of men developed chronic PTSD.

Studies of current PTSD, sometimes called "point prevalence," are important for giving us a "snapshot" of the population's well-being at a particular moment in time. Given that women are at greater risk than men for developing PTSD at some point during their lives and that, once experienced, PTSD is more lasting among women, it follows that women would also be at greater risk for current PTSD. Consistent with this reasoning, Stein et al. (1997) found current PTSD to be more prevalent among women than among men in their study of Canadian adults. Assessed for the event that currently "troubles you the most" on the basis of the Modified PTSD Symptoms Scale (MPSS), symptom criteria were met by 5% of women compared to 1.7% of men; all DSM-IV criteria, including functional impairment, were met by 2.7% of women and 1.2% of men. These sex differences were statistically significant. In a subsequent analysis of the same data set, Stein, Walker, and Forde (2000) found women to be at higher risk for PTSD even when sexual trauma was excluded. Women were at higher risk following both sexual trauma and nonsexual assaultive violence, but not following nonassaultive trauma (e.g., fire, witnessing).

Norris (1992) also studied current PTSD but used a somewhat different method for estimating conditional risk, one that did not require the respondent to select a particular event. Questions regarding intrusion and avoidance were embedded within the event inventory as probes or follow-up questions, so that they were asked for each reported event. Questions regarding numbing and arousal symptoms were asked separately and did not require respondents to make attributions of their cause. Other investigators (Resnick et al., 1993; Solomon & Canino, 1990) have also questioned whether people are able to know the reasons they feel a particular way. This approach avoids biases associated with selection of a particular index event, but it is only practical for assessing current PTSD as opposed to lifetime experience. Among persons reporting an event, 9% of women and 6% of men met all symptom criteria. The difference was strongest for the category of crime (robbery, physical assault, sexual assault), in which women's rate of current PTSD was more than twice that of men (11.5% vs. 5.5%). However, there were too few cases of male sexual assault to examine sex differences in the effects of this specific event.

Studies of Youth in Western/Developed Societies

Studies of youth and young adults suggest that the vulnerability of females begins quite early in life. Using the Detroit HMO sample of persons ages 21–30, Breslau, Davis, Andreski, Peterson, and Schulz (1997) showed that age at exposure may influence the strength of sex differences in PTSD. Using age 15 as the cutpoint, they estimated the cumulative incidence of PTSD separately for childhood and adulthood trauma. The sex difference was much greater for childhood events, for which the rates were approximately 35% for females and 10% for males, than for adulthood events, with rates of approximately 25% for females and 15% for males. These differences were not explained by differences in the types of traumas experienced. All of these rates may be overestimated given that they are based on a single-item screen for trauma, but this bias should not account for the difference between women and men.

In Wave 1 of the National Youth Survey (Boney-McCoy & Finkelhor, 1995), the effects of any prior victimization on a continuous measure of traumatic stress were somewhat, although not dramatically stronger among girls than among boys, with effect sizes of .44 and .37, respectively. In Wave 2 (Boney-McCoy & Finkelhor, 1996) the effects of victimizations occurring between Waves 1 and 2 were assessed, with Wave 1 symptoms controlled. The same pattern emerged, but this time, the sex difference was stronger, with effect sizes of .57 for girls and .34 for boys. Kilpatrick and Saunders (1999) assessed PTSD using a modified version of the DIS for DSM-III-R designed for the National Women's Survey in their sample of over 4,000 adolescents. Most items on this scale are not specific to a particular trauma, and thus do not require selection of a particular event. Girls had higher rates of PTSD than boys, both in their lifetimes (10.1% vs. 6.2%) and currently (6.2% vs. 3.7%). Youth who had experienced multiple sexual assaults were at highest conditional risk for PTSD, with lifetime rates of 34% for girls and 41% for boys. Youth who had experienced multiple physical assaults or abusive punishments were also at high risk, with rates of 40% for girls and 20% for boys. Similarly, multiple episodes of witnessing violence yielded PTSD rates of 27% in girls, 17% in boys. Giaconia et al. (1995) observed strong sex differences in data collected from a general population sample of 194 boys and 190 girls age 18, who had been studied periodically since age 5. They used the DSM-III-R version of the DIS. For both the conditional probability of PTSD (24.4% of girls vs. 4.8% of boys) and total lifetime prevalence (10.5% of girls vs. 2.1% of boys), the rates for girls exceeded those for boys by a factor of 5.

As noted earlier, Perkonigg and Wittchen (1999) included a high proportion of adolescents in their Munich sample. On the basis of DSM-IV criteria, lifetime prevalence rates of PTSD were 0.4% for all young men (0.2% for those ages 14–17 and 0.5% for those ages 18–24) and 2.2% for all young women (1.1% for those ages 14–17 and 2.8% of those ages 18–24). These rates are lower than those reported by Kessler et al. (1995) for the cohort aged 15–24 (2.8% of young men, 10.3% of young women). This difference is partially but probably not completely attributable to Criterion F in DSM-IV. Conditional risks, determined on the basis of the "most upsetting event," in the Munich sample were 2.2% for young men (1.4% of those ages 14–17; 2.4% of those ages 18–24) and 14.5% for young women (10.0% of those ages 14–17, 15.5% of those ages 18–24). Notwithstanding some differences between these results and those from the NCS, the greater vulnerability of females was just as evident as in U.S. studies.

Studies of Older Adults in Western/Developed Societies

Across most of the adult life course, gender differences appear to change little with age. Gender differences in the lifetime prevalence of PTSD were found in all age cohorts included in the NCS: 10.3% of women versus 2.8% of men for the cohort aged 15–24; 11.2% versus 5.6% for the cohort aged 25–34; 10.6% versus 5.0% for the cohort aged 35–44; and 8.9% versus 7.6% for cohort aged 45–54 (Kessler et al., 1995). As noted earlier, however, the NCS did not include adults over the age of 54. This fact, together with the fact that the maximum age for the Detroit Area Survey of Trauma was 45, has limited the availability of information about sex differences in PTSD among older people. Some data suggest that gender differences in the *point* prevalence of PTSD may dissipate in late life. Norris (1992) found strong differences overall between older adults, who showed a conditional probability of only 3%, and middle-aged and younger adults, who showed conditional probabilities, respectively, of 10% and 9%. In a reanalysis of these data, we found that age interacts with sex in predicting current PTSD. We used 55 as the cutpoint on age to complement the sampling strategy of the NCS. Women's rates were significantly higher than men's in the subsample aged 18–55 (13% vs. 8%), but women's (3%) and men's (6%) rates did not differ in the subsample over the age of 55 (see Figure 1.4).

Studies of Non-Western/Developing Societies

As noted earlier, few data exist on the prevalence of PTSD in general population samples drawn from non-Western or developing countries. If our data from Mexico (Norris et al., 2000) are any indication, this is an important area for future research. On the basis of DSM-IV criteria, lifetime rates of PTSD in Mexico were 9% for men and 16% for women, a significant difference. The rates of 10% for men and 19% for women before Criterion F was taken in account (roughly equivalent to DSM-III-R criteria) are far

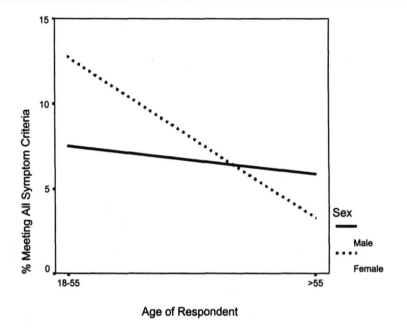

FIGURE 1.4. Conditional risk for current PTSD by sex and age in the southeastern U.S. sample.

greater than those found in the NCS (5% for men, 10% for women). Among Mexicans exposed to trauma, 11% of men and 21% of women met all criteria regarding their worst event (12% and 25% before Criterion F). These rates are again higher that those yielded by the NCS, where 8% of exposed men and 20% of exposed women met DSM-III-R criteria. Among persons meeting Criterion A2 (subjective experience of horror, terror, or helplessness), 15% of Mexican men and 26% of Mexican women met all DSM-IV criteria. Note that in Figure 1.3, men are more likely than women to meet Criterion A1, men and women are identically likely to meet Criterion A2, but women are more likely than men to meet symptom criteria and all criteria. This pattern suggests that, at least in Mexico, the source of the sex difference is the reaction to the trauma rather than the experience of trauma per se. On the other hand, the conditional risk for PTSD was very high when the worst event was sexual violence (49%) compared to, for example, 22%, when it was nonsexual violence. Of the 65 people in the sample whose worst event was sexual violence, 59 were women. This finding would tend to support the notion that their risk for sexual violence explains women's higher prevalence of PTSD. Yet whereas 31 (53%) of these 59 women met PTSD criteria, only 1 (17%) of the 6 men did so. Moreover, 28

(35%) of the 79 women who experienced nonsexual violence as their worst event met PTSD criteria compared to 9 (10%) of the 90 men whose worst event was nonsexual violence. These numbers are too small to be definitive (and surely illustrate why general population studies require such large samples), but they do not support the hypothesis that women have higher PTSD prevalence solely because they are at risk for sexual assault.

Current rates of PTSD were also significantly higher among Mexican women (3.7%) than among Mexican men (1.7%) Although the numbers are all small, these rates are nonetheless higher than those reported by Stein et al. (1997) for Canadian adults (2.7% of women, 1.2% of men). As found for the southeastern United States, sex differences in conditional probabilities were significant among adults ages 18–55 (4.7% of women vs. 1.3% of men) but not among older adults (5.8% of women vs. 6.1% of men).

With lifetime prevalence rates of only 1.1% of men and 2.2% of women, the CAPES has yielded the lowest rates of PTSD of which we aware. Recall that exposure rates in this sample (42%, 32%) were also lower than have typically been found. Because we have no experience with Chinese immigrants or expertise regarding Chinese culture, we do not speculate on the meaning of these findings. Nonetheless, it is interesting that even in this context of very low risk, the pattern of men's higher risk for exposure and women's higher risk for PTSD still held.

Summary of Sex Differences in Risk and Conditional Risk for PTSD

Although the reader may be swimming in numbers by now, it actually is not difficult to summarize these results. Regardless of whether the study described total lifetime prevalence (e.g., Kessler et al., 1995: 10% vs. 5%), conditional lifetime prevalence (e.g., Breslau et al., 1996: 13% vs. 6%), total current prevalence (e.g., Stein et al., 1997: 3% vs. 1%), or conditional current prevalence (e.g., Norris, 1992: 12% vs. 6%), women's probabilities of PTSD were significantly higher than men's. There was no exception to this rule. The data indicate that the risk associated with female gender begins in childhood (e.g., Breslau et al., 1997) and continues throughout the middle years of adulthood. Only in the specific instance of current prevalence in late life were women's and men's risk for PTSD equivalent. Moreover, women's differential risk hovered around a 2:1 ratio regardless of whether the overall rate was very low (e.g., CAPES: 2% vs. 1%) or very high (e.g., Norris et al., 2000: 21% vs. 11%).

How important was the type of exposure in explaining these effects? Not very, it appears. The NCS found men's and women's conditional risk to be the same only in the specific case of rape; for all other events, women's conditional risk was higher than men's. The Detroit Area Survey of Trauma and the Stein et al. Canadian survey showed that the effect of sex remained significant even in regression equations that controlled for type of event. Likewise, the Mexico study found that women were at greater conditional risk for PTSD following nonsexual as well as sexual violence. Nonetheless, we cannot rule out the possibility that women's experiences were *qualitatively* different from men's in a way that cannot be captured by standardized screening instruments and diagnostic measures.

SEX DIFFERENCES IN DISASTER EXPERIENCES AND EFFECTS

That said, we turn our attention to a research context that provides less opportunity for men and women to have radically different degrees or types of trauma exposure. In this section, we review findings regarding sex differences in exposure to and effects of disaster-related trauma. Although we chose not to review all studies that examined effects of specific stressors, such as motor vehicle accidents or combat, a review of results from disaster studies was in keeping with our general decision to provide a comprehensive review of sex differences in community-dwelling samples. An added benefit is that disasters represent a research context that limits variation in the timing and type of exposure. Because of our focus on community-dwelling samples, we considered only those disasters, of either natural or technological origin, that struck areas with clear geographic boundaries, where the survivor stays in or near the damaged environment. Lindy and Grace (1985) referred to disasters of this type as "centripetal" and differentiated them from "centrifugal" disasters that involve people who temporarily occupy a common space. This focus excludes events such as club or hotel fires and most transportation accidents, as well as people exposed to disasters because of emergency work in either a professional or volunteer capacity.

Exposure: Sex Differences in Disaster-Related Trauma

Studies of Adults in Western/Developed Societies

The stress associated with community-based disasters is multifaceted. Many disaster victims are exposed to acute and traumatic stressors, such as injury, threat to life, property loss, and even death, in the most serious incidents. Many also experience an array of chronic stressors, such as relocation, financial strain, and ecological stress. Because disasters impact entire communities, victims also experience a variety of vicarious stressors. Research on how gender influences the experience of disaster has focused almost solely on differential vulnerability, to the exclusion of differential exposure. Thus, our first task here was to examine the assumption that women and men should differ minimally in the nature of their objective exposure. There is some cause to question this assumption. Disasters may seem to be more random than many other traumatic events, although in actuality they are not. For example, the poor, the less educated, and ethnic minorities are generally more likely to live in undesirable, at-risk areas and reside in less safe and more vulnerable homes (Quarantelli, 1994).

Empirical data do not provide a consistent portrait of sex differences in exposure to the more traumatic elements of disasters. Gleser, Green, and Winget's (1981) in-depth report of the 1972 dam collapse in Buffalo Creek, West Virginia, represents an early and still notable examination of the stress associated with disasters. On the basis of narrative data, these investigators quantified exposure in terms of four indices: bereavement (closeness of relationship), displacement (in distance from original home), life threat during the event (physical contact with the water), and extended stress (struggle for survival during the first 2 weeks postevent). Women's and men's means did not differ on the first two indices, but men scored higher than women on the last two. Approximately 42% of the men and 32% of the women had come close to death; 33% of the men and 24% of the women scored in the *moderate* to *severe* range on extended stress. The investigators noted that women had often been sent ahead to relative safety, whereas the men stayed behind in an attempt to save others. In contrast, there were no sex differences in proportions assigned to *none, near, moderate*, and *severe* levels of exposure among the 912 adults studied 2 years after a deadly flood in Puerto Rico (Bravo, Rubio-Stipic, Canino, Woodbury, & Ribera, 1990). It might also be noted that, while based on self-reports, the indices used in both of these studies were fairly objective indicators of stress.

Lundin, Mardberg, and Otto (1993) conducted an interesting and unusual study after the Chernobyl nuclear accident in 1986. After the accident, nuclear material was carried by wind into eastern and northern Sweden, and there was considerable confusion and uncertainty about the accident's consequences for the Swedish population in either the short or long term. Lundin et al. assessed perceptions of threat within a sample of 1,000 adults in Sweden and found women to be significantly more concerned about the accident on virtually all indicators (e.g., unpleasant thoughts, preoccupation, change in personal habits). Anderson and Manuel (1994) assessed reactions of 108 male and 103 female college students to the Loma Prieta earthquake in California. After only 1 day had passed. Not only did women score significantly higher than men on the Impact of Event Scale (IES) when describing their reactions of the past 24 hours, but they also estimated that the earthquake lasted significantly longer (78 seconds) than did men (48 seconds).

Studies of Youth in Western/Developed Societies

Garrison, Weinrich, Hardin, Weinrich, and Wang (1993) examined sex differences in several different aspects of exposure to Hurricane Hugo in a sample of over 1,200 adolescents from South Carolina, most of whom were between the ages of 12 and 14. Scores on an index of exposure composed of not being with parents, relocation, injury to family or friend, injury to self, and fear of personal injury were higher, on average, among girls than among boys. A more specific analysis indicated that the difference occurred primarily because girls acknowledged a greater fear of injury during the storm.

Studies of Older Adults in Western/Developed Societies

Because relatively few studies took both gender and age into account, we reexamined available data related to Hurricanes Hugo (1989; Charleston, South Carolina, and Charlotte, North Carolina, $N = 500$) and Andrew (1992; Miami and Homestead, Florida, $N = 404$). Both samples were drawn so that younger (18–39), middle-aged (40–59), and older (60–89) men and women were all equally represented. Trauma exposure was assessed in terms of threat to life and injury; those in the highest trauma category had both of these stressors. Property damage was the individuals' assessment of the total impact of the hurricane on their property and belongings; those in the highest category assessed their losses as *much* or *enormous*. In the Hugo sample, women and men differed in their reports of trauma exposure (13% vs. 8% in the highest category) and property damage (37% vs. 24% in the highest category) only in the middle-aged group. Among adults over 60, only 6% of women and 3% of men were in the highest trauma category; 35% of women and 30% of men were in the highest loss category. In the Andrew sample, older women reported less trauma exposure than older men (18% vs. 23% in the highest category), whereas the reverse was true among younger (43% vs. 27%) and middle-aged (49% vs. 29%) adults. In each age group, the two sexes reported equivalent property damage (84%, 83%).

Studies of Non-Western/Developing Societies

We had similar data available from studies of Hurricane Paulina, which struck Acapulco, Mexico, in 1997 ($N = 200$), and the Opole flood, which devastated this city and surrounding regions in Poland in 1996 ($N = 285$). In Mexico, 56% of women were placed in the highest trauma category compared to 38% of men, but women and men did not differ in their evaluations of property damage (61% vs. 57%). In the data from Poland provided to us by Krzysztof Kaniasty, women evaluated both their trauma exposure (22% in highest category) and property damage (74% in highest category) more severely than did men (15% and 57%, respectively).

Summary of Sex Differences in Disaster Exposure

Although more research is clearly needed, our impression from these studies is that women differ from men most strongly in their self-reported experiences in disasters when the indicators are relatively subjective. In the Buffalo Creek and Puerto Rico studies, which assessed exposure relatively objectively, either men were more greatly exposed or no sex differences emerged. In the Sweden and San Francisco studies, which assessed perceptions of threat, women were affected more adversely than men. In the Hurricanes Hugo and Andrew studies, as well as in the Mexico and Poland studies, women and girls reported more trauma than men and boys. There was some indication that differences between women and men in their subjective experiences of disasters lessen in late life, but this last conclusion is based on relatively little data.

Effects: Sex Differences in Disaster-Specific PTSD

Studies of Adults in Western/Developed Societies

The literature on the overall psychological consequences of disasters is vast but considerably smaller when the focus is on PTSD specifically. A number of disaster studies were conducted in the 1980s using the DIS for DSM-III; as noted previously, this measure was later substantially revised because of its low sensitivity to PTSD. Perhaps not surprisingly, studies that used this measure have produced an array of findings that are not easy to integrate. Bravo et al. (1990) found sex to have neither a main effect nor an interaction with exposure level in predicting lifetime PTSD 2 years after the 1985 flood in Puerto Rico. The rate of PTSD found in this study was very low. Smith, Robins, Przybeck, Goldring, and Solomon (1986) also used the DIS for DSM-III to assess 500 adults in a rural area near St. Louis, Missouri, who varied in their level of exposure (none, indirect, direct) to a flood, dioxin contamination, or both. Men were more at risk than women for "any diagnosis," but because very few cases of PTSD were identified, this does not necessarily indicate that men were at greater risk for PTSD. Shore, Tatum, and Vollmer (1986) also presented combined results from the depression, generalized anxiety, and PTSD modules of the DIS for DSM-III and used date of onset to distinguish between post- and predisaster disorders. Their study of 1,025 adults conducted 38–42 months after the volcano erupted at Mt. St. Helens, in 1980, yielded results that were very different from those of Smith et al. Among women, 21% of the high-exposure group developed new disorders compared to 6% of the low-exposure group and 2% of the control group. These rates were approximately twice those of men: 11% in the high-exposure group, 3% in the low-exposure group, and 1% in the control group. As before, however, this study does not specifically tell us that women were at greater risk for PTSD.

Two studies using the DIS for DSM-III did report gender differences specifically for PTSD, in the direction of women being higher. Durkin (1993) assessed postdisaster PTSD 15 months after the 1983 earthquake in Coalinga, California. Although rates were low overall, they were substantially higher among women (3.5%) than among men (0.8%). Steinglass and Gerrity (1990) studied two communities, one (Albion, Pennsylvania) that had been struck by a devastating tornado, and another (Parsons, West Virginia) that had been seriously flooded. Both disasters occurred in 1985. Combined across the two settings, 20% of the 75 women in the study met all DSM-III criteria for postdisaster PTSD compared to 6% of the 67 men.

The data from studies that have used other measures are also mixed, but where sex differences have been found, women have always been more symptomatic. Madakasira and O(Brien (1987) collected data from 116 adults 5–8 months after a tornado in rural North Carolina. Scored on the basis of an expanded version of the Hopkins Symptom Checklist, rates of PTSD were very high overall (59%) but did not differ by sex. Freedy, Addy, Kilpatrick, Resnick, and Garrison (2000) interviewed 1,000 adults who resided in the area affected by the Loma Prieta earthquake. Two years after the event, the postdisaster prevalence of PTSD, assessed using a PTSD measure designed for use in the National Women's Survey, was 5.8% and, again, did not vary by sex. In contrast, Green et al. (1990) presented data on PTSD prevalence collected in 1974 and 1986, from 46 men and 74 women who experienced the Buffalo Creek dam collapse in 1972. Although rates decreased over the 14-year interval, rates for women (52% in 1974, 31% in 1986) were higher than rates for men (32% in 1974, 23% in 1986) at both times. Two years after Hurricane Hugo, Freedy et al. (2000) found that 5.2% of the 776 adults sampled met criteria for PTSD. In contrast to their parallel analysis of the effects of the Loma Prieta earthquake, female sex did significantly increase the odds of posthurricane PTSD (odds ratio = 3.4). In our study of Hurricane Andrew (Norris, Perilla, Ibañez, & Murphy, 2001), 21% of women met symptom criteria for PTSD compared to 13% of men. In a sample of 845 adults assessed at four points after the 1989 Newcastle earthquake in Australia, women averaged higher scores on the IES than men (Carr, Lewin, Kenardy, et al., 1997; Carr, Lewin, Webster, et al., 1997).

The research of Carol North and her colleagues, including the late Elizabeth Smith, warrants special mention, because they have used the same measure, specifically, the revised DIS for DSM-III-R, to assess PTSD in over 1,000 adults across 11 different sites (e.g., North et al., 1999; North, Nixon, & Vincent, 1998; Smith, North, & Spitznagel, 1993). In the combined database, female sex, prior psychological disorder, and type of disaster all contributed independently to the prediction of PTSD (North et al., 1998). The disaster that produced the highest prevalence of cases was the bombing of the Murray Federal Building in Oklahoma City, in 1995 (North et al., 1999). In this sample of 182 severely exposed victims, of whom 52% were female, women's rate of PTSD (45%) was twice that of men (23%).

Studies of Youth in Western/Developed Societies

Studies of youth have also yielded mixed results, but where differences have been found, girls have been more distressed. Shannon, Lonigan, Finch, and Taylor (1994) studied over 5,000 school-age children ages 9–19 (M = 14) 3 months after Hurricane Hugo in Berkely County, South Carolina, a rural area northeast of Charleston. Overall, 7% of girls met all PTSD symptom criteria compared to 4% of boys, a significant difference. Garrison et al. (1993) studied 1,264 ninth and tenth graders ranging in age from 11 to 17 (most were 12–14) 1 year after Hurricane Hugo. They classified participants by both sex and race. In ascending order of prevalence, rates of PTSD were 1.5% for black males, 3.8% for white males, 4.7% for black females, and 6.2% for white females. In logistical regressions, both female sex and white race increased odds for meeting PTSD criteria. In contrast, LaGreca, Silverman, Vernberg, and Prinstein (1996) found no effect of gender at any time point in their study of 442 children at three elementary schools in southern Dade County, Florida. The children were assessed 3, 7, and 10 months after Hurricane Andrew. Pynoos et al. (1987) also found boys and girls to be equally affected in a study of 80 boys and 79 girls ages 5–13 (M = 9) after a sniper attacked their elementary school playground in Los Angeles, California. Taken together, these data suggest, as Green et al. (1991) also speculated, that sex differences may be more pronounced in adolescents than among younger children. However, in their study of children ages 2–15 from Buffalo Creek, Green et al. found girls to be more likely to develop PTSD than boys (44% vs. 30%) regardless of age.

Studies of Older Adults in Western/Developed Societies

Disaster studies that have distinguished middle-age adults from younger and older adults have almost always found this group to be most adversely affected (e.g., Gleser et al., 1981; Shore et al., 1986; Thompson, Norris, & Hanacek, 1993). However, as we mentioned when reviewing results pertaining to differences between men's and women's exposure to disaster, there are few data regarding whether age modifies the effects of gender in adult samples. Looking at this in our Hurricane Hugo sample, we found that women had higher means on a continuous measure of posttraumatic stress symptoms than men in all age groups, but the effect size (the proportion of a standard deviation two groups differ) for this sex difference was more than twice as large in the middle-aged group (.37) as in the younger and older groups (.16). Similarly, in our Hurricane Andrew sample, differences between women and men in percentages meeting symptom criteria for PTSD were most pronounced among middle-aged participants (32% vs. 19%) and least pronounced among older participants (18% vs. 13%).

Studies of Non-Western/Developing Societies

Norris et al. (2001) conducted the only study of which we are aware that was specifically designed to compare the effects of a disaster in a developing country (Hurricane Paulina, Mexico) with the effects of a similar disaster in a developed country (Hurricane Andrew, United States). The studies were designed to be as comparable in method as possible. The same time frame (6 months postdisaster), sampling strategy (quota), and questionnaire were used in each place. Both hurricanes were Category 4 at their peak. Only the data from non-Hispanic victims of Hurricane Andrew (N = 270) were included in comparisons, because most of the Latino victims of Hurricane Andrew had immigrated to the United States from elsewhere and thus would complicate interpretations. In regression analyses that controlled for severity of exposure, age, and education, the expected sex by-country interactions emerged for continuous measures of intrusion, avoidance/numbing, and remorse (noncriterion symptoms of guilt and suicidality). The form of the interaction was such that Mexican women showed higher symptoms than explained by either their sex or country alone. A sex main effect (women higher) was found for arousal only. Overall 44% of Mexican women met symptom criteria for PTSD compared to 14% of men. This difference was much greater than that observed between U.S. women (21%) and men (13%). Also notable, in the absence of life threat or injury, no Mexican man or woman met PTSD symptom criteria, but in the presence of both of these stressors, 26% of Mexican men and 54% of Mexican women met these criteria.

Other studies of disasters in developing areas of the world have likewise found the prevalence of disaster-related PTSD to be much higher in women than men. After the Mexico City earthquake of 1985, de la Fuente (1990) assessed 573 adults living in shelters. Rates of PTSD were 18% in men and 38% in women, not strikingly different from the rates we found in Acapulco after Hurricane Paulina (14%, 44%). Durkin (1993) also found rates of post-earthquake PTSD to be substantially higher among women (26%) than among men (6%) in Santiago, Chile, 8 months after the 1985 earthquake there. These rates were much higher than those found by Durkin in Coalinga, California, using the same measure of PTSD (DIS for DSM-III).

Data provided to us by Krys Kaniasty indicated that the devastating 1996 flood in Opole, Poland ($N = 285$), was tremendously stressful for both male and female survivors. While the emotional expressiveness of the Polish people (Wierzbicka, 1994) may account, in part, for the overall high levels of symptoms, the magnitude of the sex difference (2:1) was in line with other studies. Altogether, 59% of women and 31% of men met PTSD symptom criteria. In contrast, Goenjian et al. (1994) did not find a sex difference within any of three stricken adult samples studied using the PTSD Reaction Index 18 months after the horrific 1988 earthquake in Armenia. Two of the samples were elderly, however, and all were fairly small. In a parallel study of 218 children in Armenia ($Ms = 12–13$), girls scored significantly higher than boys on the Child Version of the Reaction Index (Goenjian et al., 1995; Pynoos et al., 1993). However, the difference was relatively small and did not vary in magnitude across the three sites that differed in proximity to the epicenter.

Summary of Sex Differences in Disaster Effects

In summary, more often than not, women appear to be at greater risk than men for developing PTSD in the aftermath of disasters. The differences begin to show themselves in adolescence, possibly sooner, peak in middle age, and dissipate in late life. Traditional cultures may further exacerbate the differences, especially when they restrict the expression of emotion among men.

SEX DIFFERENCES IN COMMUNITIES TORN BY VIOLENCE

Individuals who live in areas where community or political violence is recurrent are exposed to a variety of traumatic events on a potentially daily basis. For the purposes of this chapter, "community violence" refers to a pattern of chronic exposure to multiple forms of violence, including, but not limited to, shootings, muggings, and gang chases. "Political violence" refers to trauma provoked by war and/or political unrest, and includes, but is not limited to, exposure to beatings, shootings, tear gas inhalation, severe food shortages, and raids. As with disasters, individuals living in such communities experience numerous vicarious stressors through the traumatic experiences of neighbors, friends, and family. Almost without exception, studies of community violence have been conducted with youth who live in urban America, whereas studies of political violence have been conducted with adults from eastern Europe, the Middle East, or Asia.

Exposure: Sex Differences in the Context of Community or Political Violence

Studies of Youth in Western/Developed Societies

No studies that we know of have examined sex differences in exposure to community violence outside of the United States or even among adults in the United States (a surprising gap), but several studies have examined sex differences in exposure among children and youth. In this section, all reviewed studies of youth exposed to community violence were conducted in high schools or youth-oriented programs. Sample selection was non-random, in that eligible participants were recruited and those who volunteered comprised the samples. This limitation notwithstanding, these studies suggest that boys are exposed to community violence as both victims and witnesses more frequently than girls. In a sample of 2,248 urban students in sixth through tenth grades, Schwab-Stone et al. (1995) found that 46% of the boys versus 38% of the girls had been exposed to some form of community violence. Richters and Martinez (1993) found that 88% of boys versus 25% of girls in their sample of 54 fifth- and sixth-grade urban adolescents had been the victim of a violent crime. In a study of 221 African American youth participating in a federally funded summer program, Fitzpatrick and Boldizar (1993) also concluded that boys were witnesses to and victims of community violence significantly more frequently than girls; exposure rates ranged from 70% for direct victimization to 85% for witnessing violence. However, in their study of 149 predominantly African American adolescents, Foley and Price (1999) found no sex differences in severity of (mean) exposure; every boy and girl had been exposed to at least one traumatic event.

Studies of Non-Western/Developing Societies

Many of the studies of adults' exposure to community/political violence in non-Western or developing societies have involved refugees. Mollica, Poole, and Tor (1998) used multistage area probability sampling from several campsites inhabited by Cambodian refugees. In their sample of nearly 1,000 persons, the authors found that men had been exposed to a mean of 14 traumatic events, whereas women averaged 12. Ninety-nine percent of their sample reported exposure to at least one war-related trauma. The authors commented on the nature of war violence inflicted by Khmer Rouge, noting that men were targeted to be killed by the army. In addition, there was an unusually high rate of sexual assault among males, with 1 in 4 men being a sexual assault victim. Thulesius and Hakansson (1999) found 100% exposure rates among both men and women in their study of 206 Bosnian refugees recruited from a health care clinic in Sweden. So did

Carlson and Hogan (1994) in their nonprobability sample of 50 Cambodian refugees.

Thabet and Vostanis (1999) conducted a study of 239 randomly selected Palestinian refugees, ages 6–11, living on the Gaza strip between Israel and Egypt. Gender differences were not found for the overall exposure rate of the participants. Nor were gender differences found in exposure rates among young Cambodian refugees, ages 13–25 (Sack et al., 1994). Of these youth selected randomly from a list of Khmer adolescents in Portland, Oregon, and Salt Lake City, Utah, 100% were exposed to atrocities, such as witnessing executions and being separated from family. Similarly high exposure rates have been found among children living in other war-zone areas. Kuterovac, Dyregrov, and Stuvland (1994) found an exposure rate of over 90% in a purposive sample of 134 youth, ages 10–15, living in Croatia, with no sex differences. Working in Zenica in central Bosnia, Goldstein, Wampler, and Wise (1997) identified all Bosnian children ages 6–12 living in centers for displaced families with three or more children. These 364 youth had a 100% exposure rate to war violence. None of these studies reported the mean levels of trauma exposure for the sexes. As a result, we can only conclude that there are no sex differences in proportions of youth experiencing one or more war-related stressors, and we cannot draw conclusions regarding differences in boys' and girls' overall severity of exposure.

Summary of Sex Differences in Exposure to Community/Political Violence

Whereas boys were often more highly exposed than girls in studies of community violence, and men were more exposed than women in at least one study of political violence, there were also several studies undertaken in this research context in which males and females did not differ. The explanation appears to be that overall levels of trauma were so high in these settings that individual differences exerted less of an impact than they appear to exert after disasters or within the general population. Thus sex differences may dissipate as rates of exposure approach 100%.

Effects: Sex Differences in PTSD from Community/Political Violence

Studies of Adults in Western/Developed Societies

As noted earlier, research on community violence in the United States has generally neglected adult populations, but a relevant study by Hanson, Kilpatrick, Freedy, and Saunders (1995) surveyed 1,200 randomly selected adults in Los Angeles County after the 1992 civil disturbance that began when police officers were acquitted of beating Rodney King. Of the adults, 400 lived in south-central Los Angeles, the area most affected by the riots and also known for its chronic community violence. Current prevalence of PTSD for the entire sample was 4.1%, with no sex difference; however, the article did not present sex-related results for acute versus chronic violence, or for south-central versus other Los Angeles areas separately.

Studies of Youth in Western/Developed Societies

Overall, it appears that girls exposed to community violence are at higher risk for PTSD than similarly exposed boys. To date, only one study (Berman, Kurtines, Silverman, & Serafini, 1996) did not find a sex difference in PTSD: In a nonprobability sample of 96 highly exposed youth in Miami, ages 14–18, approximately 35% of both girls and boys met criteria for PTSD based on DSM-III-R. The youth in Fitzpatrick and Boldizar's (1993) study had a combined PTSD prevalence rate of 27%, with significantly more girls than boys meeting criteria. Likewise, Berton and Stabb (1996) reported a combined prevalence rate of 29% in a sample of 97 youth, with girls again at greater risk. Foley and Price (1999) found that girls scored higher than boys on a continuous measure of PTSD symptoms in the context of community violence.

Studies of Non-Western/Developing Societies

Data pertaining to gender differences in the prevalence of PTSD among adults exposed to political violence in non-Western or developing societies are inconsistent. No sex differences emerged in Thulesius and Hakansson's (1999) sample of Bosnian refugees recruited from health clinics in Sweden, or in Cheung's (1994) census of Cambodian refugees living in Denedian, New Zealand. However, women were at greater risk for war-related PTSD in Mollica et al.'s (1998) probability sample of Cambodian refugees, and in Reppesgaard's (1997) sample of Tamil refugees from Sri Lanka who were selected randomly from camp enrollment lists.

A similarly inconsistent pattern emerges from the data on youth exposed to political violence. Thabet and Vostanis (1999) did not find sex differences in posttraumatic stress among the Palestinian refugees selected randomly from elementary schools. Nor were sex differences found in Sack et al.'s (1994) random sample of Cambodian adolescents, or in Goldstein et al.'s (1997) census of Bosnian youth living in Zenica's centers for displaced families. On the other hand, girls reported higher levels of PTSD than boys in Kuterovac et al.'s (1994) purposive sample of 134 youth from Croatia. Husain et al. (1998) also found sex differences, with girls scoring higher, in their sample of 791 students in one district in Sarajevo, as did Awadh,

Vance, El-Beblawi, and Pumariega (1998) in their random sample of youth who were in Kuwait during the war, and Macksoud and Aber's (1996) randomly selected sample of 224 youth in Lebanon.

Summary of Sex Differences in Effects of Community/Political Violence

Overall, the context of community and political violence is the least well developed of the three we have reviewed, with fewer studies overall, less consistency across the ones that exist, and large gaps in the literature. The lack of data on adult exposure to community violence makes it difficult to place the findings for youth in proper context. In contrast to the endemic violence in American inner cities, widespread political violence has been rare in the recent history of the United States, although there have been a few dramatic examples of terrorism (e.g., the bombing of the federal building in Oklahoma City and the events of 9/11/01) and increasing concern about this threat. Conversely, violence in other countries is seldom characterized as community violence. Generally, it is difficult to identify differences between the samples with and without sex differences in PTSD. There are many possible explanations for the lack of conclusive results. Even though all of the samples were highly exposed, it is possible that types, severity, and frequency of exposure may have varied greatly across these settings. Another potential explanation for the inconsistent findings involves the variety of measurement strategies employed across studies. If any conclusion can be drawn regarding sex difference in this context, it is only that when they are found, women and girls are more highly distressed than their male counterparts. Yet, notably, in contrast to studies in the two other research contexts we reviewed, a higher proportion of studies in this context did not yield sex differences. Men's and boys' risk for PTSD may thus catch up with that of women and girls when the situation becomes especially dire.

SUMMARY OF EMPIRICAL FINDINGS

The studies, although not 100% consistent, are consistent enough to warrant a number of tentative conclusions about sex differences in trauma and PTSD:

1. Men are more exposed than women to objectively defined events (Criterion A1) that are potentially traumatic, with the exception of sexual violence; this is an important exception because the event is associated with the highest conditional risk of PTSD in both men and women.

2. Being male is a risk factor for exposure primarily in adolescence and young adulthood, but, in some societies, men's greater risk may continue throughout middle age.
3. Women appear to experience comparable events as more threatening (i.e., as involving more terror, horror, or helplessness); thus, when subjective elements (Criterion A2) are taken into account, men and women differ less or not at all in trauma exposure.
4. Women are approximately twice as likely as men to develop PTSD at some point during their lives, and PTSD tends to take a more chronic course in women than men; neither the types of events experienced nor perceptions of threat fully account for these effects.
5. The risk for current PTSD associated with being female begins no later than adolescence and continues throughout young adulthood and middle age; it is not clear whether the relative comparability of men and women in late life is an aging or cohort effect.
6. Women's greater risk for PTSD clearly holds in general populations and disaster-stricken communities, and, in these cases, may be even more pronounced in the context of societies that emphasize traditional sex roles; however, it is possible that men's risk for PTSD may catch up with women's in communities torn by violence or war.

IMPLICATIONS FOR THEORY, RESEARCH, AND INTERVENTION

Implications for Theory and Research

As noted in introducing this chapter, epidemiological studies often have a descriptive rather than an explanatory purpose. Nonetheless, we have identified a number of facts that tenable theories must be able to explain: First, that being female is a risk factor, not a prerequisite, for PTSD (i.e., men can and do develop the syndrome); second, that whether described quantitatively (amount) or qualitatively (type), exposure alone cannot account for women's excess risk; third, that the differences are most clearly apparent from adolescence through middle age, and less clearly apparent in early and late life; and fourth, that societal context may amplify or diminish observed effects. Certainly, the last two "facts" are less well established than the first two, but our tentative conclusion is that both developmental and societal contexts are potentially important. More research is needed to establish with certainty the parameters in which gender exerts its effects.

Recently, Saxe and Wolfe (1999) reviewed conceptualizations pertaining to gender and PTSD, organized according to biological, feminist/ psychodynamic, and social-cognitive perspectives. Biological models may eventually provide an explanation for much of women's differential vulnerability. After all, the differences are not strictly attributable to exposure, and they were observable across cultures, developmental stages, and research contexts. Moreover, psychophysiological studies have documented sex differences in stress response. For example, Shalev, Orr, and Pitman (1993) found that women are more physiologically reactive than men to trauma stimuli on a variety of indicators, and Schaeffer and Baum (1984) reported a gender-by-exposure interaction in the production of urinary cortisol after the Three Mile Island nuclear accident, such that exposed men had higher levels than exposed women, but unexposed men and women did not differ. (Other studies show that *low* cortisol is a predictor of PTSD; see Saxe & Wolfe, 1999.) We do not have expertise in the biology of trauma and so must leave the interpretation of these epidemiological data to those who do. Suffice it to say that viable biological models will likely account for the developmental trends in sex differences across the life course; it seems entirely reasonable that some models could do so. It may be more difficult for biological models to explain why sex differences are greater in some cultures than others. (See Rassmusson & Friedman, Chapter 2, this volume, for further discussion of biological models.)

The feminist/psychodynamic perspective focuses on the important role of relationships in women's lives. From this perspective, it is important that women's heightened risk for experiencing interpersonal violence accounts for much of their higher prevalence of PTSD. Likewise, women's differential vulnerability for experiencing heightened distress following normative (as opposed to traumatic) stressful events is greatest in the sphere of network events (Kessler & McLeod, 1984). Wolfe and Kimerling (1997) noted that women may be more likely to have preexisting depression as a result of societal acceptance and perpetuation of violence against women and girls. In accord with this, Breslau et al. (1997) found that preexisting differences in the prevalence of major depressive disorder partially explained observed sex differences in the prevalence of PTSD. They also found that sex differences are greater among individuals whose first experience of trauma occurred in childhood. But can this perspective account for the finding that women are also at greater risk following events that are less obviously interpersonal, such as disasters? Actually, yes. Drawing on previous research elucidating the social consequences of disasters (see Kaniasty & Norris, 1997), we would argue with the conceptualization of disaster as an "impersonal" trauma with few implications for interpersonal relationships (Saxe & Wolfe, 1999). We have found in our own research (e.g., Norris & Kaniasty, 1996) that disaster victims often experience a deterioration in their perceptions of social support and embeddedness. Moreover, women often assume a great deal of responsibility for providing care to their families and communities when many people are simultaneously in need (Solomon, in press; Solomon, Smith, Robins, & Fischbach, 1987). Wolfe and Kimerling (1997) also speculated that the routine stressors of poverty, discrimination, and oppression may produce in women a heightened perception of threat or a reduced capacity to cope. All of these factors potentially provide explanations for the effects of sex at both the point of event perception and at the point of symptom expression. Again, stronger theories within this group will specify why these stressors or relationships vary in their explanatory power across culture and age.

The final perspective reviewed by Saxe and Wolfe (1999) was the social-cognitive perspective, according to which "an individual's gender identity is partially determined by the meanings of being a male and female in the social environment in which an individual grows up and lives" (p. 171). Culture, of course, is a critical aspect of this social environment. Saxe and Wolfe hypothesized that cognitions related to trauma, such as helplessness, are more dissonant with men's self-concepts, and that men are therefore more highly motivated to alter their thoughts about the trauma to reduce the dissonance. Thus, gender role socialization may cause men to suppress symptom experiences and women to disclose them (see also Wolfe & Kimerling, 1997). If true, we would expect these influences to be greater in cultures that foster traditional views of men and women. Overall, the social-cognitive perspective explains our findings well. It can account for the reversal of the difference between the sexes at the point where cognition and meaning come into play (Criterion A2) and can certainly account for the fact that women acknowledge the presence of symptoms more readily than men. It can account for the emergence of differences in adolescence, if less clearly for the dissipation of differences in late life.

It is admittedly frustrating that the data presented here neither support nor refute any of the various theoretical perspectives convincingly. There is a real need for research that is designed specifically to test hypotheses regarding the etiology of sex differences. There is likewise a need for research that can answer the fundamental question regarding whether these differences are "real," that is, the result of actual gender differences in perceptions and coping processes, or merely reporting biases. And finally, as noted earlier, we believe there is an urgent need for general population studies on PTSD in less developed areas of the world. Only cross-cultural studies can delineate more precisely the ways in which culture and gender combine to shape the experience of trauma and its aftermath.

Implications for Intervention

What do these findings indicate that we should do? Any answer to this question must be regarded as tentative, pending a better understanding of the etiology of PTSD. Three points, however, are rather clear. First, if trauma and PTSD are as prevalent in populations as our review suggests, then we must consider population-based solutions. A host of writers (e.g., Dohrenwend, 1978; Hobfoll, 1988; Koss & Harvey, 1991) have emphasized the need for psychosocial interventions to help people accrue or replace the resources that foster stress resistance and have furthermore shown that attention must be directed at system-level as well as individual-level resources and practices.

Second, proposed solutions must match a stress/trauma process that occurs over time, involving objective stressors or events, subjective interpretations, acute distress, and chronic disorder. Since the seminal writings of Caplan (1964), population-based solutions have distinguished between primary, secondary, and tertiary prevention. Accordingly, Norris and Thompson (1995) organized their review of the trauma prevention literature along two dimensions: (1) the *timing of the intervention*, which distinguishes between interventions taking place before the crisis (primary prevention), during the crisis (secondary prevention), or after the crisis (tertiary prevention); and (2) the *level of the intervention*, which distinguishes between interventions targeting individual-level or societal-level resources. The point here is that different approaches may be called for depending upon whether the goal is to prevent objective stressors, experienced trauma, acute posttraumatic stress, or chronic disorders. A variety of approaches—ranging from individual psychotherapy to political action—are necessary, because they tackle the problem at different points (Dohrenwend, 1978).

Third, although gender-linked risk varies across the exposure–PTSD sequence, with men more at risk at the first stage and women more at risk at the latter three stages, none of the differences documented here are so large that either gender can be neglected at any stage. To note that women are less exposed to objectively defined events is one thing, but with prevalence rates no less than 50%, women's exposure can hardly be ignored in primary prevention efforts. Perhaps no single objective would do as much to reduce the prevalence of PTSD in the population as curtailing violence. Whether political or interpersonal, sexual or nonsexual, violence is the single leading cause of PTSD in both men and women. Whereas both men and women (and both boys and girls) are frequent victims of violence, perpetrators are disproportionately male (e.g., Baker & Diaz, 2000). This is one clear, gender-linked issue: We must address the societal attitudes and practices that promote male violence.

Humans also play a role in causing, and can therefore also play a role in preventing, unintentional trauma, such as that experienced in the context of disasters. Classification schemes have almost always distinguished disasters of natural origin from those of technological origin. Human-caused events such as dam collapses and industrial accidents "represent in the eyes of victims a callousness, carelessness, intentionality, or insensitivity on the part of others" (Bolin, 1985, p. 15). Technological disasters are frequently followed by lasting disputes that fragment and politicize the community. However, the distinction between natural and technological disasters is not always clear. Human factors, such as housing quality and land use policies, may greatly exacerbate the impact of ostensibly natural phenomena. The point is that even natural disasters are often the result of individual and societal practices that are difficult, but not impossible, to alter.

The second point in the sequence is the transition from objective stressor to the subjective experience of trauma. Although women are more likely than men to experience an objective stressor as traumatic, men and women differ much less from one another in their experience of trauma (70% vs. 80%) than do events in eliciting it (67–90%). Certain events almost uniformly elicit terror, horror, or helplessness. In many ways, these are natural responses to danger that, overall, have been quite adaptive in our species and others. Suggesting that people (or women) should feel less frightened or horrified in the face of threats to life makes little sense, for that same rush of adrenalin could, in fact, save their lives. The only fruitful possibility here is to empower persons in advance of exposure in the hope of reducing the profound powerlessness that may be elicited by traumatic events (Harvey, 1990). Fostering resistance resources in at-risk populations, such as women and youth, remains an important, if elusive, goal of community psychology and psychiatry.

The next point in the chain is the transition from traumatic stress to acute posttraumatic distress. It has been said often but bears repeating that some distress is a normal reaction to abnormal events. Transient stress reactions are not, in themselves, pathological, and most people can and do "get over" stressful events (see Dohrenwend, 1978, for a fine discussion of this). It is just as accurate to say that 90% of men and 80% of women do *not* develop criterion-level psychiatric problems following trauma exposure as it is to say that 10% of men and 20% of women do. This observation bears witness to the resilience of most men and most women. In the face of crisis, social support from families, friends, and community institutions is fundamentally important for both women and men. As trauma professionals, we should search for ways to bolster and facilitate access to these naturally occurring resources.

Of course, our greatest concern is for those individuals who develop chronic, enduring PTSD. Sadly, it is here that the gender gap grows particularly large, with women being three to four times as likely as men to develop chronic conditions that in all likelihood require medical or psychotherapeutic intervention. In their review of the efficacy of current treatments for PTSD, Solomon, Gerrity, and Muff (1992) concluded that cognitive, behavioral, psychodynamic, and pharmacological therapies all hold promise, but that further research is needed to identify the most effective combinations of treatment approaches. Treatments must also be sensitive to issues of culture and gender, because a given treatment may be differentially effective for women and men. Certainly, more research on this issue is needed as well. Advances in treatment are extremely important, but we must also remember that remediation constitutes a population-level solution (tertiary prevention) only if conducted on a very large scale (Caplan, 1964).

In closing, we simply want to remind the reader that seemingly fairly low rates can produce overwhelmingly large numbers when applied to populations. If rates of PTSD in the general population are 5% for men and 10% for women, we would expect to find 25,000 male survivors and 50,000 female survivors in a metropolitan area composed of 1,000,000 adults. As important as treatment is, we will be hard pressed to alter the epidemiology of PTSD one person at a time.

ACKNOWLEDGMENTS

Preparation of this chapter was funded in part by Grant No. R01 MH51278 from the National Institute of Mental Health, Fran H. Norris, Principal Investigator. Appreciation is extended to Krzysztof Kaniasty for allowing us to include data from his study of the Opole flood in this chapter, and to David Takeuchi, Principal Investigator, NIMH Grant No. 47460, and Lisa Tracey for deriving PTSD rates by sex from the Chinese American Psychiatric Epidemiology Study in response to our request.

REFERENCES

American Psychiatric Association. (1994). *Diagnostic and statistical manual of mental disorders* (4th ed.). Washington, DC: Author.

Amir, M., & Sol, O. (1999). Psychological impact and prevalence of traumatic events in a student sample in Israel: The effects of multiple traumatic events and physical injury. *Journal of Traumatic Stress, 12*, 139–153.

Anderson, K., & Manuel, G. (1994). Gender differences in reported stress response to the Loma Prieta earthquake. *Sex Roles, 30*, 725–733.

Awadh, A., Vance, B., El-Beblawi, V., & Pumariega, A. (1998). Effects of trauma of the Gulf War on Kuwaiti children. *Journal of Child and Family Studies, 7*, 493–498.

Baker, C., & Diaz, D. (2000, April). *Relation between violence, physical and psychological indicators, and social support in a random sample of Mexicans.* Paper presented at the annual meeting of the Society for Applied Anthropology, San Francisco, CA.

Berman, S., Kurtines, W., Silverman, W., & Serafini, L. (1996). The impact of exposure to crime and violence on urban youth. *American Journal of Orthopsychiatry, 66*, 329–336.

Berton, M., & Stabb, S. (1996). Exposure to violence and post-traumatic stress disorder in urban adolescents. *Adolescence, 31*, 489–498.

Bolin, R. (1985). Disaster characteristics and psychosocial impacts. In B. T. Sowder (Ed.), *Disasters and mental health: Selected contemporary perspectives* (pp. 2–28). Rockville, MD: National Institute of Mental Health.

Boney-McCoy, S., & Finkelhor, D. (1995). Psychosocial sequelae of violent victimization in a national youth sample. *Journal of Consulting and Clinical Psychology, 63,* 726–736.

Boney-McCoy, S., & Finkelhor, D. (1996). Is youth victimization related to trauma symptoms and depression after controlling for prior symptoms and family relationships?: A longitudinal, prospective study. *Journal of Consulting and Clinical Psychology, 64,* 1406–1416.

Bravo, M., Rubio-Stipec, M., Canino, G., Woodbury, M., & Ribera, J. (1990). The psychological sequelae of disaster stress prospectively and retrospectively evaluated. *American Journal of Community Psychology, 18,* 661–680.

Breslau, N. (1998). Epidemiology of trauma and posttraumatic stress disorder. In R. Yehuda (Ed.), *Psychological trauma* (pp. 1–29). Washington, DC: American Psychiatric Press.

Breslau, N., Chilcoat, H., Kessler, R., & Davis, G. (1999). Previous exposure to trauma and PTSD effects of subsequent trauma: Results from the Detroit Area Survey of Trauma. *American Journal of Psychiatry, 156,* 902–907.

Breslau, N., & Davis, G. (1992). Posttraumatic stress disorder in an urban population of young adults: Risk factors for chronicity. *American Journal of Psychiatry, 149,* 671–675.

Breslau, N., Davis, G., & Andreski, P. (1995). Risk factors for PTSD-related traumatic events: A prospective analysis. *American Journal of Psychiatry, 152,* 529–535.

Breslau, N., Davis, G., Andreski, P., & Peterson, E. (1991). Traumatic events and posttraumatic stress disorder in an urban population of young adults. *Archives of General Psychiatry, 48,* 216–222.

Breslau, N., Davis, G., Andreski, P., Peterson, E., & Schulz, L. (1997). Sex differences in posttraumatic stress disorder. *Archives of General Psychiatry, 54,* 1044–1048.

Breslau, N., Kessler, R., Chilcoat, H., Schulz, L., Davis, G., & Andreski, P. (1998). Trauma and posttraumatic stress disorder in the community: The 1996 Detroit Area Survey of Trauma. *Archives of General Psychiatry, 55,* 627–632.

Caplan, G. (1964). *Principles of preventive psychiatry.* New York: Basic Books.

Carlson, E., & Hogan, R. (1994). Cross-cultural response to trauma: A study of traumatic experiences and posttraumatic symptoms in Cambodian refugees. *Journal of Traumatic Stress, 7,* 43–58.

Carr, V., Lewin, T., Kenardy, J., Webster, R., Hazell, P., Carter, G., & Williamson, M. (1997). Psychosocial sequelae of the 1989 Newcastle earthquake: III. Role of vulnerability factors in post-disaster morbidity. *Psychological Medicine, 27,* 179–190.

Carr, V., Lewin, T., Webster, A., Kenardy, J., Hazell, P., & Carter, G. (1997). Psychosocial sequelae of the 1989 Newcastle earthquake: II. Exposure and morbidity profiles during the first 2 years post-disaster. *Psychological Medicine, 27,* 167–178.

Cheung, P. (1994). Posttraumatic stress disorder among Cambodian refugees in New Zealand. *International Journal of Social Psychiatry, 40,* 17–26.

Davidson, J., Hughes, D., Blazer, D., & George, L. (1991). Post-traumatic stress disorder in the community: An epidemiological study. *Psychological Medicine, 21,* 713–721.

de la Fuente, R. (1990). The mental health consequences of the 1985 earthquakes in Mexico. *International Journal of Mental Health, 19,* 21–29.

Dohrenwend, B. S. (1978). Social stress and community psychology. *American Journal of Community Psychology, 6,* 1–14.

Durkin, M. (1993). Major depression and post-traumatic stress disorder following the Coalinga and Chile earthquakes. In R. Allen (Ed.), *Handbook of post-disaster intervention* (pp. 405–420). Corte Madera, CA: Select Press.

Fitzpatrick, K., & Boldizar, J. (1993). The prevalence and consequences of exposure to violence among African-American youth. *Journal of the American Academy of Child and Adolescent Psychiatry, 32*, 424–430.

Flett, R., Kazantzis, N., Long, N., MacDonald, C., & Millar, M. (2000). *Comparison of the incidence of traumatic events across Canadian, New Zealand, and North American samples.* Unpublished manuscript.

Foley, J., & Price, A. (1999). *Psychological outcomes in adolescents exposed to community violence.* Poster presented at the 7th Biennial Conference of the Society for Community Research and Action, New Haven, CT.

Freedy, J., Addy, C., Kilpatrick, D., Resnick, H., & Garrison, C. (2000). *Examination of a multivariate risk factor model for predicting post-traumatic stress disorder following two major natural disasters.* Unpublished manuscript.

Garrison, C., Weinrich, M., Hardin, S., Weinrich, S., & Wang, L. (1993). Post-traumatic stress disorder in adolescents after a hurricane. *American Journal of Epidemiology, 138*, 522–530.

Giaconia, R., Reinherz, H., Silverman, A., Pakiz, B., Frost, A., & Cohen, A. (1995). Trauma and posttraumatic stress disorder in a community population of older adolescents. *Journal of the American Academy of Child and Adolescent Psychiatry, 34*, 1369–1380.

Gleser, G., Green, B., & Winget, C. (1981). *Prolonged psychosocial effects of disaster: A study of Buffalo Creek.* New York: Academic Press.

Goenjian, A., Pynoos, R., Steinberg, A., Najarian, L., Asarnow, J., Karayan, I., Ghurabi, M., & Fairbanks, L. (1995). Psychiatric comorbidity in children after the 1988 earthquake in Armenia. *Journal of American Academy of Child and Adolescent Psychiatry, 34*, 1174–1184.

Goldstein, R., Wampler, N., & Wise, P. (1997). War experiences and distress symptoms of Bosnian children. *Pediatrics, 100*, 873–878.

Green, B., Korol, M., Grace, M., Vary, M., Leonard, A., Gleser, G., & Smitson-Cohen, S. (1991). Children and disaster: Age, gender, and parental effects on PTSD symptoms. *Journal of the American Academy of Child and Adolescent Psychiatry, 30*, 945–951.

Green, B., Lindy, J., Grace, M., Gleser, G., Leonard, A., Korol, M., & Winget, C. (1990). Buffalo Creek survivors in the second decade. *American Journal of Orthopsychiatry, 60*, 43–54.

Hanson, R., Kilpatrick, D., Freedy, J., & Saunders, B. (1995). Los Angeles County after the 1992 civil disturbances: Degree of exposure and impact on mental health. *Journal of Consulting and Clinical Psychology, 63*, 987–996.

Harvey, M. (1990, November). *An ecological view of psychological trauma and recovery from trauma.* Paper presented at the meeting of the International Society for Traumatic Stress Studies, New Orleans, LA.

Helzer, J., Robins, L., & McEvoy, L. (1987). Post-traumatic stress disorder in the general population: Findings of the Epidemiologic Catchment Area Survey. *New England Journal of Medicine, 317*, 1630–1634.

Hobfoll, S. (1988). *The ecology of stress.* New York: Hemisphere.

Hofstede, G. (1980). *Culture's consequences: International differences in work-related values.* Beverly Hills, CA: Sage.

Husain, S., Nair, J., Holcomb, W., Reid, J., Vargas, V., & Nair, S. (1998). Stress reactions of children and adolescents in war and siege conditions. *American Journal of Psychiatry, 155*, 1718–1719.

Kaniasty, K., & Norris, F. (1997). Social support dynamics in adjustment to disasters. In S. Duck (Ed.), *Handbook of personal relationships* (2nd ed., pp. 595–619). London: Wiley.

Kessler, R., & McLeod, J. (1984). Sex differences in vulnerability to undesirable life events. *American Sociological Review, 49*, 620–631.

Kessler, R., Sonnega, A., Bromet, E., Hughes, M., & Nelson, C. (1995). Posttraumatic stress disorder in the National Comorbidity Survey. *Archives of General Psychiatry, 52*, 1048–1060.

Kilpatrick, D., & Saunders, B. (1999). *Prevalence and consequences of child victimization: Results from the National Survey of Adolescents* (Final Report, Grant No. 93-IJ-CX-0023). Charleston, SC: Authors.

Koss, M., & Harvey, M. (1991). *The rape victim: Clinical and community interventions.* Newbury Park, CA: Sage.

Kuterovac, G., Dyregrov, A., & Stuvland, R. (1994). Children in war: A silent majority under stress. *British Journal of Medical Psychology, 67*, 363–375.

La Greca, A., Silverman, W., Vernberg, E., & Prinstein, M. (1996). Symptoms of posttraumatic stress in children after Hurricane Andrew: A prospective study. *Journal of Consulting and Clinical Psychology, 64*, 712–723.

Lindy, J., & Grace, M. (1985). The recovery environment: Continuing stressor versus a healing psychosocial space. In B. Sowder & M. Lystad (Eds.), *Disasters and mental health* (pp. 147–160). Washington, DC: American Psychiatric Press.

Lundin, T., Mardberg, B., & Otto, U. (1993). Chernobyl: Nuclear threat as disaster. In J. Wilson & B. Raphael (Eds.), *International handbook of traumatic stress syndromes* (pp. 431–439. New York: Plenum Press.

Macksoud, M., & Aber, J. L. (1996). The war experiences and psychosocial development of children in Lebanon. *Child Development, 67*, 70–88.

Madakasira, S., & O'Brien, K. (1987). Acute posttraumatic stress disorder in victims of a natural disaster. *Journal of Nervous and Mental Disease, 175*, 286–290.

Mollica, R., Poole, C. & Tor, S. (1998). Symptoms, functioning, and health problems in a massively traumatized population: The legacy of the Cambodian tragedy. In B. P. Dohrenwend (Ed.), *Adversity, stress, and psychopathology* (pp. 34–51). New York: Oxford University Press.

Norris, F. (1992). Epidemiology of trauma: Frequency and impact of different potentially traumatic events on different demographic groups. *Journal of Consulting and Clinical Psychology, 60*, 409–418.

Norris, F., & Kaniasty, K. (1996). Received and perceived social support in times of stress: A test of the social support deterioration deterrence model. *Journal of Personality and Social Psychology, 71*, 498–511.

Norris, F., Murphy, A., Baker, C., & Perilla, J. (2000, November). *Epidemiology of trauma and PTSD in Mexico.* Poster presented at the annual meeting of the International Society for Traumatic Stress Studies, San Antonio, TX.

Norris, F., Perilla, J., Ibañez, G., & Murphy, A. (2001). Sex differences in symptoms of post-traumatic stress: Does culture play a role? *Journal of Traumatic Stress, 14*, 7–28.

Norris, F., & Thompson, M. (1995). Applying community psychology to the prevention of trauma and traumatic life events. In J. Freedy & S. Hobfoll (Eds.), *Traumatic stress: From theory to practice* (pp. 49–71). New York: Plenum Press.

North, C., Nixon, S., Shariat, S., Mallonee, S., McMillan, J., Spitznagel, E., & Smith, E. (1999). Psychiatric disorders among survivors of the Oklahoma City bombing. *Journal of the American Medical Association, 282,* 755–762.

North, C., Nixon, S., & Vincent, R. (1998, November). *A study of the mental health effects of the Oklahoma bombing on direct survivors, compared to other disasters studied with the same methods.* Paper presented at the annual meeting of the International Society for Traumatic Stress Studies, Washington, DC.

Perkonigg, A., & Wittchen, H. (1999). Prevalence and comorbidity of traumatic events and posttraumatic stress disorder in adolescents and young adults. In A. Maercker, M. Schutzwohl, & Z. Solomon (Eds.), *Post-traumatic stress disorder: A lifespan developmental perspective* (pp. 113–133). Kirkland, WA: Hogrefe & Huber.

Pynoos, R., Frederick, C., Nader, K., Arroyo, W., Steinberg, A., Eth, S., Nunez, F., & Fairbanks, L. (1987). Life threat and posttraumatic stress in school-age children. *Archives of General Psychiatry, 44,* 1057–1063.

Pynoos, R., Goenjian, A., Tashjian, M., Karakashian, M., Manjikian, R., Manoukian, G., Steinberg, A., & Fairbanks, L. (1993). Post-traumatic stress reactions in children after the 1988 Armenian earthquake. *British Journal of Psychiatry, 163,* 239–247.

Quarantelli, E. (1994). *Future disaster trends and policy implications for developing countries.* Newark, DE: Disaster Research Center.

Reppesgard, H. (1997). Studies on psychosocial problems among displaced people in Sri Lanka. *European Journal of Psychiatry, 11,* 223–234.

Resnick, H., Kilpatrick, D., Dansky, B., Saunders, B., & Best, C. (1993). Prevalence of civilian trauma and posttraumatic stress disorder in a representative national sample of women. *Journal of Consulting and Clinical Psychology, 61,* 984–991.

Richters, J., & Martinez, P. (1993). The NIMH Community Violence Project: I. Children as victims of and witnesses to violence. *Psychiatry, 56,* 7–21.

Sack, W., McSharry, S., Clarke, G., Kinney, R., Seeley, M., & Lewinsohn, P. (1994). The Khmer Adolescent Project: I. Epidemiological findings in two generations of Cambodian refugees. *Journal of Nervous and Mental Disease, 182,* 387–395.

Saxe, G., & Wolfe, J. (1999). Gender and posttraumatic stress disorder. In P. Saigh & J. D. Bremner (Eds.), *Posttraumatic stress disorder: A comprehensive text* (pp. 160–179). Boston: Allyn & Bacon.

Schaeffer, M., & Baum, A. (1984). Adrenal cortical response to stress at Three Mile Island. *Psychosomatic Medicine, 46,* 227–237.

Schwab-Stone, M., Ayers, T., Kasprow, W., Voyce, C., Barone, C., Shriver, T., & Weissberg, R. (1995). No safe haven: A study of violence exposure in an urban community. *Journal of the American Academy of Child and Adolescent Psychiatry, 34,* 1343–1352.

Shalev, A., Orr, S., & Pitman, R. (1993). Psychophysiologic assessment of traumatic imagery in Israeli civilian patients with posttraumatic stress disorder. *American Journal of Psychiatry, 150,* 620–624.

Shannon, M., Lonigan, C., Finch, A., & Taylor, C. (1994). Children exposed to disaster: I. Epidemiology of post-traumatic symptoms and symptom profiles. *Journal of American Academy of Child and Adolescent Psychiatry, 33,* 80–93.

Shore, J., Tatum, E., & Vollmer, W. (1986). Evaluation of mental effects of disaster: Mount St. Helens eruption. *American Journal of Public Health, 76,* 76–83.

Singer, M., Anglin, T., Song, L., & Lunghofer, L. (1995). Adolescents' exposure to violence and associated symptoms on psychological trauma. *Journal of the American Medical Association, 273*, 477–482.

Smith, E., North, C., & Spitznagel, E. (1993). Post-traumatic stress in survivors of three disasters. In R. Allen (Ed.), *Handbook of post-disaster intervention* (pp. 353–368). Corte Madera, CA: Select Press.

Smith, E., Robins, L., Przybeck, T., Goldring, E., & Solomon, S. (1986). Psychosocial consequences of a disaster. In J. Shore (Ed.), *Disaster stress studies: New methods and findings* (pp. 49–76). Washington, DC: American Psychiatric Press.

Solomon, S. D. (in press). Gender differences in response to disaster. In G. Weidner, S. M. Kopp, & M. Kristenson (Eds.), *Heart disease: Environment, stress, and gender* (NATO Science Series I: Life and Behavioural Sciences, Vol. 327). Amsterdam: IOS Press.

Solomon, S. D., & Canino, G. (1990). The appropriateness of DSM-IIIR criteria for post-traumatic stress disorder. *Comprehensive Psychiatry, 31*, 227–237.

Solomon, S. D., Gerrity, E. T., & Muff, A. M. (1992). Efficacy of treatments for post-traumatic stress disorder. *Journal of the American Medical Association, 268*, 633–638.

Solomon, S. D., Smith, E., Robins, L., & Fischbach, R. (1987). Social involvement as a mediator of disaster-induced stress. *Applied Journal of Social Psychology, 17*, 1092–1112.

Stein, M., Walker, J., & Forde, D. (2000). Gender differences in susceptibility to post-traumatic stress disorder. *Behaviour Research and Therapy, 38*, 619–628.

Stein, M., Walker, J., Hazen, A., & Forde, D. (1997). Full and partial posttraumatic stress disorder: Findings from a community survey. *American Journal of Psychiatry, 154*, 1114–1119.

Steinglass, P., & Gerrity, E. (1990). Natural disasters and post-traumatic stress disorder: Short-term versus long-term recovery in two disaster affected communities. *Journal of Applied Social Psychology, 20*, 1746–1765.

Thabet, A., & Vostanis, P. (1999). Post-traumatic stress reactions in children of war. *Journal of Child Psychology and Psychiatry, 40*, 385–391.

Thompson, M., Norris, F., & Hanacek, B. (1993). Age differences in the psychological consequences of Hurricane Hugo. *Psychology and Aging, 8*, 606–616.

Thulesius, H., & Hakansson, A. (1999). Screening for posttraumtic stress disorder symptoms among Bosnian refugees. *Journal of Traumatic Stress, 12*, 167–174.

Vrana, S., & Lauterbach, D. (1994). Prevalence of traumatic events and post-traumatic psychological symptoms in a nonclinical sample of college students. *Journal of Traumatic Stress, 7*, 289–302.

Wierzbicka, A. (1994). Emotion, language, and cultural scripts. In S. Kitayama & H. Markus (Eds.) *Emotion and culture: Empirical studies of mutual influence* (pp. 133–196). Washington, DC: American Psychological Association.

Wolfe, J., & Kimerling, R. (1997). Gender issues in the assessment of posttraumatic stress disorder. In J. Wilson & T. Keane (Eds.), *Assessing psychological trauma and PTSD* (pp. 192–238). New York: Guilford Press.

World Health Organization. (1993). *The Composite International Diagnostic Interview*. Geneva, Switzerland: Author.

2 | Gender Issues in the Neurobiology of PTSD

ANN M. RASMUSSON
MATTHEW J. FRIEDMAN

$\mathbf{P}$osttraumatic stress disorder (PTSD) (American Psychiatric Association, 1994) is a relatively common psychiatric disorder, with an overall lifetime prevalence of about 8% in the general population (Kessler, Sonnega, Bromet, Hughes, & Nelson, 1995). Rates of PTSD are significantly higher in certain at-risk populations, including combat veterans, victims of rape and violent assault (e.g., Kessler et al., 1995), and adolescents exposed to high levels of community violence (e.g., Lipschitz, Rasmusson, Anyan, Cromwell, & Southwick, 2000). In addition, despite common rates of exposure to traumatic events in males and females, the incidence and prevalence rates of PTSD are reported to be at least twice as high in women and adolescent girls as in men and adolescent boys (e.g., Breslau, Davis, Andreski, Peterson, & Schultz, 1997; Deykin & Buka, 1997; Stein, Walker, Hazen, & Forde, 1997; Stein, Walker, & Forde, 2000). The reasons for this gender difference in the incidence and prevalence of PTSD are not clear. As discussed in detail elsewhere in this volume, a number of factors could contribute to increased rates of PTSD in women, including gender-related differences in neurobiology.

In this chapter, we review published studies, as well as recent data from the National Center for PTSD, regarding the neurobiology of PTSD in women. The results of these studies then are compared to previous research findings in men with PTSD. This review provides, at best, leads about neurobiological factors that may contribute to gender differences in the vulnerability for PTSD. This is due to the fact that few studies with a neurobiological focus have been done on women with PTSD, and even fewer studies have compared neurobiological responses across gender. In addition, no published studies have investigated the effects of the menstrual cycle or reproductive status on stress responsive systems in women with PTSD. Finally, methodological differences among previous studies of the neurobiology of PTSD make comparison across studies, as well as across gender, difficult.

This chapter therefore also reviews previous studies in *healthy* humans and animals that explore gender and reproductive hormone effects on stress-sensitive neurobiological systems. We hope this will provide clues about mechanisms that might increase the risk for PTSD in women. This is a challenging topic. Extensive research over the past 30 years has demonstrated that the effects of reproductive hormones on stress-sensitive systems are numerous and complex and, in some instances, gender- or species-specific. For example, estrogen appears to affect hypothalamic–pituitary–adrenal (HPA) function differently in men and women, while effects of gender on the serotonin system vary between humans and some strains of animals.

This suggests that if we really are to understand the neurobiology of PTSD in women, we must study women with PTSD—not men, and not female animals. However, research aimed at elucidating the neurobiology of PTSD has to this point focused largely on male populations, with studies in men and boys numbering over 40, where as studies in women or girls number less than 20. The reasons for this gender discrepancy in research focus are probably many and may relate in part to historical gaps in availability of money targeting research in women. For instance, the Veterans Administration, which has funded much of the past research into the neurobiology of PTSD, has focused its resources primarily on male combat veterans, because most veterans are men. Recently, though, money from public and private institutions supporting research on women has increased. The increased biological complexity of women compared to men also may contribute to the reluctance of researchers to study women. Sex hormone profiles associated with the menstrual cycle, pregnancy, and menopause have unique effects on most stress-responsive systems; thus, women must be studied in each of these states to gauge accurately the impact of stress. Short of this, research studies on women should *match* for menstrual cycle phase and hormone status. This renders clinical research on women more difficult, time-consuming, and costly. Therefore, this chapter also suggests changes in research and academic policy that may be needed to promote the execution of appropriately designed studies of the neurobiology of PTSD in women.

PREVIOUS STUDIES OF THE NEUROBIOLOGY OF PTSD IN WOMEN

The Catecholamines

Numerous studies completed over many years using a variety of methods have demonstrated hyperreactivity of the sympathetic and noradrenergic systems in men with PTSD (Southwick et al., 1999). The sympathetic and noradrenergic systems mediate the "fight-or-flight" response activated in response to threat and accompanied by intense arousal, fear, aggression, and release of stress hormones such as cortisol. Indeed, it is generally appreciated that hyperreactivity of the sympathetic and noradrenergic systems contributes to the reexperiencing and hyperarousal symptoms of PTSD, as well as to the avoidance symptoms that develop in reaction to reexperiencing and hyperarousal symptoms. Consistent with these studies, Lemieux and Coe (1995) found increased 24-hour urinary norepinephrine and epinephrine levels in premenopausal women with PTSD compared to nonabused controls. Female subjects with a history of trauma, but without PTSD, showed values intermediate between these two groups. De Bellis et al. (1999) also found increased 24-hour urinary norepinephrine and dopamine levels in a combined group of girls and boys with PTSD compared to children with overanxious disorder and healthy controls. Urinary epinephrine levels were higher in the children with PTSD compared only to those with overanxious disorder. Because gender differences were not reported in the latter study, the most conservative interpretation of these studies is that females and males with PTSD are similar in having increases in the activity of the sympathetic or noradrenergic systems.

Gender-Related Hormone Effects

Possible gender differences in the magnitude of the noradrenergic system changes in PTSD have not been well examined. In the study by De Bellis et al., (1999), boys with and without PTSD had greater 24-hour urinary norepinephrine and epinephrine levels than girls with and without PTSD. However, weight and body mass were not factored into this comparison, which is critical, because urinary norepinephrine levels increase with weight and body mass (e.g., Lemieux & Coe, 1995). Nevertheless, research in *healthy* subjects suggests that there are gender differences in the function of the noradrenergic system. In studies of students not explicitly screened for psychiatric illness, men were found to have greater urinary norepinephrine and epinephrine (e.g., Frankenhaeuser et al., 1978) responses to mental stress compared to premenopausal women, even when the analyses controlled for body weight.

The literature also suggests that fluctuations in reproductive hormones across menstrual phase and reproductive state in women influence sympathetic system reactivity (Figure 2.1). For instance, women in the luteal phase of the menstrual cycle have been shown to have increased norepinephrine levels (Goldstein, Levinson, & Keiser, 1983), increased stroke volume but lower vascular tone (Girdler, Pedersen, Stern, & Light, 1993), greater cardiovascular responses to a cold pressor test but not to mental arithmetic (Tersman, Collins, & Eneroth, 1991), and greater blood pressure and pulse changes in response to ambient environmental stress

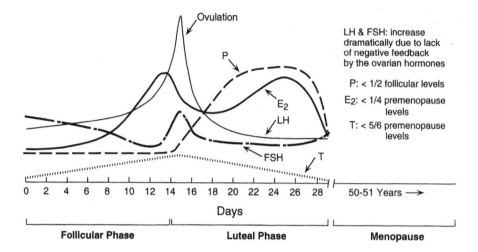

FIGURE 2.1. Reproductive hormone levels across the menstrual cycle and into menopause. Adapted from Carr and Wilson (1987). Copyright 1987 by the McGraw-Hill Companies, Inc. Adapted by permission.

(Manhem & Jern, 1994) than women in the follicular phase. Female sheep also have been shown to have greater norepinephrine and epinephrine responses to insulin-induced hypoglycemia during the luteal compared to the follicular phases of the estrus cycle (Komesaroff, Esler, Clarke, Fullerton, & Funder, 1998).

Nevertheless, estrogen levels within the luteal phase of the menstrual cycle have been found to correlate negatively with cardiac responses to stress (Sita & Miller, 1996), suggesting an inhibitory role for estrogen on sympathetic activity. Indeed, this is consistent with studies showing menopausal women to have increased cardiovascular and epinephrine responses (e.g., Saab, Matthews, Stoney, & McDonald, 1989) to mental stress compared to premenopausal women. In addition, Lindheim et al. (1992) and Komesaroff, Esler, and Sudhir (1999) reported that blood pressure and catecholamine responses to psychological stress were reduced by estrogen replacement in postmenopausal women.

Thus, if the degree of noradrenergic system hyperreactivity is considered important in mediating PTSD symptoms, menstrual phase and reproductive status should be factored into studies examining a role for the noradrenergic system in modulating PTSD risk and severity in women. On a technical note, we should also appreciate that there are more sophisticated measures of sympathetic system activity than urinary or plasma catecholamine measures, including determinations of jugular venous noradrenaline spillover and microneurography (Grassi & Esler, 1999). These methods are reported to be more accurate and can be used to discriminate between brain noradrenergic and peripheral sympathetic activity. The use of these methods is illustrated in a recent study of panic disorder (Wilkinson et al., 1998), and could potentially be extended to studies of PTSD in men and women.

Neuropeptide Y

Neuropeptide (NPY) is another sympathoadrenomedullary system neurotransmitter with probable relevance to the pathophysiology of PTSD in women. NPY, a 36-amino-acid peptide, is arguably the most abundant peptide in the peripheral and central nervous systems. NPY is stored (colocalized) with norepinephrine in most sympathetic nerve fibers involved in the mammalian fight-or-flight response. It is also present in nonadrenergic perivascular, gut, cardiac nonsympathetic, and parasympathetic nerves, as well as in the adrenal medulla (Wahlestedt & Reis, 1993). In the brain, NPY is colocalized with norepinephrine in the locus ceruleus, a brain area that mediates arousal. It is stored with a variety of other neurotransmitters in the amygdala, cortex, hippocampus, serotonergic raphe nuclei, and periaqueductal grey—also structures that play important roles in mediating the mammalian stress response (Heilig & Widerlov, 1990).

Extensive basic research has demonstrated that NPY is released when the sympathetic nervous system is intensely activated, as would be expected to occur in response to traumatic stress (e.g., Wahlestedt & Reis, 1993). Indeed, human plasma NPY levels have been shown to increase in response to activation of the sympathetic nervous system by intense exercise (Pernow 1986), electroconvulsive therapy (Richard Hauger, personal communication, March 2002), and the α_2-noradrenergic receptor antagonist, yohimbine (Rasmusson, Hauger, et al., 2000). At the synaptic level, NPY has been shown to inhibit the release of neurotransmitters with which it is colocalized, as well as to enhance the postsynaptic receptor responses to these neurotransmitters once it is released (Colmers & Bleakman, 1994). Thus, NPY appears to play a role in enhancing the efficiency of the sympathetic nervous system by increasing the threshold for stress activation of the system and enhancing signal transduction once activation occurs.

Studies of the NPY effects in the central nervous system also suggest a role for NPY in the pathophysiology of anxiety disorders such as PTSD. Intracerebroventricular injection (i.e., injection into a cerebrospinal fluid compartment within the brain) of a low dose of NPY has been shown to increase anxiety in animals via activity at brain NPY-Y_2 receptors, whereas higher doses reduce anxiety via brain NPY-Y_1 receptors (e.g., Nakajima et al., 1998). Thus a dose-dependent balance between activation of central Y_1 and Y_2 receptors may determine how much anxiety is experienced in response to the stress-induced release of

NPY. In addition, intracerebroventricular administration of NPY has been found to antagonize anxiety produced by cortiocotropin-releasing factor (CRF) (Britton, Akwa, Spina, & Koob, 2000). CRF, a peptide, has been found to be involved in generating anxiety and defensive behaviors in response to stress in animals. In addition, high levels of CRF have been found in the cerebrospinal fluid of male combat veterans with PTSD (e.g., Baker et al., 1999).

A role for NPY in the pathophysiology of anxiety disorders in humans is also supported by observations of increased behavioral anxiety in animals showing decreased NPY messenger RNA (mRNA) levels in the amygdala and cortex after exposure to chronic restraint stress (Thorsell et al., 1998). In humans, anxiety has been shown to be increased in combat veterans with PTSD treated with the α_2-antagonist, yohimbine (Southwick et al., 1993). These subjects with PTSD also showed low baseline plasma NPY levels and blunted NPY responses to yohimbine. In addition, there was a negative correlation between baseline plasma NPY levels and retrospective ratings of combat exposure, as well as activation of the sympathetic nervous system after yohimbine treatment (Rasmusson, Hauger, et al., 2000). These findings suggest that combat stress-induced decreases in plasma NPY may mediate long-term increases in the *reactivity* of the noradrenergic system in male veterans with PTSD. Indeed, these findings are consistent with animal research showing that plasma NPY decreases after chronic stress, and that these reductions are associated with increased stress activation of the noradrenergic system (Corder, Castagne, Rivet, Mormede, & Gaillard, 1992).

It is also important to note that a group of combat veterans without PTSD resembled combat veterans with PTSD in terms of decreased baseline plasma NPY. However, the combat controls showed normal NPY release and no increase in anxiety after yohimbine treatment, in contrast to PTSD subjects who exhibited reduced NPY release and elevated anxiety levels (Rasmusson et al., 2001). Thus, trauma-induced decreases in baseline NPY may increase sympathetic system reactivity, whereas maintenance of a normal capacity for NPY release in response to sympathetic nervous system stimulation may protect against the experience of pathological anxiety during stress. This possibility is supported by recent work showing that increases in plasma NPY levels are negatively correlated with dissociation (Morgan, Wang, et al., 2000) and distress (Morgan, Rasmusson, Wang, Hoyt, Hauger, & Hazlett, 2001) in male military recruits undergoing intensely stressful mock training interrogations. Further support for the impact of peripheral NPY responses on brain-mediated behavioral responses comes from the recent work of Antonijevic, Murck, Bohlhalter, Frieboes, Holsboer, and Steiger (2001) showing that the intravenous administration of NPY results in decreased nighttime ACTH and cortisol levels, as well as enhanced stage 2 and total sleep. Indeed, as outlined in Table 2.1, trauma-induced alterations in NPY physiology could contribute to several comorbid conditions associated with PTSD.

It is therefore noteworthy that we also have preliminary data in premenopausal women with PTSD showing a decrease in baseline plasma NPY levels and blunted NPY release in response to adrenocorticotropic hormone (ACTH) (Rasmusson et al., 2001). Thus, trauma-induced changes in NPY levels, or altered NPY release, may also play a role in the pathophysiology of PTSD in women, although further research is needed to verify this role.

Gender-Related Hormone Effects

Some research suggests that there may be a sexual dimorphism in the NPY response to stress. Male rats release more NPY in response to cold stress than female rats, and testosterone increases both tissue stores of NPY and NPY release (Zukowska-Grojec, 1995). These findings in rats are consistent with a study in humans showing increased exercise-induced NPY release in men compared to age-matched ovariectomized women with and without estrogen replacement (Zukowska-Grojec, 1995); indeed, testosterone levels in ovariectomized women are significantly reduced compared to levels in premenopausal women and men (Laughlin, Barrett-Connor, Kritz-Silverstein, & von Muhlen, 2000). Testosterone influences on NPY release also may account for the observed increase in exercise-induced NPY release in women in the immediate preovulatory phase of the menstrual cycle, when plasma testosterone levels in women peak (e.g., Lewandowski et al., 1998). In turn, relative decreases in NPY release during the luteal phase of the menstrual cycle may contribute mechanistically to increased norepinephrine levels observed in women during this phase (Goldstein et al., 1983).

Perhaps, then, hormone-based gender differences in NPY physiology could contribute to an increase in the rate of PTSD in women. Indeed, it seems conceivable that traumatic stress experienced during different phases of the menstrual or reproductive cycles could have different effects at a neurobiological level and thus could vary in its capacity to induce PTSD. Once chronic PTSD is established, PTSD symptoms also may vary across the menstrual and reproductive cycles in concert with changes in the capacity to restrain activation of the sympathetic nervous system by NPY. However, genetic factors may also play a role. A recently detected and relatively frequent variant in the structure of the NPY gene influences NPY release (Kallio et al., 2001) and thus might be expected to alter the adaptation of the NPY and sympathetic systems to chronic severe stress in affected individuals.

TABLE 2.1. Trauma-Induced NPY Deficits and Conditions Comorbid with PTSD

Comorbid condition	How low NPY may contribute to comorbid conditions in PTSD
Decreases in hippocampal volume (Bremner et al., 1997; Stein, Koverola, et al., 1997)	NPY inhibits glutamate release in the hippocampus (Greber et al., 1994), whereas high glutamate and cortisol levels have been found to be toxic to hippocampal neurons by contributing to metabolic energy deficits during stress (Sapolsky, 1985, 1986; McEwen et al., 1986).
Memory dysfunction (Wolfe & Schlesinger, 1997)	NPY may enhance conditioned aversive memory but interfere with working memory (Flood et al., 1987).
Poor exercise tolerance (Shalev et al., 1990)	NPY is released in response to intense exercise and increases the efficiency of the sympathetic nervous system.
Chronic pain syndromes (Beckham et al., 1997)	NPY modulates transmission along pain fibers in the spinal cord (Walker et al., 1988; Mellado et al., 1996).
Sleep disturbance	Increased reactivity of the sympathetic nervous system due to low NPY levels in PTSD may inhibit rapid eye movement (REM) sleep onset and eventuate in compensatory increases in REM density and nightmares (Mellman et al., 1997). This is supported by animal data showing that NPY reverses both CRF and psychological stress-induced shortening of pentobarbital-induced sleep (Yamada et al., 1997) and influences circadian phase shifts (Biello et al., 1997).
Blunting of positive emotions (American Psychiatric Association, 1994)	NPY mediates reward when injected into the nucleus accumbens, an important brain reward center (Josselyn & Beninger, 1993). Low levels or low release of NPY in this area may contribute to the anhedonia observed in PTSD.
Nicotine dependence (Beckham et al., 1997; Shalev et al., 1990)	Nicotine induces NPY release from the adrenal gland. Thus, high rates of smoking among patients with PTSD and traumatized individuals without PTSD may represent attempts to compensate for NPY deficits induced by trauma exposure.

The Serotonin System

The serotonin system has been implicated in a range of biobehavioral phenomena of relevance to PTSD, including anxiety, aggression, impulsivity, sleep patterns, depression and suicidality, neuroendocrine regulation, perception, and cognition (Heninger, 1997). In addition, the selective serotonin reuptake inhibitors (SSRIs) have been found to be at least partially effective in the treatment of PTSD. This is consistent with findings of serotonin system dysfunction in PTSD, including (1) decreased platelet paroxetine binding capacity and affinity, suggesting the possibility of deficient reuptake of serotonin after its release (e.g., Maes et al., 1999); (2) low platelet-poor plasma concentrations of serotonin (Spivak et al., 1999); (3) blunted prolactin response to fenfluramine, a serotonin releaser and reuptake inhibitor (Davis, Clark, Kramer, Moeller, & Petty, 1999); and (4) exaggerated reactivity to *m*-chlorophenyl piperazine (m-CPP), a serotonin 5-HT_{2c} receptor agonist, as measured by increased anxiety, panic attacks, and other PTSD symptoms in a subset of male veterans with PTSD compared to nontraumatized, healthy controls (Southwick et al., 1997). Overall, these studies suggest that there may be a decrease in serotonin availability at baseline in PTSD, accompanied by an upregulation of postsynaptic 5-HT_2 receptors that eventuates in increased behavioral responses to stress-related phasic increases in serotonin release.

Unfortunately, no studies of the serotonin system have been undertaken in women with PTSD. However, recent literature suggests that gender-related differences in serotonin system function in healthy humans could contribute to women's increased vulnerability to PTSD.

Gender-Related Hormone Effects

As discussed in detail by Rubinow, Schmidt, and Roca (1998) there are myriad effects of the gonadal hormones on all aspects of serotonin system function, including serotonin synthesis, release, reuptake, metabolism, receptor transcription, receptor number, receptor subtype, and receptor function. In addition, the serotonin system has been shown to be affected by gender, menstrual cycle phase, and reproductive state in numerous animal and human studies. However, some species-specific effects of the gonadal steroids on the serotonin system (e.g., Rubinow, Schmidt, & Roca, 1998) make it difficult to extrapolate findings from animal to humans studies. In this review then, we focus on studies of the serotonin system in humans.

In one study, Biver et al. (1996) demonstrated that there are fewer serotonergic 5-HT_2, receptors in women compared to men. Additionally, women have shown increased anxiety, prolactin, and oxytocin responses, as well as prolonged ACTH and cortisol responses to m-CPP, a serotonin 5-HT_{2c} receptor agonist (e.g., Bagdy & Arato, 1998). This suggests that women may be more vulnerable to anxiety associated with stress-induced increases in endogenous serotonin acting at 5-HT_2 receptors. In addition, Nishizawa et al. (1997) used positron emission tomography (PET) to demonstrate decreased baseline rates of serotonin synthesis in the brains of women compared to men, as well as greater decreases in brain serotonin synthesis after tryptophan depletion. Thus, it has been suggested that inadequate increases in serotonin synthesis and the availability of this neurotransmitter in response to stress may increase the vulnerability of women to depression. This may also pertain to PTSD. For example, serotonin restrains activation of the locus ceruleus (Charlety, Aston-Jones, Akaoka, Buda, & Chouvet, 1991), a brain area involved in regulation of arousal and attention (Aston-Jones, Rajkowski, & Cohen, 1999), and implicated in the pathophysiology of PTSD (Southwick et al., 1999).

Strong, recent evidence in both men and women indicates a link between neuroticism (anxiety, hostility, and depression) and a gene variant that codes for lower levels of the serotonin transporter involved in the reuptake of serotonin after its release. Interestingly, the relationship between this gene variant and neuroticism was more robust in a sample of primarily women compared to one containing primarily men (Greenberg et al., 2000). Thus, it is possible that effects of this serotonin transporter gene variant are influenced by gender or gender-related hormones. For instance, the number of serotonin transporters in the frontal lobe and brainstem is increased by estrogen (e.g., Sumner et al., 1999) and thus may vary across the menstrual cycle in women. Alternatively, a decreased capacity for serotonin synthesis in women may interact with a genetically based decrease in serotonin transporter number and affect serotonin system-mediated behavioral responses to stress.

Observed differences in serotonin system function between men and women also suggest that there may be gender differences in the responsiveness of patients with PTSD to psychotropic agents with serotonin system activity. Indeed, some, but not all, treatment studies of the SSRIs such as fluoxetine or sertraline suggest that women with PTSD may be more sensitive to their therapeutic effects (Hidalgo & Davidson, 2000). There also have been reports of the efficacy of atypical neuroleptics with a high ratio of serotonin 5-HT$_2$ to dopamine D$_2$ receptor antagonist activity, such as clozapine, risperidone, and olanzapine in PTSD (Friedman, 2000). However, studies of the efficacy of these agents in PTSD have focused on male populations, so we do not yet know how sensitive women with PTSD might be to their therapeutic effects. There may be gender differences in response to these agents given the lower number of brain 5-HT$_2$ receptors in women (Biver et al., 1996) and demonstrated effects of estrogen in upregulating 5-HT$_2$ receptor number (Sumner et al., 1999).

Thus, it is clear that studies exploring a role for the serotonin system in mediating the increased risk for PTSD in women are warranted.

The Hypothalamic–Pituitary–Adrenal Axis

The hypothalamic–pituitary–adrenal (HPA) axis is activated in response to stress and leads to the release of cortisol from the adrenal gland. Cortisol, in turn, helps mobilize energy stores to fuel the fight-or-flight response, contains sympathetic noradrenergic responses, suppresses inflammation, provides feedback to the brain to contain HPA axis activation, and has other brain effects that potentiate defense responses.

It is also important to note that high cortisol levels are thought to facilitate negative effects of stress on the structure and function of the hippocampus (e.g., Newcomer et al., 1999), locus ceruleus (Schulkin, Gold, & McEwen, 1998), and prefrontal cortex (e.g., Grundemann, Schechinger, Rappold, & Schomig, 1998), areas of the brain thought to play important roles in the production of symptoms and functional disabilities associated with chronic PTSD (e.g., Liberzon et al., 1999).

Thus, given the importance of the HPA axis in the mammalian responses to stress, there have been many investigations of HPA axis function in PTSD. However, few of these studies have focused on women. For this reason and others detailed later, it is difficult to make definitive gender-based comparisons of HPA axis function in PTSD at this time.

Tests of HPA Axis Reactivity

A recent study of HPA axis function in premenopausal women with PTSD demonstrates increased ACTH and cortisol responses to CRF, as well as increased cortisol and dehydroepiandrostefone (DHEA) responses to ACTH, in the women with PTSD compared to nontraumatized comparison subjects (Rasmusson, Lipschitz, et al., 2001; Rasmusson, Zimolo, et al., 2001). In addition, there were significant positive correlations between both the cortisol responses to CRF and ACTH, and subjects' 24-hour urinary cortisol levels and cortisol responses to CRF and ACTH stimulation ($r =$ .47–.70, with $p < .05$–.001). These data are consistent with a recent report showing that women with major depression and early life stress have increased ACTH and cortisol responses when exposed to a laboratory psychosocial stress paradigm (Heim et al., 2000). Of note, 11 of the 14 women with major depression and early life stress had current PTSD, whereas the comparison group without depression contained only 5 women with PTSD.

These studies suggest that premenopausal women with PTSD may have increased pituitary and adrenal reactivity in response to novel psychosocial stress, as well as to exogenous administration of CRF and ACTH. This is consistent with studies in male veterans with PTSD showing increased plasma cortisol reactivity during 24-hour plasma sampling (Yehuda, Teicher, Trestman, Levengood, & Siever, 1996) and increased pituitary ACTH responses to metyrapone (Yehuda, 1997). Although the latter study has been interpreted to suggest the presence of enhanced glucocorticoid negative feedback in PTSD, it is possible that greater endogenous CRF stimulation of the pituitary, or greater pituitary sensitivity to endogenous CRF, contributed to the increased ACTH responses in the PTSD subjects. This possibility is also supported by the work of Kaufman et al. (1997) showing a greater ACTH response to CRF among 13 depressed, abused children (8 with PTSD) compared to 13 depressed nonabused children (0 with PTSD) and 13 healthy controls. When the depressed, abused group was subdivided into high versus low ACTH responders, there was a trend for a greater number of subjects with PTSD to be among the high responders.

However, the findings of our CRF study in premenopausal women with PTSD contrast with a study by Smith et al. (1989) showing blunted ACTH and normal cortisol responses to CRF in 8 male veterans with PTSD, when compared to a group of 4 combat controls and 7 healthy, nontraumatized controls. It is possible that experimental confounds contributed to the findings by Smith et al. (1989). For instance, exposure to chronic stress affects HPA axis responses in healthy animals (Whitnall, 1994). Thus, combining small numbers of traumatized and nontraumatized controls into one healthy control group may not be an optimal methodological approach. In addition, psychotropic medications in that study were discontinued in male veterans with PTSD only 7 days before testing, and rates of smoking between study groups were not controlled. As outlined in Table 2.2, nicotine, antidepressants, neuroleptics, and anxiolytics can all have suppressive effects on HPA axis activity.

A recent study by Heim et al. (2000) has also produced findings unlike our results. In this study, women with childhood abuse and major depression (19/20 also had PTSD) showed lower absolute ACTH levels at 60 and 120 minutes after CRF treatment, and lower baseline and absolute cortisol levels at 5, 90, and 120 minutes compared to healthy subjects without childhood abuse. In contrast, a traumatized group without depression (4/20 subjects had PTSD) showed higher ACTH responses to CRF but lower cortisol levels at baseline and at 90 and 120 minutes after CRF treatment. During the ACTH study, the abused, depressed group showed only lower baseline cortisol levels, whereas the abused group that contained 4 subjects with PTSD showed lower cortisol levels at baseline and all time points after ACTH administration. These findings are difficult to interpret in terms of HPA axis findings in PTSD per se, because the presence of PTSD was not considered as a separate factor. However, it is possible that the presence of major depression or the severity of PTSD accounts for the different findings in the Heim et al. (2001) study. Indeed, half of the male patients with PTSD in the Smith et al. (1989) study also had major depression. However, methodological differences also make comparison of the findings difficult. In the Heim et al. (2001) study, the distribution of oral contraceptive users across groups was not reported, elapsed time since discontinuation of psychotropic medications was not reported, smoking was not ascertained, and nonabusive alcohol use by subjects during the study was allowed but not quantified. By comparison, in our recent study, smoking was matched

TABLE 2.2. Experimental Factors to Control in Neurobiology Studies of PTSD

Experimental factor	Exposure	Effects on HPA axis	Authors
Antidepressants	Chronic	Decreased hypothalamic CRF, glucocorticoid receptors, plasma cortisol.	Brady et al. (1992)
		Decreased urinary cortisol and ACTH responses to CRF.	Gold et al. (1995)
		SSRI reduced cortisol response to ACTH.	Thakore et al. (1997)
Antipsychotics	Chronic	Restored dexamethasone suppression.	Tandon et al. (1991)
Benzodiazepines	Acute	Reduced extrahypothalamic CRF, increased hypothalamic CRF, reduced plasma ACTH.	Vargas et al. (1992)
Alcohol	Acute	Increased cortisol during the subsequent period of mild withdrawal.	Sarkola et al. (1999)
	Chronic	Decreased plasma cortisol, decreased pituitary CRF binding.	Yamada et al. (1997b)
	Dependence	Decreased cortisol reactivity up to 4 weeks after abstinence.	Costa et al. (1996)
Nicotine	Acute	Increased plasma cortisol.	Sellini et al. (1989); Spohr et al. (1980)
	Chronic	Increased baseline plasma cortisol and urinary cortisol excretion, decreased baseline plasma cortisol, and stimulated plasma cortisol.	Eliasson et al. (1993); Kirschbaum et al. (1994); Sellini et al. (1989); Krishnan-Sarin et al. (1999)
Adrenal 21-hydroxylase gene mutations	Rates vary from 1/3 to 1/16 depending on ethnic group	May decrease baseline but increase reactivity of ACTH, cortisol, and its progenitor neurosteroids.	Witchel et al. (1997); Witchell & Lee (1998); Merke et al. (1999)

[a]Heterozygosity for 21-hydroxylase deficiency is frequent across all populations studied to date: 1/16 in a mixed Caucasian population, 1/3 in persons of Ashkenazi Jewish descent, 1/4 in Hispanics, 1/5 in Yugoslavians, 1/8 in Yupik Eskimos, and 1/10 in Italians (Witchel et al. (1997).

across groups, alcohol use was not allowed, subjects had been off of psychotropic medications for months to years, and reananlysis of the data excluding oral contraceptive users in the PTSD group did not alter the findings. Thus, it is clear from these studies that more work must be done to clarify the association between pituitary and adrenal reactivity patterns and PTSD in both genders.

Finally, it is interesting to note that our finding of increased DHEA release in response to ACTH in premenopausal women with PTSD is consistent with work by Lemieux and Coe (1995) showing increased 24-hour urinary 17-ketosteroid levels in premenopausal women with PTSD (17-ketosteroids are the metabolic products of DHEA). DHEA and its sulfated metabolite, DHEAS, cross into the brain, where they can act as positive modulators of the N-methy-D-aspartate (NMDA) receptor and as partial antagonists of the gamma-aminobutyric acid (GABA$_A$) receptor. In addition, oxygenated metabolites of DHEA may exert even more potent effects on brain function and behavior in brain regions such as the hippocampus (Rose et al., 1997). These compounds may affect regulation of other neurotransmitter systems thought to be involved in the generation of PTSD symptoms, increase anxiety, and influence memory or symptoms of dissociation (Chambers et al., 1999). Finally, DHEA, as well as progesterone, have antiglucocorticoid properties (e.g., Araneo, Shelby, Li, Ku, & Daynes, 1993). These compounds, therefore, could interfere with glucocorticoid negative feedback and potentially contribute to upregulation of the HPA axis in PTSD (Kudielka et al., 1998).

Dexamethasone Suppression Tests

Previous studies have shown enhanced dexamethasone suppression of plasma cortisol in postmenopausal (Yehuda et al., 1995) and premenopausal (Stein, Yehuda, & Koverola, 1997) women with PTSD. Results of these two studies in women with PTSD largely agree with studies of dexamethasone suppression performed in males (Yehuda, 1997). However, it will be important to replicate these studies before firm conclusions can be drawn. For instance, hormone replacement therapy was not monitored among participants in the study of postmenopausal women. As discussed later, estrogen administration decreases brain and pituitary glucocorticoid receptors (Chrousos, Torpy, & Gold, 1998) through which the effects of dexamethasone are exerted. In addition, it would be important to control for menstrual cycle phase in dexamethasone studies in premenopausal women. Altemus et al. (1997) found that women in the luteal phase of the menstrual cycle are more resistant to dexamethasone suppression compared to women in the follicular phase. Whether this is due to antiglucocorticoid effects exerted by high levels of progesterone during the luteal phase is not clear.

24-Hour Urinary Free Cortisol Studies

The only published study examining 24-hour urinary free cortisol levels in premenopausal women with PTSD demonstrated ~30% higher free cortisol levels in women with PTSD due to childhood sexual abuse compared to traumatized or nontraumatized controls (Lemieux & Coe, 1995). While this study has been criticized for the high free cortisol levels in all subjects, no other studies in premenopausal women have been published against which findings from this study can be compared. However, a recently presented study by Friedman, McDonough-Coyle, Jalowiec, Wang, Fournier, and McHugo (2001) also showed an approximately 30% increase in urinary free cortisol in 72 premenopausal and postmenopausal women with PTSD compared to 55 community controls, while Rasmusson, Lipschitz, et al. (2001) showed a trend for a 30% increase in the urinary free cortisol/creatinine ratio in women with PTSD in a small, underpowered study. Similarly, DeBellis et al. (1999) showed that girls and boys with PTSD had ~30% higher urinary free cortisol levels than healthy controls. In contrast, postmenopausal female Holocaust survivors with PTSD had ~30–50% lower urinary free cortisol levels than healthy, nontraumatized controls and Holocaust survivors without PTSD (Yehuda et al., 1995).

Several points must be kept in mind when interpreting the results of 24-hour urinary cortisol studies. First, 24-hour urinary free cortisol measurements reflect both baseline and reactive changes in plasma free cortisol levels. The female Holocaust survivors were confined to their homes during the study, whereas the women in our recent study and in the study by Lemieux and Coe (1995) were not. Thus, it is possible that the women and girls in the studies showing increased 24-hour urinary free cortisol levels in PTSD engaged in more physical activity or were exposed to more environmental provocations than the women in the study by Yehuda et al. (1995). If so, the effects of increased pituitary or adrenal reactivity, if characteristic of PTSD, would be more readily detected in the former two studies. It is also notable that the 24-hour urinary free cortisol levels in the Holocaust survivors correlated negatively with avoidance symptoms that in turn were very high in the survivors with PTSD. Prolonged active avoidance of traumatic reminders or employment of avoidant defenses (Mason, Wang, Yehuda, Riney, Charney, & Southwick, 2001) would be expected to minimize the frequency of stress-induced increases in ACTH, and thus may reduce trophic effects of ACTH on the adrenal gland. In time, this could reduce maximum adrenal cortisol responses to stress. Finally, a possible role for 21-hydroxylase deficiency heterozygosity should not be overlooked in producing low baseline cortisol levels in an ethnic group with high rates of functional 21-hydroxylase gene variants (see Table 2.2).

In addition, a number of other factors known to impact HPA axis function require attention in studies of 24-hour urinary free cortisol (Table 2.3). As noted in Table 2.3, differences in such factors may have contributed to the variable results of 24-hour urinary free cortisol studies in PTSD. The studies in which these variables were well controlled tended to show increased cortisol output in subjects with PTSD. In addition, no previous studies have attempted to quantify smoking rates among PTSD subjects and healthy controls. Because the prevalence and intensity of smoking is much higher among patients with PTSD and trauma controls compared to healthy, nontraumatized subjects (e.g., Beckham et al., 1997), nicotine use may have had significant unmeasured effects on the outcome of previous studies of HPA axis function in PTSD.

TABLE 2.3. 24-Hour Urinary Cortisol in PTSD: Findings and Experimental Factors Controlled

	4 weeks off medications	4 weeks off EtOH[a]/drugs	Activity matched	Nicotine matched
Reduced cortisol output in PTSD (Mason et al., 1986, male veterans;	No	No	No	No
Yehuda et al., 1990, male veterans;	No (2 weeks)	No	No	No
Yehuda et al., 1993, male veterans;	No	No	No	No
Yehuda et al., 1995, Holocaust survivors)	Yes	No? (EtOH?)	Yes	No
Cortisol output in PTSD not different (Kosten et al., 1990, male veterans;	No	No	No	No
Mason et al., 2001, male veterans;	Yes	Yes	No	No
Baker et al., 1999, male veterans)	Yes	Yes	Yes	No
Increased cortisol output in PTSD (Pitman & Orr, 1990, male veterans[b];	Yes	Yes	Yes	No?
Lemieux & Coe, 1995, females;	No	Yes	Yes	No
Maes et al., 1998, male and female burn victims;	Yes	No? (EtOH?)	Yes	No
De Bellis et al., 1999, male and female children;	Yes	Yes	Yes	Yes
Rasmusson et al., 2001, females;	Yes	Yes	Yes	Yes
Friedman et al., 2001, females)	No	No	Yes	Yes

[a]EtOH = ethanol.

[b]As male veterans with PTSD were compared to combat controls that have only somewhat lower rates and intensities of smoking (Shalev et al., 1990; Beckham et al., 1997), nicotine use was probably fairly well matched in this study.

Gender-Related Hormone Effects

Most studies in animals suggest that the HPA axis is more reactive in females than in males (e.g., Galea & McEwen, 1999). However, studies of gender differences in HPA axis functioning in healthy humans have yielded mixed results. As reviewed by Kirschbaum, Kudielka, Gaap, Schommer, and Hellhammer (1999), men have consistently shown higher ACTH and free cortisol responses to laboratory-controlled psychosocial stress than women. Men also appear to have higher circulating ACTH levels than women. On the other hand, men and women have shown comparable ACTH responses to human CRF, whereas women have shown greater ACTH responses to ovine CRF, and greater adrenal sensitivity to ACTH (Kirschbaum et al., 1999).

The neurobiological mechanisms underlying these gender differences in HPA axis responses in humans are unknown. Gender differences in "threat appraisal" could certainly contribute to the differences in HPA axis responses to laboratory psychosocial stressors between men and women. This possibility is supported by studies showing that men and women modulate their ACTH and cortisol responses differently in response to the presence of persons providing social support during exposure to laboratory psychosocial stress (Kirschbaum, Klauer, Filipp, & Hellhammer, 1995). However, there may be a more direct role for "gender-associated" hormones such as estrogen, progesterone, and testosterone as well.

For instance, estrogen has been shown to increase HPA axis reactivity to stress in men and gonadectomized or intact male animals (e.g., Chrousos et al., 1998). Urinary and plasma cortisol levels are also greater in women with increased estrogen levels due to pregnancy or high-dose estrogen replacement (Lindholm & Schultz-Moller, 1973). In addition, De Leo, la Marca, Talluri, D'Antona, and Morgante (1998) showed decreased CRF-induced ACTH release in women 8 days after ovariectomy, when estrogen levels are markedly reduced. One means by which estrogen may increase HPA axis activity is by downregulating hypothalamic and pituitary glucocorticoid Type II receptors that mediate glucocorticoid negative feedback (Chrousos et al., 1998). There is also an estrogen response element located in the region of the CRF gene that promotes its expression (Vamvakopoulos & Chrousos, 1993). Thus, it has been suggested that the increased reactivity of the HPA axis to psychosocial stress in men may be explained by the conversion of high levels of free testosterone in men to estradiol by the brain enzyme aromatase (Kirschbaum et al., 1999).

However, more recent work suggests that physiological estrogen levels may suppress HPA axis activity in women. Young, Altemus, Parkinson, and Shastry (2001) found that physiological replacement of estrogen in ovariectomized animals decreases ACTH responses to restraint stress. In addition, Komesaroff et al. (1999) have shown that physiological estrogen dosing suppresses ACTH and cortisol responses to mental stress in perimenopausal women. While these results appear to contrast with those of De Leo et al. (1998), it is important to note that the latter study lacked control subjects exposed to surgical stress but not to ovariectomy. In addition, sex steroids other than estrogen, such as progesterone and testosterone, are reduced by ovariectomy. Indeed, testosterone levels after ovariectomy are below those of normal menopause (Laughlin et al., 2000). Finally, it is important to distinguish the perimenopause from menopause, as well as to control for the time elapsed after ovariectomy or menopause in studies examining effects of estrogen or other sex steroids in women. Sex steroid and other neurotransmitter receptor systems, exposed to decreasing levels of ovarian hormones for increasing amounts of time as menopause occurs, make progressive adjustments in their number and sensitivity. Thus, estrogen could have variable effects depending on whether it was administered early or late in menopause.

Whereas testosterone is generally thought to inhibit HPA axis reactivity (Handa, Burgess, Kerr, & O'Keefe, 1994), it also may play a role in producing the enhanced ACTH and cortisol responses to novel laboratory psychosocial stress in men compared to women. Viau, Chu, Soriano, and Dallman (1999) showed that testosterone is necessary for the normal increase of arginine vasopressin (AVP) in the hypothalamus of adrenalectomized rats; AVP, in turn, is responsible for potentiation of ACTH release in response to novelty in chronically stressed rats (Aguilera, 1998). Thus, it is interesting that DHEA responses to ACTH are significantly increased in women with PTSD (Rasmusson, Zimolo, et al., 2001). Because DHEA is an immediate precursor of testosterone, it is possible that both DHEA and testosterone increase brain neurophysiological responses to novelty in women and men with PTSD. This possibility thus suggests that research into a possible role for testosterone in altering HPA axis and brain functioning in women with PTSD is needed.

Finally, a role for progesterone in increasing HPA axis function should be investigated in women. As noted earlier, progesterone has antiglucocorticoid properties and thus may interfere with glucocorticoid feedback. This possibility is supported by several studies suggesting that HPA axis reactivity is increased during the luteal phase of the menstrual cycle, when progesterone levels are markedly elevated over levels in the follicular phase. Genazzani, Lemarchand-Beraud, Aubert, and Felber (1974) demonstrated higher morning ACTH and cortisol levels during the luteal phase of the menstrual cycle in five healthy subjects, whereas Stewart et al. (1993) demonstrated decreased baseline ACTH levels during the luteal phase. Kruyt and Rolland (1982) showed a higher cortisol peak 90 minutes after ACTH administration in women tested during the luteal phase of the menstrual cycle compared to those tested during the early follicular phase. Similarly,

Kirschbaum et al. (1999) found higher salivary free cortisol, but not plasma total cortisol, responses to ACTH and psychosocial stress during the luteal compared to follicular phases of the menstrual cycle. These results, in turn, may be consistent with work by Altemus et al. (1997) demonstrating decreased sensitivity to glucocorticoid negative feedback during the luteal phase.

Nevertheless, the relative lack of studies of HPA axis function in women with PTSD, the number of experimental confounds present in earlier HPA axis studies, and the lack of studies designed explicitly to examine gender differences in HPA axis function in PTSD make it difficult to know whether there are gender differences in adaptation of the HPA axis to traumatic stress. Future research within and between genders must therefore be done with care to control for menstrual phase and reproductive status, as well as other factors with impact on HPA axis function. Only then can we determine whether alterations in HPA axis adaptations to stress contribute to the higher risk for PTSD observed in women.

Studies of Central and Peripheral Nervous System Structure and Function

There is emerging experimental evidence that women with PTSD, compared to healthy nontraumatized or traumatized controls, tend to have differences in certain types of brain-mediated abilities. For example, women with PTSD appear to exhibit (1) abnormalities in brain lateralization (Morgan, Grillon, Lubin, & Southwick, 1997); (2) increased preconscious sensitivity to changes in acoustical stimuli (Morgan & Grillon, 1999); (3) decreased conscious responses to target stimuli (Charles et al., 1995); (4) increased heart rate responses and changes in skin conductance in response to high-intensity tones, along with slower habituation of these responses; and (5) differences in blood flow in the frontal lobe and other brain areas measured by PET during the reading of personalized trauma scripts (e.g., Bremner et al., 1999).

Women with PTSD have been found to have decreases in hippocampal volume compared to healthy nontraumatized or traumatized controls (e.g., Bremner et al., 1997). They also have shown poorer performance on hippocampus-dependent cognitive tasks in one (Bremner et al., 1999), but not another (Stein, Hanna, Vacrum, & Koverola, 1999) study of explicit memory function in PTSD. It is not clear, however, whether women with PTSD have greater or lesser abnormalities in hippocampal structure or function than do men. It is also not yet clear to what extent women with PTSD, like men with PTSD, may be predisposed to the development of such abnormalities. Existing studies do not yet inform us as to whether these abnormalities are the product of traumatic stress exposure in vulnerable individuals or predate and possibly increase the risk for PTSD—very important questions for understanding PTSD, as well as the role of gender in its development.

Nevertheless, it does seem likely that gender differences in the function of any one of the neurobiological systems discussed in the preceding sections could predispose women to the development and expression of such PTSD-related brain and peripheral nervous system abnormalities. For instance, cortisol, DHEA, NPY, serotonin, and the sex steroids all play roles in the production of stress-induced changes in hippocampal structure and function. These factors also influence the function of the frontal lobe, the amygdala, and other brain areas involved in the detection and interpretation of threat, as well as the coordination of physiological or behavioral responses to threat. Thus, future research should study the means by which PTSD-associated alterations in these neurotransmitter systems may translate into the neurophysiological, cognitive, and behavioral manifestations of PTSD. Information gleaned from these studies can then be used to guide the development of improved, symptom-specific psychological and pharmacological treatment strategies.

FUTURE RESEARCH DIRECTIONS AND RESEARCH POLICY RECOMMENDATIONS

A number of methodological points should be considered in the design of future studies of the neurobiology of PTSD in women. For instance, past studies have often resorted to comparing women in either the follicular or the luteal phase of the menstrual cycle to men. However, there is no reason to think that the physiology of women in either the follicular or luteal phase of the menstrual cycle is more or less comparable to the physiology of men. Indeed, fluctuations in sex steroids across the menstrual cycle will have unique effects on neurotransmitter systems in women. In addition, sex steroids have gender-related prenatal and ongoing postnatal organizational and structural effects on the brain that persist despite the addition or subtraction of sex steroids during research studies. Therefore, we believe that parallel studies in men and women need to be conducted across developmental epochs to elucidate accurately differences in the neurobiology of PTSD between genders.

In such studies, women need to be carefully monitored for a variety of factors, including stage of menstrual cycle, oral contraceptive use, pregnancy, and menopause. Each of these states has a unique hormonal profile that may differentially affect immediate and long-term adaptations to traumatic stress. Indeed, as previously suggested by Saxe and Wolfe (1999) women may be more vulnerable to the development of PTSD during certain phases of the menstrual cycle or during different reproductive states. It is also possible that PTSD symptoms will vary across the menstrual cycle or across reproductive states. Finally, it is possible that the efficacy of medications for PTSD will vary across gender, developmental epochs, menstrual cycles, and reproductive states. Therefore, more resources need to be directed toward the study of PTSD in women. For instance, the duration of longitudinal monitoring of women in such studies may need to be lengthened to allow more time for the study of women across the stages of the menstrual cycle, as well as to allow for the recruitment of a greater number of control groups.

More attention also needs to be directed toward research in prepubertal and pubertal girls and boys exposed to trauma. Indeed, several studies have found very high rates of PTSD and partial PTSD among inner-city girls exposed to community trauma (e.g., Lipschitz et al., 2000). We thus need to address the larger socioeconomic context in which community trauma occurs and understand the spectrum of neurobiological and psychosocial factors that potentially increase the risk for PTSD among exposed children. For instance, the production of adrenal neurosteroids, such as DHEA, rises steeply at adrenarche (Genazzani, Bernardi, Monteleone, Luisi, & Luisi, 2000), a period of time before the onset of actual puberty, when adrenally derived steroids increase and induce the development of secondary sex characteristics. DHEA levels continue to rise until adulthood. Therefore, this steroid may play very different roles in the mediation of traumatic stress effects on the brain and HPA axis before and after adrenarche, and may differentially impact boys and girls. We also need to devise interventions that can alter the long-term deleterious psychiatric and psychosocial outcomes of trauma exposure in female children. For instance, Lipschitz et al. (2000) found PTSD symptoms in inner-city girls to be associated with depression, school failure, trouble with the law, smoking, and marijuana use.

Indeed, another important area for future research will be understanding how trauma, PTSD, and substance abuse disorders are interrelated. Interestingly, alcohol withdrawal in animals has been found to cause changes in brain CRF and other neurobiological factors similar to those seen after traumatic stress (Koob, 1999). Traumatic stress and PTSD, in turn, appear to be associated with neurobiological changes that predispose patients to substance abuse. Traumatic stress-induced reductions in NPY levels and/or release may be one such factor. Mice with genetically determined increases in alcohol consumption have lower brain levels of NPY, and mice with genetically engineered NPY deficits consume increased amounts of alcohol. Conversely, transgenic mice with increased brain NPY levels consume less alcohol and are more sensitive to its sedative effects (Thiele et al., 1998). We hope that further research exploring these relationships will lead to better ways to prevent or break the vicious cycle between trauma or chronic stress and substance abuse. This will be especially important for women in substance abuse treat-

TABLE 2.4. Differences in Stress System Responses between Menstrual Phases, Reproductive States, and the Sexes in Healthy Subjects

	Luteal phase versus follicular phase	Menopause versus premenopause	Women versus men
Sympathetic noradrenergic system	Increased norepinephrine (NE) levels Increased stroke volume/lower vascular tone Increased cardiovascular responses to cold pressor test Increased cardiovascular responses to environmental stress Higher estrogen levels are associated with decreased cardiovascular responding during the luteal phase	Increased cardiovascular responses to mental stress compared to menopausal women; responses are rectified by estrogen replacement	Decreased norepinephrine and epinephrine responses to mental stress
NPY	Decrease NPY release during exercise compared to the periovulatory follicular phase		Female animals release less NPY in response to the cold pressor test Testosterone increases tissue stores and release of NPY Decreased NPY release during exercise in postmenopausal women compared to age-matched men
Serotonin system	Effects of the menstrual and reproductive cycles have not been examined		Fewer serotonin 5-HT receptors Increased anxiety, prolactin, and oxytocin responses to the 5-HT agonist, m-CPP Decreased rates of 5-HT synthesis
HPA axis	Decreased cortisol suppression by dexamethsaone Increased cortisol responses to ACTH stimulation Increased cortisol responses to psychological stress		Decreased cortisol responses to the Trier Social Stress Test Similar responses to human CRF Prolonged responses to ovine CRF Increased cortisol release to ACTH

ment, who have significantly higher rates of trauma exposure than men (e.g., Najavits, Weiss, & Shaw, 1997).

Finally, genetic factors may predispose individuals to the development of PTSD or contribute to differences in the rates of PTSD across ethnic groups. Such genetic factors may become magnified in their impact by interacting with gender-specific hormonal milieus. The identification of such factors could help guide early detection and more rapid implementation of preventive or treatment approaches.

SUMMARY

As indicated in this chapter, it is not yet clear how the pathophysiology of PTSD differs between men and women. Indeed, the results of previous studies suggesting gender differences in the neurobiology of PTSD may, in part, have been influenced by differences in experimental design. However, it should also be clear that gender-related hormones, as well as hormone status within gender, influence stress-responsive systems of relevance to PTSD and probably influence short- and long-term neurophysiological adaptations to traumatic stress (summarized in Table 2.4).

Thus, future research should explore the role that such hormones may play in mediating the increased risk for PTSD in women. In addition, whereas in this chapter we suggest the importance of investigating gender differences in the noradrenergic, NPY, serotonergic, and HPA axis systems in PTSD, numerous other neurotransmitter and neuropeptide systems involved in the mediation of stress and stress-related psychiatric disorders also bear investigation. Indeed, it is possible that studying the neurobiology of PTSD in women, a group in which the neurobiological effects of trauma appear to be exaggerated, may not only help us to understand and treat PTSD in women but also may facilitate our understanding of the pathophysiology of PTSD in general.

REFERENCES

Aguilera, G. (1998). Corticotropin releasing hormone, receptor regulation and the stress response. *Trends in Endocrinology and Metabolism, 9,* 329–336.

Altemus, M., Redwine, L., Leong, Y.-M., Yoshikawa, T., Yehuda, R., Detera-Wadleigh, S., Murphy, D. L. (1997). Reduced sensitivity to glucocorticoid feedback and reduced glucocorticoid receptor mRNA expression in the luteal phase of the menstrual cycle. *Neuropsychopharmacology, 17,* 100–109.

American Psychiatric Association. (1994). *Diagnostic and statistical manual of mental disorders* (4th ed.). Washington, DC: Author.

Antonijevic, I. A., Murck, H., Bohlhalter, S., Frieboes, R. M., Holsboer, F., & Steiger,

A. (2000). Neuropeptide Y promotes sleep and inhibits ACTH and cortisol release in young men. *Neuropharmacology, 39,* 1474–1481.

Araneo, B. A., Shelby, J., Li, G.-Z. Ku, W., & Daynes, R. A. (1993). Administration of dehydroepiandrosterone to burned mice preserves normal immunologic competence. *Archives of Surgery, 128,* 318–325.

Aston-Jones, G., Rajkowski, J., & Cohen, J. (1999). Role of locus coeruleus in attention and behavioral flexibility. *Biological Psychiatry, 46,* 1309–1320.

Bagdy, G., & Arato, M. (1998). Gender-dependent dissociation between oxytocin but not ACTH, cortisol or TSH responses to m-chlorophenylpiperazine in healthy subjects. *Psychopharmacology, 136,* 342–348.

Baker, D. G., West, S. A., Nicholson, W. E., Ekhator, N. N., Kasckow, J. W., Hill, K. K., Bruce, A. B., Orth, D. N., & Geracioti, T. D. (1999). Serial CSF corticotropin-releasing hormone levels and adrenocortical activity in combat veterans with posttraumatic stress disorder. *American Journal of Psychiatry, 156,* 585–588.

Beckham, J. C., Kirby, A. C., Feldman, M. E., Hertzberg, M. A., Moore, S. D., Crawford, A. L., Davidson J. R. T., & Fairbank, J. A. (1997). Prevalence and correlates of heavy smoking in Vietnam veterans with chronic posttraumatic stress disorder. *Addictive Behaviors, 22,* 637–647.

Biello, S. M., Golombek, D. A., & Harrington, M. D. (1997). Neuropeptide Y and glutamate block each other's phase shifts in the suprachiasmatic nucleus *in vitro. Neuroscience, 77,* 1049–1057.

Biver, F., Lotstra, F., Monclus, M., Wikler, D., Damahauat, P., Mendlewicz, J., & Goldman, S. (1996). Sex differences in 5-HT$_2$ receptor in the living human brain. *Neuroscience Letters, 204,* 25–28.

Brady, L. S., Gold, P. W., Herkenham, M., Lynn, A. B., & Whitfield, H. W. (1992). The antidepressants fluoxetine, idazoxan and phenelzine alter corticotropin-releasing hormone and tyrosine hydroxylase mRNA levels in rat brain: Therapeutic implications. *Brain Research, 572,* 117–125.

Bremner, J. D., Narayan, M., Staib, L. H., Southwick, S. M., McGlashan, T., & Charney, D. S. (1999). Neural correlates of memories of childhood sexual abuse in women with and without posttraumatic stress disorder. *American Journal of Psychiatry, 156,* 1787–1795.

Bremner, J. D., Randall, P., Vermetten, E., Staib, L., Bronen, R. A., Mazure, C., Capelli, S., McCarthy, G., Innis, R. R. B., & Charney, D. S. (1997). Magnetic resonance imaging-based measurement of hippocampal volume in posttraumatic stress disorder related to childhood physical and sexual abuse—a preliminary report. *Biological Psychiatry, 41,* 23–32.

Bremner, J. D., Scott, T. M., Delaney, R. C., Southwick, S. M., Mason, J. W., Johnson, R. B., Innis, R. B., McCarthy, G., & Charney, D. S. (1995a). MRI-based measurement of hippocampal volume in combat-related posttraumatic stress disorder. *American Journal of Psychiatry, 152,* 973–981.

Breslau, N., Davis, G. C., Andreski, P., Peterson, E. L., & Schultz, L. R. (1997). Sex differences in posttraumatic stress disorder. *Archives of General Psychiatry, 54,* 1044–1048.

Britton, K. T., Akwa, Y., Spina, M. G., & Koob, G. F. (2000). Neuropeptide Y blocks anxiogenic-like behavioral action of corticotropin-releasing factor in an operant conflict test and elevated plus maze. *Peptides, 21,* 37–44.

Carr, B. R., & Wilson, J. D. (1987). Disorders of the ovaries and female reproductive tract. In E. Braunwald, K. J. Isselbacher, R. G. Petersdorf, et al. (Eds.), *Harrison's principles of internal medicine* (11th ed., pp. 1818–1837). New York: McGraw-Hill.

Chambers, R. A., Bremner, J. D., Moghaddam, B., Southwick, S. M., Charney, D. S., & Krystal, J. H. (1999). Glutamate and post-traumatic stress disorder: Toward a psychobiology of dissociation. *Seminars in Clinical Neuropsychiatry, 4*, 274–281.

Charles, G., Hansenne, M., Ansseau, M., Pitchot W., Machowski, R., Schittecatte, M., & Wilmotte, J. (1995). P300 in posttraumatic stress disorder. *Neuropsychobiology, 32*, 72–74.

Charlety, P. J., Aston-Jones, G., Akaoka, H., Buda, M., & Chouvet, G. (1991). 5-HT decreases glutamate-evoked activation of locus coeruleus neurons through 5-HT_{1a} receptors. *Comptes Rendues de l'Académie des Sciences, 312*, 421–426.

Chrousos, G. P., Torpy, D. J., Gold, P. W. (1998). Interactions between the hypothalamic–pituitary–adrenal axis and the female reproductive system: Clinical implications. *Annals of Internal Medicine 129*, 229–240.

Colmers, W., & Bleakman, D. (1994). Effects of neuropeptide Y on the electrical properties of neurons. *Trends in Neuroscience, 17*, 373–379.

Corder, R., Castagne, V., Rivet, J.-M., Mormede, P., & Gaillard, R. C. (1992). Central and peripheral effects of repeated strress and high NaCl diet on neuropeptide Y. *Physiology and Behavior, 52*, 205–210.

Costa, A., Bono, G., Martignoni, E., Merlo, P., Sances, G., & Nappi, G. (1996). An assessment of hypothalamo–pituitary–adrenal axis functioning in nondepressed, early abstinent alcoholics. *Psychoneuroendocrinology, 21*, 263–275.

Davis, L. L., Clark, D. M., Kramer, G. L., Moeller, F. G., & Petty, F. (1999). D-fenfluramine challenge in posttraumatic stress disorder. *Biological Psychiatry. 45*, 928–930.

De Bellis, M. D., Baum, A. S., Birmaher, B., Keshavan, M. S., Eccard, C. H., Boring, A. M., Jenkins, F. J., & Ryan, N. D. (1999). A. E. Bennett Research Award: Developmental traumatology: Part I. Biological stress systems. *Biological Psychiatry, 45*, 1259–1270.

De Leo, V., la Marca, A., Talluri, B., D'Antona, D., & Morgante, G. (1998). Hypothalamo–pituitary–adrenal axis and adrenal function before and after ovariectomy in premenopausal women. *European Journal of Endocrinology, 138*, 430–435.

Deykin, E. Y., & Buka, S. L. (1997). Prevalence and risk factors for posttraumatic stress disorder among chemically dependent adolescents. *American Journal of Psychiatry, 154*, 752–757.

Eliasson, M., Hagg, E., Lundblad, D., Karlsson, R., & Bucht, E. (1993). Influence of smoking and snuff use on electrolytes, adrenal and calcium regulating hormones. *Acta Endocrinologica, 128*, 35–40.

Flood, J. F., Hernandez, E. N., & Morley, J. E. (1987). Modulation of memory processing by neuropeptide Y. *Brain Research, 421*, 280–290.

Frankenhaeuser, M., von Wright, M. R., Collins, A., Wright, J. V., Sedvall, G., & Swahn, C.-G. (1978). Sex differences in psychoneuroendocrine reactions to examination stress. *Psychosomatic Medicine, 40*, 334–343.

Friedman, M. J. (1999). What might the psychobiology of posttraumatic stress disorder teach us about future approaches to pharmacotherapy? *Journal of Clinical Psychiatry, 6*(Suppl. 7), 44–51.

Friedman, M. J., McDonagh-Coyle, A. S., Jalowiec, J. E., Wang, S., Fournier, D. A., & McHugo, G. J. (2001). *Neurohormonal findings during treatment of women with PTSD due to childhood sexual abuse (CSA)*. Abstract from the 17th Annual Meeting of the International Society for Traumatic Stress Studies, New Orleans, LA.

Galea, L. A. M., & McEwen, B. S. (1999). Sex and seasonal differences in the rate of cell proliferation in the dentate gyrus of adult wild meadow voles. *Neuroscience, 89*, 955–964.

Genazzani, A. R., Bernardi, F., Monteleone, P., Luisi, S., & Luisi, M. (2000). Neuropeptides, neurotransmitters, neurosteroids, and the onset of puberty. *Annals of the New York Academy of Sciences, 900*, 1–9.

Genazzani, A. R., Lemarchand-Beraud, T. H., Aubert, M. L., & Felber, J. P. (1974). Pattern of plasma ACTH, hGH, and cortisol during menstrual cycle. *Journal of Clinical Endocrinology and Metabolism, 41*, 431–437.

Girdler, S. S., Pedersen, C. A., Stern, R. A., & Light, K. C. (1993). Menstrual cycle and premenstrual syndrome: Modifiers of cardiovascular reactivity in women. *Health Psychology, 12*(3), 180–192.

Gold, P. W., Licinio, J., Wong, M.-L., & Chrousos, G. P. (1995). Corticotropin releasing hormone in the pathophysiology of melancholic and atypical depression and in the mechanism of action of antidepressant drugs. *Annals of the New York Academy of Sciences, 771*, 716–729.

Goldstein, D. S., Levinson, P., & Keiser, H. R. (1983). Plasma and urinary catecholamines during the human ovulatory cycle. *American Journal of Obstetrics and Gynecology, 146*, 824–829.

Grassi, G., & Esler, M. (1999). How to assess sympathetic activity in humans. *Journal of Hypertension, 17*, 719–734.

Greber, S., Schwarzer, C., & Sperk, G. (1994). Neuropeptide Y inhibits postassium-stimulated glutamate release through Y2 receptors in rat hippocampal slices *in vitro*. *British Journal of Pharmacology, 113*, 737–740.

Greenberg, B. D., Li, Q., Lucas, F. R., Hu, S., Sirota, L. A., Benjamin, J., Lesch, K. P., Hamer, D., & Murphy, D. L. (2000). Association between the serotonin transporter promoter polymorphism and personality traits in a primarily female population sample. *American Journal of Medical Genetics, 96*, 202–216.

Grundemann, D., Schechinger, B., Rappold, G. A., & Schomig, E. (1998). Molecular identification of the cortisone-sensitive extraneuronal catecholamine transporter. *Nature Neuroscience, 1*, 349–351.

Handa, R. J., Burgess, L. H., Kerr, J. E., O'Keefe, J. A. O. (1994). Gonadal steroid hormone receptors and sex differences in the hypothalamo–pituitary–adrenal axis. *Hormones and Behavior, 28*, 2464–2476.

Heilig, M., & Widerlov, E. (1990). Neuropeptide Y: An overview of central distribution, functional aspects, and possible involvement in neuropsychiatric illnesses. *Acta Psychiatrica Scandinavica, 82*, 95–114.

Heim, C., Newport, D. J., Heit, S., Graham, Y. P., Wilcox, M., Bonsall, R., Miller, A. H., & Nemeroff, C. B. (2000). Pituitary–adrenal and autonomic responses to stress in women after sexual and physical abuse in childhood. *Journal of the American Medical Association, 284*, 592–597.

Heninger, G. R. (1997). Serotonin, sex, and psychiatric illness. *Proceedings of the National Academy of Sciences, 94*, 4823–4824.

Hidalgo, R. B., & Davidson, J. R. (2000). Selective serotonin reuptake inhibitors in post-traumatic stress disorder. *Journal of Psychopharmacology, 14,* 70–76.

Josselyn, S. A., & Beninger, R. J. (1993). Neuropeptide Y: Intraaccumbens injections produce a place preference that is blocked by cis-flupenthixol. *Pharmacology, Biochemistry and Behavior, 46,* 543–552.

Kallio, J., Pesonen, U., Kaipio, K., Karvonen, M., Jaakkola, U., Heinonen, O., Uusitupa, M. I. J., Koulu, M. (2001). Altered intracellular processing and release of neuropeptide Y due to leucine 7 to proline 7 polymorphism in the signal peptide of preproneuropeptide Y in humans. *FASEB Journal, 15,* 1242–1244.

Kaufman, J., Birmaher, B., Perel, J., Dahl, R. E., Moreci, P., Nelson, B., Wells, W., & Ryan, N. D. (1997). The corticotropin-releasing hormone challenge in depressed abused, depressed nonabused, and normal control children. *Biological Psychiatry, 42,* 669–679.

Kessler, R. C., Sonnega, A., Bromet, E., Hughes, M., & Nelson, C. B. (1995). Post-traumatic stress disorder in the National Comorbidity Survey. *Archives of General Psychiatry, 52,* 1048–1060.

Kirschbaum, C., Klauer, T., Filipp, S. H., & Hellhammer, D. H. (1999). Sex-specific effects of social support on cortisol and subjective responses to acute psychological stress. *Psychosomatic Medicine, 57,* 23–31.

Kirschbaum, C., Kudielka, B. M., Gaap, J., Schommer, N. C., & Hellhammer, D. H. (1999). Impact of gender, menstrual cycle phase, and oral contraceptives on the activity of the hypothalamus–pituitary–adrenal axis. *Psychosomatic Medicine, 61,* 154–162.

Kirschbaum, C., Scherer, G., & Strasburger, C. J. (1994). Pituitary and adrenal hormone responses to pharmacological, physical, and psychological stimulation in habitual smokers and nonsmokers. *Clinical Investigator, 72,* 804–810.

Komesaroff, P. A., Esler, M., Clarke, I. J., Fullerton, M. J., & Funder, J. W. (1998). Effects of estrogen and estrous cycle on glucocorticoid and catecholamine responses to stress in sheep. *American Journal of Physiology, 275,* E671–E678.

Komesaroff, P. A., Esler, M. D., & Sudhir, K. (1999). Estrogen supplementation attenuates glucocorticoid and catecholamine responses to mental stress in perimenopausal women. *Journal of Clinical Endocrinology and Metabolism, 84,* 606–610.

Koob, G. F. (1999). Stress, corticotrophin-releasing factor, and drug addiction. *Annals of the New York Academy of Sciences, 897,* 27–45.

Krishnan-Sarin, S., Rosen, M. I., & O'Malley, S. (1999). Naloxone challenge in smokers: Preliminary evidence of an opioid component in nicotine dependence. *Archives of General Psychiatry, 56,* 663–668.

Kruyt, N., & Rolland, R. (1982). Cortisol, 17α-OH-progesterone and androgen responses to a standardized ACTH-stimulation test in different stages of the normal menstrual cycle. *Acta Endocrinologica, 100,* 427–433.

Kudielka, B. M., Hellhammer, J., Hellhammer, D. H., Wolf, T. O., Pirke, K.-M., Varadi, E., Pilz, J., & Kirschbaum, C. (1998). Sex differences in endocrine and psychological responses to psychosoicial stress in healthy elderly subjects and the impact of a two-week DHEA treatment. *Journal of Clinical Endocrinology and Metabolism, 83,* 1756–1761.

Laughlin, G. A., Barrett-Connor, E., Kritz-Silverstein, D., & von Muhlen, D. (2000). Hysterectomy, oophorectomy, and endogenous sex hormone levels in older women: The Rancho Bernardo Study. *Journal of Clinical Endocrinology and Metabolism, 85,* 645–651.

Lemieux, A., & Coe, C. (1995). Abuse-related posttraumatic stress disorder: Evidence for chronic neuroendocrine activation in women. *Psychsomatic Medicine, 57,* 105–115.

Lewandowski, J., Pruszczyk, P., Elaffi, M., Chodakowska, J., Wocial, B., Switalska, H., Januszewicz, W., & Zukowska-Grojec, Z. (1998). Blood pressure, plasma NPY and catecholamines during physical exercise in relation to menstrual cycle, ovariectomy, and estrogen replacement. *Regulatory Peptides, 75–76,* 239–245.

Liberzon, I., Taylor, S. F., Amdur, R., Jung, T. D., Chamberlain, K. R., Minoshima, S., Koeppe, R. A., Fig, L. M. (1999). Brain activation in PTSD in response to trauma-related stimuli. *Biological Psychiatry, 45,* 817–826.

Lindheim, S. R., Legro, R. S., Bernstein, L., Stanczyk, F. Z., Vijod, M. A., Presser, S. C., & Lobo, R. (1992). Behavioral stress responses in premenopausal and postmenopausal women and the effects of estrogen. American. *Journal of Obstetrics and Gynecology, 167,* 1831–1836.

Lindholm, J., & Schultz-Moller, N. (1973). Plasma and urinary cortisol in pregnancy and during estrogen–gestagen treatment. *Scandinavian Journal of Clinical Laboratory Investigation, 31,* 119–122.

Lipschitz, D. S., Rasmusson, A. M., Anyan, W., Cromwell, P., & Southwick, S. M. (2000). Clinical and functional correlates of posttraumatic stress disorder in urban adolescent girls in a primary care clinic. *Journal of the American Academy of Child and Adolescent Psychiatry, 39,* 1104–1111.

Maes, M., Lin, A., Bonaccorso, S., Van Hunsel, F., Van Gastel, A., Delmeire, L., Bioddi, M., Bosmans, E., Kenis, G., & Scharpe, S. (1998). Increased 24-hour urinary cortisol excretion in patients with posttraumatic stress disorder and patients with major depression, but not in patients with fibromyalgia. *Acta Psychiatrica Scandinavica, 98,* 328–335.

Maes, M., Lin, A. H., Verkerk, R., Delmeire, L., Van Gastel, A., Van der Planken, M., & Scharpe, S. (1999). Serotonergic and noradrenergic markers of post-traumatic stress disorder with and without major depression. *Neuropsychopharmacology, 20,* 188–197.

Manhem, K., & Jern, S. (1994). Influence of daily-life activation on pulse rate and blood pressure changes during the menstrual cycle. *Journal of Human Hypertension, 8,* 851–856.

Mason, J. W., Wang, S., Riney, S., Charney, D. S., & Southwick, S. M. (2001). Psychogenic lowering of urinary cortisol levels linked to increased emotional numbing and a shame-depressive syndrome in combat-related posttraumatic stress disorder. *Psychosomatic Medicine, 63,* 387–401.

Mason, J. W., Giller, E. L., Kosten, T. R., Ostroff, R. B., & Rodd, L. (1986). Urinary-free cortisol levels in posttraumatic stress disorder patients. *Journal of Nervous and Mental Disease, 174,* 145–159.

McEwen, B., DeKloet, E., & Rostene, W. (1986). Adrenal steroid receptors and actions in the nervous system. *Physiological Reviews, 66,* 1121–1189.

Mellado, M. L., Gibert-Rahola, J., Chover, A. J., & Mico, J. A. (1996). Effect on nociception of intracerebro-ventricular administration of low doses of neuropeptide Y in mice. *Life Science, 58,* 2409–2414.

Mellman, T. A. (1997). Psychobiology of sleep disturbances in posttraumatic stress disorder. *Annals of the New York Academy of Sciences, 821,* 142–149.

Merke, D. P., Keil, M. E., Negro, P. J., Gold, P., & Chrousos, G. P. (1999). 21-

hydroxylase deficient carriers reset their hypothalamic–pituitary axis to normalize cortisol production: Potential relation to mood changes leading to a selective advantage. *Endocrine Society Meeting Poster Abstract*, PI-659.

Morgan, C. A., & Grillon, C. (1999). Abnormal mismatch negativity in women with sexual assault-related posttraumatic stress disorder. *Biological Psychiatry, 45*, 827–832.

Morgan, C. A., Grillon, C., Lubin, H., & Southwick, S. M. (1997). Startle reflex abnormalities in women with sexual assault-related posttraumatic stress disorder. *American Journal of Psychiatry, 154*, 1076–1080.

Morgan, C. A., III, Rasmusson, A. M., Wang, S., Hoyt, G., Hauger, R., & Hazlett, G. (in press). Neuropeptide Y and subjective distress in humans exposed to acute stress: Replication and extension of previous report. *Biological Psychiatry*.

Morgan, C. A., Wang, S., Southwick, S. M., Rasmusson, A., Hazlett, G., Hauger, R. L., & Charney, D. S. (2000). Plasma neuropeptide-Y concentrations in humans exposed to military survival training. *Biological Psychiatry, 47*, 902–909.

Najavits, L. M., Weiss, R. D., & Shaw, S. R. (1997). The link between substance abuse and posttraumatic stress disorder in women. A research review. *American Journal on Addictions, 6*, 273—283.

Nakajima, M., Inui, A., Asakawa, A., Momose, K., Ueno, N., Teranishi, A., Baba, S., & Kasuga, M. (1998). Neuropeptide Y produces anxiety via Y2-type receptors. *Peptides, 19*, 359–363.

Newcomer, J. W., Selke, G., Melson, A. K., Hershey, T., Craft, S., Richards, K., & Alderson, A. L. (1999). Decreased memory performance in healthy humans induced by stress-level cortisol treatment. *Archives of General Psychiatry, 56*, 527–533.

Nishizawa, S., Benkelfat, C., Young, S. N., Leyton, M., Mzengeza, S., de Montigny, C., Blier, P., & Diksic, M. (1997). Differences between males and females in rates of serotonin synthesis in human brain. *Proceedings of the National Academy of Sciences, 94*, 5308–5313.

Pernow, J. (1986). Co-release and functional interactions of neuropeptide Y and noradrenaline in peripheral symathetic vascular control. *Acta Physiologica Scandinavica* (Suppl. 568), 1–56.

Pitman, R., & Orr, S. (1990). Twenty-four hour urinary cortisol and catecholamine excretion in combat-related posttraumatic stress disorder. *Biological Psychiatry, 27*, 245–247.

Rasmusson, A. M., Hauger, R. L., Morgan, C. A. III, Bremner, J. D., Charney, D. S., & Southwick, S. M. (2000). Low baseline and yohimbine-stimulated plasma neuropeptide Y (NPY) in combat-related posttraumatic stress disorder. *Biological Psychiatry, 47*, 526–539.

Rasmusson, A. M., Lipschitz, D. S., Wang, S., Hu, S., Vojvoda, D., Bremner, J. D., Southwick, S. M., & Charney, D. S. (2001). Increased pituitary and adrenal reactivity in premenopausal women with PTSD. *Biological Psychiatry, 50*, 965–977.

Rasmusson, A. M., Zimolo, Z., Vasek, J., Lipschitz, D., Mustone, M. E., Gudmundsen, G., Southwick, S. M., Wolfe, J., & Charney, D. S. (2000). Increased drenal DHEA release in premenopausal women with PTSD. *Society for Neuroscience Abstracts, 26*, 548.

Rasmusson, A. M., Zimolo, Z., Vasek, J., Lipschitz, D. S., Mustone, M. E., Gudmundsen, G., Southwick, S. M., Wolfe, J., & Charney, D. S. (2001, December).

Increased adrenal DHEA release in premenopausal women with PTSD. Abstract from the 17th Annual Meeting of the International Society for Traumatic Stress Studies, New Orleans, LA.

Rose, K. A., Stapleton, G., Dott, K., Kieny, M. P., Best, R., Schwarz, M., Russell, D. W., Bjorkheim, I., Seckl, J., & Lathe, R. (1997). Cyp7b, a novel brain cytochrome P450, catalyzes the synthesis of neurosteroids 7a-hydroxy dehydroepiandrosterone and 7a-hydroxy pregnenolone. *Proceedings of the National Academy of Sciences, 94*, 4925–4930.

Rubinow, D. R., Schmidt, P. J., & Roca, C. A. (1998). Estrogen–serotoin interactions: Implications for affective regulation. *Biological Psychiatry, 44*, 839–850.

Saab, P. G., Matthews, K. A., Stoney, C. M., McDonald, R. H. (1989). Premenopausal and postmenopausal women differ intheir cardiovascular and neuroendocrine responses to behavioral stressors. *Psychophysiology, 26*, 270–280.

Sapolsky, R. (1985). A mechanism for glucocorticoid toxicity in the hippocampus: Increased neuronal vulnerability to metabolic insults. *Journal of Neuroscience, 5*, 1228–1232.

Sapolsky, R. (1986) Glucocorticoid toxicity in the hippocampus: Synergy with an excitotoxin. *Neuroendocrinology, 43*, 440–446.

Sarkola, T., Makisalo, H., Fukunaga, T., & Eriksson, C. J. (1999). Acute effect of alcohol on estradiol, estrone, progesterone, prolactin, cortisol, and luteinizing hormone in premenopausal women. *Alcoholism: Clinical and Experimental Research, 23*, 976–982.

Saxe, G., & Wolfe, J. (1999). Gender and posttraumatic stress disorder. In P. A. Saigh & J. D. Bremner (Eds.), *Posttraumatic stress disorder: A comprehensive text* (pp. 160–179). Boston: Allyn & Bacon.

Schulkin, J., Gold, P. W., & McEwen, B. S. (1998). Induction of corticotropin-releasing hormone gene expression by glucocorticoids: Implication for understanding the states of fear and anxiety and allostatis load. *Psychoneuroendocrinology, 23*, 219–243.

Sellini, M., Baccarini, S., Dimitriadid, E., Sartori, M. P., & Letizia, C. (1989). Effect of smoking on the hypophyseo-adrenal axis. *Medicini, 9*, 194–196.

Shalev, A., Bleich, A., & Ursano, R. J. (1990). Post-traumatic stress disorder: Somatic comorbidity and effort symptoms. *Psychosomatics, 31*, 197–203.

Sita, A., & Miller, S. B. (1996). Estradiol, progesterone and cardiovascular response to stress. *Psychoneuroendocrinology, 21*, 339–346.

Smith, M. A., Davidson, J., Ritchie, J. C., Kudler, H., Lipper, S., Chappell, P., & Nemeroff, C. B. (1989). The corticotropin-releasing hormone test in patients with posttraumatic stress disorder. *Biological Psychiatry, 26*, 349–355.

Southwick, S. M., Bremner, J. D., Rasmusson, A., Morgan, C. A., Arnsten, A., & Charney, D. S. (1999). Role of norepinephrine in the pathophysiology and treatment of posttraumatic stress disorder. *Biological Psychiatry, 46*, 1192–1204.

Southwick, S. M., Krystal, J. H., Bremner, J. D., Morgan, C. A., Nicolaou, A. L., Nagy, L. M., Johnson, D. R., Heninger, G. R., & Charney, D. S. (1997). Noradrenergic and serotonergic function in posttraumatic stress disorder. *Archives of General Psychiatry, 54*, 749–758.

Southwick, S. M., Krystal, J. H., Morgan, C. A., Johnson, D. R., Nagy, L. M., Nicolaou, A. L., Heninger, G. R., & Charney, D. S. (1993). Abnormal noradrenergic function in posttraumatic stress disorder. *Archives of General Psychiatry, 50,* 266–274.

Spivak, B., Vered, Y., Graff, E., Blum, I., Mester, R., & Weizman, A. (1999). Low platelet–poor plasma concentrations of serotonin in patients with combat-related posttraumatic stress disorder. *Biological Psychiatry, 45,* 840–845.

Spohr, U., Hengen, N., Harenberg, J., Walter, E., Augustin, J., Comberg, H. U., Morl, H., & Weber, E. (1980). The effects of nicotine on the circulation and metabolism after cigarette smoking with reference to the plasma levels of nicotine and COHb. *Munchener Medizinische Wochenschrift, 122*(Suppl. 1), 25–32.

Stein, M., Hanna, C., Vaerum, V., & Koverola C. (1999). Memory functioning in adult women traumatized by childhood sexual abuse. *Journal of Traumatic Stress, 12,* 527–534.

Stein, M., Koverola, C., Hanna, C., Torchia, M. G., & McClarty, B. (1997). Hippocampal volume in women victimized by childhood sexual abuse. *Psychological Medicine, 27,* 951–959.

Stein, M., Walker, J. R., Hazen, A. L., & Forde, D. R. (1997). Full and partial posttraumatic stress disorder: findings from a community survey. *American Journal of Psychiatry, 154,* 1114–1119.

Stein, M., Walker, J. R., & Forde, D. R. (2000). Gender differences in susceptibility to posttraumatic stress disorder. *Behaviour Research and Therapy, 38,* 619–628.

Stein, M., Yehuda, R., & Koverola, C. (1997). HPA axis functioning in adult women who report experiencing severe childhood sexual abuse. *Biological Psychiatry, 42,* 680–686.

Stewart, P. M., Penn, R., Holder, R., Parton, A., Ratcliffe, J. G., & London, D. R. (1993). The hypothalamo–pituitary–adrenal axis across the normal menstrual cycle and in polycyctic ovary syndrome. *Clinical Endocrinology, 38,* 387–391.

Sumner, B. E., Grant, K. E., Rosie, R., Hegele-Hartung, C., Fritzemeier, K. H., & Fink, G. (1999). Effects of tamoxifen on serotonin transporter and 5-hydroxytryptamine(2A) receptor binding sites and mRNA levels in the brain of ovariectomized rats with or without acute estradiol replacement. *Brain Research: Molecular Brain Research, 73,* 119–128.

Tandon, R., Mazzara, C., DeQuardo, J., Craig, K., Meador-Woodruff, J., Goldman, R., & Greden, J. F. (1991). Dexamethasone suppression test in schizophrenia: Relationship to symptomatology, ventricular enlargement, and outcome. *Biological Psychiatry, 29,* 953–964.

Tersman, Z., Collins, A., & Eneroth, P. (1991). Cardiovascular responses to psychological and physiological stressors during the menstrual cycle. *Psychosomatic Medicine, 53,* 185–197.

Thakore, J. H., Barnes, C., Joyce, J., Medbak, S., & Dinan, T. G. (1997). Effects of antidepressant treatment on corticotropin-induced cortisol responses in patients with melancholic depression. *Psychiatry Research, 73,* 27–32.

Thiele, T. E., Marsh, D. J., Ste Marie, L., Bernstein, I. L., & Palmiter, R. D. (1998). Ethanol consumption and resistance are inversely related to neuropeptide Y levels. *Nature, 396,* 366–369.

Thorsell, A., Svensson, P., Wiklund, L., Sommer, W., Ekman, R., & Heilig, M., (1998). Suppressed neuropeptide Y (NPY) mRNA in rat amygdala following restraint stress. *Regulatory Peptides, 75–76,* 247–254.

Vamvakopoulos, N. C., & Chrousos, G. P. (1993). Evidence of direct estrogenic regulation of human corticotropin-releasing hormone gene expression: Potential implications for the sexual dimorphism of the stress response and immune/inflammatory reaction. *Journal of Clinical Investigation, 92,* 1896–1902.

Vargas, M. A., Bissette, G., Owens, M. J., Ehlers, C. L., & Nemeroff, C. B. (1992). Effects of chronic ethanol and benzodiazepine treatment and withdrawal on corticotropin-releasing factor neural systems. *Annals of the New York Academy of Sciences, 654,* 145–152.

Viau, V., Chu, A., Soriano, L., & Dallman, M. F. (1999). Independent and overlapping effects of corticosterone and testosterone on corticotropin-releasing hormone and arginine vasopressin mRNA expression in the paraventricular nucleus of the hypothalamus and stress-induced adrenocorticotropic hormone release. *Journal of Neuroscience, 19,* 6684–6693.

Wahlestedt, C., & Reis, D. (1993). Neuropeptide Y-related peptides and their receptors—are the receptors potential therapeutic drug targets? *Annual Review of Pharmacology and Toxicology, 32,* 309–352.

Walker, M. W., Ewald, D. A., Perney, T. M., & Miller, R. J. (1988). Neuropeptide Y modulates neurotransmitter release and Ca^{2+} currents in rat sensory neurons. *Journal of Neuroscience, 8,* 2438–2446.

Whitnall, M. H. (1994). Regulation of the hypothalamic corticotrophin-releasing hormone neurosecretory system. *Progress in Neurobiology, 40,* 573–629.

Wilkinson, D. J., Thompson, J. M., Lambert, G. W., Jennings, G. L., Schwarz, R. G., Jefferys, D., Turner, A. G., & Esler, M. D. (1998). Sympathetic activity in patients with panic disorder at rest, under laboratory mental stress, and during panic attacks. *Archives of General Psychiatry, 55,* 511–520.

Witchel, S., & Lee, P. A. (1998). Identification of heterozygotic carriers of 21-hydroxylase deficiency: Sensitivity of ACTH stimulation tests. *American Journal of Medical Genetics, 76,* 337–342.

Witchel, S., Lee, P., Suda-Hartman, S., Trucco, M., & Hoffman, E. (1997). Evidence for a heterozygote advantage in congenital adrenal hyperplasia due to 21–hydroxylase deficiency. *Journal of Clinical Endocrinology and Metabolism, 82,* 2097–2101.

Wolfe, J., & Schlesinger, L. K. (1997). Performance of PTSD patients on standard tests of memory: Implications for trauma. *Annals of the New York Academy of Sciences, 821,* 208–218.

Yamada, Y., Tsuritani, I., Ishizaki, M., Ikai, E., Ishida, M., Noborisaka, Y., & Honda, R. (1997). Serum gamma-glutamyl transferase levels and blood pressure falls after alcohol moderation. *Clinical and Experimental Hypertension, 19,* 249–268.

Yehuda, R. (1997). Sensitization of the hypothalamic–pituitary–adrenal axis in posttraumatic stress disorder. *Annals of the New York Academy of Sciences, 821,* 57–75.

Yehuda, R., Boisoneau, D., Mason, J. W., & Giller, E. L. (1993). Relationship between lymphocyte glucocorticoid receptor number and urinary-free cortisol excretion in mood, anxiety, and psychotic disorder. *Biological Psychiatry, 34,* 18–25.

Yehuda, R., Kahana, B., Binder-Brynes, K., Southwick, S., Mason, J., & Giller, E. (1995). Low urinary cortisol excretion in Holocaust survivors with posttraumatic stress disorder. *American Journal of Psychiatry, 152,* 982–986.

Yehuda, R., Southwick, S. M., Nussbaum, G., Wahby, V., Giller, E. L., & Mason, J. W. (1990). Low urinary cortisol excretion in patients with posttraumatic stress disorder. *Journal of Nervous and Mental Disease, 178,* 366–369.

Yehuda, R., Teicher, M., Trestman, R., Levengood, R., & Siever, L. (1996). Cortisol regulation in posttraumatic stress disorder and major depression: A chrono-biological analysis. *Biological Psychiatry, 40,* 79–88.

Young, E. A., Altemus, M., Parkison, U., & Shastry, S. (2001). Effects of estrogen antagonists and agonists on the ACTH response to restraint stress in female rats. *Neuropsychopharmacology, 25,* 881–889.

Zukowska-Grojec, Z. (1995). Neuropeptide Y: A novel sympathetic stress hormone and more. *Annals of the New York Academy of Sciences, 771,* 219–233.

3 | Gender and PTSD
A Cognitive Model

DAVID F. TOLIN
EDNA B. FOA

$\mathbf{A}$s noted by Norris, Foster, and Weisshaar in this book (Chapter 1), epidemiological studies indicate that males are somewhat more likely than females to experience traumatic events (e.g., Breslau, Davis, Andreski, & Peterson, 1991; Breslau et al., 1998; Kessler, Sonnega, Bromet, Hughes, & Nelson, 1995; Norris, 1992). Despite encountering fewer traumas, however, females appear to be more likely than males to develop posttraumatic stress disorder (PTSD) (e.g., Breslau & Davis, 1992; Breslau et al., 1998; Davidson, Hughes, Blazer, & George, 1991; Helzer, Robins, & McEvoy, 1987; Kessler et al., 1995). The purpose of this chapter is to explore hypotheses about cognitive factors that influence gender differences in vulnerability to develop PTSD. We describe a cognitive model of trauma processing, discuss the potential impact of gender differences on several aspects of the cognitive model, and make recommendations for future research.

A COGNITIVE MODEL OF PTSD

To explain individual differences in recovery after a trauma, Foa and colleagues (e.g., Foa & Kozak, 1986; Foa & Riggs, 1993; Foa & Rothbaum, 1998) forwarded *emotional processing theory*, which suggests that the development of disorders such as PTSD depends on both the *content* of cognition (i.e., what the person thinks, believes, and records in memory) and the *process* of cognition (i.e., the way the person thinks, perceives, and interprets events). Adaptive cognitive features are thought to act as a buffer against the development of PTSD; trauma victims with such features are likely to process the trauma effectively. Conversely, maladaptive cognitive features are hypothesized to increase trauma victims' vulnerability to develop PTSD because they inhibit realistic processing of the traumatic event. Emotional processing theory is predicated on the following core propositions:

1. PTSD is a form of pathological fear. Thus, it is similar in many ways to the "normal" fear experienced by trauma victims who do not develop PTSD. However, it is distinguished from normal fear by the presence of specific cognitive associations, described in detail later.

2. All fear is a memory-based "program" for escaping danger. Fear helps organisms cope with imminent threat by deploying attention toward dangerous stimuli, facilitating quick assessment of danger, and activating the physiological and behavioral responses necessary to escape.

3. The fear program can be construed as a cognitive "structure" consisting of interconnected cognitive representations, and containing three kinds of information:
   a. Information about the feared *stimulus*. In the case of a trauma survivor, this information might include details about the trauma and the perpetrator.
   b. Information about verbal, physiological, and overt behavioral *responses*, including information about the victim's responses during the trauma (e.g., screaming, freezing, or running away), as well as responses that occurred after the trauma (e.g., sadness, hypervigilance, or nightmares).
   c. Interpretive information about the *meaning* of the stimulus and response elements of the structure. For trauma survivors, this may include appraisals of the perpetrator as dangerous, and also interpretations of one's own responses as appropriate (e.g., "I did what I had to do") or inappropriate (e.g., "I acted stupidly").

4. The fear structures of PTSD sufferers differ from those of individuals who recover from traumatic experience. PTSD is associated with a large number of maladaptive associations between elements of the structure. The specific associations hypothesized to increase vulnerability to develop PTSD are described later.

Figure 3.1 depicts a hypothetical fear structure of a "normal" trauma memory of a woman who was raped at gunpoint by a tall, bald man. The ovals in this model represent *stimulus* elements (e.g., "man" and "gun"). Elements related to each other are connected by lines. The rectangles represent *meaning* elements related to the self (e.g., "confused," "afraid") and to

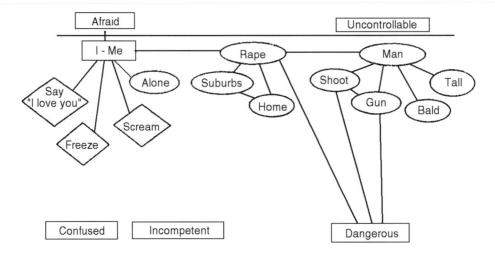

FIGURE 3.1. A schematic model of a normal rape memory. From Foa and Rothbaum (1998). Copyright 1998 by The Guilford Press. Reprinted by permission.

the world (e.g., "dangerous"). The diamonds represent *response* elements, that is, the woman's responses during the rape (e.g., "scream," "freeze").

Note that the elements of the fear structure are not isolated; rather, there is a systematic pattern of connections between elements. These connections are shown as solid lines. The concept of interconnections between cognitive elements borrows from models of cognitive psychology that conceptualize memory as a configuration of separate concepts associated with one another (e.g., Anderson & Bower, 1973). When one element is activated by an environmental trigger or an internal event, activation spreads from that element to other elements, creating new connections. Repeated activation of a connection between two elements results in a priming effect, in which thinking about one element automatically activates the related element.

In Figure 3.1, the associations between elements of the structure are realistic. For example, the stimuli "gun" and "shoot" are associated with "danger." Conversely, characteristics of the rapist such as "man," "bald," and "tall" are not associated with "danger." Thus, the woman recognizes that these attributes are not inherently dangerous. Similarly, the self is associated with the responses "freeze" and "scream," but not "incompetence." Thus, the woman recognizes that her responses during the trauma do not signify any negative meaning about herself. These realistic interelement associations indicate healthy trauma processing. We would predict that this woman would be unlikely to develop PTSD; that is, she is likely to "recover" from the trauma.

Individuals who develop PTSD, on the other hand, are hypothesized to have markedly different fear structures than do those who recover. Below, we discuss the specific elements of pathological trauma structures.

The Structure of Pathological Fear

Figure 3.2 depicts a pathological fear structure associated with PTSD, that is structurally similar to other forms of pathological fears (e.g., phobias), but differs in its large size and high number of erroneous associations (Foa, Steketee, & Rothbaum, 1989). The pathological fear structure differs from the normal fear structure in several ways (Foa & Kozak, 1986):

1. Pathological fear structures are disruptively *intense*. In other words, a pathological fear structure involves excessive response elements such as representations of avoidance and physiological arousal. In this woman's case, the diamond labeled "PTSD symptoms" depicts the excessive response elements.
2. Pathological fear structures include *unrealistic stimulus–stimulus associations* that do not accurately represent the world. As shown in Figure 3.2, this woman's fear structure contains an association between "gun" and "bald man"; that is, bald men have become associated with guns.
3. Pathological fear structures also contain *erroneous stimulus–*

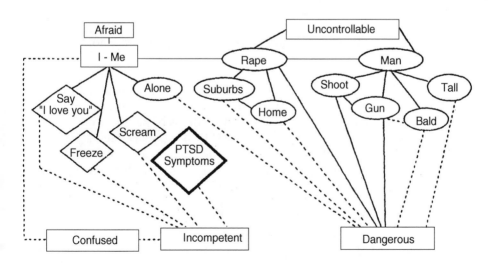

FIGURE 3.2. A schematic model of a pathological rape memory. From Foa and Rothbaum (1998). Copyright 1998 by The Guilford Press. Reprinted by permission.

meaning associations. In this woman's case, harmless stimuli such as "bald," "home," and "suburbs" have become associated with the meaning "dangerous." Similarly, her responses during and after the rape are associated with the meaning "incompetence."

4. Pathological fear structures contain *erroneous associations between harmless stimuli and escape or avoidance responses.* For example, because this woman was raped by a bald man, she is primed to avoid contact with such men.

This woman's fear structure shows a failure to process the trauma effectively. It contains excessive representations of fearful responses; she associates harmless stimuli with danger, views herself as incompetent, and tends to avoid situations that frighten her. Thus, she is less likely to recover from her trauma and is considered at high risk for developing PTSD. Below, we discuss various hypothesized reasons why some trauma survivors develop the normal fear structure depicted in Figure 3.1, whereas others develop the pathological fear structure shown in Figure 3.2.

Why Do Some Trauma Victims Recover and Others Do Not?

Foa and colleagues (e.g., Foa & Riggs, 1993; Foa & Rothbaum, 1998) posited that the following cognitive factors influence the likelihood that a person will develop PTSD:

1. *Pretrauma schemas.* Schema theory holds that an individual's set of beliefs and attitudes (schemas) influence his or her perceptions, interpretations, and memories (e.g., Beck, Emery, & Greenberg, 1985). Schema development is thought to be influenced by experiences throughout the lifespan. Thus, people's life experiences may provide them with new information that alters their beliefs and expectations. Reciprocally, schemas also influence the cognitive processing of experiences, often distorting the experience to make them schema-consistent. Thus, a person may misperceive or misremember an event as being consistent with his or her prior knowledge or beliefs. Schema-based theories of PTSD posit that trauma victims' schemas about the world and themselves prior to the trauma influence how well they will recover from the trauma. Several trauma theorists (Epstein, 1991; Horowitz, 1986; Janoff-Bulman, 1992; McCann & Pearlman, 1990) imply that trauma victims who previously viewed themselves as invulnerable and worthy, and perceived their world as benevolent, are at high risk for developing chronic emotional disturbances, because the trauma forces an extreme change in their schemas of themselves and the world. However, this view is incongruent with empirical studies indicating that multiple traumatic experiences and pretrauma psychological disturbances increase the likelihood of PTSD (Burgess & Holmstrom, 1978; Resick, 1987;

Rothbaum, Foa, Riggs, Murdock, & Walsh, 1992). Presumably, individuals with such a history do not perceive themselves as competent and the world as safe. Rather, the repeated traumas would be expected to create a strong priming effect, in which the person becomes more likely to perceive the world as extremely dangerous and him- or herself as extremely incompetent. These preexisting schemas may influence the perception or memory of the trauma, so that the trauma serves to reinforce their existing negative beliefs. To reconcile these seeming contradictions, Foa and Rothbaum (1998) suggest that it is not positive assumptions that render an individual less adept at processing a traumatic event, but rather his or her extremely *rigid* conceptions. Accordingly, they proposed that individuals who have experienced multiple traumas also hold rigid extreme views, but those views are negative rather than positive. Foa and Rothbaum further posited that trauma victims whose rules of interpretation allow finer discriminations of degree of "dangerousness" and "self-competence" will be better equipped to process the trauma as a unique event, one that should not substantially alter their evaluations of themselves or of the world. Hence, these victims will be less likely to develop PTSD. In the case of the woman raped, rigid preexisting beliefs that the world is either completely safe or completely unsafe, and that she herself is either completely competent or completely incompetent, would be thought to increase her risk of developing PTSD.

2. *Trauma memory records.* Trauma memory records consist of the memory of the trauma itself and the person's beliefs *about* the trauma. Both aspects of the record are hypothesized to influence recovery from the trauma. In the case of the woman raped by a bald man holding a gun, the trauma memory record will include representations of stimulus elements (e.g., "bald man," "gun"), response elements (e.g., "scream," "freeze"), and meaning elements (e.g., "dangerous," "helpless"). Foa et al. (1989) suggest that trauma memories differ from other fear structures in that they contain a particularly large number of stimulus elements. Thus, the trauma victim with PTSD is expected to exhibit fear of not only objectively dangerous situations (e.g., gun) but also objectively safe ones (e.g., bald men). In general, the more stressful the traumatic event, the greater its effects on emotions and behavior (Baum, 1970). Accordingly, a trauma memory of a rape would be expected to have a larger number of stimulus–danger associations than would that of a simple assault. A trauma memory with a particularly large number of stimulus–danger associations may be expected to result in the perception of the world as entirely dangerous. Such perception underlies the reluctance of the rape victim to allow others to sit behind her on a bus or subway for fear that she may be attacked from behind. Similarly, it may also lead her to view all men as potential rapists, and to sleep with the lights on in her own home.

Foa and Rothbaum (1998) also propose that trauma memories differ from other fear structures by a large number of diverse response elements.

First, the perception that the world is completely dangerous engenders a particularly large number of physiological (e.g., increased heart rate) and behavioral (e.g., escape) response elements in a fear structure. Second, a trauma memory often includes representations of trauma-related responses (e.g., freezing, screaming). Trauma victims who develop PTSD seem to interpret their responses during the trauma in a negative manner; this subsequently interferes with recovery from the trauma. The rape survivor in our example interprets her feelings and behaviors during the rape as reflecting personal incompetence. She is thus thought to be at greater risk for developing PTSD than a woman who did not reach such negative conclusions about her behavior during the trauma.

3. *Posttrauma reactions of self and others.* The third factor that can impede emotional processing is what gets recorded in memory *after* the trauma, including records of posttrauma disturbances and difficulties in resuming daily functioning. Foa and Rothbaum (1998) suggest that emotional processing of the trauma is impeded when there is a tendency to interpret initial emotional difficulties (e.g., PTSD symptoms) as a further sign of incompetence. The tendency to generate such dysfunctional interpretations can be influenced by pretrauma schemas, as well as the traumatic memory itself. Posttrauma records also include information about the reactions of others. For example, the rape survivor whose posttrauma interpersonal interactions suggest to her that the trauma was her fault, or that her reactions are inappropriate, may be at greater risk for developing PTSD than if she had experienced reasonable levels of interpersonal support after the trauma. Janoff-Bulman (1985) suggests that the reactions of others may influence the degree to which the trauma victim blames him- or herself for the event; this, in turn, is hypothesized to influence the person's recovery from the trauma. Empirical studies indicate that negative social interactions (e.g., victim blame or disbelief) have strong negative effects on victim adjustment, whereas positive reactions from others have little impact on adjustment (Davis, Brickman, & Baker, 1991; Ullman, 1995). This asymmetry may be due to a general negative interpretation of other people's reactions, and this bias creates a vicious cycle that serves to reinforce the victim's perceptions of world as dangerous and of herself as incompetent.

Thus, pretrauma schemas, trauma memory records, and records of the posttrauma reactions of self and others combine to influence the likelihood of recovery versus the development of PTSD. Figure 3.3 depicts a schematic model of these cognitive factors involved in the emotional processing of trauma. External events are symbolized by the solid rectangles, and their representations in memory are depicted by broken-line rectangles. As can be seen in Figure 3.3, the various cognitive factors can influence each other in an adaptive or maladaptive manner. For example, pretrauma records impact the person's self and world schemas. These schemas subsequently exert

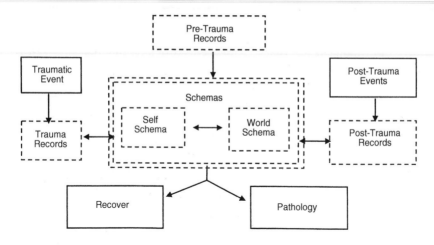

FIGURE 3.3. A cognitive model of trauma processing. From Foa and Rothbaum (1998). Copyright 1998 by The Guilford Press. Reprinted by permission.

influence on the representations of the traumatic event. Trauma records, in turn, influence the representations of posttrauma events. Pretrauma records also affect the posttrauma records, again, via their impact on self and world schemas. Thus, pretrauma and posttrauma records and schemas work in concert to determine whether a trauma victim will recover or will develop PTSD.

WHY ARE MALES LESS LIKELY TO DEVELOP PTSD THAN FEMALES?

Given the relatively high rates of trauma among males, why is the prevalence of PTSD lower in males than in females? Perhaps sex differences stem from the same factors thought to underlie individual differences in trauma recovery (see Figure 3.3): trauma memory representations (both the trauma memory itself and beliefs about the trauma), beliefs about the self, and beliefs about the world. To the extent that the cognitive factors specified by emotional processing theory do indeed play a role in sex differences in vulnerability to develop PTSD, then sex differences should be evident in one or more of these domains. In this section, we examine the empirical literature relevant to the following questions:

1. *Do males and females differ in their trauma memory records?* Emotional processing theory maintains that the trauma memory record is an important factor in recovery. As described earlier, the trauma memory re-

cord consists of the memory of the trauma itself (e.g., "what," "where," and "when" issues), as well as the person's thoughts, beliefs, and appraisals *about* the trauma (e.g., "why" issues). Accordingly, this question can be subdivided into two different inquiries:

    a. *Do females experience more severe forms of trauma on average than do males? If so, does this difference explain the differential prevalence of PTSD?* Because the trauma memory record contains the recorded details of the traumatic event, it follows that more severe kinds of trauma will lead to more intense and pathological memory records. If females are found to experience more severe forms of traumas than males, it might be concluded that differences in trauma severity (and therefore differences in the trauma memory record) underlie differences in PTSD. However, in order to isolate this factor, it is necessary to examine differences in PTSD prevalence and severity even when controlling for type of trauma. If sex differences in PTSD remain even when controlling for trauma factors, then it will be necessary to examine whether other cognitive factors can account for the remaining differences.

    b. *Do females have more negative and personalized attributions about traumatic events than do males?* The trauma memory record contains not only the details of the traumatic event but also the person's thoughts about the trauma. A trauma victim whose memory records contain an excessive amount of self-blame or guilt-related beliefs, for example, would be presumed to be at greater risk for developing PTSD. Thus, we compare males' and females' negative attributions about the trauma.

  2. *After a traumatic event, do males and females hold different beliefs about themselves and the world?* The emotional processing model also suggests that recovery from trauma is influenced by persons' schemas about themselves and the world. Normal trauma memory structures tend not to contain global, negative beliefs; rather, the trauma is viewed as a unique event without distorting the person's overall beliefs. By contrast, pathological trauma memory structures are thought to contain beliefs such as "I am completely incompetent" and "The world is completely dangerous." Thus, this question can be divided into two inquiries:

    a. *Are female trauma victims more likely than male victims to view themselves as incompetent?* If female trauma victims' self-schemas differ from those of males, then females would be expected to view themselves as more incompetent, worthless, or damaged than do males. We will examine the prevalence of these beliefs among male and female trauma victims.

    b. *Are female trauma victims more likely than male victims to view the world as dangerous?* Similarly, if females' and males' world schemas differ, then female victims should hold more beliefs that the world is a dangerous and unpredictable place than do males. We examine the degree to which males and females endorse such beliefs.

Below, we review the empirical literature relevant to each hypothesis.

Do Males and Females Differ in Their Trauma Memory Records?

Foa and Rothbaum (1998) posited that trauma records in memory influence the likelihood that the victim will develop PTSD. The trauma record consists of information not only about the trauma itself but also about the victim's interpretation of the trauma and subsequent attributions and beliefs about the trauma.

Do Females Experience More Severe Forms of Trauma on Average Than Do Males?

Judging the relative severity of different types of trauma is inherently difficult, but severity might be surmised from the rates of PTSD among both males *and* females experiencing the event. Large-scale studies suggest that rape and sexual assault (e.g., Kessler et al., 1995) and combat (e.g., Weiss et al., 1992) are associated with higher rates of PTSD among both sexes than are other types of trauma.

Another way of defining severity is the degree to which the trauma violates existing beliefs about one's self, the world, or the future. Traumas that force victims to change their global, deeply held beliefs might be judged as more severe than traumas that do not elicit such radical cognitive changes. Rape, for example, may lead victims to perceive themselves as completely incompetent or the world as completely dangerous (Foa & Rothbaum, 1998). They may also feel guilty or responsible for the rape; this attitude may be reinforced by others in the victims' environment, because many people still tend to blame the victim (e.g., Best, Dansky, & Kilpatrick, 1992). Child sexual abuse (CSA) takes place during important developmental stages and often is perpetrated by trusted caregivers; thus, CSA victims may feel particularly betrayed and powerless (Finkelhor, 1986). Combat's sustained threat of death or serious injury, along with the horror of witnessing or participating in atrocities, may lead to pervasive beliefs that one is vulnerable and that the environment is unpredictable and dangerous (Weathers, Litz, & Keane, 1995). It might be argued that traumas such as natural disasters or motor vehicle accidents, although they may be quite distressing, do not elicit the same massive disruptions of one's core beliefs and attitudes.

In their comprehensive review of studies in this book, Norris and colleagues (Chapter 1) report that females are more likely than males to experience rape and other forms of sexual assault. Males, on the other hand, are more likely than females to experience nonsexual traumas such as physical assault, combat, and accidents. This pattern of gender differences in trauma experience was observed across epidemiological and convenience-sample studies of varying ages and demographic backgrounds, spanning multiple countries.

Recently we (Tolin & Foa, 2002) completed a meta-analysis of studies showing the prevalence of various types of traumas among males and females. We calculated effect size r for differences in prevalence, weighted according to sample size. All effect size estimates were for female gender; therefore, positive effect sizes indicate a greater prevalence of trauma among females; negative effect sizes indicate a greater prevalence among males. An effect size of $r = 0$ indicates no difference between males and females; r is considered significantly different from 0 ($p < .05$) when its 95% confidence interval does not include 0. Effect size estimates of .1, .3, and .5 correspond to small, medium, and large effects, respectively.

Results of our meta-analysis, as shown in Table 3.1, suggest that the prevalence of certain types of trauma is higher among females and that the prevalence of others is higher among males. Specifically, females appear more likely than males to experience sexual assault and CSA. Males, on the other hand, appear more likely to experience nonsexual traumas such as combat, physical assault, accidents, and witnessing death or injury. Thus, the meta-analytic findings corroborate the narrative review of Norris et al. in Chapter 1 of this volume. However, it should be noted that despite the

TABLE 3.1. Meta-Analysis of the Prevalence of Different Types of Trauma among Males and Females

Trauma category	Number of comparisons	r	95% CI
Adult sexual assault	12	.17	.13–.21
Child sexual abuse	16	.15	.12–.18
Nonsexual child abuse or neglect	4	.03	.02–.05
Disaster or fire	8	−.03	−.06 − −.01
Witnessing death or injury	15	−.06	−.11–.00
Serious illness or injury	4	−.15	−.12–.03
Accident	10	−.08	−.10 − −.06
Nonsexual assault	16	−.08	−.11 − −.06
Combat, war, and terrorism	10	−.15	−.22–.07

Note. r = effect size estimate; CI = confidence interval.
[a]Females > males, $p < .05$.
[b]Males > females, $p < .05$.

large number of significant differences, most of the effect sizes are smaller than might be expected from narrative reviews of gender differences in trauma. Across studies, only the estimates for sexual assault, CSA, and combat exceeded the threshold for a "small" and significant effect.

Do females experience more severe forms of trauma than do males? The empirical results are not clear. Females are more likely to experience sexual traumas, which appear to be highly likely to elicit PTSD. On the other hand, males are more likely to experience combat, which may be equally likely to elicit PTSD. Furthermore, epidemiological studies indicate that males are approximately as likely to experience combat as females are to be raped (e.g., Kessler et al., 1995; Norris, 1992). More research is needed to link specific aspects of the traumatic experience with the onset of PTSD before this matter can be settled.

Do Differences in Trauma Type Explain Sex Differences in PTSD? In order to investigate whether gender differences in PTSD can be attributed to differential trauma experience, it is necessary to examine studies that allow gender comparisons within different types of trauma. In their review in this book, Norris et al. compared the rates of PTSD for males and females exposed to disaster and community or political violence. Females were found to be at greater risk than males for developing PTSD following disaster, although results were more ambiguous following community and political violence.

In our quantitative review (Tolin & Foa, 2002), we used meta-analysis to summarize males' and females' PTSD symptoms after several specific types of trauma. In most studies, the dependent variable was dichotomous (i.e., the presence or absence of PTSD). Some studies, however, used continuous measurement (i.e., severity of PTSD symptoms). Studies using dichotomous and continuous measurement were analyzed separately, using the effect size estimate r, weighted according to sample size. As before, all effect size estimates are for female gender. Therefore, positive effect sizes indicate a greater prevalence or severity of PTSD among females; negative effect sizes indicate a greater prevalence or severity among males.

As shown in Table 3.2, most gender differences did not reach statistical significance; that is, their 95% confidence intervals included 0. However, it is possible that some of these null results are due to small numbers of comparisons; therefore, we will consider size of the effect as well as statistical significance. Females were significantly more likely than males to meet diagnostic criteria for PTSD following disaster or fire, accident, nonsexual assault, and civilian exposure to combat, war, or terrorism (although it should be noted that the effect sizes for combat trauma did not exceed the threshold for a small effect). Effect sizes that were not significantly different from 0 but still exceeded the threshold for a small effect suggested that fe-

TABLE 3.2. Meta-Analysis of the Prevalence of PTSD among Males and Females Exposed to Specific Types of Trauma

Trauma category	Diagnosis			Continuous measurement		
	Number of comparisons	r	95% CI	Number of comparisons	r	95% CI
Adult sexual assault	3	.03	−.25–.31	0	—	
Child sexual abuse	2	.08	−.17–.32	4	.12	−.61–.28
Nonsexual child abuse or neglect	10	.17	−.13–.44	1	.24	−.04–.49
Disaster or fire	21	.10[a]	.06–.14	12	.12	−.07–.40
Witnessing death or injury	14	.06	−.01–.12	2	.14	−.01–.29
Serious illness or injury	2	−.11	−.24–.02	0	—	
Accident	18	.14[a]	.09–.20	2	.22[a]	.08–.35
Nonsexual assault	10	.30[a]	.16–.43	4	.13	−.07–.32
Combat, war, and terrorism	16	.06[a]	.01–.11	11	.12	−.03–.26
Veteran	5	.03	−.05–.12	5	0.15	−.22–.49
Civilian	11	.06[a]	.01–.11	6	0.13[a]	.11–.16

Note. r = effect size estimate; CI = confidence interval.
[a]Females > males, $p < .05$.

males were more likely than males to meet criteria for PTSD following nonsexual child abuse as well. Studies of the severity, rather than diagnosis, of PTSD indicated that females reported significantly greater symptoms of PTSD than did males following accidents and civilian exposure to combat, war, and terrorism. Effect sizes that were not significantly different from zero but still exceeded the threshold for a small effect suggested that females reported more severe PTSD symptoms than did males following CSA, nonsexual child abuse, disaster or fire, witnessing death or injury, nonsexual assault, and veteran exposure to combat. It should be noted that some of these comparisons were based on a very small number of studies and thus must be interpreted cautiously. Males, on the other hand, showed a small but nonsignificant effect for a greater probability of the PTSD diagnosis following unspecified serious illness or injury (although this finding is based on only two studies). The only trauma category in which no gender differences were found either in terms of effect size or statistical significance was adult sexual assault, although only three studies were available for this comparison. Thus, although the evidence is inconsistent, there does seem to be a general trend toward greater PTSD among females than among males exposed to the same traumas.

In interpreting these findings, it is important to bear in mind that there may be great variability in trauma severity within the same general category. For example, male Vietnam veterans typically experienced more severe combat exposure than did female veterans. Similarly, female nonsexual assault victims may be more severely injured, more frequently assaulted, or more likely to be assaulted by a friend, relative, or partner than are males. These differences in severity may lead to over- or underestimations of true gender differences in vulnerability to develop PTSD.

Substantial gender differences in trauma severity have been reported in studies of CSA. For example, the use of force is reported in 10–15% of male sexual abuse cases, compared to 19% of female cases (Finkelhor, Hotaling, Lewis, & Smith, 1990; Risin & Koss, 1987). Moreover, male victims are likely to report the use of positive coercion (reward or promised reward), whereas female victims are likely to report negative coercion (force or threats; Fritz, Stoll, & Wagner, 1981). These details are hypothesized to lead to important differences in the trauma record by creating stronger associations between the trauma and appraisals of danger. Similarly, compared to males, female CSA victims are more likely to report multiple victimizations and to have been abused by a close family member (Fischer, 1992). The greater number of victimizations is thought to increase the associative strength between elements of the trauma memory network. Victimization by a family member may create new associations between elements of danger and those representing interpersonal trust or love. Such associations may lead to impaired interpersonal relatedness, particularly when the victimization occurs during periods critical to the development of healthy cognitive representations. Thus, even within the domain of CSA, gender differences in the nature of the trauma may have far-reaching effects on the trauma memory record.

Whereas CSA severity might be greater in some aspects for females than for males, adult sexual assault may yield the opposite pattern. Male sexual assault victims may be more likely than female victims to have been assaulted by multiple perpetrators, to have been attacked multiple times, and to have been physically beaten during the sexual assault (Kaufman, Divasto, Jackson, Voorhees, & Christy, 1980; Pino & Meier, 1999). According to the cognitive model, such factors would be expected to result in stronger connections between benign stimuli and danger. The masculine gender role (e.g., Eagly, 1987) may also lead victims of such assaults to have increased connections between the trauma and cognitive elements of helplessness, vulnerability, and incompetence. These factors may have inflated PTSD rates among males, thus making it difficult to detect gender differences in trauma response.

In summary, males and females tend to experience different types of trauma, with females experiencing more sexual traumas and males tending to experience more violent, nonsexual traumas. These experiential differences create different trauma memories, which in turn influence the remainder of the memory structure. However, the results of Norris et al.'s qualitative review and our quantitative review suggest that this factor cannot fully account for the differences in PTSD. Even within trauma types, females still appear to be at somewhat greater risk for PTSD. More subtle differences in the traumatic memory might play a role, as might differences elsewhere in the cognitive structure. We next consider the potential role of beliefs *about* the traumatic event.

Do Females Have More Negative and Personalized Attributions about Traumatic Events Than Do Males?

As described earlier, the trauma memory record contains not only the details of the trauma itself but also the person's thoughts, beliefs, and appraisals *about* the trauma. This element of the trauma memory may also differ for males and females. For example, in surveys of trauma survivors, males rated motor vehicle accidents as less frightening than did females (Ehlers, Mayou, & Bryant, 1998), and described CSA as more neutral or positive and less negative than did females (Fritz et al., 1981; Nash & West, 1985; Rind, Tromovich, & Bauserman, 1998; Schultz & Jones, 1983).

Differences in trauma appraisal have been detected by epidemiological research and may confound its results. As described by Norris and colleagues (Chapter 1) in this book, most epidemiological studies have measured only the first DSM-IV (American Psychiatric Association, 1994) criterion (the person was confronted with actual or threatened death or injury to self or others) but not the second (the person responded with intense fear, helplessness, or horror). When the second criterion is added, males' trauma prevalence decreases more than does that of females; resulting in rates that are comparable across genders (Norris et al., Chapter 1, this volume; Perkonigg, Kessler, Storz, & Wittchen, 2000). This suggests that across different kinds of trauma, males are less likely to report that the trauma led them to experience extreme fear. However, these findings should be interpreted with caution, because the same sociocultural factors that lead males to underreport certain kinds of trauma may also bias their reported interpretations.

Another aspect of the trauma memory is attribution of responsibility for the trauma. Recently, Foa, Ehlers, Clark, Tolin, and Orsillo (1999) developed the Post-Traumatic Cognitions Inventory (PTCI), a measure of trauma-related thoughts and beliefs. The PTCI consists of three empirically derived scales: Negative Cognitions about Self, Negative Cognitions about the World, and Self-Blame. The first two scales are discussed in later sections; the Self-Blame scale provides additional information about elements of the trauma record. Items on the Self-Blame scale include "The event happened because of the way I acted" and "Somebody else would have stopped the event from happening." We reanalyzed Foa et al.'s (1999) data to examine gender differences on this scale. In addition to standard significance testing, for each comparison we also calculated an estimate of effect size for gender, using r.

Using data from 120 male and 183 female adults who reported a negative life event, females endorsed significantly more self-blame items than did males ($p < .05$, $r = .13$), indicating a higher degree of self-blame for the traumatic event. Similar results were found among participants reporting a trauma that met both DSM-IV trauma criteria, with females endorsing significantly more self-blame beliefs than did males ($p < .05$, $r = .14$). It should be noted, however, that this finding may confound gender with trauma type. No gender differences were found within any single trauma type, although the number of participants per cell may have been too small to detect real differences. Thus, although females may be slightly (i.e., small but significant effect) more likely than males to blame themselves after a traumatic event, it is not clear whether this difference reflects a direct effect of gender, an indirect effect of gender as a result of the type of trauma experienced, or a combination of the two.

As noted by Foa and Rothbaum (1998), erroneous trauma records stem from inappropriate stimulus–stimulus and stimulus–response pairings related to the trauma. Thus, females' greater fear may be related to an increased "conditionability" of fear-related responses. Experimental data on this issue are mixed. Stamps and Porges (1975) examined trace conditioning in newborn infants by measuring heart rate deceleration in response to a conditioned stimulus (tone) and in anticipation of an unconditioned stimulus (blinking lights). Females, but not males, showed heart rate deceleration in response to the conditioned stiumulus and in anticipation of the unconditioned stimulus. Furthermore, the gender effect appeared to be mediated by females' greater heart rate variability. These results suggest that female neonates may be more physiologically reactive, and are hence more likely to acquire learned physiological responses. However, these results should be interpreted cautiously for two reasons. First, it is not clear whether data obtained from neonates reflect processes occurring in adults. Second, the conditioned response was heart rate deceleration, not acceleration; hence, similar results might not have been found for a more fear-congruent response. In an investigation of gender differences in fear conditioning among undergraduate volunteers, Fredrikson, Hugdahl, and Öhman (1976) paired electric shock with slides of fear-congruent (snakes and spiders) and fear-incongruent (flowers and mushrooms) stimuli. Females evidenced significantly greater anticipatory electrodermal responses to phobic slides than to neutral slides, with the opposite pattern seen among males. This finding might suggest greater susceptibility to fear conditioning among females. However, the gender difference disappeared when range correction was used, suggesting that the effect may be due to greater overall physiological reactivity among females rather than genuine differences in fear conditioning. Furthermore, the gender difference disappeared altogether during an extinction phase, indicating that any gender differences were transitory. Clearly, more research is needed in gender differences in conditionability of fear responses. Nevertheless, these results provide an interesting perspective about gender differences in cognitive appraisals that we noted in our sample of trauma survivors.

After a Traumatic Event, Do Males and Females Hold Different Beliefs about Themselves and the World?

According to Foa and Rothbaum (1998), dysfunctional schemas about the self and the world underlie the development of PTSD symptoms. These schemas can be inferred by the presence of negative beliefs about the self, such as "I am totally incompetent," and negative beliefs about the world, such as "The world is completely dangerous." We next examine whether male and female trauma victims differ according to these beliefs.

Are Female Trauma Victims More Likely Than Male Victims to View Themselves as Incompetent?

To investigate gender differences in self-schemas following a trauma, we reanalyzed data from the PTCI's Negative Cognitions about Self scale (Foa et al., 1999). Items on this scale include "I am a weak person" and "I can't trust myself." Among those whose index events did not meet both DSM-IV criteria for a trauma, there was a nonsignificant trend for females to endorse more negative self-beliefs than did males ($p < .08$, $r = .13$). Among participants whose index event met criteria for a trauma, the difference was significant, with females endorsing more negative self-beliefs than did males ($p < .05$, $r = .14$). There were no gender differences when participants were separated according to type of trauma; therefore, we cannot rule out the alternative explanation that gender differences in negative self-schemas resulted from different trauma experiences.

Are Female Trauma Victims More Likely Than Male Victims to View the World as Dangerous?

To investigate gender differences in world schemas following a trauma, we reanalyzed data from the PTCI's Negative Cognitions about the World scale (Foa et al., 1999). Items from this scale include "I have to be on guard all the time" and "The world is a dangerous place." Among those whose index events did not meet DSM-IV criteria for a trauma, females endorsed significantly more negative world statements than did males ($p < .05$, $r = .17$), indicating a higher degree of negative world-related thoughts. Similar results were obtained for those whose index event met criteria for a trauma, with females endorsing significantly more negative world beliefs than did males ($p < .05$, $r = .16$). Small cell sizes prevented accurate comparisons within many types of trauma, as was the case with the Negative Cognitions about Self scale. However, there was a significant gender difference for the larger sample of participants that experienced nonsexual assault by a stranger, with females endorsing significantly more negative world beliefs than did males ($p < .05$, $r = .45$). Thus, world schemas of female trauma victims appear to be more negative (e.g., beliefs that the world is dangerous) than are those of male victims. However, as was the case with self-schemas, it is not clear whether this difference reflects a direct effect of gender or of severity of trauma. More research is needed in order to determine the extent to which this is dependent on the type of trauma experienced.

SUMMARY AND CONCLUSIONS

Several studies indicate that although males generally report a greater number of traumatic experiences than females, overall, they have a lower prevalence of PTSD. In this chapter, we have attempted to account for this gender difference using Foa and colleagues' cognitive model of trauma processing (Figure 3.3). Our first question was whether males and females differ in terms of their trauma memory record. The available data seem to indicate that this may be the case. Females are much more likely than males to experience sexual forms of assault such as rape and CSA. Males, on the other hand, are more likely than females to experience traumas such as combat, motor vehicle accidents, and nonsexual assaults. It seems reasonable to conclude that these different traumas are represented differently in memory. Indeed, rape, particularly, appears to have a high probability of eliciting PTSD in both male and female victims. However, whereas this factor seems to contribute substantially to gender differences in PTSD prevalence, it does not appear to be the sole explanation for this difference, because females are more likely than males to meet criteria for PTSD after traumas other than rape, such as a motor vehicle accident or disaster, and because combat may be as equally likely to elicit PTSD as is rape. Data from our own research and that of others suggest that females' trauma records may contain a stronger element of self-blame for the trauma. However, it is not known whether this represents a direct effect of gender or differences in the type of trauma experienced (e.g., rape may elicit more self-blame than does a motor vehicle accident in both males and females).

Next we examined whether the self- and world schemas of males and females are affected differently by trauma. Data from our own research suggest that female trauma victims hold more negative beliefs about themselves and their abilities. However, this finding was confounded by type of trauma. An alternative hypothesis is that rape victims' self-schemas are more strongly affected than are those of motor vehicle accident victims. More research is needed to parse out these factors. Our research found stronger support for the hypothesis that female trauma victims are more likely to view the world as dangerous than are male trauma victims. Preliminary evidence suggests that this cannot be attributed solely to the type of trauma experienced. Thus, the perception of the world as dangerous may mediate gender differences in PTSD. It is important to note, however, that any mediating variables appear most influential with less severe forms of traumas. With extremely severe traumas (e.g., rape, combat) the data are more mixed, with some studies showing PTSD rates among males that are comparable to or greater than those of females. Perhaps the extreme severity of some traumas can outweigh the effects of other predictor variables such as gender. More research should examine whether the pattern is linear (i.e., each incremental increase in trauma severity narrows gender differences by the same degree), or nonlinear (e.g., trauma severity overshadows other mediators only past some threshold of severity).

In conclusion, it appears that the cognitive model of PTSD can provide useful information about potential mediators of gender differences in the prevalence of PTSD. Males and females tend to be exposed to different forms of trauma; this creates differences in trauma memory records that may account for much (but not all) of the difference. Furthermore, once a trauma has been experienced, males and females differ in terms of their cognitive schemas. Specifically, females appear more likely to blame themselves for the trauma, to hold more negative views of themselves, and to view the world as more dangerous than do male trauma victims. This may be due in part to differences in the trauma itself, or it may be due to other gender-specific factors that have not yet been identified. The net effect of these cognitive differences is that males are less likely than females to develop PTSD following a trauma.

The cognitive model of gender differences in PTSD has raised at least as many questions as answers. One of the most pressing questions is whether gender differences in cognitive response are independent of gender differences in traumatic experience. Additional research is needed that assesses trauma attributions, self-schemas, world schemas, and PTSD symptoms among males and females exposed to similar traumas. Another issue concerns pretrauma beliefs about one's self and the world. Longitudinal research examining the presence of rigid, positive or negative beliefs may identify gender differences in these factors that contribute to vulnerability to develop PTSD. Finally, the cognitive model may be used to identify gender differences in posttraumatic responses other than PTSD, such as substance abuse, externalizing behaviors, and somatic problems.

REFERENCES

American Psychiatric Association. (1994). *Diagnostic and statistical manual of mental disorders* (4th ed.). Washington, DC: Author.

Anderson, J. R., & Bower, G. H. (1973). *Human associative memory.* Washington, DC: Winston.

Baum, M. (1970). Extinction of avoidance responding through response prevention (flooding). *Psychological Bulletin, 74,* 276–284.

Beck, A. T., Emery, G., & Greenberg, R. L. (1985). *Anxiety disorders and phobias: A cognitive perspective.* New York: Basic Books.

Best, C. L., Dansky, B. S., & Kilpatrick, D. G. (1992). Medical students' attitudes about female rape victims. *Journal of Interpersonal Violence, 7,* 175–188.

Breslau, N., & Davis, G. C. (1992). Posttraumatic stress disorder in an urban population of young adults: Risk factors for chronicity. *American Journal of Psychiatry, 149,* 671–675.

Breslau, N., Davis, G. C., Andreski, P., & Peterson, E. (1991). Traumatic events and posttraumatic stress disorder in an urban population of young adults. *Archives of General Psychiatry, 48,* 216–222.

Breslau, N., Kessler, R. C., Chilcoat, H. D., Schultz, L. R., Davis, G. C., & Andreski, P. (1998). Trauma and posttraumatic stress disorder in the community. *Archives of General Psychiatry, 55,* 626–632.

Burgess, A. W., & Holmstrom, L. L. (1978). Recovery from rape and prior life stress. *Research in Nursing and Health, 1,* 165–174.

Davidson, J., Hughes, D., Blazer, D., & George, L. (1991). Post-traumatic stress disorder in the community: An epidemiological study. *Psychological Medicine, 21,* 713–722.

Davis, R. C., Brickman, E. R., & Baker, T. (1991). Effects of supportive and unsupportive responses of others to rape victims: Effects on concurrent victim adjustment. *American Journal of Community Psychology, 19,* 443–451.

Eagly, A. H. (1987). *Sex differences in social behavior: A social-role interpretation.* Hillsdale, NJ: Erlbaum.

Ehlers, A., Mayou, R. A., & Bryant, B. (1998). Psychological predictors of chronic PTSD after motor vehicle accidents. *Journal of Abnormal Psychology, 107,* 508–519.

Epstein, S. (1991). Impulse control and self-destructive behavior. In L. P. Lipsitt & L. L. Mitnick (Eds.), *Self-regulatory behavior and risk taking: Causes and consequences* (pp. 273–284). Norwood, NJ: Ablex.

Finkelhor, D. (1986). *A sourcebook on child sexual abuse: New theory and research.* Beverly Hills, CA: Sage.

Finkelhor, D., Hotaling, G., Lewis, I. A., & Smith, C. (1990). Sexual abuse in a national survey of adult men and women: Prevalence, characteristics, and risk factors. *Child Abuse and Neglect, 14,* 19–28.

Fischer, G. J. (1992). Gender differences in college student sexual abuse victims and their offenders. *Annals of Sex Research, 5,* 215–226.

Foa, E. B., Ehlers, A., Clark, D. M., Tolin, D. F., & Orsillo, S. M. (1999). The Post-Traumatic Cognitions Inventory (PTCI): Development and validation. *Psychological Assessment, 11,* 303–314.

Foa, E. B., & Kozak, M. J. (1986). Emotional processing of fear: Exposure to corrective information. *Psychological Bulletin, 99,* 20–35.

Foa, E. B., & Riggs, D. S. (1993). Post-traumatic stress disorder in rape victims. In J. Oldham, M. B. Riba, & A. Tasman (Eds.), *American Psychiatric Press review of psychiatry* (Vol. 12, pp. 273–303). Washington, DC: American Psychiatric Press.

Foa, E. B., & Rothbaum, B. O. (1998). *Treating the trauma of rape: Cognitive-behavioral therapy for PTSD.* New York: Guilford Press.

Foa, E. B., Steketee, G., & Rothbaum, B. O. (1989). Behavioral/cognitive conceptualization of posttraumatic stress disorder. *Behavior Therapy, 20,* 155–176.

Fredrikson, M., Hugdahl, K., & Öhman, A. (1976). Electrodermal conditioning to potentially phobic stimuli in male and female subjects. *Biological Psychiatry, 4,* 305–314.

Fritz, G. S., Stoll, K., & Wagner, N. A. (1981). A comparison of males and females who were sexually molested as children. *Journal of Sex and Marital Therapy, 7,* 54–59.

Helzer, J. E., Robins, L. N., & McEvoy, L. (1987). Posttraumatic stress disorder in the general population: Findings of the epidemiological catchment area survey. *New England Journal of Medicine, 317,* 1630–1634.

Horowitz, M. J. (1986). *Stress response syndromes* (2nd ed.). Northvale, NJ: Jason Aronson.

Janoff-Bulman, R. (1985). The aftermath of victimization: Rebuilding shattered assumptions. In C. R. Figley (Ed.), *The study and treatment of posttraumatic stress disorder* (Vol. 1, pp. 15–35). New York: Brunner/Mazel.

Janoff-Bulman, R. (1992). *Shattered assumptions: Towards a new psychology of trauma.* New York: Free Press.

Kaufman, A., Divasto, P., Jackson, R., Voorhees, D., & Christy, J. (1980). Male rape victims: Noninstitutionalized assault. *American Journal of Psychiatry, 137,* 221–223.

Kessler, R. C., Sonnega, A., Bromet, E., Hughes, M., & Nelson, C. B. (1995). Posttraumatic stress disorder in the National Comorbidity Survey. *Archives of General Psychiatry, 52,* 1048–1060.

McCann, I. L., & Pearlman, L. A. (1990). *Psychological trauma and the adult survivor: Theory, therapy, and transformation.* New York: Brunner/Mazel.

Nash, C., & West, D. (1985). Sexual molestation of young girls: A retrospective survey. In D. J. West (Ed.), *Sexual victimization* (pp. 1–92). Brookfield, VT: Gower.

Norris, F. H. (1992). Epidemiology of trauma: Frequency and impact of potentially traumatic events on different demographic groups. *Journal of Consulting and Clinical Psychology, 60,* 409–418.

Perkonigg, A., Kessler, R. C., Storz, S., & Wittchen, H. U. (2000). Traumatic events and posttraumatic stress disorder in the community: Prevalence, risk factors, and comorbidity. *Acta Psychiatrica Scandinavica, 101,* 46–59.

Pino, N. W., & Meier, R. F. (1999). Gender differences in rape reporting. *Sex Roles, 40,* 979–990.

Resick, P. A. (1987). *The impact of rape on psychological functioning.* Unpublished manuscript, University of Missouri, St. Louis.

Rind, B., Tromovitch, P., & Bauserman, R. (1998). A meta-analytic examination of assumed properties of child sexual abuse using college samples. *Psychological Bulletin, 124,* 22–53.

Risin, L. I., & Koss, M. P. (1987). The sexual abuse of boys: Prevalence and descriptive characteristics of childhood victimizations. *Journal of Interpersonal Violence, 2,* 309–323.

Rothbaum, B. O., Foa, E. B., Riggs, D., Murdock, T., & Walsh, W. (1992). A prospective examination of posttraumatic stress disorder in rape victims. *Journal of Traumatic Stress, 5,* 455–475.

Schultz, L., & Jones, P. (1983). Sexual abuse of children: Issues for social service and health professionals. *Child Welfare, 62,* 99–108.

Stamps, L. E., & Porges, S. W. (1975). Heart rate conditioning in newborn infants: Relationship among conditionability, heart rate variability, and sex. *Developmental Psychology, 11,* 424–431.

Tolin, D. F., & Foa, E. B. (2002). *Sex differences in vulnerability for posttraumatic stress disorder.* Manuscript submitted for publication.

Ullman, S. E. (1995). Adult trauma survivors and posttraumatic stress sequelae: An analysis of reexperiencing, avoidance, and arousal criteria. *Journal of Traumatic Stress, 8,* 179–188.

Weathers, F. W., Litz, B. T., & Keane, T. M. (1995). Military trauma. In J. R. Freedy & S. E. Hobfoll (Eds.), *Traumatic stress: From theory to practice* (pp. 103–128). New York: Plenum Press.

Weiss, D. S., Marmar, C. R., Schlenger, W. E., Fairbank, J. A., Jordan, B. K., Hough, R. L., & Kulka, R. A. (1992). The prevalence of lifetime and partial posttraumatic stress disorder in Vietnam veterans. *Journal of Traumatic Stress, 5,* 365–376.

4 | The Intersection of Gender and Betrayal in Trauma

ANNE P. DePRINCE
JENNIFER J. FREYD

Many traumatic events involve some degree of social betrayal. In cases of interpersonal violence, betrayal may take the form of caregivers' or trusted partners' perpetration of violence. Some forms of trauma are less likely to involve social betrayal, such as natural disasters. This chapter explores gender differences in traumas that involve betrayal, using this framework to make predictions about gender and memory impairment in posttraumatic stress disorder (PTSD).

Childhood sexual abuse and adult betrayal traumas are gender-asymmetric. More girls than boys are abused in childhood, and more women than men are abused in intimate relationships; abusers are more likely to be men than women. Approximately one in four adult women is a survivor of childhood sexual (contact) abuse and the rates go up when adult victimization is included (Finkelhor, 1979, 1986; Kinsey, Pomeroy, Martin, & Gebhard, 1953; Koss, Gidycz, & Wisniewski, 1987; Russell, 1986;). Understanding the dynamics of response to these traumas is particularly important for understanding the role of gender in posttraumatic responses. If males and females are more likely to experience different types of traumatic events (e.g., sexual abuse vs. combat), how will this affect the posttraumatic response? How might differences in the perpetrator relationship and/or the context of traumatic events (e.g., age at time of trauma, duration of trauma) lead to alterations in cognitive processing and memory impairment?

Cognitive models of posttraumatic responses provide a framework for understanding onset and maintenance of trauma-related distress, including memory impairment. Researchers have increasingly turned to cognitive methods to examine the role of attention (e.g., DePrince & Freyd, 1999;

Freyd, Martorella, Alvarado, Hayes, & Christman, 1998; Williams, Mathews, & MacLeod, 1996) and memory (DePrince & Freyd, 1999), among other variables, in posttraumatic responses. Cognitive frameworks have also been employed to propose interventions for treatment (e.g., Rothbaum & Foa, 1996). However, the role of gender has not yet been integrated into cognitive approaches to trauma.

The current chapter considers how gender differences in the experience of and responses to trauma may relate to information processing in trauma. We first consider gender differences in rates of PTSD and in type of trauma experienced. Next, we draw on one specific cognitive model, betrayal trauma theory, to examine how the type of trauma experienced (i.e., the relationship to the perpetrator) and gender relate to one criterion of the current PTSD diagnosis: memory impairment for the traumatic event. Memory impairment is associated with PTSD in the avoidance cluster of symptoms as defined by the fourth edition of the *Diagnostic and Statistical Manual of Mental Disorders* (DSM-IV; American Psychiatric Association, 1994). Memory impairment has been well documented following trauma in samples of individuals with and without PTSD, making it an important variable for consideration following trauma (e.g., Elliott, 1997; Feldman-Summers & Pope, 1994; Freyd, 1996; Williams, 1994;). To date, theoretical models of memory impairment have not taken gender into account; this chapter focuses specifically on the interaction of gender and memory impairment in cognitive models. Through our analysis, we do not suggest that differences in information processing of traumas for men and women reflect any essential biological sex difference. Rather, we propose that gender differences in rates of interpersonal violence lead to predictable alterations in memory for women compared to men.

In considering cognitive models of memory impairment, we draw on both betrayal trauma theory and social constructionist views of gender. Betrayal trauma theory posits that psychogenic amnesia and unawareness are often necessary for survival in cases in which abuse occurs at the hands of a parent or caregiver. Information, or knowledge of the abuse that would otherwise interfere with one's ability to function within an essential relationship is blocked, for instance, that of parent and dependent child. Betrayal trauma theory is discussed in greater detail later in the chapter.

A social constructionist view focuses on the role that culture plays in ideas about gender, mental health, and trauma. Social constructionist perspectives encourage us to examine previously pathologized aspects of responses to abuse and trauma that in fact make sense as adaptations to the exploitive environment; our assumptions of sanity and insanity are often flip-flopped (Armstrong, 1994; Brown, 1994). Is it a sign of mental illness, deviance, or disorder to forget traumatic events perpetrated on a dependent child, or is such blindness instead one route to survival and thus a sign of vitality? Betrayal trauma theory, with its focus on forgetting as a way to maintain necessary systems of attachment, argues that oppressed people may be responding adaptively when they forget aspects of their own reality—it legitimizes the reaction of those who have been abused. Betrayal trauma theory extends to situations other than childhood sexual abuse. In cases of oppression by powerful others, when the victim feels dependent upon the oppressor and betrayal occurs, the theory predicts some degree of information loss about betrayal. For instance, in cases of battering and/or marital rape, when a woman feels dependent upon her male partner, some degree of unawareness of the abuse may be adaptive in maintaining an apparently, or actually, necessary system of dependence and attachment.

MEMORY IMPAIRMENT IN THE PTSD CRITERIA

Memory persistence for the traumatic event captures the central feature of PTSD—either reexperiencing phenomena, such as through flashbacks, or having periods during which memory about the trauma is unavailable. A number of studies have examined memory persistence for traumatic events, particularly in the context of childhood trauma, including sexual abuse. Across studies, roughly one-third of subjects in samples tend to report some period for which they did not have continuous access to memory for the traumatic event, though criteria for amnesia, from partial to full, vary from study to study (e.g., Elliott & Briere, 1995; Feldman-Summers & Pope, 1994; Herman & Schatzow, 1987; Loftus, Polonsky, & Fullilove, 1994; Williams, 1994). Williams (1994) conducted a prospective study in which she interviewed women 17 years after they were treated as children in the emergency room for sexual abuse. Of the women interviewed, 38% did not report memory of the emergency room visit, though the women did report other highly personal and traumatic events (such as assaults as adults, abortions, etc.), suggesting that the failure to report was due to lack of memory for the event rather than unwillingness to report.

Studies have also explored memory for other traumas, including combat. In one prospective study of veterans from the Persian Gulf War, memory was assessed at 1 month and at 2 years after return from the Gulf War (Southwick, Krystal, Johnson, & Charney, 1997). Memory assessment involved a 19-item trauma checklist in which participants endorsed experienced events that were highly traumatic in nature (e.g., seeing others killed or wounded, death of a friend). Results indicate that the vast majority of participants (88%) changed their responses on at least one item on the checklist, and 61% changed their responses on two or more items. Changes in memory report from "no" to an item at 1-month assessment to "yes" at the 2-year assessment were significantly positively correlated with PTSD severity as measured by the Mississippi Scale for Combat-Related Posttraumatic Stress Disorder. The authors suggest that these results are evidence that memory for trauma is neither fixed nor indelible, and that memory for traumatic events are amplified as PTSD symptoms increase.

PTSD AND GENDER

Research suggests that women are diagnosed with PTSD at higher rates than men (for a review, see Wolfe & Kimerling, 1997). To date, gender differences have not been thoroughly examined in light of the role that cultural and gender factors may play in the diagnosis of PTSD. Along these lines, some researchers have argued that cross-cultural issues in the diagnosis and prevalence of PTSD are poorly understood (e.g., Berberich, 1998). Willer and Grossman (1995) have suggested that women and men are treated differently in the mental health system, leading to different diagnoses for similar symptoms. For example, Willer and Grossman (1995) found that males in a Veterans Administration psychiatric outpatient clinic were given the diagnosis of PTSD more frequently than women, who tended to receive affective and schizoaffective diagnoses. Gender differences in rates of PTSD diagnosis may reflect cultural assumptions about women's mental health and realities (for a review of related issues, see Caplan, 1995).

Arguably, gender differences in PTSD may also reflect differences in the amount of trauma males and females experience. However, the literature does not clearly support the argument that women simply experience more trauma than men. Breslau and Davis (1992) reported that women were diagnosed with PTSD more frequently than men, even when men and women did not differ in the number of traumatic events experienced as measured in the study. The possibility remains that women did experience more trauma, but that such trauma was less likely to be reported because women perceived the events, or reporting of the events, as more stigmatized and secret than did men. The different rates of unreported trauma in the histories of the men and women may have had an impact on the PTSD rates.

GENDER DIFFERENCES IN TRAUMAS
EXPERIENCED AND REACTIONS

There is evidence in the literature that men and women experience different types of trauma. For example, a recent survey of 1,000 female and male active duty U.S. soldiers revealed that whereas females tended to report more sexual traumas, males tended to report more nonsexual traumas (Stretch, Knudson, & Durand, 1998). Research on sexual abuse suggests that girls tend to experience sexual abuse within the family for a longer duration of time compared to boys, who tend to experience sexual abuse by nonfamily members for a shorter duration (Dhaliwal, Gauzas, Antonowicz, & Ross, 1996; Gordon, 1990).

In addition to gender differences in types of traumatic events, there may also be gender differences in reactions to trauma. For example, sexually abused girls blamed themselves more for the assault than did boys. In a recent review, Wolfe and Kimerling (1997) noted that this difference in self-blame is likely very important to examine, and argued that girls might be at greater risk than boys for the self-blame associated with depression, shame, guilt, and social isolation following childhood sexual abuse.

INTERSECTION OF COGNITIVE MODELS AND GENDER RESEARCH

The current literature focusing on cognitive models for memory impairment and information-processing approaches to PTSD does not examine the relation between gender and memory. Though little attention has been paid to interactions between gender and PTSD, recent research suggests that women and men's experiences of trauma and emotional responses differ in some important ways. These differences appear to be important in building cognitive models for understanding posttraumatic stress responses. Betrayal trauma theory provides a framework through which to speculate on how gender may relate to memory impairment in PTSD.

BETRAYAL TRAUMA THEORY OVERVIEW

Betrayal trauma theory seeks to account for memory impairment following traumatic events. The theory posits that there is a social utility in remaining unaware of abuse when the perpetrator is a caregiver (Freyd, 1996), and it contributes to the field of traumatic stress in a number of ways. First, it accounts for memory failure in a way that can be empirically tested. Second, the theory stresses a meaning or emotion following trauma that has remained largely unexamined in research: betrayal.

BETRAYAL TRAUMA THEORY: MOTIVATION

Betrayal trauma theory draws on a variety of perspectives to explain the motivation for forgetting trauma. First, drawing on evolutionary psychology, we note that humans are excellent at detecting betrayals, which makes good sense, so that they can remove themselves from relationships in which they are being cheated. However, under some circumstances, detecting betrayals may be counterproductive to survival. Specifically, in cases when a victim is dependent on a caregiver, survival may require that she or he remain unaware of the betrayal. In the case of childhood sexual abuse, a child who is aware that her or his parent is being abusive may withdraw from the relationship (e.g., withdraw in terms of proximity, emotion, etc.). For a child who depends on a caregiver for basic survival, withdrawing may actually be at odds with survival. In such cases, children's survival would be better ensured by their being blind to the betrayal and isolating the knowledge of the event.

Betrayal trauma theory identifies attachment as an important motivation for being unaware of abuse. Infants and children depend on successful attachment to caregivers and are active in maintaining the attachment relationship. Child abuse is likely to produce a social conflict or betrayal for the victim. If the child processed the betrayal in the manner predicted by evolutionary psychology, the betrayal would be experienced as a form of emotional pain. Emotional pain, much like physical pain, can be adaptive for changing behavior. For example, physical pain caused by a broken leg provides good motivation to not walk on the leg, thereby preventing further injury. The psychic pain in detecting a betrayal would usually lead to behavior change that removes the victim from the relationship with the perpetrator. However, to withdraw from a caregiver on which the victim is dependent would create an additional threat to survival. In such a case of child abuse by a caregiver, the child may actually be better benefited for long-term survival by blocking information about the abuse from mental mechanisms that control attachment and attachment behavior. Thus, the victim would be unaware of the abuse at a conscious level.

SUPPORT FOR BETRAYAL TRAUMA THEORY

Research drawing on multiple data sets has supported betrayal trauma theory predictions that more memory impairment is found when the perpetrator is a caretaker (for a review, see Freyd, 1996). In a recent study, a sample of 202 undergraduates were asked about their experiences of physical, sexual, and emotional abuse (Freyd, DePrince, & Zurbriggen, 2001). Among those participants who reported physical and sexual abuse, more memory impairment was reported for abuse perpetrated by caretakers than by noncaretakers.

Other research indirectly provides support for betrayal trauma predictions. For example, Elliott (1997) surveyed a random sample of participants about their experiences of three types of trauma: noninterpersonal trauma (e.g., car accident, natural disaster), a witnessed trauma (e.g., witnessing domestic violence as a child), and experienced interpersonal trauma (e.g., physical assault). Participants were asked about their memory for the event, and their responses were classified into three categories of memory loss, ranging from no memory impairment to complete memory loss for some period of time. Elliott reported memory impairment across all types of trauma but particularly high rates of impairment for interpersonal victimization. Though these data do not speak directly to the victim–perpetrator relationship, they do suggest that traumas of an interpersonal nature, which have the potential for more social betrayal than noninterpersonal events, are related to higher rates of memory impairment.

BETRAYAL TRAUMA THEORY: MECHANISMS

Betrayal trauma theory implicates dissociation as a possible mechanism in blocking information about or knowledge of the trauma. Building on lessons from cognitive psychology, betrayal trauma theory suggests that dissociations or disconnections may occur between normally connected aspects of processing and memory. Via these disconnections, threatening information may be separated from awareness in the case of betrayal traumas. These cognitive dissociations, in turn, may lead to the more global symptomology of clinical dissociation.

Betrayal trauma theory does not argue that traumatic information is totally blocked from entering the nervous system. Rather, the information is blocked from mechanisms that control attachment behavior. This suggests that the information is blocked from declarative or episodic knowledge, which includes memories for which people can make statements; for example, autobiographical information, such as the names of family members, is a form of declarative knowledge. In instances when betrayal trauma information is blocked from conscious awareness, the information will be processed by other, less conscious mechanisms, such as sensory stores and/or implicit memory, which includes memories for which we do not have the ability to describe the memory verbally. For example, the process of riding a bike is a form of implicit memory; people generally cannot explain with words the procedure by which they are able to balance on a bicycle while riding.

Information about betrayal traumas may also be blocked from consciousness through the use of attention systems. Laboratory tasks have shown a relationship between attention and dissociation that may have a bearing on understanding some memory impairment seen in PTSD. Dissociation has been defined as a lack of integration of thoughts, feelings, and experiences into the stream of consciousness. Many studies have shown a relationship between PTSD and dissociation, though dissociation is not a criterion of the DSM-IV PTSD diagnosis (Bremner et al., 1992; Carlier, Lamberts, Fouwels, & Gersons, 1996; Marmar et al., 1994). Although most people show some ability to dissociate (e.g., highway hypnosis), high levels of dissociation are far less common, such as feeling states of depersonalization or derealization. The most extreme form of dissociation is dissociative identity disorder. The Dissociative Experiences Scale (DES) has been widely used to measure individual level of dissociation. In order to examine the relation between dissociation and attention, individuals who scored within the normal range on the DES (low DES) and those who scored in the clinically high range (high DES) were recruited to participate in an experiment employing selective and divided attention versions of the Stroop task (DePrince & Freyd, 1999). High DES participants performed worse on the selective attention task and better on the divided attention task when compared to low-DES participants. This finding suggests that high-DES participants may be better able to process information in divided attention structures than in selective attention environments compared to low DES participants.

In a follow-up study using a directed forgetting paradigm, DePrince and Freyd (2001) found that high-DES participants recalled fewer emotionally charged words and more neutral words under divided attention conditions when compared to low-DES participants. This finding suggests that divided attention may help high dissociators to keep threatening information from awareness and illustrates a way in which attention can be used to alter the flow of threatening information into awareness. While these studies group participants by dissociation rather than PTSD status, the relation between dissociation and PTSD suggests that these results offer possible mechanisms for some memory impairment in PTSD through dissociation. These empirical findings fit with clinical anecdotes about the frequently chaotic behavior seen in clients diagnosed with PTSD and/or dissociative disorders; that is, clients may create chaos, to some extent, in their lives in order to maintain a divided attention environment. The divided attention environment, in turn, may better enable clients to keep threatening information about trauma from awareness.

IMPORTANCE OF EMOTIONS INVOKED BY TRAUMA

Freyd (2001) suggested that traumatic events can contain both life-threatening and/or social betrayal components (see Figure 4.1). She noted that whereas some traumas may be high in fear/terror, such as a natural disaster, others traumas may be high in both fear and betrayal dimensions, such as some sadistic abuse. Still other traumatic events may be high in social betrayal but may not invoke life-threatening terror, such as some molestation by trusted others or caregivers. Betrayal trauma theory would predict more memory impairment for events that fall in the quadrants that are high in social betrayal than for events in the quadrant high in fear alone. The proposed distinction between fear and betrayal begins to tease apart how different emotions may relate to different memory and distress outcomes.

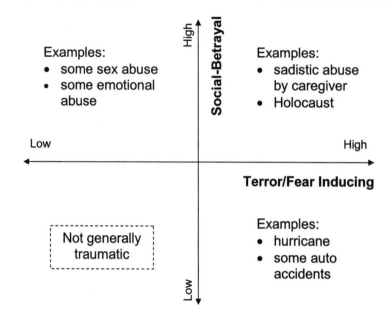

FIGURE 4.1. The two-dimensional model of trauma. Copyright 1996 by Jennifer J. Freyd. Reprinted by permission.

EXPLORING THE INTERSECTION OF
GENDER, BETRAYAL, AND MEMORY

To date, gender differences in PTSD response have not been empirically tested with respect to predictions made from cognitive models. Given evidence that women and men differ along important dimensions, such as relationship to the perpetrator, in their reports of trauma, we believe that there may be cases in which gender differences in memory impairment can be predicted from cognitive models. Specifically, we can explore predictions derived from betrayal trauma theory relevant to gender.

The research literature indicates that males and females are exposed to traumatic events that differ in important ways. Taking sexual abuse as an example, males and females differ in their relationship to the perpetrator: Girls more often tend to be abused by family members than do boys. Working within a betrayal trauma framework, this difference in perpetrator–victim relationship will lead to very different information-processing strategies. We predict that this would lead to differences in memory for the events given that the betrayal trauma framework proposes that remaining unaware of trauma helps to preserve necessary attachments. Girls who are sexually abused by caretakers will be more likely to isolate knowledge of the betrayal via information-processing mechanisms, such as alterations in attention and dissociations between normally connected aspects of consciousness. Boys, who tend to be abused more frequently by non-family members, will be less likely to isolate knowledge of the event, because it does not represent betrayal in a caretaking relationship.

Differences in the degree of betrayal and ensuing information processing may then be related to symptoms of distress. Working within the betrayal trauma theory framework, betrayal may involve dissociative mechanisms to keep threatening information from awareness. If this is the case, then betrayal via dissociative mechanisms may lead individuals to experience dissociative symptoms and problems with dissociation. For example, we predict that more betrayal would be related to higher levels of dissociation on measures of dissociation, such as the DES. Dissociating awareness of betrayals may also lead females to experience higher levels of the PTSD avoidance symptoms. If this is the case, the frequency of betrayals experienced in important attachment relationships may help us to understand in part why women receive diagnoses of PTSD and the dissociative disorders more frequently than do men.

Whereas we have proposed that females may experience more betrayal trauma than males, at least two alternative explanations can be considered in this intersection of trauma, gender, and betrayal. The first we call here the "dispositional" explanation; the second, the "situational" explanation. The dispositional explanation assumes that women may be socialized to perceive or notice betrayal more frequently than do males. The notion that females may perceive more betrayal is consistent with the idea that females are socialized to put greater value on interpersonal relationships than males (e.g., Gilligan, 1982). This socialization process may result in a disposition to notice betrayal. If females attend more to betrayal, this may lead to a compensatory mechanism that increases the likelihood that they use dissociative mechanisms to cope with the betrayal information.

The second explanation is also about perception and sensitivity to betrayal but emphasizes the situation in which women may often find themselves in society—in a role without as much power as those around them (Miller, 1986). This situational explanation assumes that the less powerful person at the time is more likely to attend to the possibility of betrayal than is the more powerful person. Less powerful individuals are likely more often in a dependent role in relationships. Being less powerful and more dependent, these individuals may perceive and notice betrayal more frequently. Betrayal trauma theory would predict that these individuals, if dependent, would then—as a compensatory reaction—be motivated to remain unaware of the betrayal.

These possibilities—that women actually experience more betrayal traumas, that they are socialized to perceive more betrayal, and that less powerful people in a given situation are more sensitive to betrayal—are not mutually exclusive. We would likely find great overlap in these categories. For example, in many cultures, females have less power than males; individuals who have less power are likely at greater risk for interpersonal trauma, which in turn leads to the first explanation—that women experience more betrayals. In this analysis, it less clear whether gender or power best explains perceptions and/or experiences of betrayal.

The notion of power as an additional variable that intersects with gender and trauma offers interesting clinical implications. It may be that individuals who are disempowered, whether male or female, will experience distress related to the betrayals they have experienced in trauma, whereas those who have access to power may experience distress related to other aspects of the event, such as the fear invoked. One reviewer of this manuscript offered the example of different reactions in Vietnam veterans, some of whom readily identify with feelings of betrayal by the government, whereas others find the notion of betrayal foreign.

FUTURE STUDY

Empirical investigation of gender differences in betrayal traumas, memory impairment and dissociative/avoidance symptoms must include methodology that gathers information about the context of the traumatic event. For example, improved questions about the victim–perpetrator relationship are needed. To date, most research has categorized interpersonal violence into two categories: family or nonfamily violence. Likely, much violence perpetrated by family members involves betrayal; however, in some cases, abuse by a family member may be perpetrated by someone on whom the victim is not dependent for survival, such as a distant relative or a parent who lives outside the home. In some nonfamily abuse, the level of betrayal of an important attachment relationship may actually be quite high. For example, a child may be abused by a trusted coach or religious leader on whom he or she is emotionally dependent. Survey and interview questions must be designed to elicit the context of the perpetrator–victim relationship in order to understand the degree of betrayal. In our laboratory, we have been developing the Betrayal Trauma Inventory, in which we ask participants whether the perpetrator was responsible for caretaking and was someone trusted.

A second methodological issue to be addressed is the inclusion of questions about betrayal in research and clinical practice. To date, the PTSD literature has been most focused on the role that fear plays in the onset and maintenance of PTSD. This is likely, because the diagnosis of PTSD was established in the context of combat survivors. Historically, the assumption was that the primary emotion invoked by combat trauma was fear or terror given the life-threatening nature of war. While asking about fear/terror makes good theoretical sense for life-threatening events, other traumatic events may be high in social betrayal components that will affect information processing, memory, and distress. These events are more likely to be experienced by females, such as those sexually abused by caregivers. Notably, social betrayal dimensions of life-threatening events such as combat should also be assessed. Shay (1994) has discussed the powerful role betrayal played in the experience and subsequent distress of many male Vietnam veterans. Vietnam veterans experienced various forms of betrayal by the military (e.g., provided with faulty weapons) responsible for their well-being, and additional betrayals upon their return to the United States, where they were frequently blamed for the war rather than celebrated, as had been veterans of previous wars. Parallels can be drawn between the veterans' experience of betrayal and interpersonal violence perpetrated by caregivers; veterans and child victims are dependent on their caregivers, the military and the family, respectively.

The proposed differences for women in cognitive processing of events related to the higher level of betrayal traumas have important implications for revictimization. If future studies support the prediction that women experience more betrayal traumas and more memory impairment, this will likely be important in understanding patterns of revictimization and relational difficulties. If compensatory processes following betrayal traumas relate to some women's failure to attend to or to process threatening information fully, these women may be at greater risk for future assault. This view is consistent with discussions in the literature of the possible role of dissociation and failures to appraise threats (e.g., Cloitre, 1998).

The role of betrayal is also critical to the examination of how women understand their own histories and make meaning of their emotions and reactions to betrayal traumas. For example, betrayal trauma theory could argue that betrayal leads women, more so than men, to avoid processing traumatic memories in a way that integrates these memories with autobiographical knowledge—keeping the memories away from awareness to preserve important attachments. However, betrayal trauma theory also posits that the event is processed at some level—an implicit level. So women may still have the experience of anxiety, fear, and shame but not have the autobiographical knowledge of its source. In these cases, in which women may feel "crazy," that image of women as "crazy" is then supported by cultural myths about women's mental health.

Finally, the role of betrayal traumas in changing how women function in relationship must be examined. Herman's (1992) complex PTSD contains a cluster of symptoms for alterations in relations with others, and many women have been labeled with borderline personality disorder diagnoses that reflect difficulties in relationships with others. Relational changes, such as withdrawal, disruptions in intimate relationships, and persistent distrust, may be related to the violations experienced in interpersonal violence. If it is the case that women experience more betrayal traumas than men, this may explain in part the differences in relational difficulties. The role of betrayals in important attachments also encourages questions about healing in relationships, such as in the context of the therapy relationship.

SUMMARY AND CONCLUSIONS

Based on the current literature, we have evidence that females experience more betrayal traumas than males, when betrayal is defined as "abuse by someone on whom the victim is dependent." We do have to be cautious in interpreting this finding. Although we have evidence of differences in men's and women's reports of trauma, we cannot determine which of these differences are explained by socialization as opposed to experience with traumatic events; that is, are women simply more willing to report abuse by caregivers than men? We do not know whether the gender differences for reported betrayal versus fear reflect gender narratives that men and women learn as they are sex-role socialized, or the experience of different traumatic events; most likely they reflect both. (An interesting, related issue is the extent to which the field of traumatic stress itself has been biased by the gendered "trauma narratives" of the researchers, clinicians, and theoreticians.) If men are on average more inclined to focus on the life-threatening aspects of trauma and less on interpersonal aspects of trauma and betrayal, this inclination may have had an impact on the field of traumatic stress studies, a field historically dominated by men. In recent years, the field has seen a substantial increase in women researchers, clinicians, and theoreticians; it has also seen a substantial increase in its focus on interpersonal trauma and events marked by betrayal. These two changes may be more than coincidental. With the important advances in the field of trauma, researchers and clinicians must maintain, as well as deepen, the commitment to examine the context of trauma, in order to understand better the influence of gender and culture on posttraumatic responses and healing.

ACKNOWLEDGMENTS

Preparation of this chapter was supported in part by the "Emotion Research Training Grant" from the National Institute of Mental Health. We wish to thank two anonymous reviewers for their comments on an earlier version of the manuscript.

REFERENCES

American Psychiatric Association. (1994). *Diagnostic and statistical manual of mental disorders* (4th ed.). Washington, DC: Author.

Armstrong, L. (1994). *Rocking the cradle of sexual politics: What happened when women said incest.* Reading, MA: Addison-Wesley.

Berberich, D. A. (1998). Posttraumatic stress disorder: Gender and cross-cultural clinical issues. *Psychotherapy in Private Practice, 17,* 29–41.

Berton, M. W., & Stabb, S. D. (1996). Exposure to violence and post-traumatic stress disorder in urban adolescents. *Adolescence, 31,* 489–498.

Bremner, J. D., Southwick, S., Brett, E., Fontana, A., Rosenheck, R., & Charney, D. (1992). Dissociation and posttraumatic stress disorder in Vietnam combat veterans. *American Journal of Psychiatry, 149*(3), 328–332.

Breslau, N. B., & Davis, D. C. (1992). Post-traumatic stress disorder in an urban population of young adults: Risk factors for chronicity. *Archives of General Psychiatry, 149,* 671–675.

Brown, L. S. (1994). *Subversive dialogues: Theory in feminist therapy.* New York: Basic Books.

Caplan, P. J. (1995). *They say you're crazy.* New York: Addison-Wesley.

Carlier, I. V. E., Lamberts, R. D., Fouwels, A. J., & Gersons, B. P. R. (1996). PTSD in relation to dissociation in traumatized police officers. *American Journal of Psychiatry, 153*(10), 1325–1328.

Cloitre, M. (1998). Sexual revictimization: Risk factors and prevention. In V. M. Follette, J. I. Ruzek, & F. R. Abueg (Eds.), *Cognitive-behavioral therapies for trauma* (pp. 278–304). New York: Guilford Press.

DePrince, A. P., & Freyd, J. J. (1999) Dissociation, attention and memory. *Psychological Science, 10,* 449–452.

DePrince, A. P., & Freyd, J. J. (2001). Memory and dissociative tendencies: The roles of attentional context and word meaning in a directed forgetting task. *Journal of Trauma and Dissociation, 2,* 67–82.

Dhaliwal, G. K., Gauzas, L., Antonowicz, D. H., & Ross, R. R. (1996). Adult male survivors of childhood sexual abuse: Prevalence, sexual abuse characteristics, and long-term effects. *Clinical Psychology Review, 16,* 619–639.

Elliott, D. M. (1997). Traumatic events: Prevalence and delayed recall in the general population. *Journal of Consulting and Clinical Psychology, 65,* 811–820.

Elliott, D. M., & Briere, J. (1995). Posttraumatic stress associated with delayed recall of sexual abuse: A general population study. *Journal of Traumatic Stress, 8,* 629–647.

Feldman-Summers, S., & Pope, K. S. (1994). The experience of "forgetting" childhood abuse: A national survey of psychologists. *Journal of Consulting and Clinical Psychology, 62,* 636–639.

Finkelhor, D. (1979). *Sexually victimized children.* New York: Free Press.

Finkelhor, D. (Ed.), (1986). *A sourcebook on child sexual abuse.* Beverly Hills, CA: Sage.

Freyd, J. J. (1996). *Betrayal trauma: The logic behind forgetting childhood abuse.* Cambridge, MA: Harvard University Press.

Freyd, J. J. (2001). Memory and dimensions of trauma: Terror may be "all-too-well" remembered and betrayal buried. In J. R. Conte (Ed.), *Critical issues in child sexual abuse: Historical, legal, and psychological perspectives* (pp. 139–173). Thousand Oaks, CA: Sage.

Freyd, J. J., DePrince, A. P., & Zurbriggen, E. L. (2001). Self-reported memory for abuse depends upon victim–perpetrator relationship. *Journal of Trauma and Dissociation, 2,* 5–16.

Freyd, J. J., Martorella, S. R., Alvarado, J. S., Hayes, A. E., & Christman, J. C. (1998). Cognitive environments and dissociative tendencies: Performance on the standard Stroop task for high versus low dissociators. *Applied Cognitive Psychology, 12,* S91–S103.

Gilligan, C. (1982). *In a different voice.* Cambridge, MA: Harvard University Press.

Gordon, M. (1990). Males and females as victims of childhood sexual abuse: An examination of the gender effect. *Journal of Family Violence, 5,* 321–332.

Herman, J. L. (1992). *Trauma and recovery.* New York: Basic Books.

Herman, J. L., & Schatzow, E. (1987). Recovery and verification of memories of childhood sexual trauma. *Psychoanalytic Psychology, 4,* 1–14.

Kinsey, A. C., Pomeroy, W. B., Martin, C. E., & Gebhard, P. H. (1953). *Sexual behavior in the human female.* Philadelphia: Saunders.

Koss, M. P., Gidycz, C. A., & Wisniewski, N. (1987). The scope of rape: Incidence and prevalence of sexual aggression and victimization in a national sample of higher education students. *Journal of Consulting and Clinical Psychology, 55,* 162–170.

Loftus, E. F., Polonsky, S., & Fullilove, M. T. (1994). Memories of childhood sexual abuse: Remembering and repressing. *Psychology of Women Quarterly, 18,* 67–84.

Marmar, C. R., Weiss, D. S., Schlenger, W. E., Fairbank, J. A., Jordan, B. K., Kulka, R. A., & Hough, R. L. (1994). Peritraumatic dissociation and posttraumatic stress in male Vietnam Theater veterans. *American Journal of Psychiatry, 151*(6), 902–907.

Miller, J. B. (1986). *Toward a new psychology of women* (2nd ed). Boston: Beacon Press.

Rothbaum, B. O., & Foa, E. B. (1996). Cognitive-behavioral therapy for posttraumatic stress disorder. In B. A. van der Kolk, A. C. McFarlane, & L. Weisaeth (Eds.), *Traumatic stress: The effects of overwhelming experience on mind, body, and society* (pp. 491–509). New York: Guilford Press.

Russell, D. E. H. (1986). *The secret trauma: Incest in the lives of girls and women.* New York: Basic Books.

Shay, J. (1994). *Achilles in Vietnam: Combat trauma and the undoing of character.* New York: Touchstone Books.

Southwick, S. M., Krystal, J. H., Johnson, D. R., & Charney, D. S. (1995). Neurobiology of post-traumatic stress disorder. In G. S. Everly & J. M. Lating (Eds.), *Psychotraumatology: Key papers and core concepts in post-traumatic stress* (pp. 49–72). New York: Plenum Press.

Stretch, R. H., Knudson, K. H., & Durand, D. (1998). Effects of premilitary and military trauma on the development of post-traumatic stress disorder symptoms in female and male active duty soldiers. *Military Medicine, 163,* 466–470.

van der Kolk, B. A., & McFarlane, A. C. (1996). The black hole of trauma. In B. A. van der Kolk, A. C. McFarlane, & L. Weisaeth (Eds.), *Traumatic stress: The ef-*

fects of overwhelming experience on mind, body, and society (pp. 3–23). New York: Guilford Press.

Willer, J. K., & Grossman, L. S. (1995). Mental health care needs of female veterans. *Psychiatric Services, 46,* 938–940.

Williams, J. M. G., Mathews, A., & MacLeod, C. (1996). The emotional Stroop task and psychopathology. *Psychological Bulletin, 120,* 3–24.

Williams, L. M. (1994). Recall of childhood trauma: A prospective study of women's memories of child sexual abuse. *Journal of Consulting and Clinical Psychology, 62,* 1182–1186.

Wolfe, J., & Kimerling, R. (1997). Gender issues in the assessment of posttraumatic stress disorder. In J. P. Wilson & T. M. Keane (Eds.), *Assessing psychological trauma and PTSD* (pp. 192–238). New York: Guilford Press.

Part II | Assessment and Diagnosis

5 | Differential Diagnosis of PTSD in Women

MARYLENE CLOITRE
KARESTAN C. KOENEN
KIM L. GRATZ
MATTHEW JAKUPCAK

The introduction of posttraumatic stress disorder (PTSD) into the psychiatric diagnostic system (DSM) in 1983 was the result of the political efforts of Vietnam veterans and the mental health workers and public policy advocates who worked with them. Thus, it is fair to say that PTSD began as a disorder belonging to men. This may have been fortunate, because the notion that environmental events could cause severe psychological problems was historically not well accepted by psychiatry or by American culture more generally. The recognition of the psychological impact of combat on men was successful in part because of the long-standing respect and appreciation for men who went to battle, in confluence with deep trepidation about the appropriateness of the Vietnam war. The recognition of PTSD as a bona fide psychiatric diagnosis might not have been so successful had it initially been framed around women and their most common traumas, such as rape and childhood sexual abuse. Nevertheless, research beginning in the mid-1980s indicated that sexually assaulted women developed symptoms identical to those of men who had been in combat. Later, the same symptoms were recognized among women survivors of childhood sexual abuse. Thus, the recognition of sexual assault and childhood abuse as traumatic events was derived by working backwards from the symptoms exhibited by the women to the events that precipitated the symptoms. PTSD became a diagnosis that was applied to women, and rape and childhood sexual abuse were recognized as traumatic events.

Investigations into the differential diagnosis of PTSD may continue to reflect gender biases, including the tendency to overlook the traumatic nature of the interpersonal violence that is typically the domain of women and, consequently, to overlook the PTSD symptoms associated with these events. This limitation in assessment may lead to the "overpathologizing" of women. For example, two reports, one with an inpatient sample (Elliot, 1995), and the other with an outpatient sample of women with history of trauma (Cloitre, 1998), indicated that when the potential diagnosis of PTSD was ignored, women were reported to have on average four Axis I diagnoses. The presence of multiple diagnoses is counterproductive and would likely interfere with the formulation of an effective treatment plan. For each disorder, there is often a specific treatment approach and pharmacological regimen. The clinician may not know which to choose or may simply select one or a subset of treatment interventions that best approximates a match to the individual's complaints. Nevertheless, the treatment cannot be comprehensive or tailored to the specific constellation of symptoms generated by trauma. As a consequence, the individual may fail to get appropriate treatment and may be perceived as failing to respond to the given treatment. The identification of the PTSD diagnosis is especially significant in that empirically supported treatments have been developed for rape victims with PTSD (Foa et al., 1991; Resick & Schnicke, 1992) and childhood abuse survivors (Chard, 2000; McDonough-Coyle et al., 2000), including those with PTSD and the associated affect dysregulation and interpersonal disturbances described within complex PTSD (see Cloitre, Konen, Cohen, & Han, 2002).

Many of the symptoms of PTSD overlap with those of other anxiety and mood disorders. In addition, the diagnosis of PTSD, like many other Axis I diagnoses, has been frequently contrasted with more enduring character traits reflected in the Axis II personality disorders. In PTSD samples, the comingling of state- and trait-like characteristics among trauma survivors who have experienced chronic and sustained traumas (e.g., childhood abuse, prisoner of war, domestic violence) have been frequently noted. Interestingly, the extant data that indicate problematic Axis I differential diagnoses have been considered and more frequently studied in male samples. In contrast, concern about problematic differential diagnoses spanning Axis I and Axis II features have been directed primarily at female trauma survivors. This may be because the types of traumas that impact personality formation are those that occur during the developmental years of childhood. And the most common childhood traumas, physical and sexual abuse, occur much more frequently among women than men (Kessler, Sonnega, Bromet, Hughes, & Nelson, 1995). Thus, there is currently an obvious gender difference in the attention allocated to specific types of differential diagnostic problems in which Axis I issues have been investigated much more frequently in male samples and Axis II issues have been more frequently considered among female trauma survivors. Cusack, Falsetti, and de Arellano (Chapter 6, this volume) suggest that there is much to be learned by exploring both types of diagnostic conundrums across the sexes.

One of the critical issues underlying problems of differential diagnosis is suspicions about or challenges to the validity and utility of the diagnosis. These concerns are not addressed in this chapter, but they are addressed elsewhere (King, Orcutt, & King, Chapter 15, this volume). While many studies have touched on the topic of problematic differential diagnoses (usually as part of the discussion section), few studies have directly focused on this issue. Fewer still discuss potential gender differences. The specific aims of this chapter are to review data that advance our understanding of the influence of gender on PTSD differential diagnosis among women, to provide practical guidelines for clinicians involved in assessing female trauma clients, and to identify fruitful directions for future research. We specifically address the issue of gender and differential diagnosis between PTSD and other Axis I disorders by considering (1) the presence and character of a traumatic stressor, (2) the ability of clinicians to discriminate between PTSD and other Axis I disorders, (3) evidence for the conceptual independence of PTSD and frequent comorbidities, and (4) the impact of PTSD compared to other disorders on functional impairment. The differential diagnosis of PTSD and the Axis II disorders also receive significant attention, including gender differences in Axis II patterns, treatment implications related to gender and Axis II diagnoses, and the relationship of complex PTSD to both PTSD and Axis II disorders.

THE NATURE OF THE TRAUMATIC STRESSOR: CRITERION A ISSUES

Gender issues in differential diagnosis also begin with the definition of the Criterion A stressor. The first challenge in the assessment of PTSD involves determining whether the specific event in an individual reports meets the definition required for a Criterion A stressor. Added to this challenge is the fact that the definition of Criterion A has changed from focusing on the type of event and its relative frequency in the general population ("an event outside the range of normal human experience") in DSM-III-R to the subjective impact of the event ("fear, helplessness, or horror") in DSM-IV. Intense debate exists about whether only certain agreed-upon event types (e.g., rape, combat) should be classified as Criterion A, or whether the definition of traumatic events should be expanded to include anything the individual defines as traumatic.

Epidemiological studies have shown that women in the general population have approximately twice the prevalence of PTSD compared to males, whereas prevalence of women's traumatic exposure is similar to or lower than that of men (see Norris et al., Chapter 1, this volume). However, the notion that female gender is a risk factor for PTSD must be critically examined (Saxe & Wolfe, 1999). It is possible that gender role socialization may impact the individual's understanding of symptoms associated with a traumatic event and/or the willingness to report traumas (Wolfe & Kimerling, 1997). Furthermore, women and men are exposed to different types of traumatic events. A gender-sensitive diagnosis of PTSD must include assessment of exposure to the full range of Criterion A events, including gender-specific events, such as miscarriage or breast cancer, that might be associated with increased risk of developing PTSD, and consideration of the social and cultural context in which the symptoms related to stress and trauma are experienced (e.g., Andrykowski, Cordova, Studts, & Miller, 1998). A review of the theoretical literature on gender differences and PTSD posits several event characteristics that might be important for gender differences in differential diagnosis. Two event characteristics are of particular importance: chronicity and attachment (Wolfe & Kimerling, 1997). Certain types of assaultive violent events (e.g., sexual abuse, domestic violence) in particular are more likely to occur in the context of an ongoing relationship and are therefore more likely to be experienced repeatedly. The impact of ongoing, repeated traumatic exposure such as that occurring in the context of domestic violence or a prisoner of war experience may have different consequences in terms of symptomatology than single-incident traumatic exposure. In particular, chronicity of the event is important to consider in the differential diagnosis of PTSD versus personality disorders and complex PTSD, an issue we return to later in the chapter (Herman, 1992).

Although the impact of traumatic events has most often been viewed in the context of life threat, its effect on interpersonal relationship may also be important in terms of likelihood of developing PTSD. Attachment theorists regard the human being's connection with others as a fundamental human need, much on the same level with food, shelter, and clothing. Attachment to others is viewed as having a biological component that is adaptive in self-preservation and in keeping young from harm (Bowlby, 1969). The role of attachment in goals and self-concept may, however, be different for men and women (Chodorow, 1978). Feminist relational theory posits that relationships have a special status for women, and that women's sense of self is organized around their ability to create and maintain relationships (Miller, 1986, p. 597). This view asserts that although relationships are important to men, men's sense of self is not as importantly defined by relationships, but rather by societal and cultural prescriptions of masculinity (Pleck, 1981, 1995). Empirical research designed to test this theory has found that men and women have different approaches to making moral judgments, with women's judgments prioritizing the preservation of relationships and men's, abstract moral principles such as justice (Gilligan,

1982). Moreover, females are more empathetic than males (Eisenberg & Lennon, 1983) and more tuned in to others' emotional states (Hall, 1978). From this perspective, women may be more vulnerable to developing PTSD following assaultive violence events because of these events' impact on the relationships that are closely tied to women's sense of self (Saxe & Wolfe, 1999). This may be particularly true in a woman's relationship with someone she trusted; in this situation, she may, in an attempt to preserve the relationship, blame herself for the violence that occurred. Alternatively, men's experience of the traditional male gender norm has been found to be related to less social support and expression of emotions (Saurer & Eisler, 1990), and a decreased likelihood to seek out help (Good, Dell, & Mintz, 1989). For men, the stress of experiencing trauma might be made more difficult by social standards that discourage help seeking and instead promote a prototypically masculine stoicism (i.e., emotional suppression).

In order understand why risk of developing PTSD appears to differ by gender even within specific types of events such as assaultive violence, future studies in this area should gather more detailed information about specific events and event characteristics associated with increased risk of developing PTSD. Studies of event characteristics and major depression have produced fruitful results (e.g., Kessler, 1991). A better understanding of the event characteristics associated with developing PTSD might provide some insight into gender differences in PTSD prevalence and/or presentation. Clinical assessments of PTSD need to be sensitive to evaluating not only the event types (e.g., rape, combat) associated with developing PTSD but also the event characteristics (e.g., perceived life threat, chronicity) that might provide information about the nature and the course of the disorder. For example, perceived life threat might strongly predict onset of PTSD following sexual assault in both men and women, but the course of the disorder in women might be influenced by whether the rape was committed by a stranger or an acquaintance, and how this factor affects current relationships. Finally, further research is needed to determine if certain gender-specific events, such as miscarriage, are associated with increased risk of developing PTSD.

DIFFERENTIAL DIAGNOSIS OF PTSD
AND OTHER AXIS I DISORDERS

A central concern in the diagnosis of PTSD is the apparent overlap of many of the diagnostic criteria with the other anxiety and mood disorders. Many symptoms of PTSD are similar to other anxiety disorders, such as intrusive thoughts (obsessive–compulsive disorder), physiological reactivity to specific stimuli (simple phobia), avoidance of people (social phobia), and irritability and hyperarousal (generalized anxiety disorder). In addition, 3 of the 17 PTSD symptoms overlap with major depressive disorder: sleep disturbance, problems with concentration, and loss of interest in previously enjoyed activity. These observations suggest that there might be significant difficulty in reliably making PTSD diagnoses.

In order to examine this issue, we reviewed literature on the discriminability between the PTSD symptom constellation and that of other disorders. First, we were uncertain whether the discriminability of the PTSD symptom constellation would be similar across the genders. Second, we wished to investigate whether rates of comorbidity were differentially high in women, and whether different patterns of comorbidity would occur by gender. Specifically, we were concerned that certain disorders strongly identified with women, such as panic disorder and depression, might be overdiagnosed, while a possible diagnosis of PTSD and perhaps even a trauma history might be overlooked. Finally, we assessed the presence of the cumulative burden of PTSD and other diagnoses. Looking at cumulative burden of functioning is an indirect empirical test of the presence of multiple disorders: One disorder should bring about a certain level of impairment (e.g., major depressive disorder); two disorders, if actually present, should be reflected in greater impairment (e.g., major depressive disorder and PTSD). This analysis allowed us to test the "reality" of PTSD versus other disorders via its impact on life functioning. We considered that PTSD might equally impair both men and women, but perhaps in different spheres of functioning. Furthermore, we were uncertain whether functional impairment in men and women would be similarly impacted by additional comorbidities.

Discriminability of PTSD Symptom Constellation

Whereas some of the symptoms of various disorders overlap in the presentation of the trauma patient, differential diagnosis is possible when all of the symptoms are viewed in unity. First, differential diagnosis hangs on the presence of "hallmark" symptoms of PTSD: symptoms of reexperiencing of the trauma, most dramatically flashbacks; nightmares; and trauma-related intrusive thoughts and images. A diagnosis of PTSD cannot be made without the presence of symptoms that specifically reference the trauma. Second, whereas it is true that a patient typically exhibits symptoms in common with many disorders (e.g., impaired concentration), the expression of such symptoms must be partnered with and fulfill the complete range of symptoms required to meet criteria for the diagnosis of PTSD compared to other disorders. For example, poor concentration can be one symptom of hyperarousal, along with others, such as startle response, suggesting a diagnosis of PTSD; but poor concentration alongside significant weight gain is more suggestive of a diagnosis of major depressive disorder.

The capacity for the full-time clinician involved in the day-to-day diagnosis of trauma patients to differentiate between PTSD symptoms and those of other disorders is an important issue in differential diagnosis. In a study by Keane, Taylor, and Penk (1997), 340 experienced clinicians, psychologists and psychiatrists were asked to rate the extent to which a common set of 90 symptoms distinctly characterized three Axis I disorders: PTSD, major depressive disorder, and generalized anxiety disorder. For the 90 symptoms, clinicians were asked to rate the extent to which each was characteristic of each of the three disorders. Clinicians rated 14 of the items predicted as unique for PTSD (i.e., the DSM-III-R criteria specific to PTSD), including reexperiencing of life-threatening conditions, remaining in a condition of heightened arousal, acting in ways that demonstrate anger and frustration about having experienced life-threatening events, suddenly acting or feeling as if an event were recurring, hypervigilance, difficulty feeling close to someone, and avoiding recollection of life-threatening events. These differences supported the hypothesis that clinicians could differentiate symptoms of PTSD from those of the other two disorders.

These analyses, in conjunction with discriminant function analyses and factor analyses of the ratings, provided more general characteristics that discriminate the three disorders. The data suggested that the PTSD symptom complex, in contrast to that of generalized anxiety disorder, tends to be situation-specific. Whereas PTSD is associated with physiological reactivity to present reminders of past traumatic events, generalized anxiety disorder is associated with reactivity to a wide variety of stimuli. Similarly, avoidance of stimuli in PTSD is associated with the trauma, whereas in generalized anxiety disorder, avoidance, if at all present, tends to be independent of any specific life event. Finally, PTSD is associated with chronic baseline hyperarousal, whereas arousal in generalized anxiety disorder tends to be more variable and to fluctuate with the ebb and flow of periods of worry.

PTSD is distinguished from major depressive disorder in that the symptoms of depression reflect low arousal and low activity across a range of situations and behaviors. This very "slowed down" presentation of the clinically depressed patient is not seen in patients with pure PTSD. Finally, PTSD differs from both generalized anxiety disorder and major depressive disorder in the expression of high level of anger or fears of acting out anger and frustration in response to both traumatic memories and symptoms of posttraumatic stress.

In this study, symptoms were "gender-neutral" in that the clinicians doing the ratings were presented only with symptoms, absent the context of a real or hypothetical case. However, because the questionnaire was circulated to clinicians who worked in the VA system, their reference point, the "prototypical PTSD patient," may have been the male combat veteran, thus potentially limiting the generalizability of results across male and female patients. The authors, in a rather innovative aspect of the study, did explore the influence of the therapist's gender on ratings. "Hit rates" in differentiating PTSD, generalized anxiety disorder, and major depressive disorder were identical, suggesting that gender-influenced perceptions, attitudes, and decision-making processes, to whatever extent they existed, did not alter the clarity with which the three diagnoses were categorized. This finding supports the reliable categorizability of the disorders.

Patterns of Axis I Comorbid Disorders

Thus far, we have argued that PTSD has unique features that discriminate it from other Axis I disorders. Nevertheless, additional considerations come to the fore with the observation of significant comorbidity associated with PTSD. Our review of this literature is limited to issues specific to differential diagnosis; gender issues and comorbidity are covered elsewhere in this volume (see Stuart, Ouimette, & Brown, Chapter 9, and Orsillo, Raja, & Hammond, Chapter 8, this volume) First, it should be noted that the central role of PTSD in posttraumatic sequelae is not in doubt. Studies that have compared trauma populations with and without PTSD have observed that PTSD is not only the most frequently diagnosed disorder but also that it is among those individuals with PTSD that other disorders are diagnosed, suggesting that PTSD is a necessary ingredient in the emergence of multiple diagnoses following a traumatic stressor. It well know that rates of PTSD are twice as high in women as in men. We wished to investigate whether rates of comorbidity were also differentially higher in women, and whether there would be differences in the patterns of comorbidity. These questions obviously have strong bearing on gender-sensitive treatment development plans.

There is, to date, only one community study and no clinical population studies that report rates of comorbidity for both men and women. In a representative national sample of 5,877 persons, Kessler et al. (1995) reported remarkably similar profiles of comorbidity in men and women, although no direct statistical comparisons were available. Major depression was the most frequent comorbid affective disorder (48% for men, and 49% for women), followed by a range of anxiety disorders, with simple phobia, social phobia, and generalized anxiety disorder being the most frequent disorders. It should be noted that the study did not use a hierarchical approach in which symptoms that overlap across diagnoses are attributed to only one predetermined disorder (e.g., PTSD). So, for example, irritability would be classified as contributing to both PTSD and to generalized anxiety disorder. In addition, the authors did not report whether the interviewers queried about overlapping symptoms to determine whether a single diagnosis would be more appropriate than multiple diagnoses. For example, a simple phobic response might be to a stimulus related to a trauma, such as an elevator for a woman raped in that situation, indicating that the symptom should be classified only under the PTSD diagnosis. The absence of a hierarchical approach or detailed queries may inflate the rates of disorders in this community-based PTSD sample. It is unclear whether this approach may also obscure gender differences or differentially inflate rates of disorders.

Studies of clinical populations, all of which have been "same-sex," show a pattern similar to this epidemiological study. Using a hierarchical, in-depth query approach with the Structured Clinical Interview for DSM (SCID), Cloitre et al. (1997) found that women with chronic PTSD related to childhood abuse were most likely to have major depressive disorder (40%) followed by an array of anxiety disorders with simple phobia, generalized anxiety disorder, and social phobia being the most common disorders. Approximately one-third of the women had a lifetime history of substance abuse. This is the only study we know of that reported systematic diagnostic assessment of comorbidities among treatment-seeking women with PTSD. Several studies of male samples are available and indicate a similar pattern of affective and anxiety disorders (see Deering, Glover, Ready, Eddleman, & Alarcon, 1996; Ford, Fisher, & Larson, 1997; Orsillo et al., 1996). One notable difference is the frequent documentation of substance abuse disorders among men, where rates of substance abuse in male, veteran PTSD samples have been reported as high as 91% (Ford et al., 1997) and are typically found above the 50% mark. However, this may be because of sample selection differences, in which many of the male samples have been studied through inpatient and long-term outpatient services reflecting the most seriously impaired of male trauma survivors. In contrast, female trauma survivors have more typically been assessed in traditional community outpatient services or in PTSD treatment research studies, which routinely exclude substance abusers. Thus, the actual rate of PTSD and comorbid substance abuse among women may be underreported. Rates of comorbid PTSD and substance abuse have recently emerged from substance abuse settings, which suggest that from 30 to 59% of women have this dual diagnosis (Najavits, Weiss, & Shaw, 1997).

Although women are diagnosed with PTSD twice as often as men, the rates and pattern of comorbid disorders seem quite similar across the genders. The only observed difference was in the rates of substance abuse. We suspect, however, that the lower rates reported for women may be the result of sampling bias. Future resources should be provided for the assessment and treatment of dually diagnosed female trauma survivors.

The Cumulative Burden of Multiple Diagnoses

PTSD has been strongly associated with decreased well-being, compromised health and quality of life, and poor psychosocial adjustment (Amaya-Jackson et al., 1999; Ferrada-Noli, Asberg, Ormstad, Lundin, & Sundbom, 1998; Kulka et al., 1990; McFarlane, Atchinson, Rafalowicz, & Papay,

1994; Zatzick et al., 1999). If PTSD is a distinct disorder, one test of its independence status would be the presence of increasing functional impairment with additional diagnoses or symptom sets; that is, impairment would be worse among persons with PTSD and some other disorder than those with either disorder alone.

Several completed mixed gender studies have examined relative functional impact of the accumulation of comorbidities. In the mixed gender study of motor vehicle accidents victims (Blanchard, Buckley, Hickling, & Taylor, 1998) mentioned earlier, persons with PTSD and depression suffered more major role impairment (work, school, or homemaking) than those with PTSD alone. Similarly, a prospective study of 211 emergency room trauma victims reported that persons who developed both major depression and PTSD experienced greater distress and dysfunction that those who developed only one or the other disorder (Shalev et al., 1998). Moreover, in a study of 534 adult Bosnia refugees, levels of functional disability were associated with comorbid symptoms of PTSD and depression, and this relationship was independent of physical health status (Mollica et al., 1999). In a recent study of 182 Oklahoma City bombing survivors, comorbidity among persons with PTSD was associated with functional impairment, dissatisfaction with work performance, and relationship problems with significant others, household members, and other relatives or friends. PTSD alone was associated only with functional impairment and relationship problems with other relatives or friends (North et al., 1999). In all of these studies, both men and women were assessed; however, no gender differences related to the relationship between number of diagnoses and functional impairment were reported or appeared to be investigated.

The most impressive study assessing the impact of PTSD and other diagnostic disorders on functional impairment concerned 4,577 members of a primary care health maintenance organization (HMO) (Shoenfeld et al., 1997). The sample size of this investigation is quite large, and gender effects concerning the impact of diagnostic status on functional impairment were conducted for all available anxiety and mood disorder diagnoses. Participants were first assessed for the presence of undetected anxiety or depressive disorders via medical records and screening interview, followed by a face-to-face interview using the Diagnostic Interview Schedule (DIS). A total of 319 men and women were identified as having one or more full-criteria anxiety or depressive disorders. Of those with a disorder, 34% were diagnosed with PTSD, the second most frequent disorder after major depression (50%). Approximately 85% of persons with PTSD had additional diagnoses, suggesting that PTSD most commonly occurs within the context of multiple disorders. PTSD was shown to be a highly impairing disorder, second only to major depression in its impact on an array of areas of functioning as measured by the Short-Form Health Survey (SF-36). As indicated in Table 5.1, PTSD as a single disorder had significant negative effects on

TABLE 5.1. Functioning and Well-Being of 4,577 HMO Patients
with Undetected/Untreated Disorders

| Effects | SF-36 functioning levels | | | | | | | |
	Physical functioning	Social functioning	Role, physical	Role, emotional	Mental health	Vitality	Bodily pain	General health
Generalized anxiety disorder	–13.9	–12.6	–21.1	–28.2	–2.9	–15.8	–12.7	–16.1
PTSD	–7.9	–18.1	–29.2	–42.0	–9.2	–23.1	–13.3	–18.8
Social phobia	–15.0	–5.0	–8.0	–22.0	–10.2	–16.8	–7.9	–12.9
Panic/agoraphobia	–14.2	–10.5	–29.7	–14.7	–16.0	–14.8	–20.1	–14.4
Major depression	–9.4	–23.3	–26.9	–46.6	–27.0	–24.4	–16.2	–22.6

Note. Data from Schoenfeld et al. (1997).

all categories of functioning and produced the second greatest impairment, after depression, on five of eight dimensions of functioning (social, physical, emotional role, and vitality and general health). The level of impairment associated with PTSD was reported as equivalent to that found for the medical diagnoses of diabetes and arthritis. Assessment of the potential interaction between PTSD diagnosis and gender found no differences on functional impairment. This is notable, especially because gender effects were associated with major depression, and, contrary to stereotypical expectations, men were found to be more impaired than women in their emotional and physical role functioning.

There has been at least one study of functional impairment in a female-only sample ($N = 67$) of childhood abuse survivors with PTSD (Han & Cloitre, 2000). PTSD symptoms impacted substantially the women's functional impairment as measured by the self-report version of the Social Adjustment Scale (SAS-SR), accounting for 33% of the impairment variance. However, other symptoms and life problems, specifically, depression, anger, and interpersonal problems, contributed an additional 23% to the explained variance for impairment. Statistical analyses controlling for the influence of each symptom set upon the others indicated that both PTSD and the symptoms of depression, anger, and interpersonal problems made a unique and significant impact on functioning.

These studies, in total, indicate that PTSD is a significantly impairing disorder and that its effects on functioning can be discriminated from those of other comorbidities and symptoms. Furthermore, as far as we can tell, PTSD per se, and as a single disorder, does not differentially impact men and women. However, it is possible that other symptoms associated with PTSD, such as depression, anger, and difficult interpersonal relations, may differentially affect men and women. These later symptoms were found to be powerful influences on impairment among women with a history of childhood abuse. They are also symptoms that are typically associated with childhood abuse survivors and overlap with the diagnosis of "complex PTSD," a characterization that is associated much more often with women than men. Thus a potentially fruitful avenue of research on trauma-related impairment would be to assess potential gender differences not only in regards to PTSD per se, but in relation to associated features of PTSD.

DIFFERENTIAL DIAGNOSIS: AXIS II PERSONALITY DISORDERS

Less research has focused on the differential diagnosis of PTSD and Axis II disorders. Most of the existing research has focused on the relationship between PTSD and antisocial personality disorder (ASPD) in Vietnam veterans (e.g., Keane & Wolfe, 1990; Kulka et al., 1990; Resnick, Foy, Donahue, & Miller, 1989; Sierles et al., 1983) and borderline personality disorder (BPD) among women with childhood sexual and/or physical abuse (e.g., Brodsky, Cloitre, & Dulit, 1995; Heffernan & Cloitre, 2000; Herman, Perry, & van der Kolk, 1989; Lubin & Johnson, 1997, Shearer, Peter, Quaytman, & Ogden, 1990; Weaver & Clum, 1993; Zanarini, 1997). The focus of this research has led to the assumption that specific personality disorders are associated with each gender following trauma. However, it is notable that this first wave of research confounds gender with type of trauma, so that it is entirely unclear whether the nature of the trauma (combat or childhood abuse) or gender generates the observed differences.

Given the assumptions and biases regarding gender differences in characterological disorders, we wished to investigate more closely whether the gender stereotype that associates ASPD with traumatized men and BPD with traumatized women was empirically supported. As is typical of new research areas, there are relatively few studies concerning trauma and personality disorders and even fewer in which gender is taken into consideration. Thus, generalizations derived from the results of these studies need to be considered with caution, due to methodological limitations such as absence of reliable measures, the evaluation of one or a few personality disorders rather than the full spectrum of Axis II diagnoses, the conflation of different traumatic events, and sample selection bias (prisons, clinical settings, VA settings).

Evidence of Trauma-Specific Influences in Personality Formation

In one of the most methodologically rigorous studies to date, the relationship between documented childhood maltreatment (physical and sexual abuse, neglect) and personality disorders in young adulthood was assessed in a representative sample of 639 children followed prospectively over 20 years (Johnson, Cohen, Brown, Smailes, & Bernstein, 1999). A history of maltreatment was strongly associated with personality disorders. Nearly 50% (46.3%) of persons who experienced some type of maltreatment as children had personality disorders compared to 11.2% of those without any maltreatment. No gender differences were found in the overall prevalence of personality disorders. Different types of maltreatment were associated with different personality disorders. Physical abuse was most frequently associated with paranoid personality disorder, followed by depressive and ASPD. The risk ratios (RRs) of developing each of these disorders among those with and without physical abuse compared to those with neglect were, respectively, 12.81, 7.26, and 10.09. Sexual abuse was most commonly associated with BPD (RR = 12.5), avoidant personality disorder (RR = 9.5) and ASPD (RR = 8.0). Neglect, in contrast, was most highly associated with narcissistic (RR = 30.33), paranoid (RR = 12.81), borderline (RR = 15.00), and depressive (RR = 9.10) personality disorders. Unfortunately, the authors did not examine whether these associations were constant across genders. However, these study data suggest that several personality disorders other than BPD and ASPD are highly overrepresented among those with childhood traumas.

This study does not exclude the possibility that ASPD is most commonly associated with abused males, while BPD is associated with abused females. ASPD was most highly associated with physical abuse; there is a known preponderance of males in physical abuse populations and, conversely, BPD was most highly associated with sexual abuse, from which girls suffer disproportionately. Thus, it is not possible to determine whether these personality disorders are more trauma- or gender-influenced. It is becoming clear, however, that both the nature of the trauma and the gender of the victim influence outcome and that some "crossover" breaks the stereotypes of gender-based personality disorders.

Evidence of Gender "Crossover" in Personality Disorder Diagnoses

Antisocial Personality Disorder in Traumatized Women

There is evidence in at least one study that the relative risk of developing ASPD is the same for women and men when the baseline comparison is to the same gender and the same type of trauma. In a prevalence study of ASPD among young adults abused and/or neglected as children (N = 416), 20.3% of boys compared to 5.3% of girls were diagnosed with ASPD (Luntz & Widom, 1994). Nevertheless, the abused girls' rate of ASPD was significantly higher than that of the female nonabused comparison group

(2.6%). The rate of ASPD among abused girls was twice that of nonabused girls, a proportion identical to that between abused and nonabused boys (20.3% and 10.1%, respectively).

Borderline Personality Disorder in Male PTSD Samples

Among PTSD combat veterans diagnosed with PTSD, BPD has frequently but not always been found to occur at high rates. In one study of treatment-seeking combat veterans with PTSD, study participants ($N = 34$) were assessed for the full range of Axis II disorders using the Personality Disorder Examination (PDE). BPD was the most frequent personality disorder (76%), followed by obsessive–compulsive (44%), avoidant (41%), and paranoid (38%) personality disorders (Southwick, Yehuda, & Giller, 1993). In contrast, in a study of a similar population of inpatient veterans in a specialized PTSD unit ($N = 107$), BPD was the least frequently occurring disorder (5.7%), while the most common disorders (in order of prevalence) were avoidant, paranoid, obsessive–compulsive, and ASPD (Bollinger, Riggs, Blake, & Ruzek, 2000). The discrepancy between these two studies may be related to differences in the presence of childhood abuse trauma. Combat veterans with PTSD are known to have high rates of childhood abuse (Bremner, Southwick, Johnson, Yehuda, & Charney, 1993), a type of trauma with which BPD is commonly associated. Because neither studies provided information about rates of childhood abuse, it is not possible to know whether the BPD was related to combat or to early childhood trauma. However, we can speculate that one reason for the discrepant rates of BPD may be related to unidentified and differing rates of childhood abuse in each of these samples.

Borderline Personality Disorder in Traumatized Men

The presence of BPD and borderline symptoms have been regularly identified in male trauma samples in clinical and community settings. Miller and Lisak (1999) found that BPD symptoms, as measured by a self-report instrument, the Personality Diagnostic Questionnaire—Revised (PDQ-R), were the only set of personality symptoms for each category of abuse (sexual, physical, or both) that distinguished college men with a history of abuse from those never abused.

Recent research on male batterers, who often have a history of childhood abuse, has suggested two distinct subtypes of batterers, one that fits the ASPD profile and the other more similar to a BPD profile (Dutton, 1998; Dutton & Golant, 1995). Both subtypes use physical violence to control their partner. However, the emotional profile and dynamics of the relationship are quite distinct. Type I batterers have ASPD features and show no remorse for their violence, are emotionally detached from their partners, and tend to use violence across situations, not just within interpersonal re-lationships. While the Type I batterer appears to become highly agitated and hostile during confrontation, his heart rate actually decreases, a psychophysiological characteristic found in sociopaths (see Gottman et al., 1995; Jacobson & Gottman, 1998).

In contrast, Type II batterers demonstrate physiological and personal-ity traits more consistent with features of BPD. They show physiological patterns of arousal and agitation, and may fear the loss of emotional con-trol as their physical arousal levels increase (Gottman et al., 1995). Type II batterers are often extremely jealous and concerned that their partner might leave the relationship. These individuals are highly insecure regard-ing their partner's loyalty. The violence appears to be restricted to interper-sonal and intimate adult relationships in which they can assert dominance (physically) and gain control through the use of intimidation. These studies suggest that the aggression and violence that can be instrumental strategies employed by men with BPD are behaviorally distinct from strategies ob-served in women with BPD but reflect the same emotional disturbances and motivation, such as emotional volatility and the desire to control and/or manipulate relationship outcomes.

Salience of Borderline Personality Disorder in Both Male and Female Trauma Samples

In the only study known to make a direct comparison of male and female trauma survivors with PTSD on personality features, Shea, Zlotnick, and Weisberg (1999) used the Personality Disorders Questionnaire—Revised (PDQ-R) in three clinical populations: combat veterans in a VA outpatient services ($N = 92$), outpatient female sexual abuse survivors ($N = 57$), and inpatient female sexual abuse survivors ($N = 83$). BPD was the second most common personality disorder across both male and female populations, with 83% of combat veterans, 53% of female childhood sexual abuse out-patients, and 92% of female childhood abuse inpatients diagnosed with the disorder. The most common personality disorder for all three groups was the same: paranoid personality disorder (89%, 83%, and 83%, respec-tively). The third most common disorder was avoidant personality disorder (50%, 63%, and 62%, respectively). These data suggest the salience of BPD in both male and female PTSD samples.

Similarities and Differences in Borderline Personality Disorder and Antisocial Personality Disorder Diagnoses

It is notable that ASPD and BPD have overlapping dimensions. For example, both disorders are characterized by impulsivity, high-risk behaviors, the ap-pearance of manipulative interpersonal traits, self-harm, and emotional dysregulation. However, these common traits may be expressed and/or interpreted within gender-associated roles, with men more often exhibiting aggressive, outwardly directed behaviors and women, internalized or self-destructive patterns of behavior (Paris, 1997). From a functional perspective, these behaviors might be interpreted as behavioral adaptations to common stressors (lack of stable family environments, neglect, and/or maltreatment) that interact with contextual demands (culturally determined gender roles) to produce overlapping but slightly disparate behaviors.

Social Influences on the Expression of Trauma-Related Personality Features

These studies suggest that trauma leads to similar emotional disturbances and needs among men and women, but that the expression of these needs has gender-specific aspects. We note very briefly the large literature suggesting that boys and girls are socialized to express their emotions quite differently. For example, a study of school-age children found that more boys expected their parents to react negatively to demonstrations of sadness, whereas more girls expected positive reactions (Fuchs & Thelen, 1988). Zeman and Garber (1996) found that children reported controlling their expressions of emotions in the presence of peers, in part due to their expectations of negative social interactions with peers following disclosure. Specifically, girls were significantly more likely than boys to expect others to be accepting and understanding of their emotional displays. Boys were significantly more likely than girls to use aggression to express both anger and sadness. These studies might suggest that males and females learn to express emotions in ways that are consistent with gender differences in the prevalence of personality disorders (i.e., BPD and ASPD). Females might be more likely to use emotion-focused coping strategies and to expect positive outcomes from expressions of emotions, whereas males might be more likely to utilize instrumental, action-based forms of coping and to have learned to exhibit aggression in response to their negative emotion states. (Folkman & Lazarus, 1980).

Social Influences on the Characterization of Trauma-Related Personality Features: Clinician Biases

Clinicians are not immune to the gender stereotyping, and appear to attend selectively to symptoms consistent with gender expectations and stereotypes. Becker and Lamb (1994) investigated gender biases in clinician's diagnoses of PTSD and personality disorders. Identical case study descriptions were sent to a clinician population of male and female social workers, psychiatrists, and psychologists ($N = 1,080$). Each case study was designed to describe both a childhood abuse history and symptoms equally representative of BPD and PTSD; the descriptions varied in the differential use of gendered pronouns. Clinicians were asked to rate the extent to which the client appeared to have each of the seven Axis I and seven Axis II diagnoses according to DSM-III-R criteria. Results indicated that, overall, BPD was the most commonly rated diagnosis given, followed by dysthymia, self-defeating personality disorder, and PTSD. However, cases described as "male" clients were significantly more likely to be diagnosed with ASPD, while "female" clients were significantly more likely to be diagnoses as having both BPD and histrionic personality disorder.

Summary

The unusually high rates of personality disorders cited in these trauma and PTSD populations should be considered with caution. First, some of the studies used the PDQ-R, a self-report measure that tends to overdiagnose personality disorders in both clinical and community samples (see Miller & Lisak, 1999). Second, the clinical studies include inpatient samples, which may represent only the most severely and chronically symptomatic trauma survivors or those currently in an acute state of disturbance. Nevertheless, the overall uniformity of the presence of borderline, avoidant, ASPD, and paranoid personality disorder symptoms among trauma survivors with and without PTSD is striking and cannot be explained away by overdiagnosis or acuity/chronicity of illness. In complementary fashion, certain disorders do not seem highly associated with trauma in either male or female samples, including dependent, histrionic, and schizoid personality disorders.

The results also suggest greater diversity or gender crossover in the BPD and ASPD disorders than has been assumed. Particularly, there is evidence that BPD is salient in both male and female samples that have experienced childhood abuse. We also suggested that BPD and ASPD reflect the same core set of emotional disturbances and differ primarily on gender-related behavioral expressions of these disturbances. The studies, despite some mixed findings and occasionally flawed methodology, suggest that clinicians might benefit from being alert to their own assumptions regarding female- and male-associated presentations of personality disorders.

PERSONALITY DISORDERS AS VARIANTS OF PTSD

There has been a long-standing discussion in the literature that BPD is actually a form of chronic PTSD (Herman, 1992). The focus on the BPD–PTSD relationship as opposed to other personality disorders may derive from the belief that BPD is the most common comorbid Axis II disorder, and that the symptoms of BPD, such as suicidal gestures, self-mutilations, and impulsive behaviors, swiftly capture the concern of clinicians. Nevertheless, as noted earlier, other personality disorders frequently co-occur with PTSD and may be subjected to the same consideration: Are they different from PTSD or are they variants? As others have noted, there is significant overlap between the symptoms of PTSD and commonly associated personality disorder (see Shea et al., 1999; Southwick et al., 1993). BPD criteria that overlap with PTSD include persistent disturbances with affect regulation (particularly anger), dissociative experiences, and identity disturbances. Feelings of alienation and social withdrawal are symptoms shared by PTSD and avoidant disorder. All of these symptoms can be understood in the context of a trauma history or, more specifically, as an adaptation to the environment posttrauma. For example, hypervigilance and or avoidance can be viewed as strategies for protecting oneself against potential dangers in the environment.

Evidence for the Distinction between PTSD and Personality Disorders

How, then, can one assess whether PTSD is distinct from these personality disorders, and might we expect to find gender differences in this process? First, it should be noted that almost all evidence of Axis II comorbidity is based on research with individuals with chronic PTSD related to sustained trauma (e.g., combat veterans, childhood abuse survivors). High rates of Axis II comorbidity have not been reported with PTSD when it is the result of other types of trauma, such as adult-onset rapes or physical assaults (Feeney, Zoellner, & Foa, 1999), suggesting that PTSD can stand alone. Further research comparing rates of Axis II comorbidity with PTSD emanating from different types of trauma is necessary.

Second, Axis II comorbidities, although appearing at high rates among men and women with chronic PTSD, are not entirely overlapping, suggesting that PTSD and personality disorders are distinct. For example, in PTSD outpatient sample studies, rates of BPD are as low as 17% and as high as 37% among women with PTSD, suggesting that PTSD frequently presents independently of BPD, and that their co-occurrence is representative of a subset of individuals, even among those chronically traumatized. Similarly, whereas the co-occurrence of ASPD is higher among individuals with PTSD than controls, the overlap not entirely identical (Gibson et al., 1999).

Third, careful assessment of the frequency, severity, and symptom patterns of PTSD with and without personality disorders can determine whether there are significant differences in the clinical presentation of Axis II comorbid PTSD. An assessment of the etiological and clinical features of women with PTSD related to childhood sexual abuse ($N = 45$) compared to women with both PTSD and BPD ($N = 26$) identified several historical and clinical differences (Heffernan & Cloitre, 2000). Those with BPD reported earlier onset of childhood sexual abuse (6.0 [$SD = 2.2$] years vs. 4.6 [$SD =$

1.8] years). They also reported the additional presence of maternal abuse and were much more likely to have experienced not only sexual abuse (most typically by the father) but also physical abuse and severe verbal abuse by the mother. Maternal verbal abuse was a particularly salient differential feature between the two groups. Women with PTSD and BPD reported verbal abuse by the mother six times more often than those with PTSD alone. These findings suggest that the additional diagnosis of BPD may be related to a more specific influence on the child's experience, namely, disruptions in attachment with a primary caregiver, the mother.

Interestingly, PTSD characterization was not affected by the presence of BPD. Total PTSD scores, as measured by the PTSD Symptom Scale— Self-Report (PSS-SR), as well as the severity and frequency of symptoms within each of the three symptom clusters (intrusion, avoidance, and arousal) did not differ between the two groups. This finding was recently replicated in a study by Feeny and colleagues (1999). The fact that BPD did not diminish, enhance, or in any way alter the PTSD presentation suggests that BPD and PTSD are independent diagnostic constructs. The women with BPD did, however, show elevations in four specific clinical measures: anger, anxiety, dissociation, and interpersonal problems. A simultaneous regression analysis in which these symptoms were forced to compete with each other revealed that increased anger was the only variable that uniquely differentiated between women with PTSD and BPD and women with PTSD alone. This suggests the key role of anger in the characterization of women dually diagnosed with PTSD and BPD.

No studies of which we are aware compare males with PTSD to males with comorbid PTSD–BPD. As mentioned earlier, males suffering from PTSD might be more likely to be diagnosed with ASPD, whereas their females counterparts are diagnosed with BPD, reflective of the gender biases in diagnosing ASPD (Becker & Lamb, 1994). However, researchers have indicated ways in which ASPD and PTSD can be differentiated, arguing that ASPD symptoms are developmentally and/or biologically determined. Bailey (1985) suggests that in working with veterans, an examination of the individual's premilitary history is important in differentiating PTSD from ASPD. Poorly defined values, truancy, and a history of institutionalization are more likely in individuals with ASPD. The presence of survivor's guilt or guilt for acts of violence is often-associated with PTSD but not present in the pure form of ASPD (Bailey, 1985). Additionally, recent studies have suggested a state of hypoarousal in cases of "pure" ASPD (e.g., Raine, Lencz, Bihrle, LaCasse, & Colletti, 2000) that contrasts with PTSD, in which presentations of hyperarousal such as exaggerated startle responses and physiological reactivity to cues are commonly found. Individuals without strong physiological arousal may actually seek out stimulation from their environment, whereas those with PTSD learn to be highly avoidant of cues that lead to reactivity.

Evidence for Distinctiveness of PTSD and Personality Disorders: Impact on Treatment

One way to determine whether personality disorders are substantially distinct from PTSD is to assess whether their presence has any impact on treatment outcome. Two PTSD treatment studies have assessed the impact of BPD on outcome: one a group modality, the other an individual treatment. Both studies included only female clients; therefore, we do not know whether the results will generalize to males with Axis II comorbid PTSD. The group treatment study used a Yalom process-oriented approach (Cloitre & Koenen, 2001) and assessed three treatment conditions: women in groups where no member had BPD (N = 18), women in groups where at least one member had BPD (N = 18), and a wait-list comparison group (N = 16). The BPD– groups showed significant improvement in PTSD and related symptoms. In contrast, the BPD+ group showed no improvement in PTSD symptoms (similar to the wait-list condition) and actual deterioration as measured by increasing problems with anger expression and interpersonal problems of control and assertiveness. Interestingly, the deterioration in the BPD+ groups was not confined to those with the BPD diagnosis; rather, all of the women in groups with BPD+ members reported more anger at the end of group than at the start of treatment. The latter findings suggest the presence of a "contagion" effect in the BPD+ groups, in which those without BPD assimilated and experienced in similar fashion the anger frequently expressed by the BPD+ women. We speculate that the women without BPD, while not as expressly angry as the BPD+ women, had significant covert anger that, once elicited, was not well managed due to relatively limited affect management and other coping skills. These data suggest that dually diagnosed PTSD patients may need to be treated separately from those with PTSD alone, or that different group treatment modalities emphasize structure and affect containment (see Lubin & Johnson, 1997; Zlotnick et al., 1997) may be more appropriate for combined PTSD–BPD groups. These data also suggest the value of individual psychotherapy in which treatment can be shaped to match the needs of the PTSD patient, taking into account level of symptom severity and available coping skills.

Nevertheless, PTSD treatment outcome differences between BPD+ and BPD– clients continue to be found even in individual psychotherapy formats. Feeney et al. (1999) assessed the presence and role of BPD in the outcome of a study of 72 women with rape-related PTSD in four different treatment conditions: prolonged exposure (PE), stress innoculation training (SIT), their combination (SIT/PE), and wait-list control (WL) . Outcome results for the women involved in the three active treatment conditions (N = 58) indicated that both the BPD+ women (N = 9) and the BPD– women (N = 49) received benefits from the treatment; however, the treatment benefits for the BPD+ women ranged from somewhat to significantly attenuated.

For example, whereas PTSD symptoms per se were significantly improved in both groups of women, other measures, particularly end-state functioning (a combination of PTSD, anxiety, and depressions symptoms), showed good end-state functioning in only 8% of women with BPD+ compared to 42% of BPD– women. This difference became more pronounced at 3-month follow-up, suggesting that the BPD+ population had greater difficulty maintaining or building upon their posttreatment gains.

The results of these two treatment studies suggest that the presence of an Axis II disorder creates additional burden in the treatment of the PTSD population, as reflected in differential (poorer) outcome. From a treatment development perspective, the results suggest that individuals with PTSD comorbid with BPD can effectively use established treatments for the resolution of PTSD symptoms, but that additional treatment interventions or strategies may be needed to address the many other symptoms that do not seem to resolve in the current PTSD-focused treatments.

Again, it is notable that the studies described here refer only to female populations, and only to those with the combined PTSD–BPD presentation. This may be because men come to treatment less frequently and among those who come to treatment for trauma-related problems, those most frequently studied have been combat veterans treated in VA settings. In these settings, the comorbid disorders most frequently gaining the attention of clinicians and provoking need for expansion of PTSD-focused treatment are the substance and alcohol abuse disorders. For example, a major study on the predictors of treatment outcome among combat veterans focused on 74 men who had completed treatment an inpatient residential rehabilitation program (Ford et al., 1997). Of the entire sample, 91% had a lifetime history of substance or alcohol abuse. Given the overwhelming presence of this comorbidity, it is not surprising that treatment was built around a multimodal rehabiliation model that included the "sobriety lifestyle" and other core areas of PTSD rehabilitation, including sleep hygiene, reentry to work or school, and relapse prevention.

DIFFERENTIAL DIAGNOSIS: COMPLEX PTSD

Despite its name, complex PTSD is actually quite distinct from PTSD and much more similar to the other personality disorders mentioned here, including BPD, avoidant, and paranoid personality disorder. Complex PTSD does not include any of the reexperiencing symptoms that are the hallmark of PTSD, nor is there emphasis on avoidant or hyperarousal symptoms. Rather, complex PTSD was developed to capture symptoms other than those included in criteria for PTSD. In addition, complex PTSD is associated specifically with a traumatic stressor of a prolonged and chronic nature, rather than a single incident or brief traumas, and is represented by traumas of human design (i.e., interpersonal), such as childhood abuse, prisoner of war or concentration camp, or domestic violence. It is more like BPD than all the other personality disorders in its emphasis on symptoms such as impulsivity, aggression, self-destructive behaviors and suicidal gestures (alterations in regulation of affect), transient dissociative episodes, and depersonalization that are independent of and distinct from flashbacks (alterations in consciousness) and difficulties in maintaining relationships (alterations in relationships). Feelings of alienation, inability to trust others, and general suspicion are all symptoms of complex PTSD that overlap with the avoidant and paranoid disorders.

Nevertheless, complex PTSD is distinguished, by definition, from all of the other personality disorders by virtue of emanating from a severe traumatic stressor. Complex PTSD symptoms, including characterological symptoms, reflect changes in functioning following traumatic exposure and need to be assessed in comparison to personality structure and symptoms prior to exposure (Jongedijk, Carlier, Schreuder, & Gersons, 1996). Additionally, complex PTSD, like simple PTSD, has some categories of symptoms that are unique to the disorder. First, the nature of the dysregulation of current interpersonal relationships reflects reenactments of victim–perpetrator dynamics that can be mapped on onto the traumatic experience. Second, the diagnosis includes the presence of a belief system in which despair and hopelessness are pervasive. Finally, some authors have also noted (Herman, 1992) that complex PTSD is characterized by somatization symptoms that distinguish it from both simple PTSD and BPD.

Controversies with Complex PTSD

Despite the strong theoretical foundation for a diagnosis of complex PTSD, empirical evidence is contradictory as to whether complex PTSD is a diagnostic category distinct from simple PTSD. Although PTSD is frequently diagnosed in the absence of complex PTSD, complex PTSD is rarely found without PTSD. For example, in the PTSD field trial for DSM-IV, complex PTSD occurred in the absence of simple PTSD in only 4–6% of the sample (Roth, Newman, Pelcovitz, van der Kolk, & Mandel, 1997). In a study of disorders of extreme stress not otherwise specified (DESNOS) and PTSD among a sample of 29 Dutch war veterans, Jongedijk et al. (1996) found that DESNOS was consistently associated with PTSD and concluded that it did not exist as a separate diagnostic category. Similarly, Newman, Riggs, and Roth (1997), in their study of 84 trauma survivors, found that only 2 subjects met criteria for complex PTSD in the absence of comorbid PTSD. In contrast to these findings, Ford (1999) found that among 84 male military veterans with documented war-related trauma exposure, veterans diagnosed with complex PTSD evidenced comorbid simple PTSD in only 54% of the cases. In addition, Ford and Kidd (1998) report that in their sample of 74 male military veterans, complex PTSD was uncorrelated with PTSD diagnosis. The discrepancy in the findings of these studies is difficult to interpret. However, it is important to note that Ford and Kidd excluded the somatization criteria when assessing complex PTSD, thereby limiting the interpretation of their results. The results do suggest the interesting notion that the relationship between simple and complex PTSD may vary by type of trauma (combat vs. childhood abuse) or by gender.

One interpretation of the preponderance of data is that complex PTSD is not a qualitatively different type of PTSD but rather a marker of severity of a posttraumatic reaction that exists on a continuum alongside simple PTSD. In support of this notion, in a study by Newman et al. (1997) an assessment of narratives by 84 trauma survivors revealed that, clients with comorbid complex PTSD and PTSD had the most unresolved themes and fewest nonrelevant themes compared to clients with and without a diagnosis of PTSD. In addition, they found that clients with comorbid complex and simple PTSD had more severe intrusive and avoidant PTSD symptoms than the other two groups. The results supported the authors' suggestion that comorbid complex and simple PTSD represent the most severe cases of PTSD, and that complex PTSD is a marker of PTSD severity.

Because complex PTSD is a relatively new area of empirical investigation, little is known about potential gender differences in the expression or symptom profile of the disorder. Gender differences are immediately observable in the frequency of the diagnosis, with women representing the large majority of those identified with complex PTSD. This is likely due to the fact that complex PTSD is defined as a disorder that emerges in the context of chronic and prolonged trauma, the prototypical example being childhood sexual abuse, a trauma experienced predominantly by women. In a report of risk factors associated with complex PTSD derived from the DSM-IV field trial data, Roth et al. (1997) reported that of the 287 study participants who had experienced sexual and/or physical abuse, only 19% were men. Because of the small size of the male sample, the authors were unable to analyze data among the men concerning risk factors such as age of onset and chronicity of abuse (both of which were predictive for women). Although the rate of complex PTSD among childhood abuse survivors was available for the total sample (50%), the breakdown by gender was not, so it remains unclear whether the 19% of men with a history of childhood trauma experienced complex PTSD at a similar rate. However, in another study of complex PTSD among combat veterans mentioned earlier (Ford & Kidd, 1998), 78% of men with childhood trauma (defined as sexual and/or physical abuse and witnessing violence) met criteria for the disorder. The higher rate of diagnosis among the men compared to the women in the Roth et al. (1997) study may be related to the fact that the men were individuals in an inpatient program, a sample biased toward severe psychopathology. Nevertheless, the results suggest that complex PTSD among men will not necessarily be found at rates lower than that obtained for women when trauma history is comparable.

PRACTICAL GUIDELINES

Assessment

Although empirical evidence on gender differences in differential diagnosis of PTSD is limited, the available data suggest several points that should be kept in mind by clinicians assessing trauma survivors. First, available evidence indicates that not only gender but also type of trauma and trauma characteristics influence whether an individual will develop "simple" PTSD, BPD, or another personality disorder or complex PTSD. Particularly severe, prolonged, and interpersonal traumatic events such as intrafamilial childhood sexual abuse and prisoner of war experiences are more likely to be associated with developing BPD and/or complex PTSD. "Simple" PTSD, or PTSD comorbid with only other Axis I disorders, is more likely to be associated with a single incident or acute traumatic event, such as a natural disaster, adult stranger rape, or a car accident. The gender-sensitive clinician will avoid gender stereotypes in assessment of trauma patients (e.g., assessing only women for BPD, men for ASPD) and consider the type and characteristics of the trauma that has occurred and assess the full range of diagnoses for both genders.

Second, an appropriate diagnosis for a client will be obtained via a thorough history of the client's difficulties and problematic behaviors, including the onset and duration of symptoms. A detailed assessment of the client's history of interpersonal relationships, childhood relationships with attachment figures and caregivers, and sense of self, both historically and currently and pre- and posttrauma is necessary. Specifically, given the characterological nature of the difficulties associated with BPD, if the client reports secure relationships and adequate emotion regulation prior to the trauma exposure, a diagnosis of PTSD or complex PTSD is likely warranted (Gunderson & Sabo, 1993). The particular PTSD diagnosis given (simple vs. complex) may in turn be determined by examining the nature of the difficulties following stressor exposure. A diagnosis of complex PTSD would be more appropriate if the client appears to experience pervasive changes in his or her sense of self and personality following exposure to the trauma.

Third, assessing the triggers of affective instability and dissociation also provide useful information to help with differential diagnosis; that is, mood swings and dissociative states may be more likely to be triggered by trauma cues in PTSD than BPD, whereas these symptoms are more often associated with perceived rejection or fear of abandonment by others in BPD. For example, Heffernan and Cloitre (2000) found that for women with PTSD alone (vs. women with PTSD and BPD), the most frequently endorsed PTSD symptom was becoming upset over reminders of abuse. Thus, for clients with PTSD alone, it appears that one of the hallmark symptoms (i.e., most frequently endorsed) is being upset by cues of the abuse. Furthermore, women with PTSD and BPD have reported higher levels of interpersonal problems than women with PTSD alone (Heffernan & Cloitre, 2000). Thus, interpersonal difficulties may suggest the possibility of a BPD or complex PTSD diagnosis, depending on the onset of the abuse and pretrauma personality organization. Finally, the presence of reexperiencing symptoms strongly suggests that a diagnosis of PTSD or complex PTSD would be more appropriate than BPD alone (Gunderson & Sabo, 1993).

Fourth, clinicians need to be sensitive to gender-specific manifestations of symptoms in differential diagnosis of PTSD. For example, the PTSD symptom "irritability and outbursts of anger" might manifest differently in men and women, with men more likely to express anger externally (e.g., physically) and women, internally (e.g., withdrawal). Similarly the self-destructive behaviors characteristics of BPD and complex PTSD might differ by gender. For women, these behaviors might more often include bingeing and purging or unsafe intimate relationships, whereas for men risk taking, such as driving fast while drinking or inciting physical fights, might be more characteristic. In addition, differences in gender roles suggest that the interpersonal difficulties characteristic of BPD and complex PTSD might present distinctly by gender. It is of note that differences in the presentation of symptoms have not been studied empirically, and research is needed in order to determine if these differences exist and impact diagnostic assessment of trauma survivors.

Treatment

As mentioned earlier in this chapter, one of the strongest motivations for the development of reliable differential diagnoses is to ensure the selection of appropriate treatment to trauma survivors. A diagnosis of PTSD or complex PTSD will likely provide a more coherent and integrated treatment than would diagnosing a client with numerous Axis I disorders such as generalized anxiety disorder, major depression, or social phobia that appear secondary to the trauma. In addition, careful diagnosis of the primacy of frequently co-ocurring trauma-related disorders can help the clinician to organize an effective treatment plan. A diagnosis of PTSD suggests that the client suffers from intrusive symptoms, emotional numbing, and hyperarousal, whereas a diagnosis of BPD suggests that the client may struggle with emotion dysregulation and impulsivity, and their impact on interpersonal functioning. The diagnosis of BPD does not suggest that the client currently struggles with intrusive memories or hyperarousal and startle symptoms.

Therefore, PTSD treatments aimed at exposing the client to the traumatic memories may be less helpful or necessary than treatments aimed at teaching interpersonal and emotion regulation skills, as well as affect tolerance (such as dialectical behavior therapy; Linehan, 1993). Finally, given the evidence that the diagnosis of complex PTSD reflects a combination of both PTSD and BPD symptoms, or that PTSD clients with childhood abuse struggle with additional burdens of affect and interpersonal regulation difficulties (Cloitre, Scarvalone, & Difede, 1997; Ford, 1999; Zlotnick, 1997), treatments that address both the reexperiencing symptoms of PTSD and characterological difficulties of emotion dysregulation and interpersonal disturbances should be considered (see Friedman, 1996; Jongedijk et al., 1996). Currently, at least one empirically supported treatment available for childhood abuse survivors specifically targets the PTSD symptoms, affect regulation and interpersonal difficulties (Cloitre et al., 2002) This two-phase treatment first provides an intensive skills training phase in affective and interpersonal regulation (STAIR), followed by a second phase comprising a modified form of prolonged exposure (PE). The treatment targets all three central problem domains typically seen in childhood abuse survivors (PTSD symptoms, affect regulation problems, and interpersonal difficulties). The sequential nature of the treatment provides clients with affect regulation skills before engaging in the exposure work, enhancing the successful use of exposure in reducing PTSD symptoms.

Finally, it should be noted that treatments may need to differ in order to attend to the behavioral manifestations of the same emotional problems. For example, clients with significant problems with substance abuse, eating disorders, and self-injurious behaviors may need a first line of treatment that immediately addresses these potentially life-threatening conditions. In a similar way, gender differences in behavioral disturbances need to be considered in treatment selection. We have suggested that some disorders have features representing different behavioral expressions of the same emotional problems (i.e., ASPD and BPD). It does not necessarily follow that the same emotional problems should be addressed with the same interventions. As noted in the previous paragraph, behavioral disturbances play a significant role in the determination of appropriate treatment. Treatment for traumatized men who engage in violent behaviors against their intimate partners needs to be different than that for traumatized women who engage in self-injury. Nevertheless, accumulating data suggest that the gender divide so commonly seen in many trauma-related treatment philosophies and interventions may narrow. For example, women prisoners tend to be highly traumatized and frequently are in prison due to drug charges. Thus, the dual presence of PTSD and substance abuse among women is highly concentrated in this setting, and the substance abuse treatments originated in VA settings may be applicable to this population. Conversely, the emerging data that variations of the BPD–PTSD combination can also be found among men with childhood trauma suggest the applicability of treatments developed and applied, at this point, only to female populations.

SUMMARY

This chapter on comorbidity and PTSD underscores the relationship between PTSD, other Axis I disorders, and the characterological or personality disorders related to reactions to stress or trauma. The high rates of comorbidity also suggest that it may be difficult to diagnose PTSD differentially from the many disorders that are often present. This is further complicated by factors related to gender. Gender biases in diagnosis, cultural prescriptions for gendered behavior, and phenomenological differences in the experiences of being a man and a woman suggest both that (1) gender differences exist in the presentation of disorders and (2) similar etiological circumstances can result in different conditions in men and women, and (3) treatment interventions may vary accordingly.

As this review indicates, much remains unknown about gender differences in the differential diagnosis of PTSD. However, one consistent finding is that whereas men and women experience equivalent numbers of traumatic stressors across the lifetime, women develop PTSD twice as often as men (10% of the female population compared to 5% of men). This difference in prevalence suggests two potentially fruitful areas of future research. First is the study of gender differences in both objective and subjective characteristics of traumatic stressors. Men experience greater exposure to life-threatening accidents and witnessing of violence, whereas women experience more interpersonal violence in the form of childhood abuse, rape, and domestic violence. Across the sexes, traumas "of human design" create greater risk for PTSD than events such as natural disasters or accidents, suggesting that women are likely to be at greater risk for the disorder by virtue of the objective characteristics of the traumatic events they experience. In addition, the meaning of traumatic interpersonal events, or their subjective characteristics, might differ between men and women. Following feminist relational theory, if women's sense of well-being and self-definition is more likely to be integrated with their capacity to develop and maintain relationships compared to men, then interpersonal violence may produce relatively greater distress and impairment to self-concept, interpersonal relatedness, and attendant functional capacity. These types of observations have important implications for the development of effective treatments, some of which might need to focus directly on the rehabilitation of a positive sense of self and the capacity to develop and maintain trusting relationships.

A related area of inquiry concerns gender-specific risk factors for violence and PTSD, including both "objective" risks, such as economic status and social mobility, and subjective or psychological risk factors, such as perceptions of control and predictability in the assessment of danger or threat. These two sets of risk factors may be interrelated. For example, women without financial resources may be less likely to leave a threatening situation (e.g., domestic violence) because there are few or no other places for them to go, which in turn increases risk for violence, or repeated violence, and the emergence of PTSD. In addition, women's sense of control and predictability may be lower relative to men's, shaped by general social mores and specific negative experiences such as domestic violence. This may lead to psychological states of "learned helplessness," in which women perceive less control or predictability than they actually have in a situation or traumatic event. The subjective features associated with traumatic events need further research, so that gender-specific understanding of trauma can be well characterized and lead to treatments with appropriate, accurate, and sensitive interventions. In addition, the study of subjective risk factors contributes to considerations of "early interventions" for at-risk adolescent or younger girls who might benefit from social interventions (e.g., school-based programs) that enhance self-esteem, sense of autonomy, and resilience.

Another area needing future research is the study of gender differences in the comorbidity of Axis II disorders. There is an assumption that ASPD is either an associated risk or consequence of trauma among men, whereas BPD fills the same role for women. However, close inspection of the data suggests that BPD is as often associated with traumatized men as with women. Further research with larger community and clinical samples, and careful measurement of personality characteristics are critical for understanding similarities and differences in men's and women's sense of self, the development of self, and the ways in which the self is compromised under the weight of trauma.

REFERENCES

Amaya-Jackson, L., Davidson, J. R., Hughes, D. C., Swartz, M., Reynolds, V., George, L. K., & Blazer, D. G. (1999). Functional impairment and utilization of services associated with posttraumatic stress disorder in the community. *Journal of Traumatic Stress, 12,* 709–724.

Andrykowski, M. A., Cordova, M. J., Studts, J. L., & Miller, T. W. (1998). Posttraumatic stress disorder after treatment for breast cancer: Prevalence of diagnosis and use of the PTSD Checklist—Civilian Version (PCL-C) as a screening instrument. *Journal of Consulting and Clinical Psychology, 66,* 586–590.

Bailey, J. E. (1985). Differential diagnosis of posttraumatic stress and antisocial personality disorders. *Hospital and Community Psychiatry, 36,* 881–883.

Becker, D., & Lamb, S. (1994). Sex bias in the diagnosis of borderline personality disorder and posttraumatic stress disorder. *Professional Psychology: Research and Practice, 25,* 55–61.

Blanchard, E., Buckley, T., Hickling, E. J., & Taylor, A. E. (1998). Posttraumatic stress disorder and comorbid major depression: Is the correlation an illusion? *Journal of Anxiety Disorders, 12,* 21–37.

Bollinger, A. R., Riggs, D. S., Blake, D. D., & Ruzek, J. I. (2000). Prevalence of personality disorders among combat veterans with posttraumatic stress disorder. *Journal of Traumatic Stress, 13,* 255–270.

Bowlby, J. (1969). *Attachment.* New York: Basic Books.

Bremner, J. D., Southwick, S. M., Johnson, D. R., Yehuda, R., & Charney, D. S. (1993). Childhood physical abuse and combat-related posttraumatic stress disorder in Vietnam veterans. *American Journal of Psychiatry, 150,* 235–239.

Brodsky, B. S., Cloitre, M., & Dulit, R. A. (1995). Relationship of dissociation to self-mutilation and childhood abuse in borderline personality disorder. *American Journal of Psychiatry, 152,* 1788—1792.

Chard, K. (2000, November). Cognitive processing therapy for sexual abuse (CPT-SA). In M. Cloitre (Chair), *Empirically supported treatments for chronic PTSD related to childhood abuse and multiple traumatization.* Symposium presented at the meeting of the International Society for Traumatic Stress Studies, San Antonio, TX.

Chodorow, N. (1978). *The reproduction of mothering.* Berkeley: University of California Press.

Cloitre, M. (1998, May). Interpersonal violence in the lives of men and women. Plenary session at the conference *Posttraumatic stress syndromes: Practical strategies for evaluation and treatment,* New York Hospital–Cornell Medical Center, Westchester Division.

Cloitre, M., & Koenen, K. C. (2001). Interpersonal group process treatment for CSA-related PTSD: A comparison study of the impact of borderline personality disorder on outcome. *International Journal of Group Psychotherapy, 51,* 379–398.

Cloitre, M., Koenen, K. C., Cohen, L., & Han, H. (2002). Skills training in affective and interpersonal regulation followed by exposure: A two-phase treatment for PTSD related to childhood abuse. *Journal of Consulting and Clinical Psychology.*

Cloitre, M., Scarvalone, P., & Difede, J. (1997). Posttraumatic stress disorder, self and interpersonal dysfunction among sexually retraumatized women. *Journal of Traumatic Stress, 10,* 435–450.

Deering, C. G., Glover, S. G., Ready, D., Eddleman, H. C., & Alarcon, R. D. (1996). Unique patterns of comorbidity in posttraumatic stress disorder from different sources of trauma. *Comprehensive Psychiatry, 37,* 336–346.

Dutton, D. (1998). *The abusive personality: Violence and control in intimate relationships.* New York: Basic Books.

Dutton, D., & Golant, S. K. (1995). *The batterer.* New York: Basic Books.

Eisenberg, N., & Lennon, R. (1983). Sex differences in empathy and related capacities. *Psychological Bulletin, 94,* 100–131.

Elliot, D. (1995). *Severe early trauma: I. Therapy for adult survivors.* Nevada City, CA: Cavalcade Productions.

Feeney, N. C., Zoellner, L., & Foa, E. (1999). Treatment outcome for PTSD among female assault victims with comorbid personality disorders. In M. Cloitre (Chair), *The role of personality disorders in the assessment and treatment of PTSD.* Symposium presented at the meeting of the Association for Advancement of Behavior Therapy, Toronto, Canada.

Ferrada-Noli, M., Asberg, G. M., Ormstad, K., Lundin, T., & Sunbom, E. (1998). Suicidal behavior after severe trauma: Part 1. PTSD diagnoses, psychiatric comorbidity, and assessments of suicidal behavior. *Journal of Traumatic Stress*, *11*, 103–112.

Foa, E. B., Olasov-Rothbaum, B., Riggs, D. S., & Murdock, T. B. (1991). Treatment of post-traumatic stress disorder in rape victims: Comparison between cognitive-behavioral procedures and counseling. *Journal of Consulting and Clinical Psychology*, *59*, 715–723.

Folkman, S., & Lazarus, R. S. (1980). An analysis of coping in a middle-aged community sample. *Journal of Health and Social Behavior*, *21*, 219–239.

Ford, J. (1999). Disorders of extreme stress following war-zone military trauma: Associated features of posttraumatic stress disorder or comorbid but distinct syndromes? *Journal of Consulting and Clinical Psychology*, *67*, 3–12.

Ford, J., & Kidd, P. (1998). Early childhood trauma and disorders of extreme stress as predictors of treatment outcome with chronic posttraumatic stress disorder. *Journal of Traumatic Stress*, *11*, 743–761.

Ford, J., Fisher, P., & Larson, L. (1997). Object relations as a predictor of treatment outcome with chronic posttraumatic stress disorder. *Journal of Consulting and Clinical Psychology*, *65*, 547–559.

Friedman, M. J. (1996). PTSD diagnosis and treatment for mental health clinicians. *Community Mental Health Journal*, *32*, 173–189.

Fuchs, D., & Thelen, M. (1988). Children's expected interpersonal consequences of communicating their affective state and reported likelihood of expression. *Child Development*, *59*, 1314–1322.

Gibson, L. E., Holt, J. C., Fondacaro, K. M., Tang, T. S., Powell, T. A., & Turbitt, E. L. (1999). An examination of antecedent traumas and psychiatric comorbidity among male inmates with PTSD. *Journal of Traumatic Stress*, *12*, 473–484.

Gilligan, C. (1982). *In a different voice: Psychological theory and women's development*. Cambridge, MA: Harvard University Press.

Good, G. E., Dell, D. M., & Mintz, L. B. (1989). Male role and gender role conflict: Relations to help-seeking in men. *Journal of Counseling Psychology*, *36*, 295–300.

Gottman, J. M., Jacobson, N. S., Rushe, R. H., Shortt, J. W., Babcock, J., La Taillade, J. J., & Watlz, J. (1995). The relationship between heart rate reactivity, emotionally aggressive behavior, and general violence in batterers. *Journal of Family Psychology*, *9*, 227–248.

Gunderson, J. G., & Sabo, A. N. (1993). The phenomenological and conceptual interface between borderline personality disorder and PTSD. *American Journal of Psychiatry*, *150*, 19–27.

Hall, J. A. (1978). Gender effects in decoding nonverbal cues. *Psychological Bulletin*, *85*, 845–858.

Han. H., & Cloitre, M. (2000, November). *Functional Impairment among women with PTSD related to childhood abuse*. Poster presented at the meeting of the International Society for Traumatic Stress Studies, San Antonio, TX.

Heffernan, K., & Cloitre, M. (2000). A comparison of PTSD with and without borderline personality disorder among women with childhood sexual abuse: Etiological and clinical characteristics. *Journal of Nervous and Mental Disease*, *188*, 589–595.

Herman, J. L. (1992). *Trauma and recovery.* New York: Basic Books.

Herman, J. L., Perry J. C., & van der Kolk, B. A. (1989). Childhood trauma in borderline personality. *American Journal Psychiatry, 146,* 490–495.

Jacobson, N. S., & Gottman, J. M. (1998). *When men batter women.* New York: Simon & Schuster.

Johnson, J. G., Cohen, P., Brown, J., Smailes, E., & Bernstein, D. P. (1999). Documented childhood maltreatment increases risk for personality disorders during young adulthood. *Archives of General Psychiatry, 56,* 600–606.

Jongedijk, R. A., Carlier, I. V. E., Schreuder, B. J. N., & Gersons, B. P. R. (1996). Complex posttraumatic stress disorder: An exploratory investigation of PTSD and DES NOS among Dutch war veterans. *Journal of Traumatic Stress, 9,* 577–586.

Keane, T. M., Taylor, K. L., & Penk, W. E. (1997). Differentiating post-traumatic stress disorder (PTSD) from major depression (MDD) and generalized anxiety disorder (GAD). *Journal of Anxiety Disorders, 11,* 317–328.

Kessler, R. C. (1995). The epidemiology of psychiatric comorbidity. In M. T. Tsuang, M. Tohen, & G. E. P. Zahner (Eds.), *Textbook in psychiatric epidemiology* (pp. 179–198). New York: Wiley.

Kessler, R. C., Sonnega, A., Bromet, E., Hughes, M., & Nelson, C. (1995). Posttraumatic stress disorder in the national comorbidity survey. *Archives of General Psychiatry, 52,* 1048–1060.

Kulka, R. A., Schlenger, W. E., Fairbank, J. A., Hough, R. L., Jordan, B. K., Marmar, C. R., & Weiss, D. S. (1990). *Trauma and the Vietnam War generation: Report of the findings from the National Vietnam Veterans Readjustment Study.* New York: Brunner/Mazel.

Linehan, M. M. (1993). *Cognitive-behavioral treatment of borderline personality disorder.* New York: Guilford Press.

Lubin, H., & Johnson, D. R. (1997). Interactive psychoeducational group therapy for traumatized women. *International Journal of Group Psychotherapy, 47,* 271–290.

Luntz, B. K., & Widom, C. S. (1994). Antisocial personality disorders in abused and neglected children grown up. *American Journal of Psychiatry, 151*(5), 670–674.

McDonough-Coyle, A., Friedman, M. J., McHugo, G., Ford, J., Mueser, K., Demment, C. C., Schnurr, P., Descamps, M., & Fournier, D. (2000, November). Cognitive restructuring and exposure for CSA survivors with PTSD. In M. Cloitre (Chair), *Empirically supported treatments for chronic PTSD related to childhood abuse and multiple traumatization.* Symposium presented at the meeting of the International Society for Traumatic Stress Studies, San Antonio, TX.

McFarlane, A. C., Archinson, M., Rafalowicz, E., & Papay, P. (1994). Physical symptoms in post-traumatic stress disorder. *Journal of Psychosomatic Research, 38,* 715–726.

Miller, J. B. (1986). *Toward a new psychology of women* (2nd ed.). Boston: Beacon Press.

Miller, P., & Lisak, D. (1999). Association between childhood abuse and personality disorder symptoms in college males. *Journal of International Violence, 14,* 642–656.

Mollica, R. F., McInnes, K., Sarajlic, N., Lavelle, J., Sarajlic, I., & Massagli, M. P. (1999). Disability associated with psychiatric comorbidity and health status in

Bosnia refugees living in Croatia. *Journal of the American Medical Associations*, *282*, 433–439.

Najavits, L. M., Weiss, R. D., & Shaw, S. R. (1997). The link between substance abuse and posttraumatic stress disorder in women: A research review. *American Journal on Addictions*, *6*, 273–283.

Newman, E., Riggs, D. S., & Roth, S. (1997). Thematic resolution, PTSD, and complex PTSD: The relationship between meaning and trauma-related diagnoses. *Journal of Traumatic Stress*, *10*, 197–213.

North, C. S., Nixon, S. J., Shariat, S., Mallonee, S., McMillen, J. C., Spitznagel, E. L., & Smith, E. M. (1999). Psychiatric disorders among survivors of the Oklahoma City bombing. *Journal of the American Medical Association*, *282*, 755–762.

Orsillo, S. M., Weathers, F. W., Litz, B. T., Stainber, H. R., Huska, J. A., & Keane, T. M. (1996). Current and lifetime psychiatric disorders among veterans with war-zone related posttraumatic stress disorder. *Journal of Nervous and Mental Disease*, *184*(5), 307–313.

Paris, J. (1997). Predispositions, personality traits, and posttraumatic stress disorder. *Harvard Review of Psychiatry*, *8*, 175–183.

Pleck, J. (1981). *The myth of masculinity*. Cambridge, MA: MIT Press.

Pleck, J. (1995). The gender role strain paradigm: An update. In R. Levant & W. Pollack (Eds.), *A new psychology of men* (pp. 11 -32). New York: Basic Books.

Raine, A., Lencz, T., Bihrle, S., LaCasse, L., & Coletti, P. (2000). Reduced prefrontal gray matter volume and reduced autonomic activity in antisocial personality disorder. *Archives of General Psychiatry*, *57*, 119–127.

Resick, P. A., & Schnicke, M. K. (1992). Cognitive processing therapy for sexual assault victims. *Journal of Consulting and Clinical Psychology*, *60*, 748–756.

Resnick, H. S., Foy, D. W., Donahue, C. P., & Miller, E. N. (1989). Antisocial behavior and post-traumatic stress disorder in Vietnam veterans. *Journal of Clinical Psychology*, *45*, 860–866.

Roth, S., Newman, E., Pelcovitz, D., van der Kolk, B., & Mandel, F. (1997). Complex PTSD in victims exposed to sexual and physical abuse: Results from the DSM-IV field trial for posttraumatic stress disorder. *Journal of Traumatic Stress*, *10*, 539–555.

Saurer, M. K., & Eisler, R. M. (1990). The role of masculine gender role stress in expressivity and social support network factors. *Sex Roles*, *23*, 261–271.

Saxe, G., & Wolfe, J. (1999). Gender and posttraumatic stress disorder. In P. A. Saigh & J. D. Bremner (Eds). *Posttraumatic stress disorder: A comprehensive text* (pp. 160–179). Needham Heights, MA: Allyn & Bacon.

Schoenfeld, W. H., Verboncoeur, C. J., Fifer, S. K., Lipschutz, R. C., Lubeck, D. P., & Buesching, D. P. (1997). The functioning and well-being of patients with unrecognized anxiety disorders and major depressive disorder. *Journal of Affective Disorders*, *43*, 105–119.

Shalev, A., Freedman, S., Peri, T., Brandes, D., Sahar, T., Orr, S., & Pitman, R. (1998). Prospective study of posttraumatic stress disorder and depression following trauma. *American Journal of Psychiatry*, *155*, 630–637.

Shea, T., Zlotnick, C., & Weisberg, R. B. (1999). Commonality and specificity of personality disorder profiles in subjects with trauma histories. *Journal of Personality Disorders*, *13*, 199–210.

Shearer, S. L., Peter, C. P., Quaytman, M. S., & Ogden R. L. (1990). Frequency and correlates of childhood sexual and physical abuse histories in adult female borderline inpatients. *American Journal Psychiatry, 147,* 214—216.

Southwick, S. M., Yehuda, R., & Giller, E. L. (1993). Personality disorders in treatment-seeking combat veterans with posttraumatic stress disorder. *American Journal of Psychiatry, 150,* 1020–1023.

Weaver, T. L., & Clum, G. A. (1993). Early family environments and traumatic experiences associated with borderline personality disorder. *Journal of Consulting and Clinical Psychology, 61,* 1068–1075.

Wolfe, J., & Kimerling, R. (1997). Gender issues in the assessment of posttraumatic stress disorder. In J. P. Wilson & T. M. Keane (Eds.), *Assessing psychological trauma and PTSD.* New York: Guilford Press.

Zanarini, M. C. (1997). *Role of sexual abuse in the etiology of borderline personality disorder.* Washington, DC: American Psychiatric Press.

Zatzick, D. F., Marmar, C. R., Weiss, D. S., Metzler, T. J., Golding, J. M., Steward, A., Sclenger, W. E., & Wells, K. B. (1999). Posttraumatic stress disorder and functioning and quality of life outcomes in a nationally representative sample of male veterans. *American Journal of Psychiatry, 154,* 1690–1695.

Zeman, J., & Garber, J. (1996). Display rules for anger, sadness, and pain: It depends on who is watching. *Child Development, 67,* 957–973.

Zlotnick, C. (1997). Posttraumatic stress disorder (PTSD), PTSD comorbidity, and childhood abuse among incarcerated women. *Journal of Nervous and Mental Disease, 185,* 761–763.

Zlotnick, C., Shea, T. M., Rosen, K., Simpson, E., Mulrenin, K., Begin, A., & Pearlstein, T. (1997). An affect-management group for women with posttraumatic stress disorder and histories of childhood sexual abuse. *Journal of Traumatic Stress, 10,* 425–436.

6 | Gender Considerations in the Psychometric Assessment of PTSD

KAREN CUSACK
SHERRY FALSETTI
MICHAEL DE ARELLANO

Over the last 10 years, there has been an explosion of measures developed for assessing posttraumatic stress disorder (PTSD). As a clinician or researcher interested in trauma and PTSD, choosing which assessment instrument to use with a particular population can be overwhelming. In this chapter, we review several of the most widely used instruments for assessing traumatic events and PTSD, and make some recommendations based on sensitivity to gender and suitability with different populations. The vast majority of available instruments were initially developed and validated using male combat veteran samples. We feel it is important to address what, if any, implications this may have for using these instruments to assess traumatic events and PTSD accurately with both men and women who have experienced a range of traumatic events.

It is our hope that this chapter will provide information for researchers and clinicians alike to help determine the most appropriate measures to use, as well as the empirical work needed in order to advance our understanding of gender differences in PTSD. The measures that we review in this chapter are generally well known and in most cases have well-established psychometric properties. Although some of the newer measures have been only preliminarily evaluated in terms of psychometrics, we felt that this was not reason to exclude them. Instead, we review the instruments, evaluating them in terms of strengths and weaknesses, with a focus on gender. This chapter also provides recommendations for further types of needed psychometric evaluation. Each of the measures reviewed here can easily be obtained. Several excellent chapters or review articles already exist on the general topic of psychometric assessment of PTSD or trauma (see

Carlson, 1997; Norris & Riad, 1997; Resnick, Falsetti, Kilpatrick, & Freedy, 1996; Solomon, Keane, Newman, & Kaloupek, 1996; Weathers & Keane, 1999). We discuss, when relevant, features of these instruments that have incorporated cultural factors or gender-specific knowledge of trauma and PTSD in their construction. Although this has not generally been a practice in the development of trauma and PTSD assessments, some examples include the Potential Stressful Events Interview (Kilpatrick, Resnick, & Freedy, 1991), which has included features such as normalizing the experience of traumatic events and providing behaviorally specific definitions for sexual abuse; the Harvard Trauma Questionnaire (Mollica et al., 1992), which includes culture-specific items for the assessment of traumatic events and/or trauma-related symptomatology; and the Composite International Diagnostic Interview (World Health Organization, 1993), which has been developed and validated using cross-cultural samples. We also discuss features that make their use more or less appropriate for a specific gender.

THE RELEVANCE OF RELIABILITY AND VALIDITY

In evaluating the usefulness of any instrument, the two most important considerations concern its *reliability* and *validity*. Reliability is the extent to which scores on an instrument are free of measurement error (i.e., it measures the consistency of responses). Three types of reliability are important to look at when evaluating an instrument. Test–retest reliability refers to the consistency of responses over time (generally 1–2 weeks apart). Internal reliability refers to consistency across items in the same measure. Interrater reliability refers to consistency across different interviewers/scorers of the instrument. For evaluating trauma assessment instruments, test–retest and interrater reliability are important to examine. Internal reliability is not as relevant here, because the experience of one event is assumed to be independent of the other events being assessed. In evaluating PTSD assessments, each of these types of reliability is important. The several potential sources of threats to reliability of trauma assessment measures include ambiguity in items. For example, an item that asks a woman "Have you ever been raped?" has been shown to underestimate greatly the true rates of sexual assault. Many stereotypes exist regarding what the term "rape" means. Therefore, use of more behaviorally specific items (e.g., "forced you to have intercourse [anal, oral, vaginal] against your will") is likely to yield more accurate estimates. A culturally relevant example of this is asking a refugee from a war-torn region, "Have you ever been physically assaulted?" This may be very confusing or is likely to yield inconsistent responses from individuals who have experienced ongoing violence in their community. Defining a physical assault in behavioral terms is likely to yield more accurate results. For example, wording the question "Have you ever experienced intentional harm from another person that resulted in physical injury to yourself?" is likely to be more sensitive in detecting the events of interest.

Having a measure that produces consistent results is important but certainly not sufficient. The validity of a measure refers to how accurately the intended construct is assessed. Three types of validity are examined: content, criterion-related, and construct validity. Content validity is the most complex and refers to how well the domain of interest is reflected. This is established by careful definition of the construct, generating items that are reviewed and revised, and using expert judgment. Measures with good content validity *for a specific population* are those that were developed using focus groups and expert consensus during item generation. Demonstrating validity across groups is especially important when there is reason to expect differences between groups based on gender or cultural group. Knowing that a scale is "psychometrically mature" is not helpful if the population for which we wish to use it is likely to have a different interpretation of the items.

Criterion-related validity includes the relation between scores on an instrument and some variable of interest, such as a diagnosis or an outcome. When the score on an instrument is used to predict a score on another measure administered at the same time, this criterion-related validity is known as concurrent validity. If the criterion is measured at some later date (e.g., using test scores to predict diagnosis), it is referred to as predictive validity. The *sensitivity* of a measure is the proportion of individuals with a positive diagnosis who have a positive test. The *specificity* refers to the proportion of individuals with a negative diagnosis who have a negative test.

Construct validity demonstrates that the test measures what it is supposed to, and does not measure constructs it is not supposed to. Often, when a scale is developed, it is desirable to show that it correlates strongly with another measure of the same construct (convergent validity) and weakly with measures of other constructs (discriminant or divergent validity).

For purposes of evaluating traumatic event instruments, content validity is particularly important. For example, if the queried types of events are restrictive, then the information obtained and subsequent PTSD data will be restricted as well. For research purposes, the implications may be that the prevalence of trauma is highly underestimated. Clinically, the implications could include missing a PTSD diagnosis that would otherwise be a focus of treatment. The item that queries about "rape" also demonstrates a content validity problem. Although forced sexual intercourse is the intended construct, what is really being assessed is a subset of these cases that acknowledges the experience as rape. Careful research in interviewing women and using expert consensus has resulted in changes in the wording of many measures. Finally, with both trauma and PTSD assessments, the proliferation of instruments makes it especially important to look at criterion-related validity.

ASSESSMENT OF TRAUMATIC EVENTS

The assessment of potentially traumatic events is essential in a thorough assessment of PTSD. According to DSM-IV, the necessary criterion for a traumatic event requires that the individual has experienced an event that may include threatened death, threat to physical integrity, actual injury, or witnessing any of these events. The person's response also must involve intense fear, helplessness, or horror (American Psychiatric Association, 1994). Typical events include physical and sexual assaults, combat, natural disasters, accidents, and war. When assessing for history of traumatic events, effective assessment should include queries of experience with a variety of stressful events, qualities of events that may be risk factors for PTSD, and subjective reactions to the events (Kimerling, 1996; Resnick et al., 1996).

Evidence suggests that women may experience higher rates of certain *qualitative* features of trauma (e.g., more repetitive events, greater life threat, more intense subjective reactions) that put them at greater risk for PTSD. With the changes in PTSD criteria in DSM-IV, greater attention has been given to the victim's reaction to the event by acknowledging that the person must react with "intense fear, helplessness, or horror" (American Psychiatric Association, 1994). This area could benefit from further investigation in the literature on gender differences in PTSD. It is possible that women, for various reasons, experience greater subjective reactions at the time of the trauma, which results in higher rates of PTSD. Studies that incorporate solid assessment of these factors may highlight gender differences that provide greater understanding of differential PTSD rates. Another plausible hypothesis is that women experience traumas with more recurrences of the same trauma type (e.g., multiple domestic violence assaults or greater severity of trauma). Trauma assessment instruments that inquire about repetitive events and severity indicators may help to increase our understanding of how these events affect gender rates of PTSD.

The following section reviews several instruments that assess traumatic experiences. Included for each instrument is a description of the types of events assessed, as well as any information on reliability and validity. The instruments differ considerably in their interpretations of what constitutes a traumatic event. In reviewing these measures, we were most interested in looking at how well the instruments queried about traumas, or aspects of traumas, that are relevant to the gender differences noted in the literature. These areas include the number of traumatic events, the duration of the event, severity, age at the time of occurrence, whether the event was interpersonal in nature, and the relationship to the perpetrator (Resnick et al.,

1996). Many of these variables have been found to be highly associated with the development of chronic PTSD. Interestingly, they also to be especially relevant to traumatic experiences in women. In evaluating the instruments, we also paid special attention to those that used a preface to normalize the experience of sexual assault. This is important, because the use of such a preface increases the likelihood that sexual abuse victims will admit to their experience and also recognize certain events as sexual assault. We also paid particular attention to instruments that used behaviorally specific terms to define events. Epidemiological studies using such instruments achieved significantly higher prevalence rates over previous studies (Resnick, Kilpatrick, Dansky, Saunders, & Best, 1993). Table 6.1 (see p. 158) summarizes the instruments based on these important features. For each instrument, the initial population for which the scale was validated with is reported in terms of gender and type of population. Instruments are summarized according to whether the questions regarding sexual assault use behaviorally specific wording rather than terms requiring respondents to label their experience as rape or sexual assault. The heading "Chronicity/duration" refers to whether the instrument has queries for repeated events, or the duration of the events. "Severity" refers to any queries that indicate the severity of the trauma (e.g., life threat, physical injury, intense fear). Finally, the instruments are compared on their use of a preface that describes and normalizes sexual assault experiences.

Many of the instruments for assessing trauma history lack complete psychometric data to support their use, which is unfortunate, because many of the instruments have strong features. In terms of psychometric data, information on the reliability and validity of the trauma assessment instruments is somewhat limited. In many cases, these measures were designed for use in specific studies, and psychometric data were not reported. It is strongly recommended that future studies using these instruments provide such psychometric data.

Potential Stressful Events Interview (PSEI)

The PSEI (Kilpatrick, Resnick, & Freedy, 1991) is a structured interview that evolved from two previous trauma measures, the National Women's Study PTSD Module (Kilpatrick, Resnick, Saunders, & Best, 1989), and the previous Incident Report Interview (Kilpatrick et al., 1987). The instrument was normed on the DSM-IV Field Trial population of male and female community and psychiatric populations. The PSEI takes approximately 60–90 minutes to complete, and is therefore one of the lengthiest of the trauma assessment measures. It was designed in response to findings that only about one-half of women who have had sexual assault experiences that meet the legal definition of rape actually respond positively when asked if they had been raped (Kilpatrick, Best, et al., 1989; Koss, 1985). The PSEI, administered as a structured interview, uses an introductory preface that normalizes the types of potential traumatic events, and includes behaviorally specific descriptions for events such as "Has a man or boy ever made you have sex by using force or threatening to harm you or someone close to you? Just so there is no mistake, by sex, we mean putting a penis in your vagina." The PSEI also includes queries for age at the time of event, indications of severity of the event, and the relationship to the perpetrator (when relevant). On the sexual assault section of the instrument, there are separate sections that are non-gender-specific, a section for women only, and a section for men only. The instrument also takes into account both objective characteristics and subjective reactions. Thirteen potentially traumatic events are assessed. The instrument allows for description of both low- and high-magnitude stressors, which are categorized into first (only), most recent, and worst high-magnitude events. There are also queries for whether the trauma involved multiple events. Although explicit psychometric data are not available on the instrument, findings of comparable rates of trauma prevalence with other measures and across cities in the DSM-IV Field Trial for PTSD, as well as the behaviorally specific wording, provide confidence in its reliability. Concordance with the DSM-IV Criterion A for PTSD supports its validity. This instrument is appropriate for use with both men and women. It is a good choice for the assessment of women because of the behaviorally specific sexual assault questions.

Traumatic Assessment for Adults (TAA)

The TAA (Resnick, Best, Kilpatrick, Freedy, & Falsetti, 1993) is a briefer interview that was based on the PSEI and retains many of the same features. It contains an opening preface regarding traumatic events, followed by questions that assess lifetime history of 13 events, including combat, accident, disaster, molestation, rape, aggravated assault, witnessing violence, other situations that include injury, and other situations that include fear of being killed or seriously injured. The TAA also includes an introductory preface to the sexual assault questions, indicating that the perpetrator may have been someone known to the victim, that the event may not have been reported, and that it may have occurred at any point in his or her lifetime. Each event is assessed in terms of the age of first/ only and last occurrence. Severity of the event is assessed through questions about suffering injury or fearing death at the time of the event. The TAA does not actually assess chronicity of events; instead, it assesses the ages of the first and most recent event. The TAA was validated with male and female adult mental health center clients. The validity of the measure was supported by trauma exposure that was highly consistent with rates previously reported in this population using a different trauma assessment measure (Saunders, Kilpatrick, Resnick, & Tidwell, 1989). The instrument also performed well in a study with archival clinic data in which every case was positively identified using the TAA. Similar to the PSEI, this instrument is appropriate for use with both men and women. It retains the behaviorally specific questions regarding sexual assault and therefore is particularly useful for assessing women.

Traumatic Stress Schedule (TSS)

The TSS (Norris, 1990), a brief screening device for traumatic events, also includes questions regarding the individual's subjective response to the event(s). The instrument is administered as a structured interview, yet is straightforward enough to be administered by nonclinicians. The scale has 10 items assessing potentially traumatic events, including physical assault, robbery, sexual assault, loss of a loved one through accident/homicide/suicide, personal injury or property loss through natural disaster, forced evacuations, motor vehicle accident with injury, and other terrifying or shocking experiences. One drawback of the instrument is that there is no preface to normalize the occurrences of traumatic events. In addition, Norris and Riad (1997) and Resnick et al. (1996) have noted that a shortcoming of the instrument is the use of only a single item for assessing sexual assault that is not behaviorally specific, and no items that specifically inquire about childhood sexual or physical abuse. Further, the question regarding sexual assault is restricted to the use of force or threat of harm. This would exclude many cases of childhood sexual abuse that occur without explicit force or threat. Based on a community sample of men and women in six southeastern U.S. cities, the instrument appears to have good reliability. Test–retest reliability for the TSS was reported to be .868 across administrations of the measure given 1 week apart. The concurrent validity of the measure is demonstrated by the identical agreement between the TSS and the National Women's Study PTSD Module (Norris & Riad, 1997). Self-report versions of a combined TSS/Civilian Mississippi Scale have been developed in English and Spanish. The Spanish version was created using back translation and centering, and was tested with 94 male and female victims of Hurricane Andrew in Dade County, Florida. Test–retest reliability was found to be .88 following a 1-week interval. The concurrent validity of both language versions of the measure is demonstrated by the identical agreement between the TSS and the National Women's Study PTSD Module (Norris & Riad, 1997). This instrument may not be as sensitive at assessing childhood sexual and physical abuse; thus, when used with women, it may be helpful to supplement with questions from another instrument such as the PSEI or the TAA.

Life Stressor Checklist (LSC)

The LSC (Wolfe & Kimerling, 1997) can be administered in either interview or self-report format. The instrument queries a total of 30 varied traumatic experiences, including both DSM-IV-consistent experiences and those empirically identified as stressful experiences for women. Examples of unique items include the assessment of abortion, sexual harassment, domestic violence, and sexual assault. Although some of the stressors that are asked about in this instrument would not qualify as DSM-IV traumatic stressors, it is important to recognize the potentially stressful nature of these more female-specific experiences. The LSC inquires about subjective reactions to stressors, and also includes global measures of current distress. The instrument does not specifically inquire about repetition of events and, similar to the TAA, inquires about the age of the individual when the event began and ended. If an event was repeated, the respondent is asked to describe the event that had the "largest impact on you." For items that assess childhood sexual experiences, the wording only allows for childhood sexual experiences that involved subjects being forced in some way, or threatened with harm if they did not comply. However, in the case of childhood sexual abuse, it is not necessary that force or threat be present in order to constitute a criterion A traumatic event. Although reliability studies have not been conducted with the LSC, the authors noted using the LSC in studies with female veterans and finding endorsement of Criterion A items to be highly correlated with PTSD diagnosis. Several in-process studies are currently being conducted with the LSC. With the exception of the assessment of childhood sexual assault experiences, this instrument is highly recommended for use with women because of the many items specifically focused on traumatic event that have higher prevalence rates in women, such as domestic violence and sexual harassment.

Trauma History Questionnaire (THQ)

The THQ (Green, 1996) is a self-report measure created from the DSM-IV field trial Potential Stressful Events Interview (reviewed earlier in the chapter). It begins with a preface that normalizes the occurrence of traumatic events. Twenty-four behaviorally specific items assess a range of traumatic events, including crime-related trauma, disaster, and physical and sexual assault. Six items are devoted to physical and sexual experiences, and include a query for whether an event was repeated. This information is useful for determining the differential impact of having been physically assaulted on one occasion compared to being in an abusive relationship in which the physical assaults were ongoing. Each of the sexual experiences questions inquire about the relationship to the perpetrator. The items that assess for sexual experiences are each described by the use of force, which again, may exclude child sexual abuse victims who were coerced. Frequency data are collected for each event, as well as age at the time of each occurrence. Dimensions of the stressors, such as life threat, are indirectly assessed by counting all items expected to include life threat. In this way, the instrument does not appear to attend to subjective responses to the trauma. Good overall test–retest reliability has been reported for the THQ on a sample of college women. For items that assess traumas such as seeing dead bodies, robbery, or being attacked with a weapon, the correlations ranged from .90 to 1.00. For items such as "other unwanted sex," the correlations were much lower (.47). The author reported data from two mixed-gender samples using the THQ (Green, 1996). Within a college student population, men reported more mugging, serious injury, seeing others injured/killed, and being attacked with a weapon. Women reported more forced intercourse, sexual touching, and other forced sexual experiences. Among a sample of psychiatric outpatients, men reported more mugging, serious accidents, seeing others killed/injured, and combat. Women reported more of any sexual experience, break-ins while at home, being attacked without a weapon, and being beaten. It appears that this instrument is appropriate for use with both men and women. However, when used in a population with potentially high prevalence rates of childhood sexual abuse, another, more sensitive instrument in assessing child sexual abuse may be needed as a supplement.

PTSD ASSESSMENT INSTRUMENTS

Several interview and self-report measures have been developed in recent years to assess symptoms of PTSD. According to the current diagnostic conceptualization of PTSD, the components of the disorder include (1) reexperiencing the event which involves intrusive, unintended daytime

TABLE 6.1. Instruments for Assessing Traumatic Events

Scale	Validation population	Administration time	Behaviorally specific	Chronicity/ duration	Reliability	Severity	Sexual assault preface
PSEI	M/F	60–90 min	Yes	Yes	N/C	Yes	Yes
TAA	M/F outpatients	10–15 min	Yes	No—only age first and last	N/C	Yes	Yes
TSS	M/F community	10–30 min	No	No	T-R .88	No	No
LSC	F—veterans	15–30 min	Yes	Yes	N/C	Yes	No
THQ	F—general	5–10 min	Yes	Yes	T-R .47–.92	No	Yes

Note. T-R, Test–retest reliability; N/C, not completed; M, male; F, female.

recollections, nightmares, or dissociative episodes; (2) behavioral avoidance of external cues or situations that the individual associates with the event, and emotional numbing or a restricted range of affect; and (3) autonomic disturbance, usually hyperarousal, exaggerated startle response, or pronounced irritability (American Psychiatric Association, 1994).

Many of the PTSD measures reviewed here were initially developed with men in the study of combat-related PTSD. As a result, the reliability and validity of some of these instruments have only been documented with male populations. While this may appear to pose a significant problem for using these instruments with female populations, our opinion is that it does not. The reasons for this are that (1) the majority of these measures are stringently tied to DSM criteria for PTSD, which has been shown to apply universally to both men and women; (2) the few measures that were developed on an exclusively female population (e.g., PTSD Symptom Scale–Interview [PSS-I]; Foa, Riggs, Dancu, & Rothbaum, 1993) do not differ significantly in content or form from the male-validated measures; and (3) the male-validated measures have been used in both male and female populations across a variety of traumatic events, frequently yielding very similar results.

To further examine any potential gender and ethnic differences in symptom reporting, we analyzed a subset of the data collected for the DSM-IV field trials (Kilpatrick, Resnick, Saunders, & Best, 1998) using the SCID. For a full description of the methodology of the DSM-IV field trials, refer to Kilpatrick et al. (1998). Included in current analyses were 238 subjects assessed in St. Louis, Missouri, and Charleston, South Carolina. In this sample, 182 people were white, 53 were African American, 1 person was Hispanic, and 2 people reported race/ethnicity other than the above. With regard to gender, 29.8% of the sample was male, and 70.2% was female. When we examined the rates of current and lifetime PTSD using the SCID, we found that women were more likely to have both lifetime (61.1% vs. 18.4%) and current (48.5% vs. 14.7%) PTSD compared to the men in the sample. However, of those individuals who had PTSD, there were no differences in the endorsement of specific symptom items based on gender or race. This finding is interesting, because it demonstrates that although multiple factors may lead to differential rates of PTSD, the PTSD construct itself appears to be universal.

Gender differences in responses on the CAPS were also examined in a study with Holocaust survivors (Yehuda, Schmeidler, Siever, Binder-Brynes, & Elkin, 1997). In the analysis of the data, each of the 17 symptoms of PTSD were examined individually by gender. Results showed no gender differences in overall PTSD scores. However, two items on the CAPS, psychogenic amnesia and sense of foreshortened future, were found to be significantly higher for women (men: $M = .85$, $SD = 1.64$; women: $M = 2.55$, $SD = 2.63$, $t(98) = 3.37$, $p < .001$). Further studies that address differential posttraumatic responses between the sexes would help in understanding what role gender plays in PTSD. From these data, we can conclude that from a gender perspective the use of a sensitive trauma assessment measure may be a more important issue than the PTSD symptom item assessment. Without a gender-appropriate trauma assessment measure, PTSD may not be assessed at all and will go undetected.

Having said this, we do not view all the PTSD instruments as being equivalent, and in fact believe that several factors make some PTSD measures better suited for use with women. First, women have often been exposed to traumatic events that involve repeated episodes, such as childhood sexual abuse, domestic violence, and sexual assault in adulthood. Therefore, instruments that allow for assessment of multiple traumas will be most appropriate for women. In many cases, however, distinguishing between specific incidents of abuse may be impossible, and the abuse as a whole may need to be considered before proceeding with the assessment. Second, it is not uncommon for many women to have trauma histories that have never been reported, let alone even discussed with others. For this reason, instruments with prefaces to help put the respondent at ease were rated more highly for women. Another factor to consider is that child sexual abuse, which is more prevalent in women, may pose difficulties for respondents in identifying a "change" since the event, because the event may have occurred at a very young age. In these instances, it may be confusing to inquire about a symptom by having the individual link it to a particular event (most relevant with Criteria C and D). Instead, a measure that does not force the respondent to tie the two together is recommended.

As mentioned earlier, all of the structured interviews for PTSD described below correspond closely with DSM criteria. The structured interviews are summarized in Table 6.2 (see p. 165). The structured interviews are compared based on (1) the type of population on which the scale was validated; (2) whether the instrument allows for assessing multiple events; (3) whether the respondent is required to link Criteria C and D symptoms to a particular trauma; (4) test–retest reliability; (5) sensitivity and specificity; (6) whether the instrument yields a continuous or dichotomous diagnostic output (or both); and (7) whether the responses are rated with behavioral anchors for greater precision.

Self-report measures of PTSD symptoms fall under two categories: (1) those that correspond directly with DSM criteria in order to make diagnostic decisions, and (2) those that are not DSM-correspondent and provide general information regarding PTSD symptoms. Instruments in the latter category should not be used as stand-alone instruments for assessment and diagnosis of PTSD. Their use is recommended for screening purposes or in conjunction with other measures. The self-report measures for PTSD presented in Table 6.3 (see p. 170) are described using the same criteria as PTSD interviews.

Interviews

Structured Clinical Interview for DSM-IV (SCID)

The SCID (Spitzer, Williams, Gibbon, & First, 1995) is a structured interview used for diagnosing a variety of disorders based on DSM Axis I and Axis II disorders, and includes a PTSD module that may be administered separately. It is particularly useful when a thorough assessment of comorbidity is desired, and for comparison with other studies, as it has been frequently used in PTSD studies. The PTSD module was created for use in the National Vietnam Veterans Readjustment Study (NVVRS; Kulka et al., 1990) and has since been used with a variety of military and civilian populations, representing a wide range of traumatic stressors. The SCID includes 17 items corresponding to DSM criteria, plus two items pertaining to guilt. It has demonstrated good reliability and validity in a male combat-veteran population. Test–retest reliability of .93 was reported for the SCID when audiotaped interviews were scored independently by a trained clinician (Kulka et al., 1991). It has been validated against other measures of PTSD, including the Mississippi Scale (.53) and the PK scale of the Minnesota Multiphasic Personality Inventory (MMPI) (.48). Against a composite PTSD diagnosis, sensitivity was .81, and specificity was .98. The SCID is primarily intended for diagnostic purposes only and, as a result, does not provide continuous symptom scores that can be used to detect changes in symptom severity. Another disadvantage is that the instrument does not assess for the frequency or severity of symptoms. Although the SCID does assess multiple traumatic experiences, it asks the individual to respond to the symptom questions regarding the "worst" event experienced. This may potentially result in a loss of important information regarding the effects of other traumas, and therefore result in a significant underestimation of PTSD rates. Also, the SCID includes trauma screening that is not behaviorally specific or sensitive, and is therefore likely to result in many respondents "skipping out" of the PTSD portion of the instrument. A study conducted by Falsetti et al. (1996) found that the SCID traumatic events portion missed a significant number of traumatic events that were otherwise identified by the TAA. Based on these findings, we would recommend using a separate traumatic event assessment measure in conjunction with the SCID PTSD interview. A final disadvantage of the SCID is the emphasis on using only a trained clinician for administering the interview. This can impose serious limitations for research purposes or use in busy clinical settings such as family practice offices.

Diagnostic Interview Schedule (DIS)

The DIS (Robbins, Helzer, Croughan, & Ratcliff, 1981), a more highly structured interview than the SCID, is therefore more suited for use by lay interviewers. Several large-scale epidemiological studies have used variants of the DIS (Breslau, Davis, Andreski, & Peterson, 1991; Kessler et al., 1995; Resnick, Kilpatrick, et al., 1993). The initial validation study with a mixed-gender community sample reported a sensitivity of .87 and a specificity of .73. Subsequently, Kulka and colleagues (1991) examined the validity with combat veterans and found that, against a SCID-based PTSD diagnosis, the specificity was .98 but sensitivity was .22. Although some concerns were raised about the diagnostic utility of this instrument, Weathers and Keane (1999) noted that modifications made by some researchers appear to have successfully improved its diagnostic capability (e.g., Kessler et al., 1995; Resnick, Kilpatrick, et al., 1993). Resnick, Kilpatrick, et al. (1993) modified the DIS for use in an epidemiological study of trauma and PTSD in women by adding several symptom queries to include all DSM-III-R symptoms; eliminating DIS follow-up probes used to determine exclusionary criteria, and did not require respondents to link symptoms to specific traumas. A test–retest reliability coefficient of .45 was reported at a 1-year interval. Like the SCID, the DIS is most useful for studies of comorbidity and cross-study comparisons. The DIS is capable of handling multiple traumas and addresses this by interviewing the respondent on up to three traumas separately. A criticism of this approach is that it requires respondents to decide from which trauma they experience symptoms such as increased irritability and loss of interest in activities. Because of the strict wording and dichotomous score format of interviews like the DIS, it does not appear to be one of the more sensitive measures for addressing the complexities of interviews with female trauma victims.

Composite International Diagnostic Interview (CIDI)

The CIDI (World Health Organization, 1993) is the product of a joint project undertaken by the World Health Organization and the former U.S. Alcohol, Drug Abuse, and Mental Health Administration. It is a comprehensive, standardized instrument for assessment of mental disorders according to the definitions and criteria of ICD-10 and DSM-IV. It is intended for use in epidemiological and cross-cultural studies, as well as for clinical and research purposes. Revisions to the CIDI are carried out by an international advisory committee, both to keep abreast of updates in the diagnostic classification schemes and to improve the reliability and validity of the instrument. The PTSD module of the CIDI was based on the structure of the DIS PTSD module, and is therefore similar in content and format. It is also highly structured, allowing for administration by paraprofessionals. The CIDI inquires about PTSD symptoms for up to three events and provides a dichotomous scoring output. Many of the same criticisms of the DIS apply to the CIDI as well. The instrument was tested in five sites: Amsterdam, Bangalore, Melbourne, St. Louis, and Zagreb (Peters et al., 1996). The validation sample included both men and women who were survivors of natural disasters, accidents, and war, and a general population sample. The internal consistency was .86. The concurrent validity against a PTSD diagnosis made by a clinician was low (kappa = .26). However, the authors reported that this was due to the clinicians' diagnosis being independent of the 1-month time frame required by the DSM-III-R. When the duration criterion was removed, the kappa increased to .55. Further validation studies are recommended with this instrument, because it shows great promise through its multicultural development and validation. However, as with other structured interviews that lack behavioral descriptions, continuous scoring, and clinical judgment, the resulting information provided is limited. The CIDI would be most appropriate for use in conjunction with other measures, and not as a screen for PTSD, due to its potential to underdiagnose.

PTSD Symptom Scale–Interview (PSS-I)

The PSS-I (Foa, Riggs, Dancu, & Rothbaum, 1993) is a structured interview designed to assess DSM-III-R symptoms of PTSD. Excellent reliability and validity have been reported for the PSS-I. Test–retest reliability for the total severity score was .80, and for the diagnosis of PTSD, .91. Compared with the SCID, the PSS-I diagnosed PTSD with a sensitivity of .88, a specificity of .96, and an overall efficiency of .94. The 17 items assess the severity of symptoms that correspond to the diagnostic criteria for PTSD. The scale was initially validated on a population of rape victims but has been used with general clinical samples as well. In addition to the instrument's solid psychometric properties, it has the advantage of being easy to administer and providing dichotomous and continuous scores. The PSS-I was designed to be used by paraprofessional interviewers. A disadvantage is that, like most of the PTSD interviews, the PSS-I requires respondents to link their Criteria C and D symptoms to a particular event. The PSS-I assesses symptoms over just the past 2 weeks, rather than persisting for at least 1 month, which the PTSD diagnostic criteria specify. The instrument does not allow for assessment of lifetime diagnoses and limits the respondent to one event.

Structured Interview for PTSD (SI-PTSD)

The SI-PTSD (Davidson, Smith, & Kudler, 1989) is a structured interview that assesses all 17 PTSD symptoms with an initial prompt question that is followed by behaviorally specific examples for clarification. Behavioral anchors help to reduce ambiguity and potential discrepancies in ratings. Symptoms are rated on a 4-point scale, with items rated as 2 or higher counted as present. The scale allows for making a diagnosis of PTSD, as well as summing severity scores for each item. It can be administered by clinicians or appropriately trained paraprofessionals. Test–retest reliability was reported at .71 and interrater reliability ranged from .97 to .99 within cluster. Diagnostic agreement across raters was 100%. The strong interrater correlations support the idea that using behaviorally specific anchors results in greatly increased agreement. Against the SCID, the sensitivity was .96, and the specificity .80. The reported psychometric data were obtained using a population of war veterans, and no further validation studies have been reported in the literature. The SI-PTSD has, however, been used with various traumatized populations that include both men and women. Although this scale allows for a lifetime diagnosis to be made, presence of lifetime symptoms are based on items that ask for the "worst ever" experience, which does not necessarily imply that all "worst ever" symptoms occurred at the same point in time. A drawback of this instrument is that it is not designed to assess multiple events. It also requires respondents to link Criteria C and D to the one identified event.

Clinician-Administered PTSD Scale (CAPS)

The CAPS (Blake et al., 1990, 1995) was developed at the National Center for PTSD in Boston. The instrument was intended for use by clinicians experienced with PTSD and structured interviewing, but there is some evidence that it can be used by appropriately trained paraprofessionals (Blake et al., 1995). Similar to the SI-PTSD, the CAPS contains behaviorally anchored prompt questions and rating scales that increase the reliability and the confidence in being able to train paraprofessionals in the use of a structured clinical interview. The CAPS assesses up to three events and is the only interview that does not require respondents to link Criteria C and D symptoms to a particular event, which can become quite confusing or impossible with multiple/chronic events. The CAPS was initially validated on a population of combat veterans, although it is commonly used with both males and females. The psychometric properties of the instrument are excellent. An internal consistency of .94 was reported for the 17 PTSD items. Test–retest reliability measured 2–3 days apart varied from .90 to .98. When measured against the SCID PTSD module, the sensitivity was .84 and the specificity .95. The CAPS also correlated .91 with the Mississippi Scale for Combat-Related PTSD. In addition, subscale and total scores for the CAPS have been found to be comparable for African Americans and Caucasians. The CAPS was recently revised to correspond to the DSM-IV. The two versions of this scale include the CAPS-DX, which assesses both past month, current, and lifetime diagnosis, and the CAPS-SX, which is the 1-week symptom status version.

PTSD–Interview (PTSD-I)

The PTSD-I (Watson, Juba, Manifold, Kucala, & Anderson, 1991) is a structured interview that provides queries of the 17 PTSD symptoms with

TABLE 6.2. Structured Interviews for PTSD

Scale	Validation population	Multiple traumas	C and D symptoms linked	Test–retest reliability >.75	Sensitivity and specificity >.80	C/D	Behavioral anchors
SCID	M—veteran	No	Yes	Yes	Yes	D	No
DIS	M/F community	Yes—3	Yes	N/C	No	D	No
CIDI	M/F trauma and community	Yes—3	Yes	No Yes—IC	N/C	D	No
PSS-I	F—rape victims	No	Yes	Yes	Yes	Both	No
SI-PTSD	M—veterans	No	Yes	No IR .97–.99	Yes	Both	Yes
CAPS	M—veterans	Yes—3	No	Yes	Yes	Both	Yes
PTSD-I	M—veterans	No	Yes	Yes	Yes	Both	No

Note. IC, internal consistency reliability; IR, interrater reliability; C/D, continuous/dichotomous diagnostic score; N/C, not completed.

a single prompt question, using a severity rating on a 7-point scale from "no/never" to "extremely/always." Symptoms with ratings of 4 or higher are considered to be present. This interview uses a format that has the respondent make the severity ratings, and therefore more resembles a self-report measure than a structured interview. There is also no rating for lifetime versus current presence of the disorder. Strong reliability and validity has been reported for this scale with male combat veterans. The internal consistency for all 17 items was .92. Test–retest reliability for a 1-week interval was .95. Against a PTSD diagnosis based on the DIS, the sensitivity was .89, the specificity, .94, the efficiency, .92, and the kappa, .84. The PTSD-I has been validated and used primarily with veteran populations. The PTSD-II, designed to correspond with the DSM-IV, is currently under development.

DSM-Correspondent Self-Report Measures

PTSD Symptom Scale—Self-Report (PSS-SR)

The PSS-SR (Foa et al., 1993) is a self-report instrument that is almost identical to the PSS-I, with slight changes in wording. The 17 items corresponding directly to DSM-III-R criteria are scored on a 4-point scale. Like the interview format, this scale assess symptoms over the past 2 weeks. This self-report version has also demonstrated good reliability and validity in a sample of rape victims. Internal consistency of .91 was reported for the 17 items. Test–retest reliability for the total severity over a 1-month period was .74. Against a SCID-based PTSD diagnosis, the sensitivity was .62, the specificity was 1.00, and the efficiency was .86. The authors reported a kappa of .73 for diagnostic agreement between the interview and self-report formats.

Modified PTSD Symptom Scale—Self-Report (MPSS)

The MPSS (Falsetti, Resnick, Resick, & Kilpatrick, 1993) is a modification of the PSS-I developed by Foa et al. (1993). This modified version assesses both frequency and severity of symptoms. The scale consists of 17 items that correspond to DSM-III-R and DSM-IV symptom criteria. Good reliability and validity were reported for the scale in both a community and a clinic sample of men and women. Evidence for internal consistency includes Cronbach's alphas of .96 for the treatment sample and .97 for the community sample. Compared with the SCID, the sensitivity rate was .93 for the treatment sample and .91 for the community sample. The specificity of the scale was .62 in the treatment sample and .84 in the community sample.

The MPSS has been used in many countries outside of the United States and has been translated into several languages including Spanish, French, Arabic, German, Polish, Hindi, and Japanese.

Posttraumatic Stress Diagnostic Scale (PDS)

The PDS (Foa, Cashman, Jaycox, & Perry, 1997) is the first self-report measure to assess all six of the criteria for DSM-IV PTSD. The first two sections include questions regarding possible traumatic events and whether these events qualify as DSM-IV Criterion A stressors. The next section covers all 17 DSM PTSD symptoms, rating each on a 4-point scale of frequency. Following this, the impact of symptoms on various aspects of social and occupational functioning is assessed. The scale allows for both continuous scoring and a dichotomous diagnostic output. The PDS was developed on a population of both males and females who had undergone a variety of traumatic events, including combat, accidents, natural disasters, sexual and nonsexual assault, and other traumatic experiences. The scale has demonstrated good reliability and validity. Internal consistency was demonstrated with an alpha of .92 for the Total Symptom Severity, .78 for Reexperiencing, .84 for Avoidance, and .84 for Arousal. Test–retest reliability was .83 over a 2- to 3-week interval. Against a SCID PTSD diagnosis, sensitivity was reported at .89 and specificity at .75.

PTSD Checklist (PCL)

The PCL (Weathers, Litz, Herman, Huska, & Keane, 1993; Weathers & Ford, 1996) is a 17-item instrument initially based on DSM-III-R criteria but subsequently revised to correspond with DSM-IV criteria. Each item is rated on a 5-point scale that asks how much the respondent was bothered by the symptom in the past month. Three different versions allow for different trauma reference: the civilian version (PCL-C) refers to a stressful experience from the past; the military version (PCL-M) refers to a stressful military experience; and the specific version (PCL-S) refers to a specific stressor identified by the respondent. Excellent reliability and validity have been reported for the scale. Test–retest reliability was .96, with an alpha of .97 over the 17 items. Against a PTSD diagnosis based on the SCID, a cutoff score of 50 on the PCL yielded a sensitivity of .82, a specificity of .83, and a kappa of .64. The scale has been validated with male and female veterans, with 23% of the sample being African American. Comparisons across the two racial groups did not yield significant differences on PCL scores, nor was race by PTSD status interaction significant. These findings provide some support for the comparable use of the PCL with white and African American veteran populations. The scale has been successfully used with other traumatized populations, including breast cancer survivors and motor vehicle accident survivors.

Non-DSM-Correspondent Self-Report Measures

Impact of Event Scale (IES)

The IES (Horowitz, Wilner, & Alvarez, 1979) was the first scale created to assess posttraumatic symptoms. This 15-item instrument assesses symptoms of intrusion and avoidance. The IES items ask the respondent to rate the frequency of symptoms on a 4-point scale. The scale has been validated with a variety of populations, including combat veterans, male and female assault survivors, female sexual assault survivors, natural disaster victims, and accident victims. As with all scales in this section, the IES does not correspond directly with the DSM criteria and therefore cannot be used to make diagnostic decisions. The instrument can be extremely useful as a screener, or to measure symptom changes over time. Good test–retest reliability of .87 for intrusion and .79 for avoidance was reported. Similarly, the internal consistency was demonstrated with an alpha of .79 for intrusion and .82 for avoidance. A revised version of the instrument developed by Weiss and Marmar (1997) added 7 items that assess symptoms of hyperarousal. The revised version assesses 14 of the 17 DSM-IV PTSD symptoms. Construct validity was demonstrated by correlations between the scales of .74 and .87. Although the revisions allow for assessing all three of the PTSD symptom clusters, the revised instrument is not recommended as a stand-alone instrument for making diagnostic decisions, but rather as a screening measure or a tool to measure change in therapy.

Mississippi Scale for Combat-Related PTSD (Mississippi Scale)

The Mississippi Scale (Keane, Caddell, & Taylor, 1988) has been widely used to measure combat related PTSD. It was used in the NVVRS. The scale consists of 35 items rated on a 5-point scale of frequency. Items measure intrusion, avoidance, arousal, and self-persecution. Very good psychometric properties have been reported for the Mississippi Scale. Studies of the psychometric properties of the Mississippi Scale with combat veterans, which have included oversampling for African Americans, have found no racial differences in validity or reliability measures. Although the Mississippi Scale has been used widely with various ethnic populations in the United States, it is unclear whether its psychometric properties are similar for other ethnic minority groups. Internal consistency for the combat-related form was reported to be .94, with a 1-week test–retest reliability of .97. Using a cutoff score of 107, the instrument's sensitivity was .93, and specificity, .89.

A Civilian version of the scale has been developed and mainly includes changes to items that reference military experiences (Vreven, Gudanowski, King, & King, 1995). Twenty-four of the 35 items are identical; for 8 items on the Civilian version, the wording "in the military" or "in the service" was changed to "in the past," and for 3 items, phrases that refer to the military are simply dropped. The civilian version has four additional items that allow for greater correspondence with the DSM-III-R criteria. The instrument is available in English, Dutch, and Spanish. The Civilian version was validated on a community-based sample of 668 nonveterans from the NVVRS. Although reliability of the scale is reportedly good (internal consistency = .86), some questions have been raised regarding convergent and discriminant validity. A revised version of the Civilian Mississippi Scale (R-CMS), developed by Norris and Perilla (1996), is available and validated in English and Spanish. The instrument was validated with two bilingual community samples exposed to Hurricane Andrew. Internal consistency for both the English and Spanish versions is demonstrated by Cronbach's values of .86–.88 for the English, and .88–.92 for the Spanish version. Some support for the instrument's validity comes from findings that rates of PTSD based on the R-CMS increased if the victim had injury or life threat (20% vs. 9%), and increased even more if the victim experienced both (37%).

Crime-Related PTSD Scale (CR-PTSD)

The CR-PTSD (Saunders, Arata, & Kilpatrick, 1990) was empirically derived from the Symptom Checklist 90—Revised (SCL-90-R). Saunders et al. identified 28 items from the SCL-90-R that were capable of discriminating female crime victims with and without PTSD. The CR-PTSD has been reported to have an alpha of .93 and correctly classified 89% of female crime victims as having PTSD. Although not a diagnostic measure, the CR-PTSD can be useful as a supplementary measure of PTSD or in the analysis of archival data.

Harvard Trauma Questionnaire (HTQ)

The HTQ (Mollica et al., 1992) assesses both potentially traumatic events and trauma-related symptoms. The first section assesses 17 different types of potentially traumatic events, including torture, rape, murder, brainwashing, combat situation, and serious lack of food or water. The traumatic events portion of the HTQ is sensitive to many of the traumatic events that refugees and individuals from war-torn regions are likely to have experienced. These events are consistent with the DSM-IV Criterion A, yet are not picked up by the many other available trauma assessment instruments. Originally developed in English, the HTQ has been translated and validated in Vietnamese, Laotian, and Khmer versions. The authors used both forward and backward translation procedures to maximize linguistic equivalence, and discussion groups to enhance the validity of the instrument. This is one of the few instruments developed specifically for each population and culture. Rather than merely translating the items, Mollica et al. recommend approaches that emphasize using clinical expertise, ethnographic studies, and focus groups to identify items. The "core" PTSD items are kept equivalent, yet other features specific to the culture are introduced. Mollica et al. reported good reliability (test–retest = .89; interrater = .93; coefficient alpha = .96) and demonstrated the HTQ's effective use in the field.

ASSOCIATED FEATURES OF THE PTSD CONSTRUCT

Some clinical researchers have argued that the current measures and, in fact, the DSM-IV criteria for PTSD do not fully capture the range of post-traumatic symptomatology, especially for chronic forms of trauma, such as domestic violence, physical abuse, and sexual abuse (Herman, 1992). In addition, others argue that the core beliefs that traumatic events impact, particularly chronic forms of trauma or childhood trauma, are relevant aspects of posttraumatic problems that need to be addressed (Janoff-Bulman, 1992). The core symptoms of PTSD do appear to describe a universal response to trauma, regardless of gender or cultural group. However, the extent to which there are differences for various populations of victimization type, gender, and culture is an area that needs to be more fully examined in the PTSD literature.

TABLE 6.3. Self-Report Measures of PTSD

Scale	Validation population	Multiple traumas	C and D symptoms linked	Reliability >.75	Sensitivity and specific- ity >.80	C/D
PSS-SR	F—rape victims	No	Yes	No	No	Both
MPSS	F—crime victims, community	Unspecified[a]	Yes	Yes	Yes— community	Both
PDS	M/F mixed trauma	No	Yes	Yes	No	Both
PCL	M/F—veterans	Unspecified	No	Yes	Yes	Both
IES	M/F mixed trauma	No	No	Yes	N/A	C
Mississippi	M—veterans	Unspecified	No	Yes	Yes	C
CR-PTSD	F—crime victims	No	Yes	Yes—IC	No	C
HTQ	M/F refugees	Unspecified	No	Yes	No	C

Note. IC, internal consistency reliability; C/D, continuous/dichotomous diagnostic score.

[a]"Unspecified" refers to instruments that do not specify any trauma, so that the symptoms being reported could come from multiple trauma.

There is evidence to indicate that women with a history of incestuous abuse are significantly more likely to dissociate than those without such a history (Dancu, Riggs, Hearst-Ikeda, Shoyer, & Foa, 1996; Strick & Wilcoxon, 1991). Certain characteristics of trauma that are more often present for women (i.e., greater number of perpetrators, greater severity of sexual abuse, more frequent physical abuse, and incest) have been found to relate to higher levels of dissociation (Gershuny & Thayer, 1999). These findings emphasize the need to examine dissociative symptoms in females with a history of incest as well as PTSD. PTSD assessments that include dissociative symptoms as an additional feature are recommended in order to better understand this aspect of incest.

There is also some evidence to indicate that cognitive attributions related to trauma may differ as a function of gender. Two studies have found that victimized women or girls seem to be less likely to attribute blame to the perpetrator and, in fact, are more likely to attribute causal implications to themselves (Fischer, 1992; Hunter, Goodwin, & Wilson, 1992; Janoff-Bulman, 1979; Meyer & Taylor, 1985). Resick (1993) reported findings from a previous study indicating that attributions of self-blame for the rape predicted higher self-criticism scores on a measure of self-esteem. Identification of self-blame early on may have important implications for treatment. Instruments such as the Rape Attribution Questionnaire (Frazier, 1997) can be useful in providing a detailed description of victims' beliefs. Core beliefs about the meaningfulness and benevolence of the world, and self-worth can be assessed with a measure such as the World Assumptions Scale (Janoff-Bullman, 1979). Other important attributional factors to assess in rape victims include the appraisal of safety and the subjective appraisal of threat (Resick, 1993). Rape victims who appraised the situation as safe before the rape occurred report higher fear and depression than those women who perceived the situation as dangerous from the beginning. It has also been noted that a factor *more important* than the presence of weapons, threats, or injuries is the subjective appraisal of threat. This finding is consistent with the DSM-IV changes in Criterion A2, which emphasize the importance of victims' subjective reactions.

CONCLUSIONS AND RECOMMENDATIONS

This chapter has reviewed some of the available instruments for assessing potentially traumatic events and PTSD, in order to help clinicians and researchers evaluate instruments in terms of gender and cultural sensitivity. Several factors have been identified that are important to address when using these measures with both men and women. For the assessment of traumatic events, these include dimensions of the event such as number of occurrences, whether chronic in nature, severity, age, whether interpersonal in nature, and relationship to the perpetrator. In assessing PTSD, we have pointed out dimensions of interviews and self-report instruments that are important when assessing men or women, including rating scales with behavioral anchors, assessment of multiple traumas, and not requiring the respondent to link Criteria C and D symptoms to the trauma.

We have reviewed the specific instruments based on the extent to which they incorporate these criteria and have indicated what we believe are their strengths and weaknesses for men and women. For the assessment of trauma history, although no single instrument fulfills each of the recommended criteria, the TAA, LSC, and THQ address the majority of issues relevant to women. The TAA is unique in its use of event prefaces, as well as multiple questions to capture sexual trauma, and queries that are sensitive to childhood sexual trauma. The LSC is unique in its query of additional experiences (e.g., sexual harassment, witnessing domestic violence) that may prove important for capturing the full range of experiences leading to PTSD, particularly for women. The THQ is very brief and used as a self-report instrument, yet it manages to capture important features such as the relationship to the perpetrator and repetition of events.

For measures of PTSD symptoms, a few of the reviewed measures incorporate those features that are especially relevant to women. For the structured interviews, the CAPS does an excellent job of capturing most of these features. The CAPS addresses multiple traumas, does not require the DSM-IV Criteria C and D symptoms to be linked to a particular trauma, provides both continuous and dichotomous scoring outputs, and uses behavioral anchors in its symptom rating. If a briefer interview is desired, especially when assessing symptoms in response to only one event, instruments such as the PSS-I may be useful. When self-report instruments are used, either in addition to a structured interview or to assess symptom change, the majority of the reviewed instruments are useful with diverse populations. The PCL and MPSS, two instruments that are especially recommended, both have good psychometric properties and can incorporate multiple traumas. In addition, the PCL does not require respondents to link C and D symptoms to their trauma. The MPSS, with its attention to both frequency and severity of symptoms, is unique among the self-report instruments and may be especially helpful as a screener when a complete structured interview is not possible. The HTQ has proven highly useful for assessing the unique experiences of both male and female refugees and displaced persons. The authors' careful attention to language and cultural issues in the development and validation of the instrument provides strong confidence in the HTQ's ability to detect cases of PTSD in this population.

In addition to these recommendations, our review of trauma and PTSD instruments leads us to conclude that further validation of these instruments with diverse populations is warranted. There are currently a number of widely used instruments for both trauma and PTSD. We strongly recommend that what is needed at this time is further psychometric evaluation with these instruments, and to refine them accordingly. We feel that, rather than creating new measures with different populations, there is merit in testing how well the current instruments perform in various populations.

An additional recommendation is the further exploration of associated features of PTSD. While the construct of PTSD does appear to apply universally, it does not appear to incorporate the entire spectrum of disorders commonly seen in both women and men. We believe that future assessment studies should address factors such as attributions regarding the event and beliefs concerning trust, safety, and self-esteem. These factors may differ between men and women. Whereas no single variable will likely explain the gender differences in PTSD, the identification of several powerful moderator variables may increase our understanding of this phenomenon and help to identify how treatment of PTSD should be approached in males and females.

As trauma assessment instruments continue to become more sophisticated in their inclusion of factors associated with greater PTSD risk, questions surrounding gender differences will begin to be answered. Direct comparisons of male and female responses on the same measure, and from the same trauma population, will also add to our understanding of how gender influences response to trauma. Knowing that the same gender differences are not found across trauma types, and that, in fact, among some trauma populations, little or no difference is found, appears to confirm that it is not female gender that is the risk factor for PTSD, but rather some other unique variables. Further advances in the psychometric assessment of trauma and PTSD will hopefully account for findings such as women being 15 times more likely than men to develop PTSD following physical assault (Kessler et al., 1995). Assessing for whether the perpetrator is known (or romantically involved), whether the assault is chronic versus discrete, the degree of injury sustained, and how strongly victims believed they would be seriously hurt or killed may all be important questions that should be included in assessment of trauma and PTSD.

REFERENCES

American Psychiatric Association. (1994). *Diagnostic and statistical manual of mental disorders* (4th ed.). Washington, DC: Author.

Blake, D. D., Weathers, F. W., Nagy, L. M., Kaloupek, D. G., Gusman, F. D., Charney, D. S., & Keane, T. M. (1995). The development of a Clinician-Administered PTSD Scale. *Journal of Traumatic Stress, 8*, 75–90.

Blake, D. D., Weathers, F. W., Nagy, L. M., Kaloupek, D. G., Klauminzer, G., Charney, D. S., & Keane, T. M. (1990). A clinician rating scale for assessing current and lifetime PTSD: The CAPS-1. *Behavior Therapist, 18*, 187–188.

Breslau, N., Davis, G. C., Andreski, P., & Peterson, E. L. (1991). Traumatic events and posttraumatic stress disorder in an urban population of young adults. *Archives of General Psychiatry, 48*, 216–222.

Carlson, E. B. (1997). *Trauma assessments: A clinician's guide.* New York: Guilford Press.

Dancu, C. V., Riggs, D. S., Hearst-Ikeda, D., Shoyer, B. G., & Foa, E. B. (1996). Dissociative experiences and posttraumatic stress disorder among female victims of criminal assault and rape. *Journal of Traumatic Stress, 9(2)*, 253–267.

Davidson, J. R. T., Smith, R. D., & Kudler, H. S. (1989). Validity and reliability of the DSM-III criteria for post-traumatic stress disorder: Experience with a structured interview. *Journal of Nervous and Mental Disease, 177*, 336–341.

Falsetti, S., Resnick, H., Resick, P., & Kilpatrick, D. (1993). The modified PTSD symptom scale: A brief self-report measure of posttraumatic stress disorder. *Behavior Therapist, 16*, 161–162.

Falsetti, S. A., Johnson, M. R., Ware, M. R., Emmanuel, N. J., Mintzer, O., Book, S., Ballenger, J. C., & Lydiard, R. B. (1996, March). *Beyond PTSD: Prevalence of trauma in an anxiety disorders sample.* Paper presented at the 16th annual conference of the Anxiety Disorders Association of America, Orlando, FL.

Fischer, G. J. (1992). Gender differences in college student sexual abuse victims and their offenders. *Annals of Sex Research, 5*, 215–226.

Foa, E. B., Cashman, L., Jaycox, L., & Perry, K. (1997). The validation of a self-report measure of posttraumatic stress disorder: The Posttraumatic Diagnostic Scale. *Psychological Assessment, 9(4)*, 445–451.

Foa, E. B., Riggs, D. S., Dancu, C. V., & Rothbaum, B. O. (1993). Reliability and validity of a brief instrument for assessing post-traumatic stress disorder. *Journal of Traumatic Stress, 6*, 459–473.

Frazier, P. (1997). *Rape Attribution Questionnaire.* Unpublished manuscript.

Gershuny, B. S., & Thayer, J. F. (1999). Relations among psychological trauma, dissociative phenomena, and trauma-related distress: A review and integration. *Clinical Psychology Review, 19*(5), 631–657.

Green, B. (1996). Trauma History Questionnaire. In B. H. Stamm & E. M. Varra (Eds.), *Measurement of stress, trauma and adaptation* (pp. 366–368). Lutherville, MD: Sidran Press.

Herman, J. (1992). *Trauma and recovery.* New York: Basic Books.

Horowitz, M. J., Wilner, N., & Alvarez, W. (1979). Impact of Event Scale: A measure of subjective stress. *Psychosomatic Medicine, 41,* 209–218.

Hunter, J. A., Goodwin, D. W., & Wilson, R. J. (1992). Attributions of blame in child sexual abuse victims: An analysis of age and gender influences. *Journal of Child Sexual Abuse, 1,* 75–89.

Janoff-Bulman, R. (1979). Characterological versus behavioral self-blame: Inquiries into depression and rape. *Journal of Personality and Social Psychology, 37,* 1798–1809.

Janoff-Bulman, R. (1992). *Shattered assumptions: Towards a new psychology of trauma.* New York: Free Press.

Keane, T. M., Caddell, J. M., & Taylor, K. L. (1988). Mississippi Scale for Combat-Related Posttraumatic Stress Disorder: Three studies in reliability and validity. *Journal of Consulting and Clinical Psychology, 56,* 85–90.

Kessler, R. C., Sonnega, A., Bromet, E., Hughes, M., & Nelson, C. B. (1995). Posttraumatic stress disorder in the National Comorbidity Survey. *Archives of General Psychiatry, 52,* 1048–1060.

Kilpatrick, D., Resnick, H., & Freedy, J. (1991). *The Potential Stressful Events Interview.* Unpublished instrument, Medical University of South Carolina, Charleston, SC.

Kilpatrick, D., Resnick, H., Saunders, B., & Best, C. (1989). *The National Women's Study PTSD module.* Unpublished instrument, Medical University of South Carolina, Charleston, SC.

Kilpatrick, D., Resnick, H., Saunders, B., & Best, C. (1998) Rape, other violence against women, and posttraumatic stress disorder. In B. P. Dohrenwend (Ed.), *Adversity, stress, and psychopathology* (pp. 161–176). New York: Oxford University Press.

Kilpatrick, D. G., Saunders, B., Amick-McMullen, A., Best, C. L., Veronen, L., & Resnick, H. (1989). Victim and crime factors associated with the development of posttraumatic stress disorder. *Behavior Therapy, 20,* 199–214.

Kilpatrick, D. G., Veronen, L. J., Saunders, B. E., Best, C. L., Amick-McMullen, A., & Paduhovich, J. (1987). *The psychological impact of crime: A study of randomly surveyed crime victims* (Final report, Grant No. 84–IJ-CX-0039). Washington, DC: National Institute of Justice.

Kimerling, R. (1996). Clinical assessment and diagnosis of traumatic experiences in women. *Journal of Psychological Practice, 2*(4), 34–46.

Koss, M. P. (1985). The hidden rape victim: Personality, attitudinal, and situational characteristics. *Psychology of Women Quarterly, 9,* 193–212.

Kulka, R. A., Schlenger, W. E., Fairbank, J. A., Hough, R. L., Jordan, B. K., Marmar, C. R., & Weiss, D. S. (1990). *Trauma and the Vietnam War generation: Report on the findings from the National Vietnam Veterans Readjustment Study.* New York: Brunner/Mazel.

Kulka, R. A., Schlenger, W. E., Fairbank, J. A., Hough, R. L., Jordan, B. K., Marmar, C. R., & Weiss, D. S. (1991). Assessment of posttraumatic stress disorder in the community: Prospects and pitfalls from recent studies of Vietnam veterans. *Psychological Assessment, 3,* 547–560.

Meyer, C. B., & Taylor, S. E. (1985). Adjustment to rape. *Journal of Personality and Social Psychology, 50,* 1226–1234.

Mollica, R. F., Caspi-Yavin, Y., Bollini, P., Truong, T., Tor, S., & Lavelle, J. (1992). The Harvard Trauma Questionnaire: Validating a cross-cultural instrument for measuring torture, trauma, and posttraumatic stress disorder in Indochinese refugees. *Journal of Nervous and Mental Disease, 180*(2), 111–116.

Norris, F. H. (1990). Screening for traumatic stress: A scale for use in the general population. *Journal of Applied Social Psychology, 20*(2), 1704–1718.

Norris, F. H., & Perilla, J. L. (1996). The revised Civilian Mississippi Scale for PTSD: Reliability, validity, and cross-language stability. *Journal of Traumatic Stress, 9*(2), 285–298.

Norris, F. H., & Riad, J. K. (1997). Standardized self-report measures of civilian trauma and posttraumatic stress disorder. In J. P. Wilson & T. M. Keane (Eds.), *Assessing psychological trauma and PTSD* (pp. 7–42). New York: Guilford Press.

Peters, L., Andrews, G., Cottler, L. B., Chatterji, S., Janca, A., & Smeets, R. M. W. (1996). The Composite International Diagnostic Interview Post-Traumatic Stress Disorder module: Preliminary data. *International Journal of Methods in Psychiatric Research, 6*(3), 167–174.

Resick, P. A. (1993). The psychological impact of rape: Special section: Rape. *Journal of Interpersonal Violence, 8,* 223–255.

Resnick, H. S., Best, C. L., Freedy, J. R., Kilpatrick, D. G., & Falsetti, S. A. (1993). *Trauma Assessment for Adults (TAA).* Unpublished assessment interview.

Resnick, H. S., Falsetti, S. A., Kilptrick, D. G., & Freedy, J. R. (1996). Assessment of rape and other civilian trauma-related PTSD: Emphasis on assessment of potentially traumatic events. In T. Miller (Ed.), *Theory and assessment of stressful life events* (International Universities Press Stress and Health Series, pp. 235–271). Madison, CT: International Universities Press.

Resnick, H. S., Kilpatrick, D. G., Dansky, B. S., Saunders, B. E., & Best, C. L. (1993). Prevalence of civilian trauma and posttraumatic stress disorder in a representative national sample of women. *Journal of Consulting and Clinical Psychology, 61*(6), 984–991.

Robbins, L. N., Helzer, J. E., Croughan, J., & Ratcliff, K. S. (1981). National Institute of Mental Health Diagnostic Interview Schedule: Its history, characteristics, and validity. *Journal of Applied Social Psychology, 16,* 464–481.

Saunders, B. E., Arata, C. M., & Kilpatrick, D. G. (1990). Development of a Crime-Related Posttraumatic Stress Disorder Scale for women within the Symptom Checklist—90–Revised. *Journal of Traumatic Stress, 3,* 439–448.

Saunders, B. E., Kilpatrick, D. G., Resnick, H. S., & Tidwell, R. P. (1989). Brief screening for lifetime history of criminal victimization at mental health intake: A preliminary study. *Journal of Interpersonal Violence, 4,* 267–277.

Solomon, S. D., Keane, T. M., Newman, E., & Kaloupek, D. G. (1996). Choosing self-report measures and structured interviews. In E. B. Carlson (Ed.), *Trauma research methodology.* Lutherville, MD: Sidran Press.

Spitzer, R. L., Williams, J. B. W., Gibbon, M., & First, M. B. (1995). *Structured Clini-*

cal Interview for DSM-IV—Patient Version. New York: Biometric Research Department, New York State Psychiatric Institute.

Strick, F. L., & Wilcoxon, S. A. (1991). A comparison of dissociative experiences in adult female outpatients with and without histories of early incestuous abuse. *Dissociation, 4*(4), 193–199.

Vreven, D. L., Gudanowski, D. M., King, L. A., & King, D. W. (1995). The Civilian version of the Mississippi PTSD Scale: A psychometric evaluation. *Journal of Traumatic Stress, 8,* 91–109.

Watson, C. G., Juba, M. P., Manifold, V., Kucala, T., & Anderson, P. E. D. (1991). The PTSD interview: Rationale, description, reliability, and concurrent validity of a DSM-III-based technique. *Journal of Consulting and Clinical Psychology, 47,* 179–188.

Weathers, F., & Ford, J. (1996). Psychometric review of PTSD Checklist. In B. H. Stamm (Ed.). *Measurement of stress, trauma, and adaptation.* Lutherville, MD: Sidran Press.

Weathers, F. W., & Keane, T. M. (1999). Psychological assessment of traumatized adults. In P. A. Saigh & J. D. Bremner (Eds.), *Posttraumatic stress disorder: A comprehensive text* (pp. 219–247). Boston, MA: Allyn & Bacon.

Weathers, F. W., Litz, B. T., Herman, D. S., Huska, J. A., & Keane, T. M. (1993). *The PTSD Checklist (PCL): Reliability, validity, and diagnostic utility.* Paper presented at the 9th annual conference of the ISTSS, San Antonio, TX.

Weiss, D. S., & Marmar, C. R. (1997). The impact of event scale-revised. In J. P. Wilson & T. M. Keane (Eds.), *Assessing psychological trauma and PTSD* (pp. 399–411). New York: Guilford Press.

Wolfe, J., & Kimerling, R. (1997). Gender issues in the assessment of PTSD. In J. P. Wilson & T. M. Keane (Eds.), *Assessing psychological trauma and PTSD* (pp. 192–238). New York: Guilford Press.

World Health Organization. (1993). *Composite international diagnostic interview—Version 1.1.* Geneva: Author.

Yehuda, R., Schmeidler, J., Siever, L. J., Binder-Brynes, K., & Elkin, A. (1997). Individual differences in posttraumatic stress disorder symptom profiles in Holocaust survivors in concentration camps or in hiding. *Journal of Traumatic Stress, 10*(3), 453–463.

7 | Gender and Psychophysiology of PTSD

JESSICA M. PEIRCE
TAMARA L. NEWTON
TODD C. BUCKLEY
TERENCE M. KEANE

For many men and women, traumatic life events exact a dramatic and sometimes enduring toll on emotional functioning. As one example, even when encountered months or years after a traumatic event, life experiences that are reminiscent of the event may revivify traumatic emotion and generate increases in heart rate, muscle tension, and other autonomic functions. Indeed, elevated autonomic responses to trauma-reminiscent "cues" are a hallmark characteristic of posttraumatic stress disorder (PTSD) that develops in the wake of overwhelming life events such as combat or rape (e.g., Kardiner, 1941).

Historically, psychophysiological studies of autonomic responses played a critical role in the emerging science of PTSD, providing empirical validation for patients' clinical reports of heightened physical stress and tension (Blanchard & Buckley, 1999). Psychophysiology is likely to play an equally important role in shaping future scientific inquiry into some of the central questions about PTSD, including its clinical course, responsiveness to clinical interventions, and accompanying medical comorbidities. For instance, psychophysiological responses are recognized as potentially important prospective predictors of emotional sequelae and clinical status following traumatic exposure (e.g., Blanchard et al., 1996), and preliminary evidence suggests they may be valuable process indicators of psychological treatment efficacy (e.g., Pitman et al., 1996). In addition, exaggerated cardiovascular responses to psychological stressors are identified as potential contributors to physical morbidity and mortality, particularly cardiovascular diseases such as atherosclerosis and elevated blood pressure (e.g., Barnett, Spence,

Manuck, & Jennings, 1997). Thus, psychophysiology may be central to mapping the processes that contribute to the emerging links among traumatic stress exposure, PTSD, and compromised physical health status (e.g., Schnurr & Jankowski, 1999). Finally, and perhaps most fundamentally, psychophysiological responses are one element of a more broadly integrated construct of emotional functioning, making them key to any comprehensive understanding of the alterations in basic emotional dynamics that are so pervasive in PTSD, particularly in its chronic forms.

Within this context, the present chapter considers the scientific literature on gender and psychophysiology of PTSD among adults. Although there is a sizable empirical literature on the psychophysiological responses of men with PTSD, empirical study of the psychophysiology of PTSD among women is relatively new. Thus, one aim of this present chapter is to comprehensively review studies of the psychophysiology of adult women with PTSD, including the few studies that have included both men and women. In addition, drawing upon the stress and emotion literature more broadly, we consider a triad of biopsychosocial factors important for a comprehensive understanding of the gender and psychophysiology of PTSD. This biopsychosocial triad—reproductive hormones, emotions and coping, and chronic environmental strain—has implications for understanding the autonomic consequences of trauma-reminiscent experiences and the health consequences of exaggerated autonomic responding, and for investigations designed to illuminate gender differences in the psychophysiology of PTSD. Finally, drawing from this literature review, we make recommendations for the next generation of research on gender and the psychophysiology of PTSD.

PSYCHOPHYSIOLOGY OF PTSD: A BRIEF HISTORY AND OVERVIEW

Prior to formal recognition of PTSD as a diagnostic entity, the sequelae of combat trauma exposure were described as irritable heart, shell shock, or war neurosis. Many reports of these disorders referred to elevated autonomic arousal as part of the symptom profile. Dobbs and Wilson (1960) provided the seminal laboratory examination of this phenomenon when they examined heart rate (HR), respiration rate, and electroencephalograph (EEG) responses of World War II and Korean combat veterans, and a comparison group of university students, while participants were exposed to simulated combat sounds. The combat veterans had higher baseline levels of HR and respiration rate and also showed a greater magnitude of cardiac response to the combat sounds than the students.

Subsequent studies explored the relationship between PTSD diagnostic status and physiological reactivity in cue reactivity paradigms with a PTSD group, a trauma-exposed non-PTSD comparison group, and occasionally, a non-trauma-exposed comparison group. Procedurally, participants in these studies were presented with a variety of trauma- and non-trauma-related stimuli while their peripheral physiological responses were recorded. Independent laboratories replicated the general finding that, relative to those in comparison groups, individuals diagnosed with PTSD showed elevated physiological responses to trauma-related stimuli. This was observed across multiple physiological indicators, including cardiovascular, electrodermal, and muscle tension reactivity (e.g., Pitman, Orr, Forgue, de Jong, & Claiborn, 1987). As a whole, these early studies indicated that the elevated autonomic arousal associated with PTSD was fairly specific to trauma-related stimuli and did not generalize to all classes of stimuli (e.g., Pitman et al., 1987).

In the ensuing years, empirical studies across populations, laboratories, and experimental methods have consistently demonstrated that when compared to PTSD diagnoses obtained through the use of structured interviews, autonomic reactivity measures discriminate between cases and noncases with sensitivity and specificity greater than .70. Thus, researchers have argued that physiological responses to trauma-related cues may be a useful adjunct to standard assessment procedures (e.g., Blanchard & Buckley, 1999).

More recently, investigators pursuing an independent line of research have sought to validate the clinical observation that individuals diagnosed with PTSD demonstrate an enhanced *startle* response to external stimuli. The evidence for this phenomenon has been less persuasive than the cue reactivity research; some studies have found evidence for exaggerated startle responses (Orr, Lasko, Shalev, & Pitman, 1995), whereas others fail to find support for the phenomenon (Grillon, Morgan, Southwick, Davis, & Charney, 1996). Recent work has focused on how the startle response, which is primarily mediated by brainstem neural circuitry (LeDoux, 1990), is modulated by higher cortical influences, such as negative emotional states induced by the presence of explicit threat cues (Grillon, Morgan, Davis, & Southwick, 1998). It may be that elevated startle responses and autonomic reactivity to trauma-related cues are functionally related. For example, priming negative affective states with exposure to trauma-related cues may potentiate startle responses to neutral stimuli.

APPLICATIONS OF PSYCHOPHYSIOLOGY: CLINICAL STATUS, TREATMENT EFFICACY, AND CARDIOVASCULAR HEALTH

In addition to its role in assessment and symptom validation, psychophysiological measurement has the potential to yield important information in applied domains, including predicting the clinical course of PTSD and indexing the efficacy of clinical interventions designed to ameliorate its symptoms. In addition, because exaggerated cardiovascular responses to psychological stressors have been identified as potential contributors to physical morbidity and mortality, psychophysiological studies of PTSD may be essential to understanding linkages among traumatic stress exposure, PTSD, and compromised physical health status (Schnurr & Jankowski, 1999).

Prediction of Clinical Status and Response to Treatment

Assessment of physiological responses may have utility in predicting at-risk individuals immediately after trauma exposure. For example, Blanchard et al. (1996) found that cardiac response to trauma-related cues in the months shortly after a motor vehicle accident (MVA) predicted future clinical PTSD status 12 months posttrauma. MVA survivors who showed the greatest cardiac reactivity to trauma cues shortly after a traumatic event were those with the highest probability of meeting diagnostic criteria for PTSD at a 12-month follow-up. Similarly, elevated resting HR assessed during the acute posttrauma period predicted PTSD at 1 month (Shalev et al., 1998) and 6 months after the trauma (Bryant, Harvey, Guthrie, & Moulds, 2000).

In addition to predicting follow-up clinical status, physiological response to trauma-related cues may also index treatment response. Many contemporary behavioral and cognitive-behavioral accounts of anxiety or PTSD assert that physiological arousal and diminution of response to trauma-related cues are key markers for monitoring the efficacy of intervention (e.g., Foa, Steketee, & Rothbaum, 1989). Accordingly, some investigators have examined whether physiological reactivity to relevant cues and reduction in such responses during the course of treatment are associated with positive clinical outcomes with PTSD patients. Although the data are limited, existing studies suggest that psychophysiological responses measured during the course of treatment may have predictive utility (Blanchard & Buckley, 1999). Preliminary data suggest that combined within- and between-session reductions in physiological responses to trauma-related stimuli may predict more favorable improvements in clinical status (Pitman et al., 1996).

Cardiovascular Health

PTSD has been associated with increased incidence of myocardial infarction and elevated frequency of atrioventricular conduction problems (Boscarino & Chang, 1999), along with lower HR variability (Cohen et al., 1997), a risk factor for increased risk for mortality from cardiovascular events (Odemuyiwa et al., 1991). The potential for psychophysiological assessment to illuminate linkages between PTSD and cardiac disease, and perhaps other medical conditions, is highlighted by laboratory and epidemiological investigations outside the domain of traumatic stress studies.

For example, elevated resting HR and blood pressure have been linked with future cardiovascular morbidity and mortality (e.g., Greenland et al., 1999). Other prospective, longitudinal studies have documented associations between elevated cardiovascular reactivity to mental and behavioral stressors, and occurrence of future blood pressure elevations (Matthews, Woodall, & Allen, 1993), hypertension (Menkes et al., 1989), coronary heart disease (Keys, Taylor, Blackburn, Anderson, & Somonson, 1971), and progression of carotid artery disease (Barnett et al., 1997). Exaggerated reactivity may also play a role in poor health more generally, including increased occurrence of minor infectious illnesses among otherwise healthy young adults (Dembroski, MacDougall, Slatts, Eliot, & Buell, 1981). These findings do not conclusively establish that cardiovascular parameters play a causal role in disease (e.g., reactivity may be a biological diathesis that promotes disease only when accompanied by stress exposure, or a marker for other cardiovascular disease risks), but they nonetheless highlight the role of psychophysiological assessment in evaluating pathways leading from stress to health outcomes (e.g., Boyce et al., 1995).

Results of these studies with nontraumatized populations suggest that connections among PTSD, cardiovascular parameters, and relevant health outcomes should be explored. When compared to individuals in control groups, both men and women diagnosed with PTSD show elevated cardiovascular responses to trauma-reminiscent cues (Pitman et al., 1987), along with elevated ambulatory and resting cardiovascular levels, particularly HR and, to a lesser extent, blood pressure (e.g., Keane et al., 1998; Orr, Lasko, et al., 1998). Although other studies have not found statistically significant group mean differences (e.g., Orr, Meyerhoff, Edwards, & Pitman, 1998), a recent meta-analysis of 34 studies found that, relative to individuals without PTSD, individuals diagnosed with PTSD have elevated resting HR and diastolic blood pressure (DBP) levels (Buckley & Kaloupek, 2001).

Speculatively, recurrent adrenergic response to stressful environmental cues and chronic physiological hyperactivation among individuals with PTSD may contribute to cardiovascular disease risk, perhaps by generating functional and morphological changes in the cardiovascular system (e.g., Blascovich & Katkin, 1993). Researchers are also beginning to examine the effect of PTSD on health outcomes in a variety of organ systems besides the cardiovascular system (e.g., Schnurr, Spiro, & Paris, 2000). Psychophysiological investigations that assess the impact of PTSD on sympathetic nervous system and neuroendocrine responses to environmental demands will clearly have a role in ascertaining the functional mechanisms by which PTSD becomes associated with poor health outcomes.

PSYCHOPHYSIOLOGY OF PTSD IN WOMEN

The assessment of physiological responses to both trauma-related and neutral stimuli has enhanced understanding of PTSD symptom presentation and can be a meaningful component of the comprehensive assessment of PTSD (Keane, Weathers, & Foa, 2000). In addition, emerging areas of inquiry highlight the relevance of psychophysiological assessment for understanding the course of PTSD, its responsiveness to mental health interventions, and its physical health correlates. However, the vast majority of psychophysiological studies of PTSD have been conducted with adult male participants; psychophysiological studies of women with PTSD began to appear in the early 1990s (e.g., Resnick, Kilpatrick, & Lipovsky, 1991). To date, approximately eight studies have examined autonomic reactivity and acoustic startle response in adult women with PTSD. We review this literature with a focus on two questions: (1) Do women with PTSD demonstrate elevated psychophysiological responding when compared to women without PTSD? (2) Do women with PTSD demonstrate the same pattern and magnitude of psychophysiological response as men with PTSD?

Psychophysiological Responding in Women with and without PTSD

Overall, when exposed to trauma-related cues, women with current PTSD demonstrate heightened psychophysiological levels (i.e., absolute response levels during cue exposure) and reactivity (i.e., increase from resting baseline) compared to women with lifetime occurrence of PTSD (i.e., women who once met but no longer meet diagnostic criteria), or women who never developed PTSD. As detailed later, group differences are exhibited in response to both trauma cues and startle probes, and across a variety of psychophysiological channels, including HR, skin conductance (SC), blood pressure, and muscle tension. A few studies, however, have failed to replicate group differences in psychophysiological responding.

In a study of women exposed to war-zone stressors in Vietnam, HR, SC, and systolic (SBP) and diastolic blood pressure (DBP) were measured during presentation of neutral and standardized Vietnam war-zone cues (Wolfe et al., 2000). On average, women with current war-zone-related PTSD exhibited significantly greater SC levels and SBP reactivity to the war-related cues than women who had never developed PTSD. The psychophysiological responses of the lifetime PTSD group generally fell between those of the other two groups. In another study of women Vietnam veterans, Carson et al. (2000) limited their sample to nurses who witnessed severe injury or death. Women with current PTSD were compared to women with no history of PTSD on HR, SC, and lateral frontalis and corrugator electromyogram (EMG) responses to audiotaped scripts of personalized and standard war-zone nursing scenes, as well as scripts with positive and neutral content. The PTSD group demonstrated greater HR, SC, and lateral frontalis EMG reactivity to both the personalized and standard trauma scripts than the group with no history of PTSD. Furthermore, women with PTSD showed greater HR and corrugator EMG reactivity to the personalized scripts than women without PTSD, despite both groups reporting equivalent emotional responses to the scripts (e.g., sadness and disgust). In addition, using an a priori discriminant function derived from psychophysiological studies conducted primarily with male participants (e.g., Pitman et al., 1987), the authors successfully classified 76% of the women with PTSD as responders (sensitivity) and 81% of women without PTSD as nonresponders (specificity).

Examining the effects of PTSD related to childhood sexual abuse, Orr, Lasko, et al. (1998) recorded the HR, SC, and EMG of women with current PTSD, women with lifetime PTSD, and women with a history of childhood sexual abuse who had never developed PTSD. Women with current PTSD exhibited higher HR during individually tailored imagery of their sexual abuse than did women in the other groups; they also manifested higher corrugator EMG levels than the women who never developed PTSD. Utilizing the same discriminant function described earlier, the authors found moderate levels of sensitivity (66%) and high levels of specificity (78%).

In contrast to these studies, two cue reactivity investigations failed to find consistent patterns of psychophysiological responding to trauma-related stimuli in women. Peirce et al. (1996) examined HR, SBP and DBP, SC, skin temperature, and lateral frontalis EMG response to standardized sexual assault cues in women with lifetime sexual assault-related PTSD, and women with no history of sexual assault-related PTSD (although some had sexual assault histories). There were no group differences in reactivity or absolute levels of any psychophysiological variable, although the lifetime PTSD group reported stronger negative emotional responses (e.g., angry, unhappy) to the trauma cues than did the control group. Lifetime rather than current PTSD status, use of standardized as opposed to idiographic cues, and population characteristics (e.g., all women had taken methadone prior to the study session) may account for the absence of group differences. Kilpatrick, Best, Ruff, and Veronen (1984) studied rape victims' HR and SC responses to rape-related fear scenes (e.g., walking past men, etc.). They found little elevation in HR or SC arousal to these scripts, perhaps because the scripts were not sufficiently potent cues.

Finally, several studies have examined the acoustic startle reflex in women with PTSD, with mixed results. In a study comparing women with current sexual assault–related PTSD to women who were never assaulted and had no history of PTSD, women with PTSD exhibited greater eyeblink responses in the left eye than the right, whereas women in the comparison group exhibited symmetrical eyeblink responses (Morgan, Grillon, Lubin, & Southwick, 1997). In addition, women with recent PTSD (from adult sexual assault) exhibited greater left eyeblink reflexes than those with long-standing PTSD (from childhood or adolescent sexual assault). The authors suggested that the effects of PTSD on startle reflex pathways may subside over time. Another interpretation is that early trauma may affect the development of startle reflexes differently than later trauma. In contrast, eyeblink responses to acoustic startle probes did not differentiate women with current childhood sexual abuse-related PTSD, women with lifetime PTSD, and women with childhood sexual abuse who never developed PTSD (Metzger et al., 1999). However, women with current or lifetime PTSD had greater HR reactivity and slower habituation of SC responses to startling tones than women who never developed PTSD (Metzger et al., 1999). Among former Vietnam War nurse veterans, eyeblink response, SC reactivity, and SC habituation rate in response to startling tones failed to differentiate women with war-zone-related PTSD, women with lifetime PTSD, and women who never developed PTSD (Carson et al., 1999). Women with current PTSD demonstrated greater HR reactivity to startling tones than did the other two groups.

Psychophysiological Responding in Men and Women with PTSD

Most investigators who have included both men and women in psycho-physiological studies of PTSD have neither compared men's and women's responding nor reported results by gender (e.g., Blanchard et al., 1996). To our knowledge, only two studies of the psychophysiology of PTSD have compared results by gender.

In a study of Israeli men and women, HR, SC, and frontalis EMG reactivity to personalized scripts involving trauma-related imagery were assessed in individuals with current non-combat-related PTSD, and individuals with no history of PTSD (Shalev, Orr, & Pitman, 1993). Across gender, participants with PTSD showed greater HR and EMG reactivity to the trauma imagery than participants with no history of PTSD. Although gender comparisons were not statistically significant, women with PTSD exhibited 33% higher physiological responding than men with PTSD (differences on specific physiological channels were not reported). A second study also assessed Israeli civilians, with and without PTSD, who had experienced repeated Iraqi missile attacks during the Gulf War (Laor et al., 1999). Compared to individuals without PTSD, those with PTSD demonstrated greater HR, SBP, and DBP reactivity to a standardized, trauma-related script (i.e., a radio transmission broadcast during the original missile attack). Participants with PTSD did not respond differently from those without PTSD to positive (i.e., ocean waves), action (i.e., police car chase), neutral (i.e., party chatter) or fear (i.e., child screaming with dogs barking) scripts. The authors found neither a main effect of gender nor an interaction of PTSD with gender on psychophysiological responding. Although limited to two studies, these findings suggest that men and women with PTSD respond similarly to trauma cues across psychophysiological systems.

Summary and Conclusions

Psychophysiological studies suggest that women with current PTSD do experience heightened responding compared to trauma-exposed women who never developed PTSD, as well as women without trauma histories. In some cases, women with current PTSD showed greater reactivity than did women with lifetime PTSD. The majority of these small studies support the presence of HR and SC reactivity, both in response to traumatic event cues (e.g., Wolfe et al., 2000) and to acoustic startle probes (e.g., Metzger et al., 1999). Preliminary evidence suggests that facial EMG may be another useful indicator of differences between women with and without PTSD (e.g., Orr, Lasko, et al., 1998).

Although two studies did not find PTSD group differences in HR and SC responding (e.g., Peirce et al., 1996), several possibilities might explain this discrepancy. Both studies were hampered by methodological limitations, including unique population characteristics and the use of cues that were standardized or otherwise not specific to PTSD events. Furthermore, these two disconfirming studies may mirror the literature on men, in which approximately 30–40% of men with PTSD are "nonresponders" who fail to exhibit psychophysiological reactivity to trauma-related cues (Keane et al., 1998). The relatively new research on the nonresponse phenomenon has examined the influence of participants' psychological traits, symptoms, and comorbid conditions, any of which could be operative in psychophysiological studies of women.

Acoustic startle studies have so far been inconsistent in their results, with some finding that women with PTSD demonstrate exaggerated eyeblink response to startle stimuli (Morgan et al., 1997) and others finding no group differences (e.g., Metzger et al., 1999). Previous research with men has produced similarly inconsistent results, although researchers have begun to suggest factors that may contribute to this inconsistency (Shalev, Peri, Orr, Bonne, & Pitman, 1997).

With regard to gender comparisons—whether men and women with PTSD exhibit similar patterns of psychophysiological responding—the two relevant studies reviewed found no statistically significant gender differences (Laor et al., 1999; Shalev et al., 1993). Furthermore, two other studies provide indirect support of gender similarities: Carson et al. (2000) and Orr, Lasko, et al. (1998) cross-validated their psychophysiological assessment in women using a discriminant function drawn from a male-dominant sample. In summary, preliminary evidence indicates that both men and women exhibit similarly enhanced psychophysiological reactivity when presented with trauma-reminiscent cues, but relevant studies are few in number and additional research is needed to substantiate these findings.

GENDER AND THE BIOPSYCHOSOCIAL TRIAD: REPRODUCTIVE HORMONES, EMOTION AND COPING, AND CHRONIC ENVIRONMENTAL STRAIN

It is well established that psychophysiological responses are influenced by the combined effects of biological, psychological, and social factors (e.g., Jackson, Treiber, Turner, Davis, & Strong, 1999). Drawing on the stress and emotion literature more broadly, we consider a triad of gender-linked biopsychosocial factors that are important for a thorough understanding of gender and the psychophysiology of PTSD: (1) reproductive hormones, (2) emotions and coping, and (3) chronic environmental strain. This biopsychosocial triad has implications for the autonomic consequences of trauma-reminiscent experiences and the health consequences of exaggerated autonomic responding, and may also be important in investigations designed to illuminate potential gender differences in the psychophysiology of PTSD.

Hormonal Correlates of Women's Cardiovascular Stress Responses

Among healthy adults, there are both similarities and differences in men's and women's cardiovascular and neuroendocrine responses to acute laboratory stressors (Stoney, Davis, & Matthews, 1987). In general, men and women show similar DBP, urinary norepinephrine, and cortisol responses. In contrast, gender differences are apparent for HR, SBP, and urinary epinephrine; women show the higher resting HRs and tend to show greater HR reactivity, whereas men show the higher resting SBP, SBP reactivity, and urinary epinephrine. It has been hypothesized that differences in men's and women's levels of circulating reproductive hormones (i.e., estrogen, progesterone) may provide a plausible basis for these observed gender differences in cardiovascular reactivity; for example, there are estrogen receptors in the myocardium, and estrogen potentiates certain mechanisms of vasodilation (Gilligan, Quyyumi, & Cannon, 1994; Legato, 1997). This hypothesis has been evaluated by a number of studies that directly and indirectly examined the role of reproductive hormones in cardiovascular reactivity.

Menstrual Cycle

The normal female menstrual cycle, with its cyclic alterations in estrogen, progesterone, follicle-stimulating and luteinizing hormones, has been used as a natural experiment to assess the role of hormones in women's cardiovascular reactivity. The most rigorous investigations verify menstrual cycle phase by using serum assays of multiple hormones, as opposed to less reliable approaches, such as basal body temperature, self-report, or estradiol assays only (Stoney, Owens, Matthews, Davis, & Caggiula, 1990).

In general, studies that have employed this stringent method find no significant menstrual cycle phase effects (luteal vs. follicular, or vs. menstrual, or both) for blood pressure or HR reactivity to laboratory stressors (e.g., Stoney et al., 1990), although there are exceptions (e.g., Miller & Sita, 1994). However, these null effects for menstrual cycle phase do not mean that reproductive hormones are unrelated to women's acute cardiovascular stress responses. When serum estradiol and progesterone were directly assayed, higher levels of circulating progesterone were associated with lower DBP reactivity, and higher levels of estradiol were associated with lower HR and SBP reactivity (Sita & Miller, 1996). At the same time, there were no main effects of menstrual cycle phase on cardiovascular responses. Thus, there are relationships between reproductive hormones and cardiovascular responses to stress, but these relationships do not appear to culminate in reliable menstrual cycle phase effects on reactivity. One possible exception to this concerns hemodynamic measures (e.g., cardiac output, total peripheral resistance). Some evidence suggests that these measures do vary by menstrual cycle phase (although the reasons for this are unclear), even when BP and HR are statistically equivalent across phases (e.g., Miller & Sita, 1994).

Natural, Surgical, and Experimentally Induced Menopause

Biologically, natural menopause refers to the cessation of menses and is characterized by various hormonal changes, including declines in estradiol levels. A number of studies have tested associations between naturally occurring menopausal status and psychophysiological reactivity to acute laboratory stressors among normal women. The most rigorous studies ascertain menopausal status via serum hormone assays. Two studies reported no association between menopausal status and either cardiovascular resting levels (Blumenthal et al., 1991; Saab, Matthews, Stoney, & McDonald, 1989), or reactivity to laboratory stressors (Blumenthal et al., 1991), whereas Stoney (1999) reported higher resting and task HR among premenopausal women as opposed to postmenopausal women. In contrast, other evidence suggests that postmenopausal women exhibit greater HR and blood pressure reactivity than premenopausal women, but effects are contingent on the laboratory stressor employed (e.g., Saab et al., 1989). In the one study that included men, there was evidence that postmenopausal women's SBP and DBP responses exceeded those of men (Owens, Stoney, & Matthews, 1993). This suggests that women's postmenopausal status may reverse the well-documented gender patterns for SBP (i.e., that men's reactivity is greater than women's) and DBP reactivity (i.e., no gender differences; Stoney et al., 1987). In summary, there is conflicting evidence regarding associations between menopausal status and stress reactivity, but only a few studies have examined this issue. Inconsistencies could reflect a number of factors, including age differences between selected groups of pre- and postmenopausal women, the effects of early versus late menopause, or unobserved differences in underlying hormonal status.

In other approaches to assessing the role of women's reproductive hormones in cardiovascular responses, the effects of either surgically or pharmacologically induced menopause have been examined. In one study, women who underwent a hysterectomy with removal of the ovaries showed greater blood pressure reactivity than women who underwent a hysterectomy without removal of the ovaries (Stoney, Owens, Guzick, & Matthews, 1997). This provides indirect support for the role of reproductive hormones in cardiovascular reactivity, because surgical removal of the ovaries results in a greater decline in circulating ovarian hormones than does hysterectomy alone. Contrasting results were obtained in a study that examined effects of pharmacological suppression of ovarian hormones on stress reactivity of premenopausal women (Matthews, Berga, Owens, & Flory, 1998). Contrary to expectations, experimental suppression of ovarian hormone levels was not related to variations in cardiovascular responses to acute laboratory stressors.

Exogenous Estrogens: Oral Contraceptives and Hormone Replacement

Women's oral contraceptive use has been associated with altered resting cardiovascular parameters, including lower DBP and total peripheral resistance, and higher cardiac output, stroke volume, and SBP (Davis, 1999). Cardiovascular reactivity does not appear to be associated with oral contraceptive use among nonsmokers. However, the combined effects of being a smoker and using oral contraceptives are associated with significantly higher blood pressure reactivity (Davis, 1999). One study did fail to replicate the increase in cardiovascular reactivity among women who smoke and use oral contraceptives (Girdler, Jamner, Jarvik, Soles, & Shapiro, 1997). Interestingly, however, this study examined smokers and nonsmokers of both genders, and found that being a smoker was related to cardiovascular reactivity only among females; the cardiovascular responses of male smokers and nonsmokers did not differ. This is consistent with other reports that women's heart rate and blood pressure responses to smoking exceed those of men's (Stone, Dembroski, Costa, & MacDougall, 1990).

With regard to hormone replacement therapy (HRT) among postmenopausal women, some studies suggest that HRT is associated with attenuated cardiovascular reactivity (e.g., Collins et al., 1982), whereas other studies report that HRT is associated with greater reactivity (Burleson et al., 1998). Inconsistencies could be due to a variety of methodological factors, including duration of HRT use and differences in HRT administration (oral vs. transdermal patch) that affect delivery and metabolic pathways (Burleson et al., 1998).

Summary and Implications

Among healthy adults not selected for trauma exposure, there is preliminary evidence that certain reproductive hormones affect women's cardiovascular reactivity to acute stressors. Higher circulating levels of estrogen and progesterone have been associated with blunted reactivity. When hormonal levels are reduced due to menopause, women show cardiovascular hyperreactivity in some cases, and one commonly observed gender difference (i.e., SBP reactivity greater among men than women) reverses. With regard to exogenous hormones, oral contraceptive use increases acute reactivity among women who also smoke. The acute reactivity consequences of HRT are harder to evaluate, because the few studies that have been conducted vary greatly in important methodological parameters.

These studies raise a number of important substantive and methodological considerations for research on gender and the psychophysiology of traumatic exposure and PTSD. For example, among women with PTSD, cardiovascular reactivity to trauma-related stimuli may be magnified postmenopause, and with the use of certain exogenous hormones. To the extent that elevated reactivity plays a role in subsequent cardiac disease (e.g., Barnett et al., 1997), these life transitions and health behaviors could contribute to elevated risks for poorer health among women with traumatic stress exposures (e.g., Golding, 1994). This hypothesis should be explored empirically. In addition, smoking status may be particularly relevant to the cardiovascular regulation of women with PTSD, and even more so among women who use oral contraceptives. This topic deserves increased attention given the high prevalence of smoking among women with histories of victimization and PTSD (Acierno, Kilpatrick, Resnick, Saunders, & Best, 1996).

Another consideration of particular relevance for women with PTSD concerns the role of hormonal and menstrual cycle irregularities in cardiovascular dysregulation. In the studies cited earlier, potential participants with hormonal and self-reported menstrual cycle irregularities were carefully identified and excluded from participation. For example, Stoney et al. (1990) had participants evaluate their menstrual cycle patterns for 3–6 months prior to the laboratory session. One-fourth of the women initially eligible were eventually excluded due to menstrual cycle irregularities observed during this presession monitoring. Consequently, the generally null effects of menstrual cycle phase and reactivity cannot safely be generalized to women with detectable menstrual irregularities, including alterations in both hormonal level and time course. This is particularly relevant to women with histories of trauma exposure given the documented associations between trauma exposure and menstrual irregularities; community surveys indicate that these problems are up to twice as prevalent among women who have been sexually victimized (Golding, 1996). Moreover, provocative preliminary data suggest that women's premenstrual syndromes, including premenstrual dysphoric disorders, are associated with cardiovascular dysregulation characterized by a mixed pattern of hyper- and hyporeactivity compared to controls (e.g., Girdler et al., 1998). Notably, one such study showed a significant positive association between premenstrual dysphoric disorder and history of sexual abuse. Taken together, these studies highlight the importance of examining links between cardiovascular dysregulation and traumatic stress exposure, including the potential mediating role of altered reproductive hormone profiles.

Finally, there are important methodological implications related to the behavioral and hormonal factors reviewed earlier (i.e., menstrual irregularities and menstrual syndromes, menopausal status, smoking status, and oral contraceptive use). If not assessed or controlled in psychophysiological studies of PTSD and gender, these factors represent potential threats to internal validity. Observed cardiovascular differences between groups could be due to differences in menstrual dysfunction, or menopausal or smoking status, for example, rather than to gender, diagnostic, or stress exposure status. Future studies should assess both psychiatric and control groups on these factors, or, where relevant and feasible, consider matching groups.

Gender Differences in Emotion and Coping

Gender differences in emotional experience, expression, and coping are well documented and may contribute to differences in how men and women respond to events that revivify traumatic affect and how they manage the emotional aftermath of such events. In this section, we consider the potential role of gender-linked affective and cognitive processes in the psychophysiology of PTSD.

Emotional Experience and Expression

Compared to men, women are more likely to express emotion (Kring & Gordon, 1998) and to report a greater intensity of feeling (Brody & Hall, 1993). Specifically, women report more negative, inwardly directed emotions than do men (e.g., shame, guilt, sadness, fear, and anxiety; Kring & Gordon, 1998). In addition, although reports of absolute levels of happiness are equivalent across gender, women report less happiness than men when happiness is considered as a proportion of total emotional experience

(Mirowsky & Ross, 1995). These gender differences in emotional experience and expression are thought to be due to socialization factors rather than to innate biological differences (Manstead, 1992).

On the basis of overall gender differences in emotion, one might expect women, as compared to men, to exhibit stronger verbal, facial, and psychophysiologic responsivity to negative emotion cues. To the contrary, studies of the psychophysiology of emotion reveal that although women's verbal and facial emotion expressions tend to be at least equal to men's responses, men tend to be more physiologically reactive than women (Kring & Gordon, 1998; Lai & Linden, 1992). Furthermore, triggers for physiological reactivity tend to be differentially salient for men and women; women respond more to affective valence, and men respond more to arousal (Lang, Greenwald, Bradley, & Hamm, 1993). With regard to specific emotions, women exhibit greater psychophysiological reactivity to sadness and disgust, whereas men exhibit greater reactivity to anger and fear (Kring & Gordon, 1998). Furthermore, after experiencing intense emotion, men's physiological recovery is faster if they express the emotion, whereas women's recovery is more dependent on their use of a preferred method of managing strong emotion (Lai & Linden, 1992). Many of these gender differences may be due to women being particularly attuned and responsive to emotional aspects of interpersonal relationships.

Although gender differences in emotion research suggest that, overall, women may be less psychophysiologically reactive, the majority of research has been conducted using anger as the target emotion. In these studies, women tend to exhibit less reactivity, or patterns that differ from men (Earle, Linden, & Weinberg, 1999). Women may be more, or differentially, reactive to cues of interpersonal traumatic events that arouse emotions such as sadness or disgust. This scenario is consistent with results of Carson et al. (2000), wherein nurse veterans asked to imagine their Vietnam experiences were both psychophysiologically reactive and reported intense sadness. Women are more likely than men to be exposed to interpersonal traumatic events, such as sexual assault, which typically precipitate high levels of inwardly directed negative emotion (i.e., sadness and shame). Thus, reminders of sexual assault and other interpersonal traumas—whether in the laboratory or in everyday experience—may predispose women to exhibit stronger psychophysiological responses than men. Future research should explore the possibility that psychophysiological reactivity in men and women with PTSD will be amplified in the context of gender-salient cues and emotions.

Coping

Although the relationship between coping and psychophysiological responding is not yet clear, evidence suggests that each influences the other. An avoidant coping style, characterized by denial and repression of thoughts or emotions, is generally understood to be less effective in reducing distress. In studies conducted primarily with men, adherence to an avoidant coping style predicts increased SBP reactivity to stressful tasks in the laboratory (Morrison, Bellack, & Manuck, 1985) and delayed recovery of normal HR after stressful tasks (Vitaliano, Russo, Paulsen, & Bailey, 1995). Women who report that they often use an avoidant coping style also exhibit greater blood pressure reactivity to laboratory tasks than those who use avoidance less often (Fontana & McLaughlin, 1998). Furthermore, suppression of strong emotion blunts cardiovascular responding during a stressor but increases the likelihood of stronger responding to a later stressor (Larkin, Semenchuk, Frazer, Suchday, & Taylor, 1998). Psychophysiological suppression research mirrors research on thought suppression, which has demonstrated that women with rape-related PTSD experience a rebound in rape-related thoughts after suppressing them for a short time (Shipherd & Beck, 1999). Future research on coping and psychophysiological responding should address this issue by including extended recovery periods to evaluate the effect of rebound thoughts and emotions.

However, gender differences do exist in certain aspects of coping and psychophysiological responding. Although men who suppress their anger demonstrate greater blood pressure reactivity to stressful laboratory tasks, there are no differences in reactivity between women who do and do not suppress anger (Vögele, Jarvis, & Cheeseman, 1997), suggesting that the effects of some coping strategies may be less applicable to women than others. The meaning of the stressor itself may also play a role, in that differences in reactivity may not be detectable when tasks presented in the laboratory are less relevant to women (Lash, Gillespie, Eisler, & Southard, 1991). Thus, although coping has not been fully evaluated in studies of psychophysiological responding in PTSD, use of avoidance to cope with a personally relevant trauma cue might alter the pattern of psychophysiological reactivity. Because women are generally more likely to use emotion-focused coping, including avoidance (Ptacek, Smith, & Dodge, 1994), the alterations may be more evident in women.

It should also be noted that in cue reactivity paradigms employed in the study of PTSD, lab stressors that involve exposure to trauma-related cues typically require passive coping (e.g., listening to a trauma-reminiscent script; Carson et al., 1999). In contrast, "control" stressors include both passive coping (e.g., listening to an emotionally neutral script; Carson et al., 1999) and active coping tasks (e.g., mental arithmetic; Orr, Meyerhoff, et al., 1998). In general, active and passive coping tasks generate qualitatively different physiological loads, with the former eliciting elevated SBP and HR (a presumed ß-adrenergic load), and the latter eliciting increases in DBP (a presumed α-adrenergic load; e.g., Saab & Schneiderman, 1993). On the whole, however, trauma-cued physiological reactivity has been evaluated only in tasks producing an α-adrenergic load, on which men and women typically demonstrate equivalent reactivity, leaving an entire dimension of physiological responding unevaluated. This is clearly an area for future research.

Gender differences in coping and psychophysiological responding may be even more complex, involving hormonal status or mood, or both. One study reported a relationship between coping style and blood pressure reactivity in female participants that was evident only during the premenstrual phase, suggesting a complex influence of hormonal status on coping and psychophysiological reactivity (Fontana & McLaughlin, 1998). Alternatively, coping style may not directly affect psychophysiological responding; the relationship may instead be mediated by mood and one's response to his or her mood. Preliminary work demonstrates that dysphoric women are more likely than nondysphoric women to use both avoidance coping and rumination in response to depressed mood (Sigmon, Hotovy, & Trask, 1996). Although coping is not independently correlated to SC levels after exposure to a negative social scene, rumination is positively correlated, suggesting the possibility of a mediational effect (Sigmon et al., 1996). Women report more rumination in response to depressed mood than men (Nolen-Hoeksema, Parker, & Larson, 1994), and so may exhibit greater reactivity when in that mood state.

Psychophysiological changes may themselves trigger coping responses. Studies drawn from the larger anxiety literature reveal that individuals readily identify and process interoceptive cues. Accurate feedback about (nontraumatic) fear-induced physiological responding increases fear habituation and produces lower absolute levels of fear (Telch, Valentiner, Ilai, Petruzzi, & Hehmsoth, 2000). Interestingly, individuals with anxiety disorders are more accurate than nondisordered individuals in their assessment of interoceptive cues, and acute anxiety is positively correlated with accuracy (Zoellner & Craske, 1999). Although coping strategies are not typically assessed in interoception studies, we speculate that participants process their own physiological information and cope with it in such a way that both their reactivity and fear decrease. Indeed, the process may be circular, wherein an attempt to cope with emotions focuses attention on physiological cues and improves accuracy, which then engages attendant coping strategies and reduces physiological responding. Future research should attempt to extend these findings to PTSD populations, because the results have important implications for the treatment of hyperarousal in PTSD.

Although we know little about gender differences in coping with PTSD, studies have found that male veterans with PTSD use more emotion-focused coping strategies (especially avoidance) in general and in response to a trauma reminder than veterans without PTSD (e.g., Fairbank, Hansen, & Fitterling, 1991). In general, greater use of emotion-focused coping in response to trauma is associated with greater distress in both men and women (e.g., Valentiner, Foa, Riggs, & Gershuny, 1996).

In summary, avoidant coping is associated with reactivity to stressful tasks in men and women not selected for trauma exposure or PTSD. The relationship may be further mediated by type of task, hormonal status, or mood. Psychophysiological responding may also engage coping systems, although the potential for gender differences is unknown in this field. The predominant use of emotion-focused strategies in women with PTSD places them at greater risk of continued distress when compared to men, and may affect their psychophysiological reactivity differentially.

Chronic Environmental Strain

Chronic environmental strain refers to ongoing "background" stressors that tax one's coping abilities and resources. The sources of chronic strain are myriad; examples include ongoing interpersonal conflict, excessive workplace demands, poverty, unstable or unsafe housing, and exposure to racist, sexist, or other environments that are hostile to aspects of one's core identity.

With regard to psychophysiology, some evidence suggests that chronic environmental strain significantly potentiates physiological reactivity to acute stressors (Matthews, Gump, Block, & Allen, 1997). Importantly, exposure to traumatic stressors appears to contribute to some sources of chronic strain; trauma survivors may experience increased occupational instability, more frequent periods of unemployment, and reduced incomes (Fairbank, Ebert, & Zarkin, 1999). For some individuals, chronic strain may be an equal or larger contributor than trauma to later distress or PTSD (e.g., Sundquist, Bayard-Burfield, Johansson, & Johansson, 2000). To date, however, no studies have examined how chronic background strain might contribute to the psychophysiological reactivity of individuals with PTSD.

The inclusion of measures of chronic strain may be particularly important for psychophysiological studies of women with PTSD; recent studies reveal that, compared to men, women experience more chronic strain and are exposed to more minor and major (nontraumatic) life stressors, including workplace and interpersonal stressors (Davis, Matthews, & Twamley, 1999). Chronic strain associated with being a woman in the military increases risky health behavior such as illicit drug use and smoking (Bray, Fairbank, & Marsden, 1999). Several authors have concluded that women experience greater chronic stress related to their gender role socialization than men, which, in turn, precipitates greater overall psychological distress and physical health impairment (Watkins & Whaley, 2000).

Chronic strain is also relevant to psychophysiology of minority group members. Research with healthy individuals in the United States documents the presence of ethnic differences and interactions between ethnicity and gender on psychophysiological responsivity. For example, African Americans manifest greater overall cardiovascular reactivity to laboratory stressors compared to Caucasians (Anderson, McNeilly, & Myers, 1992). Additionally, cardiovascular reactivity in African Americans is mediated by peripheral resistance factors, whereas reactivity in Caucasians stems from changes in cardiac factors (Anderson et al., 1992; Light, Turner, Hinderliter, & Sherwood, 1993). Chronic stress exposure in the lives of African Americans due to the consequences of social inequality (e.g., higher unemployment and poverty rates) is thought to cause subtle physiological impairment (Anderson et al., 1992). Although the mechanism is not yet known, chronic strain may increase the magnitude of cardiovascular reactivity or lower the threshold for a cue to provoke a physiological response.

Notably, ethnic differences previously documented in men have not always generalized to women (e.g., Light et al., 1993). For example, using a public speaking stressor, Saab et al. (1997) found that African American men were less reactive on measures of HR, SBP, and cardiac output than were African American women and Caucasian men and women. Due to a similar interaction on measures of psychosocial functioning (e.g., coping, hostility), the authors concluded that the differences probably stem from environmental and social rather than biological factors. Because some research groups have found no interaction between ethnicity and gender on cardiovascular reactivity (Jackson et al., 1999), however, the question still remains to be fully addressed.

Chronic strain could conceivably exacerbate minority group members' physiological reactivity to trauma-related experiences. Although this specific hypothesis has not been tested, two psychophysiological studies of Cambodian refugees may shed light on the pertinent issues, in spite of mixed results. In the first study, refugees with PTSD demonstrated greater HR increases to both trauma and nontrauma stimuli than did American Vietnam veterans with PTSD, Cambodians without current PTSD, veterans without current PTSD, or Americans with no history of trauma or PTSD symptoms (Kinzie et al., 1998). Although analyses were not conducted by gender, the authors reported that the strongest subjective emotional reactions were evident in Cambodian women both immediately following and a week after the experimental session. In contrast, one startle reflex study of young adult Cambodian American male and females found that, overall, Cambodians were less physiologically reactive on SC and eyeblink measures than Caucasians (Wright, Masten, Northwood, & Hubbard, 1997). In addition, although male and female Caucasians were similar in reactivity, male and female Cambodians differed significantly in eyeblink and SC reactivity. Although chronic environmental strain may be influential in studies of gender and the psychophysiology PTSD, research in this area is still developing and, as yet, inconclusive. Clearly, the impact of trauma-related loss of resources, as well as race- and gender-related strain, should continue to be evaluated.

SUMMARY AND DIRECTIONS FOR FUTURE RESEARCH

Overall, the research on gender and psychophysiology of PTSD is lacking, as is a coherent conceptual framework for the existing research. In this chapter, we not only reviewed the current literature but also outlined a triad of biopsychosocial factors that may serve as a guide for future research in this area.

Given the paucity of research on gender and the psychophysiology of PTSD, the most pressing need is for the inclusion of women in psychophysiological studies of PTSD. If the research reviewed here is an indication, there may be few or no gender differences in cardiovascular and SC reactivity to trauma-related stimuli. However, the support for this conclusion is not yet substantial. One obvious difficulty with conducting gender comparisons in trauma and PTSD research is that men and women are likely to have PTSD in response to different types of trauma (i.e., sexual assault–related PTSD is more prevalent among women, whereas combat-related PTSD is more prevalent in men), as well experience trauma and PTSD at different ages (e.g., sexual assault is likely to occur at an earlier age than war-zone exposure). When trauma type is confounded with gender, it is very difficult to determine the basis of any gender-related differences. To address this issue, researchers should focus on PTSD from traumas experienced with equivalent frequency, and at equivalent ages, in both genders (e.g., natural or perpetrated disaster). After substantial research has documented the presence or absence of a gender difference in psychophysiological reactivity, further exploration is necessary to determine whether mechanisms by which reactivity is expressed differ by gender.

Even if the results of future investigations support the conclusion that there are no gender differences in reactivity to trauma cues in men and women with PTSD, the end result may be influenced by factors that exhibit gender differences, such as reproductive hormones, emotions and coping, and chronic environmental strain. The associations noted between levels of estrogen and progesterone, and cardiovascular reactivity suggest that hormonal factors should be studied in women with PTSD. Women with current PTSD have high rates of some of the risk factors for reproductive dysfunction, such as menstrual cycle irregularity, natural or induced menopause, smoking, and oral contraceptive use (Acierno et al., 1996; Golding, 1996). These factors are known to alter cardiovascular reactivity, but their influence on reactivity in women with PTSD is unknown. Future psychophysiological studies of PTSD might examine the influence of these risk factors by matching groups on these variables. When matching is not feasible (e.g., because hormonal or health behavior factors are strongly correlated with trauma exposure and PTSD), efforts to measure these related factors and assess their contribution to physiological responding are encouraged.

Emotional and coping factors need to be explored as potential sources of gender differences in the psychophysiology of PTSD. There are reliable gender differences in the expression and psychophysiological correlates of emotion, and because different trauma types and characteristics are likely to elicit different emotions, distinct patterns of psychophysiological arousal may emerge for men and women. Studies could be conducted in which subjective experience of emotion, and facial expressions of emotion, are coupled with psychophysiological assessment in men and women with PTSD and trauma-exposed individuals without PTSD. We also recommend that future research in the psychophysiology of PTSD build on basic interpersonal psychophysiology paradigms (e.g., Newton, Bane, Flores, & Greenfield, 1999) to examine interpersonal processes that may trigger reactivity among individuals with histories of interpersonal violence. These processes may have particular relevance to gender-related outcomes, because women are particularly reactive to and affected by negative characteristics of the social environment, perhaps in part due to gender role socialization.

Coping and psychophysiological reactivity processes may well influence each other in healthy adults, but little is known about their relationship in men and women with PTSD. Examining the association between dominant coping styles and reactivity, and the influence of interoception may prove to be fruitful. Future studies would also benefit from the use of a variety of active and passive coping tasks, as well as measures of the effect of hormonal status and mood on psychophysiological reactivity to trauma-related cues.

Finally, the influence of chronic environmental strain on psychophysiological reactivity in PTSD is, as yet, unstudied. Measurement of chronic strain has implications for psychophysiological responses, especially for women and ethnic minorities, but poses conceptual and methodological challenges similar to those posed by gender comparisons per se; that is, trauma type, severity, and age at exposure may be confounded with ethnicity and gender, making unambiguous interpretations difficult, if not impossible. Nonetheless, pursuing areas such as responses to natural, accidental, or perpetrated disasters, as well as measuring the strain incurred by exposure to these traumas, may be one way to approach this topic. In addition, ethnic comparisons within gender may be feasible (e.g., assessing responses to sexual assault among women of different ethnicities, and responses to combat among men), and would make an important contribution to this understudied area.

Finally, it should be noted that interactions between all the biopsychosocial factors may prove influential in psychophysiological studies of PTSD. For example, individuals under chronic strain due to racism may have to engage coping strategies more often, with fewer resources. The greater resulting physiological load may lead to exaggerated psychophysiological reactivity when they are exposed to stressful cues (Clark, Anderson, Clark, & Williams, 1999). Research that successfully measures and evaluates all three factors will ultimately be the most productive.

In summary, trauma takes a dramatic toll on the mental and physical well-being of men and women throughout the world. Continued study of the psychophysiology of trauma and PTSD will enhance understanding of adaptation to catastrophic stressors and support efforts to treat associated psychological and physiological sequelae. Inclusion of men and women and people of color in these psychophysiological studies will greatly increase the applicability of this research and enhance the scientific understanding of trauma and PTSD.

REFERENCES

Acierno, R., Kilpatrick, D. G., Resnick, H. S., Saunders, B. E., & Best, C. L. (1996). Violent assault, posttraumatic stress disorder, and depression: Risk factors for cigarette use among adult women. *Behavior Modification, 20,* 363–384.

Anderson, N. B., McNeilly, M., & Myers, H. (1992). Toward understanding race difference in autonomic reactivity: A proposed contextual model. In J. R. Turner, A. Sherwood, & K. C. Light (Eds.), *Individual differences in cardiovascular response to stress: Perspectives on individual differences* (pp. 125–145). New York: Plenum Press.

Barnett, P. A., Spence, J. D., Manuck, S. B., & Jennings, J. R. (1997). Psychological stress and the progression of carotid artery disease. *Journal of Hypertension, 15,* 49–55.

Blanchard, E. B., & Buckley, T. C. (1999). Psychophysiological assessment and PTSD. In P. A. Saigh & J. D. Bremner (Eds.), *Posttraumatic stress disorder: A comprehensive text* (pp. 248–266). Boston: Allyn & Bacon.

Blanchard, E. B., Hickling, E. J., Buckley, T. C., Taylor, A. E., Vollmer, A. J., & Loos, W. R. (1996). The psychophysiology of motor vehicle accident related posttraumatic stress disorder: Replication and extension. *Journal of Consulting and Clinical Psychology, 64,* 742–751.

Blascovich, J., & Katkin, E. S. (1993). Cardiovascular reactivity to psychological stress and disease: Conclusions. In J. Blascovich & E. S. Katkin (Eds.), *Cardiovascular reactivity to psychological stress and disease* (pp. 225–237). Washington, DC: American Psychological Association.

Blumenthal, J. A., Frederikson, M., Matthews, K. A., Kuhn, C. M., Schniebolk, S., German, D., Rifai, N., Steege, J., & Rodin, J. (1991). Stress reactivity and exercise training in premenopausal and postmenopausal women. *Health Psychology, 10,* 384–391.

Boscarino, J. A., & Chang, J. (1999). Electrocardiogram abnormalities among men with stress-related psychiatric disorders: Implications for coronary heart disease and clinical research. *Annals of Behavioral Medicine, 21,* 227–234.

Boyce, W. T., Chesney, M., Alkon, A., Tschann, J. M., Adams, S., Chesterman, B., Cohen, F., Kaiser, P., Folkman, S., & Wara, D. (1995). Psychobiologic reactivity to stress and childhood respiratory illnesses: Results of two prospective studies. *Psychosomatic Medicine, 57*, 411–422.

Bray, R. M., Fairbank, J. A., & Marsden, M. E. (1999). Stress and substance use among military women and men. *American Journal of Drug and Alcohol Abuse, 25*, 239–256.

Brody, L. R., & Hall, J. A. (1993). Gender and emotion. In M. Lewis & J. M. Haviland (Eds.), *Handbook of emotions* (pp. 447–460). New York: Guilford Press.

Bryant, R. A., Harvey, A. G., Guthrie, R. M., & Moulds, M. L. (2000). A prospective study of psychophysiological arousal, acute stress disorder, and posttraumatic stress disorder. *Journal of Abnormal Psychology, 109*, 341–344.

Buckley, T. C., & Kaloupek, D. G. (2001). A meta-analytic examination of basal cardiovascular activity in posttraumatic stress disorder. *Psychosomatic Medicine, 63*, 585–594.

Burleson, M. H., Malarkey, W. B., Cacioppo, J. T., Poehlmann, K. M., Kiecolt-Glaser, J. K., Berntson, G. G., & Glaser, R. (1998). Postmenopausal hormone replacement: Effects on autonomic, neuroendocrine, and immune reactivity to brief psychological stressors. *Psychosomatic Medicine, 60*, 17–25.

Carson, M. A., Metzger, L. J., Lasko, N. B., Paulus, L. A., Pitman, R. K., & Orr, S. P. (1999, November). *Physiologic reactivity to startling tones in female Vietnam nurse veterans.* Poster session presented at the annual meeting of the International Society for Traumatic Stress Studies, Miami, FL.

Carson, M. A., Paulus, L. A., Lasko, N. B., Metzger, L. J., Wolfe, J., Orr, S. P., & Pitman, R. K. (2000). Psychophysiologic assessment of posttraumatic stress disorder in Vietnam nurse veterans who witnessed injury or death. *Journal of Consulting and Clinical Psychology, 68*, 890–897.

Clark, R., Anderson, N. B., Clark, V. R., & Williams, D. R. (1999). Racism as a stressor for African Americans: A biopsychosocial model. *American Psychologist, 54*, 805–816.

Cohen, H., Kotler, M., Matar, M. A., Kaplan, Z., Miodownik, H., & Cassuto, Y. (1997). Power spectral analysis of heart rate variability in posttraumatic stress disorder patients. *Biological Psychiatry, 41*, 627–629.

Collins, A., Hanson, U., Eneroth, P., Hagenfeldt, K., Lundberg, U., & Frankenhaeuser, M. (1982). Psychophysiological stress responses in postmenopausal women before and after hormonal replacement therapy. *Human Neurobiology, 1*, 153–159.

Davis, M. C. (1999). Oral contraceptive use and hemodynamic, lipid, and fibrinogen responses to smoking and stress in women. *Health Psychology, 18*, 122–130.

Davis, M. C., Matthews, K. A., & Twamley, E. W. (1999). Is life more difficult on Mars or Venus?: A meta-analytic review of sex differences in major and minor life events. *Annals of Behavioral Medicine, 21*, 83–97.

Dembroski, T. M., MacDougall, J. M., Slatts, S., Eliot, R. S., & Buell, J. C. (1981). Challenge-induced cardiovascular response as a predictor of minor illnesses. *Journal of Human Stress, 7*, 2–5.

Dobbs, D., & Wilson, W. P. (1960). Observations on persistence of war neurosis. *Diseases of the Nervous System, 21*, 1–6.

Earle, T. L., Linden, W., & Weinberg, J. (1999). Differential effects of harassment on cardiovascular and salivary cortisol stress reactivity and recovery in women and men. *Journal of Psychosomatic Research, 46,* 125–141.

Fairbank, J. A., Ebert, L., & Zarkin, G. A. (1999). Socioeconomic consequences of traumatic stress. In P. A. Saigh & J. D. Bremner (Eds.), *Posttraumatic stress disorder: A comprehensive text* (pp. 80–198). Boston: Allyn & Bacon.

Fairbank, J. A., Hansen, D. J., & Fitterling, J. M. (1991). Patterns of appraisal and coping across different stressor conditions among former prisoners of war with and without posttraumatic stress disorder. *Journal of Consulting and Clinical Psychology, 59,* 274–281.

Foa, E. B., Steketee, G., & Rothbaum, B. O. (1989). Behavioral/cognitive conceptualizations of post-traumatic stress disorder. *Behavior Therapy, 20,* 149–154.

Fontana, A., & McLaughlin, M. (1998). Coping and appraisal of daily stressors predict heart rate and blood pressure levels in young women. *Behavioral Medicine, 24,* 5–16.

Gilligan, D. M., Quyyumi, A. A., & Cannon, R. O. (1994). Effects of physiological levels of estrogen on coronary vasomotor function in postmenopausal women. *Circulation, 89,* 2545–2551.

Girdler, S. S., Jamner, L. D., Jarvik, M., Soles, J. R., & Shapiro, D. (1997). Smoking status and nicotine administration differentially modify hemodynamic stress reactivity in men and women. *Psychosomatic Medicine, 59,* 294–306.

Girdler, S. S., Pedersen, C. A., Straneva, P. A., Leserman, J., Stanwyck, C. L., Benjamin, S., & Light, K. C. (1998). Dysregulation of cardiovascular and neuroendocrine responses to stress in premenstrual dysphoric disorder. *Psychiatry Research, 81,* 163–178.

Golding, J. M. (1994). Sexual assault history and physical health in randomly selected Los Angeles women. *Health Psychology, 13,* 130–138.

Golding, J. M. (1996). Sexual assault history and women's reproductive and sexual health. *Psychology of Women Quarterly, 20,* 101–121.

Greenland, P., Daviglus, M. L., Dyer, A. R., Liu, K., Huang, C. F., Goldberger, J. J., & Stamler, J. (1999). Resting heart rate is a risk factor for cardiovascular and noncardiovascular mortality: The Chicago Heart Association Detection Project in industry. *American Journal of Epidemiology, 149,* 853–862.

Grillon, C., Morgan, C. A. III, Davis, M., & Southwick, S. M. (1998). Effects of experimental context and explicit threat cues in acoustic startle in Vietnam veterans with posttraumatic stress disorder. *Biological Psychiatry, 44,* 1027–1036.

Grillon, C., Morgan, C. A. III, Southwick, S. M., Davis, M., & Charney, D. S. (1996). Baseline startle amplitude and prepulse inhibition in Vietnam veterans with PTSD. *Psychiatry Research, 64,* 169–178.

Jackson, R. W., Treiber, F. A., Turner, J. R., Davis, H., & Strong, W. B. (1999). Effects of race, sex, and socioeconomic status upon cardiovascular stress responsivity and recovery in youth. *International Journal of Psychophysiology, 31,* 111–119.

Kardiner, A. (1941). *The traumatic neuroses of war.* New York: Harper & Row.

Keane, T. M., Kolb, L. C., Kaloupek, D. G., Orr, S. P., Blanchard, E. B., Thomas, R. G., Hsieh, F. Y., & Lavori, P. W. (1998). Utility of psychophysiology measurement in the diagnosis of posttraumatic stress disorder: Results from a department of Veterans Affairs cooperative study.*Journal of Consulting and Clinical Psychology, 66,* 914–923.

Keane, T. M., Weathers, F. W., & Foa, E. B. (2000). Diagnosis and assessment. In E. B. Foa, T. M. Keane, & M. J. Friedman (Eds.), *Effective treatments for PTSD* (pp. 18–36). New York: Guilford Press.

Keys, A., Taylor, H. L., Blackburn, J., Anderson, J. T., & Somonson, E. (1971). Mortality and coronary heart disease among men studied for 23 years. *Archives of Internal Medicine, 128,* 201–214.

Kilpatrick, D. G., Best, C. L., Ruff, M. H., & Veronen, L. J. (1984, November). *Psychophysiological assessment in the treatment of rape-induced anxiety.* Paper presented at the annual meeting of the Association for Advancement of Behavior Therapy, Washington, DC.

Kinzie, J. D., Denney, D., Riley, C., Boehnlein, J., McFarland, B., & Leung, P. (1998). A cross-cultural study of reactivation of posttraumatic stress disorder symptoms: American and Cambodian psychophysiological response to viewing traumatic video scenes. *Journal of Nervous and Mental Disease, 186,* 670–676.

Kring, A. M., & Gordon, A. H. (1998). Sex differences in emotion: Expression, experience, and physiology. *Journal of Personality and Social Psychology, 74,* 686–703.

Lai, J. Y., & Linden, W. (1992). Gender, anger expression style, and opportunity for anger release determine cardiovascular reaction to and recovery from anger provocation. *Psychosomatic Medicine, 54,* 297–310.

Lang, P. J., Greenwald, M. K., Bradley, M. M., & Hamm, A. O. (1993). Looking at pictures: Affective, facial, visceral, and behavioral reactions. *Psychophysiology, 30,* 261–273.

Laor, N., Wolmer, L., Wiener, Z., Sharon, O., Weizman, R., Toren, P., & Ron, S. (1999). Image vividness as a psychophysiological regulator in posttraumatic stress disorder. *Journal of Clinical and Experimental Neuropsychology, 21,* 39–48.

Larkin, K. T., Semenchuk, E. M., Frazier, N. L., Suchday, S., & Taylor, R. L. (1998). Cardiovascular and behavioral response to social confrontation: Measuring real-life stress in the laboratory. *Annals of Behavioral Medicine, 20,* 294–301.

Lash, S. J., Gillespie, B. L., Eisler, R. M., & Southard, D. R. (1991). Sex differences in cardiovascular reactivity: Effects of the gender relevance of the stressor. *Health Psychology, 10,* 392–398.

LeDoux, J. E. (1990). Information flow from sensation to emotion plasticity in the neural computation of stimulus value. In M. Gabriel & J. Moore (Eds.), *Learning and computational neuroscience: Foundations of adaptive networks* (pp. 3–52). Cambridge, MA: Bradford Books/MIT Press.

Legato, M. J. (1997). Gender-specific physiology: How real is it? How important is it? *International Journal of Fertility, 42,* 19–29.

Light, K. C., Turner, J. R., Hinderliter, A. L., & Sherwood, A. (1993). Race and gender comparisons: I. Hemodynamic responses to a series of stressors. *Health Psychology, 12,* 354–365.

Manstead, A. S. R. (1992). Gender differences in emotion. In A. Gale & M. W., Eysenck (Eds.), *Handbook of individual differences: Biological perspectives* (pp. 355–387). Chichester, UK: Wiley.

Matthews, K. A., Berga, S. L., Owens, J. F., & Flory, J. D. (1998). Effects of short-term suppression of ovarian hormones on cardiovascular and neuroendocrine reactivity to stress in women. *Psychoneuroendocrinology, 23,* 307–322.

Matthews, K. A., Gump, B. B., Block, D. R., & Allen, M. T. (1997). Does background stress heighten or dampen children's cardiovascular responses to acute stress? *Psychosomatic Medicine, 59,* 488–496.

Matthews, K. A., Woodall, K. C., & Allen, M. T. (1993). Cardiovascular reactivity to stress predicts future blood pressure status. *Hypertension, 122,* 479–485.

Menkes, M. S., Matthews, K. A., Krantz, D. S., Lundberg, U., Mead, L. A., Qaqish, B., Liang, K. Y., Thomas, C. B., & Pearson, T. A. (1989). Cardiovascular reactivity to the cold pressure test as a predictor of hypertension. *Hypertension, 14,* 524–530.

Metzger, L. J., Orr, S. P., Berry, N. J., Ahern, C. E., Lasko, N. B., & Pitman, R. K. (1999). Physiologic reactivity to startling tones in women with posttraumatic stress disorder. *Journal of Abnormal Psychology, 108,* 347–352.

Miller, S. B., & Sita, A. (1994). Parental history of hypertension, menstrual cycle phase, and cardiovascular response to stress. *Psychosomatic Medicine, 56,* 61–69.

Mirowsky, J., & Ross, C. E. (1995). Sex differences in distress: Real or artifact? *American Sociological Review, 60,* 449–468.

Morgan, C. A., Grillon, C., Lubin, H., & Southwick, S. M. (1997). Startle reflex abnormalities in women with sexual assault–related posttraumatic stress disorder. *American Journal of Psychiatry, 154,* 1076–1080.

Morrison, R. L., Bellack, A. S., & Manuck, S. B. (1985). Role of social competence in borderline essential hypertension. *Journal of Consulting and Clinical Psychology, 53,* 248–255.

Newton, T. L., Bane, C. M., Flores, A., & Greenfield, J. (1999). Dominance, gender, and cardiovascular reactivity during social interaction. *Psychophysiology, 36,* 245–252.

Nolen-Hoeksema, S., Parker, L. E., & Larson, J. (1994). Ruminative coping with depressed mood following loss. *Journal of Personality and Social Psychology, 67,* 92–104.

Odemuyiwa, O., Malik, M., Farrel, T., Bashir, Y., Poloniecki, J., & Camm, J. (1991). Comparison of the predictive characteristics of heart rate variability index and left ventricular ejection fraction for all-cause mortality, arrhythmic events and sudden death after acute myocardial infarction. *American Journal of Cardiology, 68,* 434–439.

Orr, S. P., Lasko, N. B., Metzger, L. J., Berry, N. J., Ahern, C. E., & Pitman, R. K. (1998). Psychophysiological assessment of women with posttraumatic stress disorder resulting from childhood sexual abuse. *Journal of Consulting and Clinical Psychology, 66,* 906–913.

Orr, S. P., Lasko, N. B., Shalev, A. Y., & Pitman, R. K. (1995). Physiologic responses to loud tones in Vietnam veterans with posttraumatic stress disorder. *Journal of Abnormal Psychology, 104,* 75–82.

Orr, S. P., Meyerhoff, J. L., Edwards, J. V., & Pitman, R. K. (1998). Heart rate and blood pressure resting levels and responses to generic stressors in Vietnam veterans with posttraumatic stress disorder. *Journal of Traumatic Stress, 11,* 155–164.

Owens, J. F., Stoney, C. M., & Matthews, K. A. (1993). Menopausal status influences ambulatory blood pressure levels and blood pressure changes during mental stress. *Circulation, 88,* 2794–2802.

Peirce, J. M., Brown, J. M., Long, P. J., Nixon, S. J., Borrell, G. K., & Holloway, F. A. (1996, November). *Comorbidity and subjective reactivity to meaningful cues in female methadone maintenance patients.* Paper presented at the annual meeting of the Association for Advancement of Behavior Therapy, New York, NY.

Pitman, R. K., Orr, S. P., Altman, B., Longpre, R. E., Poire, R. E., Macklin, M. L., Michaels, M. J., & Steketee, G. S. (1996). Emotional processing and outcome of imaginal flooding therapy in Vietnam veterans with chronic posttraumatic stress disorder. *Comprehensive Psychiatry, 37,* 409–418.

Pitman, R. K., Orr, S. P., Forgue, D. F., de Jong, J. B., & Claiborn, J. M. (1987). Psychophysiological assessment of posttraumatic stress disorder imagery in Vietnam combat veterans. *Archives of General Psychiatry, 44,* 970–975.

Ptacek, J. T., Smith, R. E., & Dodge, K. L. (1994). Gender differences in coping with stress: When stressor and appraisals do not differ. *Personality and Social Psychology Bulletin, 20,* 421–430.

Resnick, H. S., Kilpatrick, D. G., & Lipovsky, J. A. (1991). Assessment of rape-related posttraumatic stress disorder: Stressor and symptom dimensions. *Psychological Assessment, 3,* 561–572.

Saab, P. G., Llabre, M. M., Schneiderman, N., Hurwitz, B. E., McDonald, P. G., Evans, J., Wohlgemuth, W., Hayashi, P., & Klein, B. (1997). Influence of ethnicity and gender on cardiovascular responses to active coping and inhibitory–passive coping challenges. *Psychosomatic Medicine, 59,* 434–446.

Saab, P. G., Matthews, K. A., Stoney, C. M., & McDonald, R. H. (1989). Premenopausal and postmenopausal women differ in their cardiovascular and neuroendocrine responses to behavioral stressors. *Psychophysiology, 26,* 270–280.

Saab, P. G., & Schneiderman, N. (1993). Biobehavioral stressors, laboratory investigation, and the risk of hypertension. In J. J. Blascovich & E. S. Katkin (Eds.), *Cardiovascular reactivity to psychological stress and disease* (pp. 49–82). Washington, DC: American Psychological Association.

Schnurr, P. P., & Jankowski, M. K. (1999). Physical health and post-traumatic stress disorder: Review and synthesis. *Seminars in Clinical Neuropsychiatry, 4,* 295–304.

Schnurr, P. P., Spiro, A., & Paris, A. H. (2000). Physician-diagnosed medical disorders in relation to PTSD symptoms in older male military veterans. *Health Psychology, 19,* 91–97.

Shalev, A. Y., Orr, S. P., & Pitman, R. K. (1993). Psychophysiologic assessment of traumatic imagery in Israeli civilian patients with posttraumatic stress disorder. *American Journal of Psychiatry, 150,* 620–624.

Shalev, A. Y., Peri, T., Orr, S. P., Bonne, O., & Pitman, R. K. (1997). Auditory startle responses in help-seeking trauma survivors. *Psychiatry Research, 69,* 1–7.

Shalev, A. Y., Sahar, T., Freedman, S., Peri, T., Glick, N., Brandes, D., Orr, S. P., & Pitman, R. K. (1998). A prospective study of heart rate response following trauma and the subsequent development of posttraumatic stress disorder. *Archives of General Psychiatry, 55,* 553–559.

Shipherd, J. C., & Beck, J. G. (1999). The effects of suppressing trauma-related thoughts on women with rape-related posttraumatic stress disorder. *Behaviour Research and Therapy, 37,* 99–112.

Sigmon, S. T., Hotovy, L. A., & Trask, P. C. (1996). Coping and sensitivity to aversive events. *Journal of Psychopathology and Behavioral Assessment, 18,* 133–151.

Sita, A., & Miller, S. B. (1996). Estradiol, progesterone and cardiovascular response to stress. *Psychoneuroendocrinology, 21,* 339–346.

Stone, S. V., Dembroski, T. M., Costa, P. T., Jr., & MacDougall, J. M. (1990). Gender differences in cardiovascular reactivity. *Journal of Behavioral Medicine, 13,* 137–156.

Stoney, C. M. (1999). Plasma homocysteine levels increase in women during psychological stress. *Life Sciences, 64,* 2359–2365.

Stoney, C. M., Davis, M. C., & Matthews, K. A. (1987). Sex differences in physiological responses to stress and in coronary heart disease: A causal link? *Psychophysiology, 24,* 127–131.

Stoney, C. M., Owens, J. F., Guzick, D. S., & Matthews, K. A. (1997). A natural experiment on the effects of ovarian hormones on cardiovascular risk factors and stress reactivity: Bilateral salpingo oophorectomy versus hysterectomy only. *Health Psychology, 16,* 349–358.

Stoney, C. M., Owens, J. F., Matthews, K. A., Davis, M. C., & Caggiula, A. (1990). Influences of the normal menstrual cycle on physiologic functioning during behavioral stress. *Psychophysiology, 27,* 125–135.

Sundquist, J., Bayard-Burfield, L., Johansson, L. M., & Johansson, S. E. (2000). Impact of ethnicity, violence and acculturation on displaced migrants: Psychological distress and psychosomatic complaints among refugees in Sweden. *Journal of Nervous and Mental Disease, 188,* 357–365.

Telch, M. J., Valentiner, D. P., Ilai, D., Petruzzi, D., & Hehmsoth, M. (2000). The facilitative effects of heart-rate feedback in the emotional processing of claustrophobic fear. *Behaviour Research and Therapy, 38,* 373–387.

Valentiner, D. P., Foa, E. B., Riggs, D. S., & Gershuny, B. S. (1996). Coping strategies and posttraumatic stress disorder in female victims of sexual and nonsexual assault. *Journal of Abnormal Psychology, 105,* 455–458.

Vitaliano, P. P., Russo, J., Paulsen, V. M., & Bailey, S. L. (1995). Cardiovascular recovery from laboratory stress: Biopsychosocial concomitants in older adults. *Journal of Psychosomatic Research, 39,* 361–377.

Vögele, C., Jarvis, A., & Cheeseman, K. (1997). Anger suppression, reactivity, and hypertension risk: Gender makes a difference. *Annals of Behavioral Medicine, 19,* 61–69.

Watkins, P. L., & Whaley, D. (2000). Gender role stressors and women's health. In R. M. Eisler & M. Hersen (Eds.) *Handbook of gender, culture, and health* (pp. 43–62). Mahwah, NJ: Erlbaum.

Wolfe, J., Chrestman, K. R., Ouimette, P. C., Kaloupek, D., Harley, R. M., & Bucsela, M. (2000). Trauma-related psychophysiological reactivity in women exposed to war-zone stress. *Journal of Clinical Psychology, 56,* 1371–1379.

Wright, M. O., Masten, A. S., Northwood, A., & Hubbard, J. J. (1997). Long-term effects of massive trauma: Developmental and psychobiological perspectives. In D. Cicchetti & S. L. Toth (Eds.), *Developmental perspectives on trauma: Theory, research, and intervention* (pp. 181–225). Rochester, NY: University of Rochester Press.

Zoellner, L. A., & Craske, M. G. (1999). Interoceptive accuracy and panic. *Behaviour Research and Therapy, 37,* 1141–1158.

Part III | Comorbidity

8 | Gender Issues in PTSD with Comorbid Mental Health Disorders

SUSAN M. ORSILLO
SHEELA RAJA
CHARITY HAMMOND

$\mathbf{P}$osttraumatic stress disorder (PTSD) is associated with a significant psychological, social, and financial burden for the men and women who experience the disorder, their friends and family, and for society as a whole (Greenberg et al., 1999; Kulka et al., 1990; Murray & Lopez, 1996). However, PTSD is rarely the only psychological disorder present among individuals with a history of exposure to a traumatic event. Data from the United States National Comorbidity Survey (NCS) established that among individuals with a lifetime history of PTSD, 88.3% of men and 79.0% of women also reported a lifetime history of at least one other disorder (Kessler et al., 1999). Anxiety, mood, somatoform, and personality disorders frequently co-occur with PTSD, impacting virtually every aspect of the disorder. Research has demonstrated that comorbidity is related to a chronic course of PTSD (Blanchard, Buckley, Hickling, & Taylor, 1998; Breslau & Davis, 1992; McFarlane & Papay, 1992), more severe psychopathology related to the comorbid conditions (Sautter et al., 1999; Shalev et al., 1998; Zimmerman & Mattia, 1999a), and significantly more functional impairment or disability (Mollica et al., 1999; Shalev et al., 1998). Comorbid conditions often mask the presence of PTSD symptoms, decreasing the likelihood that the diagnosis is accurately identified and treated (e.g., Mueser et al., 1998; Zimmerman & Mattia, 1999b). Thus, it is critical to attend to issues of comorbidity with PTSD when assessing and treating trauma-exposed individuals.

Gender issues related to comorbidity with PTSD have scarcely been considered. Yet, gender-specific patterns of comorbidity are likely, given the demonstrated gender differences in the prevalence and patterns of psychopathology in the population. Significant gender differences in the prevalence of several specific psychological disorders were found in the NCS (Kessler, 1998). Although a number of theories have been advanced to explain these gender differences, including biological differences, differential socialization, and discrimination in assessment and diagnostic nomenclature, the implications for assessment and treatment are still not fully understood.

Our purpose in this chapter is to examine the nature of comorbidity of psychological disorders with PTSD, with a specific emphasis on potential gender differences. Because substance use and somatoform disorders are covered in separate chapters, studies focusing primarily on these disorders are excluded from our review and discussion. We first briefly consider why gender study is important and relevant to the study of comorbidity with PTSD. Next we provide an overview of the literature to date on PTSD and comorbid conditions by gender. Given the relatively sparse literature on gender and comorbidity with PTSD, we provide some recommendations for future research, paying significant attention to the complex issues that potentially obscure the nosological and clinical implications of the cumulative literature. Finally, we discuss potential treatment implications.

GENDER AND PSYCHOPATHOLOGY

Significant gender differences in the prevalence of psychological disorders have been consistently documented in clinical practice and research. An examination of these differences and the theories that have been advanced to explain them provides a foundation for exploring the role of gender in PTSD comorbidity. Interestingly, recent epidemiological studies confirm that men and women are equally likely to be diagnosed with a psychological disorder (Kessler, 1998). In other words, men and women do not differ in their probability of being diagnosed with some psychological condition. However, there are differences in the pattern of *specific* disorders across genders. In particular, women are more likely than men to be diagnosed with mood and anxiety disorders, whereas men are much more likely to be diagnosed with substance use, conduct disorders, and adult antisocial behavior (Kessler, 1998).

Several theories have been advanced to attempt to explain these gender differences. Sociocultural influences have been portrayed as potentially important in understanding the development of panic disorder and agoraphobia. Barlow (1988) proposed that the perception of stressful events as unpredictable and uncontrollable is a psychological vulnerability that increases an individual's risk for developing panic disorder. This perceptual style is likely based on a person's learning history and direct experience with stressors. Traditional sex roles may influence perception of, and experience with, stressors (Barlow, 1988). Men are traditionally socialized to be independent, masterful, and assertive, which likely increases their perception of controllability, whereas women are expected to be more passive and dependent, behavioral patterns that lead to the perception of uncontrollability over one's environment. Coping styles that are consistent with traditional sex roles may also influence the development of agoraphobia. Barlow proposed that the incidence of panic symptoms may be similar among men and women, but that the genders may differ in their primary method of coping with these experiences. Specifically, Barlow argued that perhaps it is more culturally acceptable for women to cope by avoiding situations that elicit panic, which increases their risk of developing agoraphobia. In contrast, men may be more likely to use drugs or alcohol as a mean of avoiding their internal experiences, which increases their risk for substance abuse rather than an anxiety disorder. Data support the notion that parenting styles encouraging stereotypical gender roles are significantly related to the later development of anxiety disorders (Chorpita & Barlow, 1998).

Physiological factors have also been identified as potentially important in explaining gender differences in the prevalence of various psychological disorders. Based on a recent review of the literature, Merikangas and Pollock (2000) argued that the most compelling explanation for higher rates of anxiety disorders among women is that women have higher levels of arousal, psychophysiological response to stress, and somatic stress, as well as a greater awareness of somatic anxiety than men. Fluctuations in female reproductive hormones across the lifespan are also thought to impact on the underlying vulnerability for anxiety disorders in women. For instance, anxiety in response to a biological challenge (carbon dioxide intake) has been shown to be significantly stronger in the early follicular phase than in the midluteal phase for women with panic disorder (Perna, Brambilla, Arancio, & Bellodi, 1995). Furthermore, women with generalized anxiety disorder and premenstrual syndrome reported a significant increase in their anxiety symptoms during the premenstrual phase of their cycle (McLeod, Hoehn-Saric, Foster, & Hipsley, 1993). Panic symptoms also seemed to be linked to hormonal changes associated with pregnancy. For instance, a majority of women with preexisting panic disorder reported an improvement in their symptoms during pregnancy (Villeponteaux, Lydiard, Laraia, Stuart, & Ballenger, 1992), but a significant subgroup is at risk for a return of symptoms during the postpartum period (Cohen, Sichel, Dimmock, & Rosenbaum, 1994a, 1994b). Clearly, more research is needed to further elucidate how these hormonally mediated neurobiological changes impact on increased risk of development of anxiety disorders in women (Merikangas & Pollock, 2000).

There have also been a number of theories directed at explaining the higher rates of mood disorders, particularly major depressive disorder, among women. Research has indicated that gender differences in depression do not seem to emerge until after the age of 15 (Nolen-Hoeksema & Girgus, 1994), suggesting that this developmental stage may include important biological or sociological events related to the differential development of depression. While biological, and particularly hormonal, etiologies have been examined as potential contributory factors, their importance has not been substantiated (Hankin & Abramson, 1999; Strickland, 1992).

Stronger evidence exists implicating cognitive factors in the differential rate of depression between the genders. Women seem to be more likely to develop a ruminative response style that increases their vulnerability to becoming depressed (Hankin & Abramson, 1999). Also, the value women place on intimate relationships might also put them at risk when disruptions in the relationship occur (Fincham, Beach, Harold, & Osborne, 1997; Hammen, Marks, Mayo, & DeMayo, 1985), although some data suggest that divorce presents a higher risk of depression for men (cf. Bruce & Kim, 1992).

However, these gender differences in cognitive style likely develop among girls before adolescence and thus do not fully explain the gender shift that occurs at this developmental stage. Nolen-Hoeksema and Girgus (1994) reviewed the existing literature and concluded that these risk factors only lead to depression in the face of gender-related challenges that commonly begin in early adolescence. Specifically, as a result of their gender, girls and women are more likely to be confronted with abuse, harassment, restrictions on their choice, devaluation (Nolen-Hoeksema & Girgus, 1994), negative events in their families (Hankin & Abramson, 1999), and discrimination and stress related to caretaking of children and older relatives (Strickland, 1992). The differential risk by gender for direct experience with these negative, stressful events seems to be a strong explanatory factor for the difference in prevalence of depression among men and women.

There is also evidence that gender is linked to substance use (see Stewart, Ouimette, & Brown, Chapter 9, this volume) and personality disorders. For instance, Paris (1997) argued that the behavioral differences in the diagnostic criteria of antisocial and borderline personality disorders are influenced by traditional gender roles. Hamburger, Lilienfeld, and Hogben (1996) demonstrated that gender moderates the relationship between psychopathy and antisocial and histrionic personality disorders, such that psychopathic males exhibit antisocial patterns, whereas psychopathic females exhibit histrionic patterns.

In summary, gender seems to play a significant role in the development of general psychopathology. Thus, it is reasonable to expect that men and women seeking treatment for PTSD may differ significantly in the their specific comorbid presentation. Given the documented impact of comorbidity with PTSD on symptom severity, course, and functional impairment, a better knowledge and understanding of these potential gender differences may inform and improve treatment delivery. Thus, we provide a review of the literature on comorbidity and PTSD, and explore what is currently known about gender specific patterns.

PSYCHIATRIC COMORBIDITY

Although a number of studies describe the psychological symptoms and disorders that often develop following exposure to a trauma, far fewer studies on the specific comorbidity between PTSD and other psychological disorders have been conducted. Furthermore, the findings that have emerged from controlled research are influenced by a variety of important factors, such as the nature of the traumatic event experienced by individuals in the sample, length of time that has passed since the trauma, type of assessment instrument used, and a number of other methodological variations (discussed more fully later) that make it difficult to generalize findings beyond a specific sample. As a result, prevalence rates of some comorbid disorders vary widely from study to study. However, despite these issues, some patterns are still fairly consistent across most studies, and some interesting theories have been advanced to potentially explain these relationships. We review some of the more consistent findings based on controlled studies to elucidate typical patterns of comorbidity and briefly discuss the conceptual relationship between these disorders and PTSD. In our review, we only include estimates of comorbidity that have been shown to be significantly related to PTSD diagnostic status. Furthermore, because we are most interested in provided gender-specific rates of psychopathology, we have excluded any studies that do not report prevalence rates by gender.

For most disorders, we report rates of both current and lifetime comorbidity. Current comorbidity typically refers to the current co-occurrence of two psychological disorders, whereas lifetime comorbidity usually reflects a history of additional disorders among individuals who currently meet criteria for the index disorder (e.g., PTSD). While rates of current comorbidity may provide the most clinically relevant information for clinicians working with PTSD, lifetime comorbidity also has implications for the course of symptoms over time among individuals who experience traumatic events.

Mood Disorders

Across studies of varying design, mood disorders have been found to co-occur quite commonly among individuals with a diagnosis of PTSD. Although little is known about the interrelationship between PTSD and depression/dysthymia, it has been suggested that these disorders may develop as a complicated grieving response to the loss associated with experiencing a traumatic event (Deering, Glover, Ready, Eddleman, & Alarcon, 1996). Major depressive disorder (MDD) is the most commonly occurring problem, with current rates of 17–23% among women (Cascardi, O'Leary, & Schlee, 1999; Kulka et al., 1988) and 10–55% among men (Gibson et al., 1999; Green, Grace, Lindy, Gleser, & Leonard, 1990; Green, Lindy, Grace, & Gleser, 1989; Hryvniak, 1989; Kulka et al., 1988; McFarlane & Papay, 1992; Orsillo, Weathers, et al., 1996). Lifetime rates of comorbid depression range from 42 to 49% among women (e.g., Breslau, Davis, Peterson, & Schulz, 1997; Kessler et al., 1995; Kulka et al., 1988) and 26 to 70% (Engdahl, Speed, Eberly, & Schwartz, 1991; Gibson et al., 1999; Kessler et al., 1995; Kulka et al., 1988; Orsillo, Weathers, et al., 1996) among men diagnosed with PTSD.

One issue of concern regarding the comorbidity of PTSD and MDD is that the significant symptom overlap between the two disorders may artificially inflate rates of comorbidity. As defined in DSM-IV (American Psychiatric Association, 1994), five of the nine depressive symptoms are necessary to meet Criterion A for MDD. Three of these nine symptoms (diminished interest in activities, difficulty sleeping, and difficulty concentrating) are also symptoms of PTSD. However, research has discounted the influence of these shared symptoms and has confirmed that the presence of both disorders reflects two unique symptom patterns (Blanchard et al., 1998; Orsillo, Litz, Weathers, Steinberg, & Keane, 1994).

Dysthymia is also fairly prevalent, with approximately 23–33% of women (Kessler et al., 1995; Kulka et al., 1988) and 21–29% of men (Gibson et al., 1999; Kessler et al., 1995; Kulka et al., 1988) with PTSD meeting criteria at some point during their lifetime. Although bipolar disorder co-occurs less frequently with PTSD than the other mood disorders, the prevalence rate is still significantly higher among individuals with PTSD compared to those without PTSD. Specifically, current rates of manic episodes are estimated to be about 4% among men (Gibson et al., 1999; Kulka et al., 1988) and 2.5% among women (Kulka et al., 1998) with PTSD. Lifetime rates of comorbid manic episodes range from 3 to 6% among women (Kessler et al., 1995; Kulka et al., 1988) and 6 to 12% among men (Gibson et al., 1999; Kessler et al., 1995; Kulka et al., 1988).

Anxiety Disorders

Individuals with PTSD also commonly meet criteria for additional anxiety disorders, including generalized anxiety disorder (GAD), social phobia, panic disorder, obsessive–compulsive disorder (OCD), and specific phobia. Many of these anxiety disorders have been functionally linked with PTSD, underscoring their potential importance in the development of an adequate treatment plan.

For example, Roemer (1997) proposed that GAD and PTSD are functionally related, in that worry, the primary feature of GAD, serves to suppress emotional reactions to internal and external trauma-related cues. It has been documented that individuals with GAD worry to distract themselves from emotional distress and physiological arousal (e.g., Borkovec & Roemer, 1995). Thus, the chronic worry associated with GAD may develop as a coping strategy among individuals with PTSD used to manage symptoms of intrusion and arousal.

Although the data currently supporting this theory are preliminary, several studies have demonstrated that GAD co-occurs with PTSD at a rate of about 38% among women (Kulka et al., 1988) and 7–20 % among men (e.g., Engdahl et al., 1991; Kulka et al., 1988; Orsillo, Weathers, et al., 1996). Lifetime rates of GAD range from 5 to 15% among women (e.g., Breslau et al., 1997; Kessler et al., 1995; Kulka et al., 1988). Estimates ranging from 16 to 94% have been found among male samples (Engdahl et al., 1991; Gibson et al., 1999; Kessler et al., 1995; Kulka et al., 1988), making it difficult to determine the specific prevalence of this comorbidity among men. Significant changes in the diagnostic criteria of GAD over the last decade and differential application of exclusionary criteria across studies may account for some of this variability. Current diagnostic criteria mandate that GAD should not be diagnosed as a comorbid condition with PTSD if the anxiety/worry occurs exclusively during the course of PTSD (American Psychiatric Association, 1994). It may be that this distinction is harder to make with male compared to female patients.

Social phobia has also been conceptually linked with interpersonal, trauma-related PTSD (Orsillo, Heimberg, Juster, & Garrett, 1996; Orsillo, 1997). It is common for victims of interpersonal traumas, such as rape, domestic violence, and combat, to experience shame about their involvement in the traumatic experience and to be rejected or blamed by others. Shame and interpersonal rejection have also been theoretically linked to the development of social phobia (Barlow, 1988; Buss, 1980), raising the possibility of a shared etiology for the two disorders. Preliminary research supports the hypothesis that trauma-related shame and negative responses from others play a significant role in the development of social phobia among individuals with PTSD (Orsillo, Heimberg, et al., 1996). While few studies have directly assessed the comorbidity of social phobia and PTSD, lifetime rates of 26–28% have been found among women with PTSD (Breslau et al., 1997; Kessler et al., 1995), and 17–28% among men (Kessler et al., 1995; Orsillo, Weathers, et al., 1996).

It has been theorized that panic disorder develops comorbidly with PTSD through classical conditioning (Falsetti, Resnick, Dansky, Lydiard, & Kilpatrick, 1995). Falsetti and her colleagues suggest that unconditioned fear responses to the traumatic event can pair with internal trauma-related cues, leading the individual to develop fear and avoidance of the physical sensations associated with the fear response. When the individual develops both a generalized fear of having panic attacks, and fear and avoidance of specific trauma-related cues, then comorbid diagnoses of PTSD and panic disorder should be assigned. Studies suggest that panic disorder co-occurs with PTSD in 13% of women (Kulka et al., 1988) and 5% of men (Kulka et al., 1988), with lifetime rates of 7–21% among women (Breslau et al., 1997; Kessler et al., 1995; Kulka et al., 1988) and 7–28% in men (Kessler et al., 1995; Kulka et al., 1988; Orsillo, Weathers, et al., 1996).

De Silva and Marks (1999) conceptually linked PTSD and OCD, presenting 8 cases in which a severe traumatic experience led to the development of OCD in addition to full-blown PTSD or significant PTSD symptomatology. In some, but not all, of the cases, the content of the obsessions and compulsions was directly linked to the trauma. For instance, a victim of sexual assault, who reported feeling "dirty" following the attack, developed concerns about contamination and ritualistic cleaning behavior of her clothes and apartment. Current rates of OCD have been estimated at about 8% among women (Kulka et al., 1988) and 9–13% among men (e.g., Gibson et al., 1999; Kulka et al., 1988; McFarlane & Papay, 1992) diagnosed with PTSD. Lifetime rates are approximately 13% among women (Kulka et al, 1988) and 6–10% among men (Kulka et al., 1988; Orsillo, Weathers, et al., 1996).

Specific phobia commonly co-occurs with PTSD, despite diagnostic criteria suggesting that a comorbid diagnosis should not be assigned if the anxiety and fear associated with the phobic object are better accounted for by the PTSD diagnosis (American Psychiatric Association, 1994). Thirty-six percent of women (Breslau et al., 1997) and 12–31% of men with PTSD also meet criteria for specific phobia during their lifetime (Kessler et al., 1995; Orsillo, Weathers, et al., 1996).

Additional Disorders

While several other individual disorders have been linked to trauma exposure in men and women, comorbidity studies have primarily focused on rates of additional anxiety and mood disorders. Furthermore, whereas the prevalence of some additional comorbid conditions, such as schizophrenia, antisocial personality disorder (ASPD), and eating disorders, have been empirically derived, they have been primarily examined in gender-specific samples. For instance, current comorbid rates of schizophrenia from 10 to 16% have been found among men diagnosed with PTSD (Gibson et al., 1999; Hryvniak, 1989). However, the rates among women are unknown. On the other hand, a history of eating disorders has been found to be relatively common (25%) among females with PTSD (e.g., Lipschitz, Winegar, Hartnick, Foote, & Southwick, 1999), whereas rates for men have not been reported. While current rates of ASPD have been found to range from 12 to

15% among male veterans with PTSD (e.g., Orsillo, Weathers, et al., 1996; Southwick, Yehuda, & Giller 1993), similar rates have been found among veterans without PTSD (e.g., Orsillo, Weathers, et al., 1996). Furthermore, the association between ASPD and PTSD among women has not been established.

Summary

In summary, a number of studies have confirmed significant comorbidity, particularly between PTSD, mood, and other anxiety disorders. Although specific prevalence rates vary widely, some emergent patterns can potentially inform the assessment and treatment of traumatized individuals. Of particular note, for most disorders, the prevalence rates did not differ dramatically between men and women. As discussed earlier, in nontraumatized samples, women are more likely to be diagnosed with mood and anxiety disorders. However, in the studies reviewed earlier, men and women with PTSD had similar rates of comorbid dysthymia, social phobia, lifetime panic disorder, OCD, and specific phobia. With regard to MDD and GAD, it is difficult to draw conclusions about potential gender differences given the wide variability in the prevalence rates found across samples of men. However, a preliminary analysis of this literature suggests that the pattern and form of comorbid psychopathology may be quite similar for men and women with PTSD.

Unfortunately, the majority of the studies we reviewed did not allow direct comparisons between genders, and comparing prevalence rates by gender across studies should be done with caution given the significant methodological variations across studies (e.g., trauma type, method of deriving diagnosis, clinical vs. community population). Thus, studies that directly compare rates between men and women within a particular sample are needed to provide accurate gender-specific information. Among the studies that we reviewed for this chapter, including a non-PTSD comparison group, only three of them statistically compared comorbidity patterns across the genders (Helzer, Robins, & McEvoy, 1987; Hubbard, Realmutto, Northwood, & Masten, 1995; Shalev et al., 1998). However, an analysis of these three studies, and a close examination of studies that include prevalence rates by gender, without statistically testing gender differences, may still be informative to clinicians treating individuals with PTSD.

GENDER COMPARISONS OF COMORBIDITY WITH PTSD

The three studies that directly compared comorbidity patterns among men and women with PTSD revealed minimal gender differences. Within a community sample, Helzer et al. (1987) found that women with PTSD had a greater likelihood of being diagnosed with comorbid panic disorder and simple phobia than men. The only gender difference in comorbidity with PTSD found in a small sample of 59 Cambodian American youth who survived civil conflict was that only women with PTSD experienced increased prevalence of somatoform pain disorder compared to controls (Hubbard et al., 1995). Finally, no gender differences in comorbidity of depression were evident in a sample of 211 Israeli ER patients with PTSD (Shalev et al., 1998). While these studies are valuable in that they directly compare comorbidity across gender, their results are severely limited due to changes in diagnostic criteria because of the large community study conducted (Helzer et al., 1987), the specialized nature of the samples (e.g., Hubbard et al., 1995; Shalev et al., 1998), and the limited range of comorbid diagnoses assessed (Shalev et al., 1998).

Several other studies, including large epidemiological surveys, have included men and women in their samples but have not statistically compared the genders. For example, Kessler and colleagues (1995) examined the comorbid disorders reported by men and women with PTSD derived from the NCS. In contrast to findings in the general population, men and women with PTSD did not differ in their likelihood of being assigned a comorbid diagnosis of a depressive mood disorder. Specifically, 48% of men and 49% of women with PTSD were also assigned a lifetime history of depression, and 21% of men and 23% of women with PTSD were assigned a lifetime history of dysthymia. In contrast, there did seem to be gender differences with regard to the presence of manic episodes among individuals with PTSD. Interestingly, men with PTSD were assigned a history of mania at twice the rate of women with PTSD (12% vs. 6%), whereas in the general population, no gender difference in prevalence was apparent (Kessler et al., 1998).

The absence of a gender difference in depressive disorders among trauma-exposed individuals with PTSD is striking given the consistent finding over time that adult women are much more likely to be at risk for the development of depression. If replicated, this finding lends significant support to the proposed etiological role of stressful and traumatic life events in the development of depression (e.g., Hankin & Abramson, 1999; Nolen-Hoeksema & Girgus, 1994; Strickland, 1992).

Consistent with findings from the general population, women with PTSD were more likely to be assigned a lifetime diagnosis of panic disorder (men = 7%, women = 13%) and agoraphobia (men = 16%, women = 22%) than men with PTSD. However, in contrast to general population findings (Kessler et al., 1994), rates of other anxiety disorders were roughly comparable across genders in the PTSD sample.

Men with PTSD were more likely to report lifetime histories of conduct disorder compared to women (men = 43%, women = 15%; Kessler et al., 1995), which is consistent with gender patterns in the general community (Kessler et al., 1994). However, conduct disorder appeared to be linked more strongly to the traumatic event for women than for men. Specifically, men with conduct disorder were less likely to experience a traumatic event before the onset of their conduct disorder symptoms, whereas women were more likely to develop conduct disorder posttrauma (Kessler et al., 1995).

The National Vietnam Veterans Readjustment Survey (NVVRS) conducted over 3,000 interviews with male and female veterans of the Vietnam Era (Kulka et al., 1988). Again, direct gender comparisons have not been statistically examined in this sample, but the data reveal certain patterns. Interestingly, some gender differences in this sample are consistent with findings from the community PTSD sample, and others are not. For example, in contrast to women with PTSD in the community, women in this military sample were more likely than men to have been assigned an additional diagnosis of depression both within the past 6 months (men = 16%, women = 23%) and over the course of their lifetime (men = 26%, women = 42%). Dysthymia was also more prevalent as a comorbid diagnosis for women (men = 21%, women = 33%). Interestingly, in contrast to population estimates (Kessler et al., 1994), but consistent with the PTSD subsample of the NCS study (Kessler et al., 1995), male veterans with PTSD were more likely than female veterans to have experienced a manic episode in the past 6 months (men = 4%, women = 3%) and within their lifetime (men = 6%, women = 3%) (Kulka et al., 1988).

With regard to the anxiety disorders, women with PTSD were more likely to have been assigned a diagnosis of panic disorder with the past 6 months (men = 5%, women = 13%) and over the course of their lifetime (men = 8%, women = 21%) (Kulka et al., 1988). Rates of GAD were roughly comparable across genders, with about 20% of both men and women being assigned a diagnosis within the past 6 months, and 44% of men and 38% of women carrying a lifetime diagnosis (Kulka et al., 1988).

It is difficult to draw any specific conclusions about gender differences in the specific patterns of comorbidity that occur with PTSD. More research is needed to determine whether men and women with PTSD differ in their likelihood of presenting with an additional anxiety disorder. Both studies described here suggest that women are more likely to present with an additional diagnosis of panic disorder, underscoring the importance of considering this diagnosis when treating women with PTSD. More information is needed to determine potential gender differences in the prevalence of the other anxiety disorders.

With regard to mood disorders, in both studies reviewed, men were more likely to have manic experiences than women, a pattern that is inconsistent with prevalence findings in the general population. One possibility is that symptoms of hypervigilance and arousal may be misattributed to mania in men with PTSD. However, more research is needed to determine potential etiological and treatment implications of this pattern.

In the nonmilitary sample, men and women with PTSD did not appreciably differ in their rates of comorbid depression and dysthymia. This findings needs to be replicated and examined statistically. However, if the finding remains consistent, it may have important implications for understanding the etiology of the two classes of disorders. One possibility is that depressed men are more at risk to become victims of traumatic events and/or to develop PTSD in response to trauma exposure. Data from the NCS confirm that whereas both men and women with a history of major depression are at heightened risk for developing PTSD, the risk is greater for men (Kessler et al., 1999). Another possible explanation for the lack of a gender differences in comorbid depression, briefly discussed earlier, is that both depression and PTSD develop as the result of trauma exposure. Research is needed to explore more fully these hypotheses and to elucidate their treatment implications. Furthermore, additional research is needed to determine why this pattern did not emerge within the military sample. Nonetheless, clinicians should be aware that in both the men and women they treat with PTSD, depression will likely be a prominent part of the presenting symptom picture.

RESEARCH IMPLICATIONS

Although a multitude of studies have examined additional disorders associated with PTSD, the research on gender, comorbidity, and PTSD thus far is significantly limited. Comorbidity, a complex issue to study, is often examined in a cursory manner. A number of issues need to be addressed in future research on this topic if the results are to be used in a way that can inform treatment.

Inclusion of Women in Studies

The majority of studies directed at comorbidity and PTSD include only male participants, and few studies statistically compare comorbidity rates between the genders. Because so few studies have included men and women, it is difficult to determine if the same patterns of comorbidity apply to both genders.

Type of Trauma

A related issue is that, in general, women experience different types of trauma than men. Women are more likely to be exposed to rape, sexual molestation, and childhood parental neglect and physical abuse, whereas men are more likely to be exposed to life-threatening accidents, fires, floods, natural disasters, combat, physical attack, or the injury or death of another

(Kessler et al., 1995). These qualitative differences in the nature of the traumas experienced likely impact on the symptoms reported by men compared to women (Deering et al., 1996). For instance, there is some evidence that GAD symptoms are associated with most types of trauma, panic symptoms may be linked to unpredictable and sudden events (e.g., rape), and somatic symptoms may be the result of physically brutal events (Deering et al., 1996). The potential influence of trauma type on gender and comorbidity is apparent in the comparison of the military and nonmilitary samples described earlier.

Use of an Appropriate Control Group

The studies reviewed in this chapter compare individuals with and without PTSD on rates of comorbid psychopathology to determine if the high rates of additional disorders are specifically due to PTSD. However, comparisons with other patient groups could be helpful in determining if the rates and patterns of comorbidity among individuals with PTSD are unique in any way to this population. Overall rates of comorbidity with PTSD do not seem to be particularly higher than rates of comorbidity with most other psychological disorders (Kessler et al., 1994). However, there may be differences in comorbidity patterns that have thus far not been studied. Research in this area could inform our understanding and treatment of the nature of posttrauma psychopathology.

Coverage of Disorders

It is uncommon for studies of comorbidity with PTSD to include the full range of Axis I and II disorders in their assessment. Often, the decision about what disorders to include in the assessment is guided by previous findings. For instance, since depression is frequently found to be comorbid with PTSD, most studies include depression in their assessment. Whereas this approach builds on preexisting findings, it may unintentionally bias the conclusions drawn from the literature. In other words, it is difficult to know if disorders such as avoidant personality disorder or social phobia infrequently present with PTSD, or if they are simply not assessed.

Sample

The results of studies on comorbidity are likely to be highly influenced by whether the sample is drawn from a clinical setting or the community. Epidemiological studies are generally considered the best design to provide accurate estimates of comorbidity with good generalizability. However, diagnoses in these studies are typically made by laypersons, who may inaccurately label transient responses to internal and external stressors as psychological disorders (Regier et al., 1998). Furthermore, in order to make predictions about course and prognosis, and to choose appropriate interventions, we are most interested in how comorbidity occurs within a clinical or treatment-seeking sample. Clinical samples assessed in comorbidity studies to date have not always been representative of the general PTSD population (e.g., samples of inpatient adolescents, ER patients, male inmates) and, as a result, may vary widely in reported levels of psychological distress. For example, inpatient veterans (e.g., Hryvniak, 1989) may be lower functioning and suffer from more comorbid disorders than nonhospitalized PTSD victims. Thus, carefully designed clinical studies are needed to best inform mental health professionals about the nature of comorbidity likely to be present among patients with PTSD.

Careful Consideration of the Onset of Disorders

In order to understand the clinical and theoretical significance of comorbidity as it relates to PTSD, research that elucidates the temporal pattern of comorbidity is needed. Many of the theories on the comorbidity of PTSD and other disorders suggest that the comorbid disorders develop as a result of exposure to the traumatic event (e.g., Deering et al., 1996; De Silva & Marks, 1999; Falsetti et al., 1995; Orsillo, 1997; Roemer, 1997). However, several studies have revealed that preexisting psychopathology increases an individual's risk for developing PTSD (Green et al., 1990; Kessler et al., 1999; Mirza, Bhadrinath, Goodyer, & Gilmour, 1998).

Examining the onset of comorbid conditions is a particularly relevant gender issue. The comorbid disorders that frequently predate the development of PTSD, depression, and other anxiety disorders are consistently more prevalent among women (e.g., Kessler et al., 1994). Furthermore, there is some evidence that preexisting disorders differentially increase risk for developing PTSD for men compared to women. For instance, within the NCS sample, Kessler et al., (1999) found that panic disorder was a significant risk factor for developing PTSD for men but not for women. Furthermore, within a sample of individuals exposed to a mass shooting, a history of predisaster diagnosis (excluding PTSD) significantly predicted the development of PTSD for women but not for men (North, Smith, & Spitznagel, 1994).

To complicate an already complex picture, gender and onset of comorbid disorders may be further influenced by the relationship of type of trauma and gender, as discussed earlier. The onset of a traumatic event may vary systematically across the genders. Rape, sexual molestation, and childhood parental neglect, traumas that are most common among women (Kessler et al., 1995), may occur earlier in life.

Future studies that examine age of onset must consider a prospective design that takes into account both the participant's entire life history of traumatic events and the development of PTSD-related disorders as they precede, coexist with, or follow the onset of PTSD (Deering et al., 1996). Many studies that have examined the onset of comorbid conditions utilize a retrospective design that is fraught with bias. These studies frequently produce conflicting results (e.g., Mellman et al., 1992; O'Toole, Marshall, Schureck, & Dobson, 1998).

Accuracy of Assessment

Studies that assess comorbidity must use "gold standard" assessment procedures for deriving diagnoses. The instruments used should be demonstrated to be valid and reliable, and researchers must show some interrater reliability within their specific study sample. Many studies have assessed PTSD and comorbid disorders using the Diagnostic Interview Schedule (DIS; e.g., Helzer et al., 1987; Kessler et al., 1995; Lipschitz et al., 1999; North et al., 1994), an instrument designed to be administered by laypersons that does not allow for use of clinical judgment. Other studies have based diagnosis on the clinician-administered version of the Structured Clinical Interview for DSM (SCID; e.g., Shalev et al., 1998), patient-report version of the SCID (e.g., Hubbard et al., 1995), or chart reviews of clinician notes (e.g., Hryvniak, 1989). The lack of consistent measurement methods makes drawing conclusions across studies difficult, particularly because research has documented that the type of assessment instrument used in a particular study has profound effects on the prevalence of disorders revealed (e.g., Wittchen, 1996; Zimmerman & Mattia, 1999b).

The use of non-clinician-administered scales is perhaps most problematic. Whereas these assessment strategies make epidemiological studies feasible, the findings may lack a clinical context. Making accurate diagnoses requires use of clinical judgment and, as such, it is important that the criteria in DSM-IV not be applied mechanically by untrained individuals (American Psychiatric Association, 1994). For example, a patient may have a primary diagnosis of PTSD, and a clinician may conclude that additional GAD symptoms are better accounted for by the hypervigilance symptoms of PTSD. However, in some standard interview formats (e.g., the DIS), this patient would be diagnosed with both PTSD and GAD, even if a clinician would not conceptualize the symptoms in this manner.

Furthermore, DSM-IV includes several exclusion criteria that are necessary to establish boundaries between disorders. For instance, for many conditions, the presence of an underlying physical disorder that could potentially contribute to the expression of symptoms must be ruled out. Thyroid, adrenal, pituitary, parathyroid, and seizure disorders, and multiple sclerosis and mitral valve prolapse can all produce symptoms that may be attributed to a psychological disorder. The importance of ruling out potential medical complications may be particularly relevant for women. Because so many physical disorders manifest in symptoms of depression, anxiety, and somatization disorder, which are much more common among women, the misdiagnosis of physical disorders as psychiatric in part accounts for women's higher rate of these disorders (Klonoff & Landrine, 1997).

Gender biases in assessment must also be considered in determining comorbidity with PTSD. Ford and Widiger (1989) demonstrated that clinicians might be influenced by stereotyping and sex bias when assigning personality disorders to patients. They found that psychologists significantly failed to diagnose histrionic personality disorder more often in male than in female patients. Furthermore, they failed to diagnose ASPD in female patients more often than in male patients. And, these apparent sex biases were more evident for the female cases. For a fuller discussion on gender issues, assessment, and PTSD, see Cusack et al. (Chapter 6, this volume).

Socioeconomic Status and Ethnicity

Data derived from general psychopathology research underscore the importance of examining mental illness in the context of ethnicity and socioeconomic status. Rates of almost all disorders have been found to decline monotonically with increases in income and education; furthermore, rates of general psychopathology differ across ethnic groups (Kessler et al., 1994). Specifically, African Americans are less likely to be diagnosed with mood disorders, substance use, and lifetime comorbidity compared to Caucasians. In contrast, Hispanics have a higher prevalence of current mood disorders and comorbidity than non-Hispanic whites.

None of the studies in our review on comorbidity included socioeconomic status or ethnicity as factors to consider in making gender comparisons, despite the fact that these attributes likely influence symptom presentation, detection of psychological disorders, likelihood of seeking and receiving treatment, and response to intervention. Future research on diverse populations to address these issues is sorely needed.

Summary

In conclusion, although comorbidity with PTSD has been assessed in a number of studies, gender has been largely ignored, and several complex methodological issues deserve significant attention in future research. Although careful scientific control is needed to determine specific comorbidity with PTSD, these diagnostic issues are important only if they impact treatment in a meaningful and significant way. Thus, we now discuss the potential treatment implications of comorbidity with PTSD among men and women.

TREATMENT IMPLICATIONS

As mentioned earlier, comorbidity of psychological disorders with PTSD has been linked with a more chronic course of the PTSD (Blanchard et al., 1998; Breslau & Davis, 1992; Mcfarlane & Papay, 1992; Zlotnick et al., 1999), more severe comorbid symptoms (Blanchard et al., 1998; Sautter et al., 1999 Shalev et al., 1998; Zimmerman & Mattia, 1999a), and significant functional role impairment (Blanchard et al., 1998; Mollica et al., 1999; Shalev et al., 1998). However, given the lack of research on gender, PTSD, and comorbidity, potential gender differences in these complications have not been fully explored. Given that this area is in its infancy, the delineation of specific treatment recommendations for men compared to women with PTSD and comorbid conditions would be premature, particularly because our review of the literature detected few differences. Instead, in this section, we briefly consider recommendations and findings from other contexts, such as studies on gender differences in psychological treatment in general and recommendations for treating comorbidity with PTSD regardless of gender, that may be potentially important for clinicians who treat men and women with PTSD.

The Impact of Gender on Treatment Delivery

General population studies underscore the importance of considering patient gender in order that a disorder be identified and appropriately treated. Women diagnosed with a psychological disorder are more likely to seek health services than men, despite their relative disadvantage in access to health insurance (Kessler, 1998). Women may also be more likely to be targeted for treatment in primary care settings. Badger et al. (1999) found that male physicians were significantly more likely to explore symptoms of depression and discuss a diagnosis with female compared to male patients.

Given the relatively high rate of comorbid depression in men with PTSD, this gender bias in detection and treatment may be particularly problematic in this population. Health care providers need to be educated about the high rate of depression among traumatized male patients in order to facilitate the detection and appropriate treatment of these disorders. It is recommended that practitioners consider administering a brief screening for depression (e.g., the Beck Depression Inventory–II; Beck, Steer, & Brown, 1996, or the Reynolds Depression Screening Inventory; Reynolds & Kobak, 1998) to the male and female clients they treat for trauma-related disorders.

There is also some evidence for gender bias in the type of treatment offered to men and women in the general population. For instance, gender influences the type of medications prescribed to individuals with psychological disorders. National survey data reveal that women in general are more likely than men to receive prescriptions for anxiolytics and antide-pressants (Hohmann, 1989; Sclar, Robison, Skaer, & Galin, 1998) but are equally likely to receive prescriptions for hypnotics/barbituates and anti-psychotics. These gender differences persist even when the influence of symptoms, physician diagnosis, and sociodemographic and health service factors is controlled (Hohmann, 1989). Gender also impacts the probabil-ity that a patient in primary care will be referred for mental health treat-ment. Badger and colleagues (1999) found that both male and female phy-sicians in this setting recommended therapy more often for female than male patients who presented with the same somatic depression.

Potential gender biases in treatment recommendations need to be ex-plored in a PTSD population. It may be that depression in males with PTSD is undertreated. Physicians and mental health care providers should care-fully explore the potential utility of antidepressants and psychotherapy among men with a trauma history who present for treatment.

A Functional Approach to Treatment of Comorbid Disorders

Although little is known about the impact of gender on the psychological treatment of comorbid conditions associated with PTSD, the course of treatment will likely be influenced by the conceptual and functional rela-tionship between the comorbid disorders. Formal definitions of comorbidi-ty, based on a medical model, assume that two independent disorders are present simultaneously in an individual and that they each require specific treatment; yet clinical judgment frequently suggests that this is not the case. Many of the theories of comorbidity, as discussed earlier, assume that the trauma plays an important conceptual role in the development of both dis-orders. These issues (both within PTSD and among other disorders) have led theorists to propose a functional, dimensional alternative to our current classification system (Hayes, Wilson, Gifford, Follette, & Strosahl, 1996). The goal of this approach is to identify functional processes that underlie the identifiable signs and symptoms expressed by patients. Thus, the topo-graphical characteristics of a patient's behavior are not the basis for classifi-cation; instead, there is a focus on the functional processes thought to have produced and maintained the behaviors.

Wasler and Hayes (1998) proposed that experiential avoidance might be a functional dimension underlying the myriad psychological problems reported by men and women with a history of trauma exposure. Experien-tial avoidance refers to the attempted avoidance of internal experiences, such as thoughts, feelings, and memories. Wasler and Hayes argue that the symptoms of the disorders that co-occur with PTSD, including, for in-stance, self-injurious behavior, avoidance, disordered eating, and substance use, might be best understood as attempts to control and avoid internal ex-periences such as sadness, anxiety, fear, thoughts of worthlessness, and painful memories.

Research on experiential avoidance suggests that there may some gender differences in this construct among clinical samples, with women reporting significantly more avoidance then men (Hayes, Bergan, et al., 1996). However, it is even more likely that the methods used to exert experiential control (e.g., behavioral avoidance, use of substances, disordered eating) will differ between men and women as a result of learning history and gender socialization, although our preliminary investigation suggests fewer gender differences in comorbidity than would be expected. Thus, it may be that the underlying process that produces psychopathological behaviors in men and women is similar, and that treatment directed at this process will be more successful than symptom-based, gender-influenced approaches.

Alarcon, Glover, and Deering (1999) also proposed a model to account for the comorbidity seen with chronic PTSD that does not assume the presence of discrete independent disorders. These authors developed a cascade model of stress response, suggesting that the symptoms expressed by individuals with a history of trauma exposure constantly change over time in response to a variety of interrelated factors operating at different stages. Thus, designating specific comorbid disorders may be an unnecessary and perhaps misleading characterization of the symptom expression of men and women with a trauma history. In other words, comorbidity, in this case, may simply reflect a number of interrelated symptoms that arise from a patient's perceived need to cope with the traumatic event, and the internal and external stressors that have arisen from the experience.

These theories suggest that the function of comorbid conditions and their interrelationship with exposure to the traumatic event require attention when developing a treatment plan for a patient with PTSD and comorbid conditions. Although the development of such treatment approaches has not been extensively discussed in the literature, few important issues have been raised in the literature based on the conceptual models discussed earlier that can guide clinical work in this area. For instance, Falsetti and Resnick (1997) suggested that additional treatment may be indicated before engaging in trauma processing with patients diagnosed with comorbid PTSD and panic disorder. If the patient's fear and avoidance of physical sensations are directly addressed, he or she might be more willing to engage in a trauma processing therapy, such as exposure therapy. Given the gender differences in the prevalence of comorbid panic disorder discussed earlier, addressing this potential fear before initiating a trauma-focused intervention may be particularly warranted for female patients.

Roemer (1997) discussed the potential obstacles to treatment that can be associated with comorbid GAD and PTSD. Based on the findings discussed earlier, GAD appears to be present as a comorbid condition with similar frequencies among men and women with PTSD. Like panic disorder, GAD is associated with a tendency toward wanting to avoid emotional experiences. Thus, a patient with comorbid GAD and PTSD may present with superficial worries and concerns in a subtle attempt to avoid processing more threatening, trauma-related emotional material in session (Roemer, 1997). Clinicians must be vigilant to observe these avoidance responses and address them directly in order to facilitate the treatment of both disorders.

Men and women with comorbid social phobia and PTSD may also pose distinct treatment challenges. For instance, they may be less likely to accept referral into a PTSD therapy group given their fear of being exposed to the scrutiny of others and speaking in front of a group (Orsillo, 1997). Once in the group, an individual with both social phobia and PTSD may be less likely to actively participate or may be at risk for dropping out prematurely. Addressing these social concerns directly and relating them back to the shame and social rejection associated with the traumatic event may facilitate trauma-focused treatment.

SUMMARY

It has been established that PTSD rarely occurs as a single disorder. Instead, the presence of comorbid psychopathology is the norm. Based on our review of the more general comorbidity literature, there are a number of important gender differences that one might anticipate as impacting the course and treatment of PTSD. The literature on gender issues in PTSD with comorbid mental health disorders is in its infancy. Although a number of studies describe psychological disorders that occur within specific populations (e.g., rape victims, individuals with PTSD), carefully controlled studies are absent. Given the complex methodological issues associated with studying comorbidity, this absence of studies is not surprising. Furthermore, comorbidity may, in some cases, be better understood from a functional rather than a structural viewpoint. Regardless of the classification issues, the multiplicity of symptoms coexisting with PTSD requires more study. Researchers are encouraged to include men and women of varying ethnicities and socioeconomic status in order to expand more fully our understanding of this area.

REFERENCES

Alarcon, R. D., Glover, S. G., & Deering, C. G. (1999). The cascade model: An alternative to comorbidity in the pathogenesis of posttraumatic stress disorder. *Psychiatry, 62,* 114–124.

American Psychiatric Association. (1994). *Diagnostic and statistical manual of mental disorders* (4th ed.). Washington, DC: Author.

Badger, L. W., Berbaum, M., Carney, P. A., Dietrich, A. J., Owen, M., & Stem, J. T.

(1999). Physician–patient gender and the recognition and treatment of depression in primary care. *Journal of Social Service Research, 25,* 21–39.

Barlow, D. H. (1988). *Anxiety and its disorders: The nature and treatment of anxiety and panic.* New York: Guilford Press.

Beck, A. T., Steer, R. A., & Brown, G. K. (1996). *Manual for the BDI-II.* San Antonio, TX: Psychological Corporation.

Blanchard, E. B., Buckley, T. C., Hickling, E. J., & Taylor, A. E. (1998). Posttraumatic stress disorder and comorbid major depression: Is the correlation an illusion? *Journal of Anxiety Disorders, 12,* 21–37.

Borkovec, T. D., & Roemer, L. (1995). Perceived functions of worry among generalized anxiety disorder subjects: Distraction from more emotional topics? *Journal of Behavior Therapy and Experimental Psychiatry, 26,* 25–30.

Breslau, N., & Davis, G. C. (1992). Posttraumatic stress disorder in an urban population of young adults: Risk factors for chronicity. *American Journal of Psychiatry, 149,* 671–675.

Breslau, N., Davis, G. C., Peterson, E. L., & Schultz, L. (1997). Psychiatric sequelae of posttraumatic stress disorder in women. *Archives of General Psychiatry, 54,* 81–87.

Bruce, M. L., & Kim, K. M. (1992). Differences in the effects of divorce on major depression in men and women. *American Journal of Psychiatry, 149,* 914–917.

Buss, A. H. (1980). *Self-consciousness and social anxiety.* New York: Freeman.

Cascardi, M., O'Leary, D. O., & Schlee, K. (1999). Co-occurrence and correlates of posttraumatic stress disorder and major depression in physically abused women. *Journal of Family Violence, 14,* 227–249.

Chorpita, B. F., & Barlow, D. H. (1998). The development of anxiety: The role of control in the early environment. *Psychological Bulletin, 124,* 3–21.

Cohen, L. S., Sichel, D. A., Dimmock, J. A., & Rosenbaum, J. F. (1994a). Impact of pregnancy on panic disorder: A case series. *Journal of Clinical Psychiatry, 55,* 284–288.

Cohen, L. S., Sichel, D. A., Dimmock, J. A., & Rosenbaum, J. F. (1994b). Postpartum course in women with preexisting panic disorder. *Journal of Clinical Psychiatry, 55,* 289–292.

Deering, C. G., Glover, S. G., Ready, D., Eddleman, H. C., & Alarcon, R. D. (1996). Unique patterns of comorbidity in posttraumatic stress disorder from different sources of trauma. *Comprehensive Psychiatry, 37,* 336–346.

De Silva, P., & Marks, M. (1999). The role of traumatic experiences in the genesis of obsessive–compulsive disorder. *Behaviour Research and Therapy, 37,* 941–951.

Engdahl, B., Speed, N., Eberly, R. E., & Schwartz, J. (1991). Comorbidity of psychiatric disorders and personality profiles of American World War II prisoners of war. *Journal of Nervous and Mental Disease, 179,*181–187.

Falsetti, S. A., & Resnick, H. S. (1997). Frequency and severity of panic attack symptoms in a treatment seeking sample of trauma victims. *Journal of Traumatic Stress, 10,* 683–689.

Falsetti, S. A., Resnick, H. S., Dansky, B. S., Lydiard, R. B., & Kilpatrick, D. G. (1995). The relationship of stress to panic disorder: Cause or effect? In C. M. Mazure (Ed.), *Does stress cause psychiatric illness?* (pp. 111–147). Washington, DC: American Psychiatric Press.

Fincham, F. D., Beach, S. R. H., Harold, G. T., & Osborne, L. N. (1997). Marital satisfaction and depression: Different causal relationships for men and women? *Psychological Science, 8,* 351–357.

Ford, M. R., & Widiger, T. A. (1989). Sex bias in the diagnosis of histrionic and antisocial personality disorders. *Journal of Consulting and Clinical Psychology, 57,* 301–305.

Gibson, L. E., Holt, J. C., Fondacaro, K. M., Tang, T. S., Powell, T. A., & Turbitt, E. L. (1999). An examination of antecedent traumas and psychiatric comorbidity among male inmates with PTSD. *Journal of Traumatic Stress, 12,* 473–485.

Green, B. L., Grace, M. C., Lindy, J. D., Gleser, G. C., & Leonard, A. (1990). Risk factors for PTSD and other diagnoses in a general sample of Vietnam veterans. *American Journal of Psychiatry, 147,* 729–733.

Green, B. L., Lindy, J. D., Grace, M. C., & Leonard, A. C. (1992). Chronic posttraumatic stress disorder and diagnostic comorbidity in a disaster sample. *Journal of Nervous and Mental Disease, 180,* 760–766.

Greenberg, P. E., Sisitsky, T., Kessler, R. C., Finkelstein, S. N., Berndt, E. R., Davidson, J. R. T., Ballenger, J. C., & Fyer, A. J. (1999). The economic burden of anxiety disorders in the 1990s. *Journal of Clinical Psychiatry, 60,* 427–435.

Hamburger, M. E., Lilienfeld, S. O., & Hogben, M. (1996). Psychopathy, gender, and gender roles: Implications for antisocial and histrionic personality disorders. *Journal of Personality Disorders, 10,* 41–55.

Hammen, C., Marks, T., Mayo, A., & DeMayo, R. (1985). Depression self-schemas, life stress, and vulnerability to depression. *Journal of Abnormal Psychology, 94,* 308–319.

Hankin, B. L., & Abramson, L. Y. (1999). Development of gender differences in depression: Description and possible explanations. *Annals of Medicine, 31,* 372–379.

Hayes, S. C., Bergan, J., Strosahl, K., Wilson, K. G., Polusny, M., Naugles, A., McCurry, S., Parker, L., & Hart, P. (1996, November). *Measuring psychological acceptance: The Acceptance and Action Questionnaire.* Paper presented at the meeting of the Association for Advancement of Behavior Therapy, New York, NY.

Hayes, S. C., Wilson, K. G., Gifford, E. V., Follette, V. M., & Strosahl, K. (1996). Experiential avoidance and behavioral disorders: A functional dimensional approach to diagnosis and treatment. *Journal of Consulting and Clinical Psychology, 64,* 1152–1168.

Helzer, J. E., Robins, L. N., & McEvoy, L. (1987). Post traumatic stress disorder in the general population: Findings of the epidemiologic catchment area survey. *New England Journal of Medicine, 317,* 1630–1634.

Hohmann, A. A. (1989). Gender bias in psychotropic drug prescribing in primary care. *Medical Care, 27,* 478–490.

Hryvniak, M. R. (1989). Concurrent psychiatric illness in inpatients with posttraumatic stress disorder. *Military Medicine, 184,* 399–401.

Hubbard, J., Realmutto, G. M., Northwood, A. K., & Masten, A. S. (1995). Comorbidity of psychiatric diagnoses with posttraumatic stress disorders in survivors of childhood trauma. *Journal of the American Academy of Child and Adolescent Psychiatry, 34,* 1167–1173.

Kessler, R. C. (1998). Sex differences in the DSM-III-R psychiatric disorders in the United States: Results from the National Comorbidity Survey. *Journal of the American Medical Women's Association, 53,* 148–158.

Kessler, R. C., McGonagle, K. A., Zhao, S., Nelson, C. B., Hughes, M., Eshleman, S., Hans-Ulrich, W., & Kendler, K. S. (1994). Lifetime and 12–month prevalence of DSM-III-R psychiatric disorders in the United States: Results from the National Comorbidity Survey. *Archives of General Psychiatry, 51,* 8–19.

Kessler, R. C., Sonnega, A., Bromet, E., Hughes, M., & Nelson, C. B. (1995). Posttraumatic stress disorder in the National Comorbidity Study. *Archives of General Psychiatry, 52,* 1048–1060.

Kessler, R. C., Sonnega, A., Bromet, E., Hughes, M., Nelson, C. B., & Breslau, N. (1999). Epidemiological risk factors for trauma and PTSD. In R. Yehuda (Ed.), *Risk factors for posttraumatic stress disorder* (pp. 23–59). Washington, DC: American Psychiatric Press.

Klonoff, E., & Landrine, H. (1997). *Preventing misdiagnosis of women: A guide to physical disorders that have psychiatric symptoms.* Thousand Oaks, CA: Sage.

Kulka, R. A., Schlenger, W. E., Fairbank, J. A., Hough, R. L., Jordan, B. K., Marmar, C. R., & Weiss, D. S. (1988). *Contractual report of findings from the National Vietnam Veterans Readjustment Study: Vol. II. Tables of findings.* Research Triangle Park, NC: Research Triangle Institute.

Kulka, R. A., Schlenger, W. E., Fairbank, J. A., Hough, R. L., Jordan, B. K., Marmar, C. R., & Weiss, D. S. (1990). *Trauma and the Vietnam War generation.* New York: Brunner/Mazel.

Lipschitz, D. S., Winegar, R. K., Hartnick, E., Foote, B., & Southwick, S. M. (1999). Posttraumatic stress disorder in hospitalized adolescents: Psychiatric comorbidity and clinical correlates. *Journal of American Academy of Child and Adolescent Psychiatry, 38,* 385–392.

McFarlane, A. C., & Papay, P. (1992). Multiple diagnoses in posttraumatic stress disorder in the victims of a natural disaster. *Journal of Nervous and Mental Disease, 180,* 498–504.

McLeod, D., Hoehn-Saric, R., Foster, G., & Hipsley, P. (1993). The influence of premenstrual syndrome on ratings of anxiety in women with generalized anxiety disorder. *Acta Psychiatrica Scandinavica, 88,* 248–251.

Mellman, T. A., Randolph, C. A., Brawman-Mintzer, O., Flores, L. P., & Milanes, F. J. (1992). Phenomenology and course of psychiatric disorders associated with combat-related posttraumatic stress disorder. *American Journal of Psychiatry, 149,* 1568–1574.

Merikangas, K. R., & Pollock, R. A. (2000). Anxiety disorders in women. In M. B. Goldman, & M. C. Hatch (Eds.), *Women and health* (pp. 1010–1023). San Diego: Academic Press.

Mirza, K. A. H., Bhadrinath, B. R., Goodyer, I. M., & Gilmour, C. (1998). Post-traumatic stress disorder in children and adolescents following road traffic accidents. *British Journal of Psychiatry, 172,* 443–447.

Mollica, R. F., McInnes, K., Sarajlic, N., Lavelle, J., Sarajlic, I., & Massagli, M. P. (1999). Disability associated with psychiatric comorbidity and health status in Bosnian refugees living in Croatia. *Journal of the American Medical Association, 282,* 433–439.

Mueser, K. T., Goodman, L. B., Trumbetta, S. L., Rosenberg, S. D., Osher, F. C., Vidaver, R., Auciello, P., & Foy, D. W. (1998). Trauma and posttraumatic stress disorder in severe mental illness. *Journal of Consulting and Clinical Psychology, 66,* 493–499.

Murray, C. J. L., & Lopez, A. D. (Eds.). (1996). *The global burden of disease.* Cambridge, MA: Harvard University Press.

Nolen-Hoeksema, S., & Girgus, J. S. (1994). The emergence of gender differences in depression during adolescence. *Psychological Bulletin, 115,* 424–443.

North, C. S., Smith, E. M., & Spitznagel, E. L. (1994). Posttraumatic stress disorder in survivors of a mass shooting. *American Journal of Psychiatry, 151,* 82–88.

Orsillo, S. M. (1997). Social avoidance and PTSD: The role of comorbid social phobia. *NC-PTSD Clinical Quarterly, 7*(3), 54–57.

Orsillo, S. M., Heimberg, R. G., Juster, H. R., & Garrett, J. (1996). Social phobia and PTSD in Vietnam veterans. *Journal of Traumatic Stress, 9,* 235–252.

Orsillo, S. M., Litz, B. T., Weathers, F. W., Steinberg, H. R., & Keane, T. M. (1994, November). *Defining the boundaries of PTSD: A symptom-level analysis of the comorbidity of PTSD and major depression.* Poster session presented at the annual meeting of the Association for Advancement of Behavior Therapy, San Diego, CA.

Orsillo, S. M., Weathers, F. W., Litz, B. T., Steinberg, H. R., Huska, J. A., & Keane, T. M. (1996). Current and lifetime psychiatric disorders among veterans with war zone related posttraumatic stress disorder. *Journal of Nervous and Mental Disease, 184,* 307–313.

O'Toole, B. I., Marshall, R. P., Schureck, R. J., & Dobson, M. (1998). Posttraumatic stress disorder and comorbidity in Australian Vietnam veterans: Risk factors, chronicity, and combat. *Australian and New Zealand Journal of Psychiatry, 32,* 32–42.

Paris, J. (1997). Social factors in the personality disorders. *Transcultural Psychiatry, 34,* 421–452.

Perna, G., Brambilla, F., Arancio, C., & Bellodi, L. (1995). Menstrual cycle-related sensitivity to 35% CO_2 in panic patients. *Biological Psychiatry, 37,* 528–532.

Reynolds, W. M., & Kobak, K. A. (1998). *Reynolds Depression Screening Inventory: Professional manual.* Odessa, FL: Psychological Assessment Resources.

Regier, D. A., Kaelber, C. T., Rae, D. S., Farmer, M. E., Knauper, B., Kessler, R. C., & Norquist, G. S. (1998). Limitations of diagnostic criteria and assessment instruments for mental disorders. *Archives of General Psychiatry, 55,* 109–115.

Roemer, L. (1997). Treatment of worry in trauma-exposed individuals: Reducing cognitive avoidance to facilitate trauma-focused emotional processing. *NC-PTSD Clinical Quarterly, 7*(3), 58–60.

Sautter, F. J., Brailey, K., Uddo, M. M., Hamilton, M. F., Beard, M. G., & Borges, A. H. (1999). PTSD and comorbid psychotic disorder: Comparison with veterans diagnosed with PTSD or psychotic disorder. *Journal of Traumatic Stress, 12,* 73–88.

Sclar, D. A., Robison, L. M., Skaer, T. L., & Galin, R. S. (1998). What factors influence the prescribing of antidepressant pharmacotherapy?: An assessment of national office-based encounters. *International Journal of Psychiatry in Medicine, 28,* 407–419.

Shalev, A. Y., Freedman, S., Peri, T., Brandes, D., Sahar, T., Orr, S. P., & Pitman, R. K. (1998). Prospective study of posttraumatic stress disorder and depression following trauma. *American Journal of Psychiatry, 155,* 630–637.

Southwick, S. M., Yehuda, R., & Giller, E. L. (1993). Personality disorders in treatment-seeking combat veterans with posttraumatic stress disorder. *American Journal of Psychiatry, 150,* 1020–1023.

Strickland, B. R. (1992). Women and depression. *Current Directions in Psychological Science, 1,* 132–135.

Villeponteaux, V. A., Lydiard, B., Laraia, M. T., Stuart, G. W., & Ballenger, J. C. (1992). The effects of pregnancy on preexisting panic disorder. *Journal of Clinical Psychiatry, 53,* 201–203.

Wasler, R. D., & Hayes, S. C. (1998). Acceptance and trauma survivors: Applied issues and problems. In V. M. Follette, J. I. Ruzek, & F. R. Abueg (Eds.), *Cognitive-behavioral therapies for trauma* (pp. 256–277). New York: Guilford Press.

Wittchen, H. U. (1996). Critical issues in the evaluation of comorbidity of psychiatric disorders. *British Journal of Psychiatry, 168*(Suppl. 30), 9–16.

Zimmerman, M., & Mattia, J. I. (1999a). Psychotic subtyping of major depressive disorder and posttraumatic stress disorder. *Journal of Clinical Psychiatry, 60,* 311–314.

Zimmerman, M., & Mattia, J. I. (1999b). Psychiatric diagnosis in clinical practice: Is comorbidity being missed? *Comprehensive Psychiatry, 40,* 182–191.

Zlotnick, C., Warshaw, M., Shea, M. T., Allsworth, J., Pearlstein, T., & Keller, M. B. (1999). Chronicity in posttraumatic stress disorder (PTSD) and predictors of course of comorbid PTSD in patients with anxiety disorders. *Journal of Traumatic Stress, 12,* 89–100.

9 | Gender and the Comorbidity of PTSD with Substance Use Disorders

SHERRY H. STEWART
PAIGE OUIMETTE
PAMELA J. BROWN

Research on the association between posttraumatic stress disorder (PTSD) and substance use disorders (SUDs) began with studies of male combat veterans in Veterans Administration (VA) settings (see reviews by Keane & Wolfe, 1990; Kofoed, Friedman, & Peck, 1993). Although early research on comorbid PTSD–SUDs focused almost exclusively on male veterans whose pathology arose in the context of combat trauma, research on women with comorbid PTSD–SUDs has expanded over the last decade, suggesting potential different etiological pathways for men and women (Najavits, Weiss, & Shaw, 1997). A review of gender and PTSD–SUD comorbidity is important, because patient gender may confer differential treatment implications (Kimerling, Ouimette, & Cronkite, 1998).

The major purpose of this chapter is to examine gender as a potentially important individual-difference variable with respect to the co-occurrence of PTSD and SUDs. We begin with a review of studies that have examined comorbidity rates in both general and patient populations to demonstrate that PTSD–SUD comorbidity is an important issue in both nonclinical and clinical samples of both genders. We then examine similarities and differences in the predictors of comorbidity in male and female samples. In the next section, we review the research examining potential functional relations between these two forms of behavioral pathology to determine whether there may be gender differences in the ways that PTSD and SUDs are interrelated. For example, we look at evidence suggesting that women may be more susceptible than men to a form of comorbidity in which the PTSD precedes the development of the SUD. Although prior research suggests that patients with comorbid PTSD–SUDs are a particularly severely affected group relative to those patients with either of these disorders alone, little previous research has attended to gender as a possible moderator of these effects. Thus, we present new data from treatment-seeking men and women with SUDs to demonstrate that gender moderates PTSD status effects on aspects of service utilization and treatment course. We conclude with a section on the implications of observed gender differences for the treatment of women versus men with comorbid PTSD–SUDs.

GENDER AND PTSD–SUD COMORBIDITY IN GENERAL AND CLINICAL POPULATIONS

In this section, we review several large-scale epidemiological and clinical studies of PTSD–SUDs. We begin with studies conducted with nationally representative samples of men and women exposed to a variety of traumatic events. After establishing that gender may influence prevalence of PTSD–SUDs in general population studies, we then turn to samples of treatment seeking populations. By virtue of the nature of the traumas involved, many of the clinical samples are exclusively male or exclusively female. Nevertheless, such studies allow for an estimation of the scope of this problem in treatment settings.

Comorbidity in Men and Women in Unselected General Population Samples

The strongest evidence for PTSD and SUDs signaling increased risk for the other disorder comes from the National Comorbidity Survey (NCS; Kessler, Sonnega, Bromet, Hughes, & Nelson, 1995; Kessler et al., 1997). In that study, Kessler et al. (1995) examined rates of comorbid SUDs among those with and without PTSD. The DSM-III-R (American Psychiatric Association, 1987) PTSD module from the Diagnostic Interview Schedule (DIS; Robins, Helzer, Croughan, & Ratcliff, 1981), and the World Health Organization (WHO) Composite International Diagnostic Interview (CIDI; World Health Organization, 1990), were administered to a nationally representative sample of 5,877 Americans (2,812 men, 3,065 women). Among the men with PTSD, rates of comorbid SUDs were approximately 52% for alcohol disorders and 35% for drug disorders. Among the women with PTSD, rates of comorbid SUDs were approximately 28% for alcohol disorders and 27% for drug disorders. Because SUDs are more prevalent among men than among women in the general population (Kessler et al., 1997), it is important to examine rates of SUDs in those with and without PTSD separately by gender (see Stewart, 1996). In fact, statistically significant odds ratios (ORs) of having an alcohol use disorder in the presence of PTSD were obtained for both the men (OR = 2.06) and the women (OR = 2.48) in the Kessler et al. (1995) study. Similarly, significantly increased odds of having a drug use disorder in the presence of PTSD were seen among both men (OR = 2.97) and women (OR = 4.46).

The ORs obtained in the Kessler et al. (1995) study suggest trends for SUDs to be more commonly comorbid with PTSD for women than for men when compared with SUD rates among gender-matched controls without PTSD. This trend is consistent with findings for alcohol use disorder comorbidity from the St. Louis site of the Epidemiologic Catchment Area Survey (Helzer, Robins, & McEvoy, 1987). In this study, women showed a trend toward higher risk for alcohol use disorder–PTSD comorbidity relative to men (although the opposite trend was found for drug use disorders).

In another analysis of data from the NCS, Kessler et al. (1997) examined rates of lifetime co-occurrence of DSM-III-R (American Psychiatric Association, 1987) alcohol dependence with other psychiatric disorders (including PTSD) in a community sample of 8,098 men and women. Among those with lifetime alcohol dependence, 10.3% of men and 26.2% of women met criteria for PTSD. Because PTSD is more prevalent among women than among men in the general population (Breslau, Davis, Andreski, & Peterson, 1991; Kessler et al., 1995), it is important to examine rates of PTSD in those with and without alcohol use disorders separately by gender (see Stewart, 1996). The significantly increased odds of PTSD in the presence of lifetime alcohol *dependence* did not vary significantly by gender (ORs = 3.60 and 3.20 for women and men, respectively). However, the odds of PTSD in the presence of lifetime alcohol *abuse* were significantly greater among women than among men (ORs = 1.01 and 0.45 for women and men, respectively).

Comorbidity in Men and Women in Clinical Samples

A study by Keane, Caddell, Martin, Zimering, and Fairbank (1983) was one of the first identifying high rates of SUDs in male, treatment-seeking combat veterans with PTSD. Many subsequent studies with clinical samples of male combat veterans have confirmed high rates of comorbid SUDs among those with PTSD. In these studies, rates of comorbid alcohol use disorders among male veterans with PTSD have ranged from 64 to 84%, and rates of comorbid drug use disorders have ranged from 40 to 44% (see review by Stewart, Pihl, Conrod, & Dongier, 1998). Conversely, according to reviews by Keane, Gerardi, Lyons, and Wolfe (1988) and Stewart (1996), VA samples of combat-exposed males receiving treatment for SUDs show high rates of comorbid PTSD (e.g., 46–62% with current PTSD; McFall, Mackay, & Donovan, 1991; Sharkansky, Brief, Peirce, Meehan, & Mannix, 1999).

Studies of women with assault-related PTSD have demonstrated that high rates of PTSD–SUD comorbidity are not limited to combat-exposed males. A review by Keane and Kaloupek (1997) reports comorbidity rates of 25–39% for SUDs in assaulted women with PTSD. According to a review by Najavits et al. (1997), samples of women with SUDs show high rates of comorbid PTSD, most commonly deriving from a history of repetitive childhood physical and/or sexual violence. PTSD diagnoses in female samples of patients with SUDs indicate high prevalence rates in the range of 30–59% (e.g., Brady, Killeen, Saladin, Dansky, & Becker, 1994; Dansky, Saladin, Brady, Kilpatrick, & Resnick, 1995; Fullilove et al., 1993; Kovach, 1986).

Summary

Taken together, these studies converge in suggesting that PTSD and SUDs are commonly co-occurring disorders among men and women in both general and clinical populations. In mental health treatment settings geared for SUDs or trauma-related problems, approximately half of the men and one-third of the women will evidence this dual diagnosis. Studies that have examined gender-specific risk ratios for one disorder in the presence of the other (i.e., PTSD in the presence/absence of SUD, and vice versa) suggest somewhat increased risk for this form of dual diagnosis among women relative to men. However, more research involving statistical comparisons of risk ratios across gender is needed to draw firmer conclusions.

PREDICTORS OF PTSD–SUD COMORBIDITY IN MEN AND WOMEN

The data reviewed suggest that a diagnosis of PTSD, or of SUD, confers risk for developing the other disorder among both men and women. The next step is to identify which individuals are at risk to develop this form of comorbidity. In this section, we review studies that have investigated variables associated with PTSD–SUD comorbidity among men and women to examine whether there are gender-specific risk factors. This information can help clinicians target at-risk individuals to prevent the development of this dual diagnosis.

Predictors of PTSD–SUD Comorbidity in Men

Among male war veterans, numerous studies suggest a significant positive association between combat trauma severity and substance abuse (e.g., Branchey, Davis, & Lieber, 1984; Green, Lindy, Grace, & Gleser, 1989; Kulka et al., 1990; McFall et al., 1991; Yager, Laufer, & Gallops, 1984). In this population, severity of combat trauma also appears to be a useful predictor of comorbid PTSD–SUDs. For example, in a study of 489 male Vietnam veterans in treatment for SUDs, severity of war combat experiences, as determined by scores on the Revised Combat Scale (RCS; Gallops, Laufer, & Yager, 1981), was the best predictor of a comorbid diagnosis of PTSD (McFall et al., 1991). Another study demonstrated that exposure to extremely severe combat stressors, such as mutilation and grotesque death, was predictive of the dual diagnosis of PTSD–SUDs in male veterans (Green et al., 1989).

Some emerging evidence suggests that childhood trauma may also be involved in the occurrence of comorbid PTSD–SUDs in male war veterans—a group in which the emphasis has largely been on understanding this form of dual diagnosis within the context of combat trauma. For example, Triffleman, Marmar, Delucchi, and Ronfeldt (1995) conducted a pilot study to examine the prevalence of childhood trauma and PTSD in 38 male veteran inpatients with SUDs. Five dimensions of childhood trauma were assessed: loss/separation; physical abuse; witnessing intrafamilial violence; sexual abuse; and emotional neglect. Seventy-seven percent of these male veteran substance abusers reported having been exposed to severe childhood trauma, and 48% had experienced two or more types of severe trauma. The most common combination (40%) involved both witnessing intrafamilial violence and experiencing physical abuse. Number of childhood trauma exposures was positively correlated with lifetime PTSD, and lifetime PTSD was positively correlated with the number of lifetime substance abuse disorders. Moreover, number of childhood trauma exposures was found to be strongly positively correlated with the number of lifetime substance abuse disorders. This latter relation remained significant after controlling for a number of possible third variables, including demographics, family history of alcohol problems, combat exposure, and combat-related PTSD.

Predictors of PTSD–SUD Comorbidity in Women

More recent studies have examined predictors of comorbid PTSD–SUDs in female samples (e.g., Brady et al., 1994; Fullilove et al., 1993; Najavits, Weiss, & Shaw, 1999; Ouimette, Wolfe, & Chrestman, 1996). Fullilove et al. (1993) examined associations between the experience of violent events, other trauma, and PTSD among 105 women seeking treatment for an SUD at an outpatient, inner-city program. Ninety-nine percent of the sample reported trauma in one or more of 14 categories of traumatic events, with 87% reporting lifetime exposure to a violent trauma. Among women with comorbid PTSD, 97% reported one or more violent traumas compared with 73% of women substance abusers without PTSD. The likelihood of a comorbid PTSD diagnosis was strongly associated with having been exposed to multiple violent traumas.

Brady et al. (1994) explored the relations between PTSD, substance abuse, and traumatic victimization histories in 55 women receiving treatment for an SUD. Thirty of the women were diagnosed with comorbid PTSD, and the remaining 25 did not meet criteria for a comorbid PTSD diagnosis. The comorbid and SUD-only groups were compared on variables such as degree of addiction severity. Substance abusing women with comorbid PTSD were more likely to have been victims of sexual and physical abuse, particularly childhood abuse, than women with SUDs alone. Comorbid women also had significantly higher scores on the Addiction Severity Index (ASI; McLellan et al., 1992).

Ouimette et al. (1996) compared three non-treatment-seeking groups of American women who had served in the Vietnam war to clarify characteristics associated with comorbid PTSD–alcohol use disorders in women. The three groups were those with comorbid PTSD and alcohol abuse (N = 12), those with PTSD only (N = 13), and those with neither PTSD nor alcohol abuse (N = 22). The comorbid group reported greater severity of PTSD symptoms than the other two groups, more sexual abuse as children (cf. Brady et al., 1994), as well as more adult sexual assault. Degree of sexual abuse in childhood was significantly correlated with greater self-reported problem drinking. The authors concluded that the cumulative effects of lifetime trauma exposure (particularly sexual victimization) might be important in accounting for comorbid PTSD–alcohol abuse in women.

A similar study was conducted by Najavits et al. (1999) to assess the clinical characteristics of civilian women with comorbid PTSD–SUDs. These authors compared 28 women with both disorders to 29 women with PTSD alone. The majority of women in both groups had sought treatment. Of the total sample, 95% reported a history of physical or sexual abuse, with virtually all (98%) reporting their first trauma prior to age 18 years. Unlike the findings of Ouimette et al. (1996), the two groups of women in the Najavits et al. (1999) study did not differ in number or types of lifetime traumas, or current PTSD severity. Instead, the two groups consistently differed on a number of childhood and adulthood protective factors (e.g., having a sense of purpose in life, the presence of a strong adult during childhood) known to be associated with resilience from trauma. In each case, the comorbid women obtained lower scores on these protective factors. The authors concluded that the absence of such protective factors might be important in accounting for dual diagnoses of PTSD–SUDs in women with lifetime histories of victimization.

Does Gender Moderate the Effect of Abuse History on SUD–PTSD Status?

One theme emerging from the majority of these studies is that more severe trauma of an interpersonal nature (e.g., sexual abuse) is predictive of PTSD–SUD comorbidity. A recent study examined whether the relationship between a history of interpersonal trauma and PTSD–SUD status differed for men and women (Ouimette, Kimerling, Shaw, & Moos, 2000). In other words, does a history of abuse confer greater or lesser risk for this dual diagnosis for men compared to women? A total of 24,959 adult patients (745 females, 24,206 males) seeking treatment at the Department of Veterans Affairs (VA) for SUDs were assessed with the ASI (McLellan et al., 1992). Physical and sexual abuse histories were assessed with two relevant items from the ASI. Specifically, within the ASI family/social domain, respondents are queried about any "serious problems getting along with mother, father, brothers/sisters, sexual partner/spouse, children, other significant family, neighbors, co-workers." This is followed by the questions: "Did any of these people abuse you (1) physically (cause you physical harm)? Or (2) sexually (force sexual advances or sexual acts)?" Among patients with SUDs, gender emerged as a moderator of the abuse history effect in moderated multiple regression analyses (Baron & Kenny, 1986). Specifically, the relationship between abuse and PTSD diagnosis was stronger for female than for male patients with SUDs. Among women, 23% with abuse histories compared to only 7% without abuse histories met criteria for PTSD. Among men, 14% with abuse histories and 12% without met criteria for PTSD.

Summary

The majority of studies reviewed in this section converge in suggesting that severity of trauma exposure appears to be an important predictor of comorbid PTSD–SUDs in men and women alike. Specifically, comorbid individuals appear to have been exposed to more severe trauma than individuals with either PTSD or SUDs alone. Among male veterans, severity of combat exposure relates to comorbidity, and among clinical samples of women, severity of victimization histories (e.g., childhood sexual abuse, rape, or exposure to violence) has been related to comorbidity. A history of sexual and physical abuse may place women more at risk for this dual diagnosis than men. The study by Najavits et al. (1999) does not support this position, but it does suggest that the absence of certain "protective factors" may be important in the development of comorbidity in women. The relevance of the relative absence of such protective factors in accounting for comorbid PTSD–SUDs in men remains to be investigated.

Although comorbidity in men has tended to be understood in terms of severity of combat trauma exposure, emerging evidence suggests that PTSD secondary to a history of childhood abuse may be a prevalent problem among men as well as women seeking treatment for SUDs. Comorbid PTSD–SUDs deriving from a history of childhood abuse is commonly seen among both female and male clinical samples of substance abusers. These findings are consistent with reviews of the literature on the long-term correlates of childhood sexual and physical abuse. Such reviews converge in suggesting that both PTSD and SUDs are among the more common psychiatric disorder correlates of childhood sexual and physical abuse (e.g., Briere & Runtz, 1993; Kendall-Tackett, Meyer Williams, & Finkelhor, 1993; Malinosky-Rummell & Hansen, 1993; Polusny & Follette, 1995). It should be cautioned, however, that none of the studies reviewed earlier have included control groups matched for important third variables.

FUNCTIONAL RELATIONS BETWEEN PTSD AND SUDs IN MEN AND WOMEN

Several potential functional relations have been suggested to explain the high rates of comorbidity between PTSD and SUDs (see review by Stewart et al., 1998). PTSD could increase the risk of development of a SUD if PTSD patients are using substances in an attempt to self-medicate their PTSD symptoms (Khantzian, 1985). Conversely, SUDs could increase risk for development of PTSD by increasing the likelihood of exposure to certain types of trauma. Finally, a SUD could (1) increase the chances of the development of PTSD following exposure to a traumatic event or (2) exacerbate the symptoms of PTSD over the longer term (e.g., as a consequence of heightened arousal secondary to repeated substance withdrawal experiences). In this section, we review studies that have used various methodologies to investigate potential functional relations between PTSD and SUD symptoms among men versus women. We examine evidence on whether any of these pathways may be more applicable to one gender than the other. Understanding these pathways will help tailor treatments more specifically for men and women.

"Gradient of Effect"

In determining whether a causal relationship exists that might explain the frequent comorbidity of PTSD and SUDs, one suggested criterion has been to establish a "gradient of effect" (see review by Chilcoat & Breslau, 1998). This causal criterion suggests that as the level of exposure to a causal agent increases, the effect on the causal outcome should be greater. If PTSD and SUD are causally related, then as levels of symptoms of one disorder increase, so should levels of symptoms of the other disorder. In this section, we review three studies to examine the degree to which this criteria is met across genders, with respect to the potential causal relationship between PTSD and SUDs.

McFall, Mackay, and Donovan (1992) used a correlational design to examine potential functional relations between the various DSM-III-R (American Psychiatric Association, 1987) PTSD symptom clusters and severity of alcohol use disorder symptoms in a clinical sample of 108 male Vietnam Theater veterans presenting for treatment of a SUD. Approximately 92% presented with an alcohol use disorder, 60% with a drug use disorder, and 53% with both alcohol and drug use disorders. Severity of PTSD symptoms was assessed with the Mississippi Scale for Combat-Related PTSD (M-PTSD; Keane, Caddell, & Taylor, 1988). Severity of alcohol use disorder symptoms was assessed with the Michigan Alcoholism Screening Test (MAST; Selzer, 1971). M-PTSD items were conceptually divided into the DSM-III-R (American Psychiatric Association, 1987) symptom clusters: intrusions, numbing/avoidance, and arousal. MAST scores were significantly positively correlated with M-PTSD arousal and intrusions scores, but not with avoidance/numbing scores. These findings suggest a "gradient of effect" with respect to PTSD arousal and intrusion symptoms with alcohol use disorder symptoms among men.

Stewart, Conrod, Pihl, and Dongier (1999) used a correlational design to examine potential functional relations between the various DSM-IV (American Psychiatric Association, 1994) PTSD symptoms and severity of alcohol use disorder symptoms in a community-recruited sample of 295 women substance abusers. Lifetime substance dependence diagnoses were assessed with the Computerized Diagnostic Interview Schedule (C-DIS Management Group, 1991). Approximately 83% of the sample was diagnosed with alcohol dependence, and the rest with a drug use disorder with or without alcohol dependence. About 49% of the sample met lifetime criteria for two or more dependence diagnoses. Severity of PTSD symptoms was assessed with the PTSD Symptoms Scale—Self-Report (PSS-SR; Foa, Riggs, Dancu, & Rothbaum, 1993). Severity of alcohol use disorder symptoms was assessed with the Physical Dependence (Ph) scale of the Comprehensive Drinker Profile (CDP; Miller & Marlatt, 1984). PSS-SR items were divided into four symptom clusters based on the results of a principal components factor analysis: intrusions, numbing, avoidance, and arousal. These four categories approximate the organization of PTSD symptoms outlined in the DSM-IV (American Psychiatric Association, 1994), except that numbing and avoidance symptoms were examined separately. Consistent with the findings of McFall et al. (1992) with males for alcohol, severity of women's alcohol use disorder symptoms was significantly positively correlated with severity of PTSD arousal symptoms, but not with numbing or avoidance symptoms. Inconsistent with the findings of McFall et al. (1992) for men, among the women in the Stewart, Conrod, Pihl, et al. (1999) study, PTSD intrusion symptoms were unrelated to severity of the alcohol use disorder symptoms. These findings suggest a "gradient of effect" with respect to PTSD arousal symptoms and alcohol use disorder symptoms among women. However, comparing the McFall et al. (1992) and the Stewart, Conrod, Pihl, et al. (1999) findings suggests a greater specificity of relation of alcohol disorder symptoms to the PTSD arousal symptoms cluster among women than among men. Caution should nonetheless be exerted in interpreting the meaning of these differences, because several methodological differences between the McFall et al. and the Stewart, Conrod, Pihl, et al. study might account for these apparent gender differences (e.g., different assessment tools; community vs. clinical samples of individuals with SUDs).

The findings of Stewart, Conrod, Pihl, et al. (1999) regarding "gradient of effect" relations between particular PTSD symptom clusters and severity of alcohol use disorder symptoms in women substance abusers are highly consistent with the results of a study by Saladin, Brady, Dansky, and Kilpatrick (1995; Study 1). In this study, the pattern of PTSD symptoms in 28 women seeking treatment for a SUD comorbid with PTSD was compared with the symptom pattern of 28 women with PTSD only. Consistent with previous findings for men (McFall et al., 1992) and women (Stewart, Conrod, Pihl, et al., 1999), Saladin et al.'s (1995) women with comorbidity evidenced significantly more symptoms in the PTSD arousal cluster (DSM-IV; American Psychiatric Association, 1994) than the PTSD-only women. In particular, the women with comorbidity reported significantly more sleep disturbance than the PTSD-only women. Consistent with Stewart, Conrod, Pihl, et al.'s (1999) previous findings with women, but inconsistent with the findings of McFall et al. (1992) for men, the two groups of women in the Saladin et al. (1995) study did not differ in the number of symptoms from the intrusion cluster.

An even stronger argument for the "gradient of effect" criterion in assessing a causal relationship between PTSD and SUDs could be made if patients perceive that the two disorders are "psychologically connected" (Rachman, 1991). Brown, Stout, and Gannon-Rowley (1998) examined perceptions of functional associations between PTSD and SUDs among 42 patients with comorbidity (26 women, 16 men) receiving treatment for an SUD at a private hospital. The large majority of these patients reported feeling that their SUD symptoms worsened when their PTSD symptoms worsened (77%), and that their SUD symptoms improved when their PTSD symptoms improved (79%). In addition, over half the patients with comorbidity reported feeling that their PTSD symptoms worsened when their SUD symptoms worsened (51%), and that their PTSD symptoms improved when their SUD symptoms improved (52%). This pattern of findings regarding patient perceptions is consistent with a "vicious cycle" being operative between symptoms of these two disorders, such that one disorder sustains the other (Stewart, 1996). Moreover, it strongly supports the "gradient of effect" criteria. However, the sample sizes of men and women in the Brown et al. (1998) study were insufficient to test potential moderating effects of gender. In fact, no research to date has examined patient perceptions of functional associations separately by gender. Future studies should examine gender as a moderator of the Brown et al. findings to determine whether the perception that a worsening of PTSD symptoms leads to a worsening of SUD symptoms is stronger among women than among men.

The findings reviewed in this section show that a gradient of effect exists between certain sets of PTSD symptoms and severity of SUD symptoms in both men and women, consistent with the position that a causal relation may exist between these two commonly comorbid disorders. In addition, male and female patients perceived that their SUD and PTSD symptoms were functionally related. However, if a causal relation exists, the direction of causality remains unclear: PTSD could cause SUDs, or vice versa. The findings are consistent with notions that PTSD arousal symptoms motivate patients with PTSD to abuse alcohol/drugs in an attempt to self-medicate their hyperaroused state. This self-medication could involve attempts to aid in sleep, reduce irritability, reduce concentration difficulties, reduce hypervigilance, or to control excessive startle response (cf. LaCoursiere, Godfrey, & Ruby, 1980; Stewart, 1997). These findings are also consistent with suggestions that chronic heavy use of alcohol or other drugs may ultimately exacerbate PTSD arousal symptoms over the longer term (see LaCoursiere et al., 1980). For example, Stewart et al. (1998) have reviewed evidence that chronic alcohol abuse and/or alcohol withdrawal might lead to an intensification of certain PTSD arousal symptoms (e.g., heightened startle) over time. Although these potential functional associations between PTSD arousal symptoms and substance abuse appear to be operative among both men and women, the findings of Stewart, Conrod, Pihl, et al. (1999) and Saladin et al. (1995) highlight the primacy of arousal symptoms in the PTSD–SUD relationship among women. Lab-based psychophysiological studies suggest that both male veterans with combat-related PTSD and women with PTSD from childhood sexual abuse show equivalently heightened startle response when sober, relative to male and female non-PTSD controls (Carson & Orr, 1999). Future experimental research might focus on examining gender as a potential moderator variable in the dampening effects of alcohol on indices of PTSD arousal symptoms (e.g., startle response) and/or on alcohol withdrawal–induced arousal enhancement.

"Temporality"

In determining whether a causal relationship exists that might explain the frequent comorbidity of PTSD and SUDs, one criterion that has been suggested is establishing "temporality" (see review by Chilcoat & Breslau, 1998). This criterion suggests that a causal factor must precede the effect temporally. If PTSD causes SUDs, then the onset of PTSD must precede the development of the SUD. If SUDs cause PTSD (e.g., by increasing risk of exposure to traumatic events or by inducing a state in which PTSD is more likely to develop following trauma exposure), then the onset of the SUD must precede the development of the PTSD. Chilcoat and Breslau (1998) note that temporal order is the only undisputed criterion of causality. In this section, we review studies that have examined the degree to which the "temporality" criterion is met across genders with respect to the potential causal relationship between PTSD and SUDs.

Using data from the NCS, Kessler et al. (1995, 1997) examined the relative order of onset of PTSD versus SUDs in comorbid cases. Kessler et al.'s (1995) results suggest that PTSD was the primary disorder (in the sense of having an earlier age at onset) more often than not with respect to comorbid SUDs among both men and women. Among the comorbid men, the majority (i.e., 53–65%) developed the PTSD prior to the SUD. Among the comorbid women, the percentage who developed the PTSD prior to the SUD was even higher (i.e., 65–84%). These results thus suggest trends for PTSD to develop prior to SUDs more often among comorbid women than among comorbid men.

This trend was confirmed in a later study by Kessler et al. (1997) that focused on individuals with alcohol use disorders. With respect to relative order of onset of PTSD and alcohol use disorders in comorbid cases, Kessler et al. noted significant gender differences in the retrospective temporal ordering of alcohol dependence and other disorders. Men were more likely to report their alcohol dependence as temporally primary, and women more likely to report theirs as temporally secondary or occurring in the same year as their PTSD. Specifically, 53% of comorbid males compared to only 35% of comorbid females reported that their alcohol dependence preceded their PTSD. In contrast, 65% of comorbid women compared to only 47% of comorbid men reported that their PTSD preceded or began within the same year as their alcohol dependence. Similar findings have been obtained in adolescents. Deykin and Buka (1997) examined relative order of onset of PTSD and SUDs in a large sample of adolescents in treatment for SUDs. More of the comorbid females than comorbid males developed PTSD prior to the SUD (59% vs. 28%, respectively).

To investigate differences between comorbid patients whose PTSD preceded their SUD and vice versa, Brady, Dansky, Sonne, and Saladin (1998) divided 33 adult patients with comorbid PTSD and cocaine dependence into two groups. In the first group (i.e., the "primary PTSD" group), the PTSD developed before the onset of cocaine dependence. In the second group (i.e., the "primary cocaine" group), the PTSD developed after cocaine dependence was established. In the primary PTSD group, the precipitating trauma was generally childhood abuse, whereas in the primary cocaine group, the trauma exposure was generally associated with using or obtaining cocaine. In the primary PTSD group, there were significantly more women, and more use of benzodiazepines and opiates (i.e., prescription depressant drugs). Thus, Brady et al.'s findings are consistent with the findings of Kessler et al. (1995, 1997) in suggesting that women may be more susceptible than men to a form of comorbid PTSD–SUD in which the PTSD develops prior to the SUD.

Breslau, Davis, Peterson, and Schultz (1997) used the DIS (Robins et al., 1981) to measure lifetime DSM-III-R (American Psychiatric Association, 1987) psychiatric disorders in a stratified random sample of 801 adult American women. Cox proportional hazards models with time-dependent covariates were used to calculate the hazard ratios of first onset of other disorders following PTSD. The presence of PTSD was found to signal significantly increased risks for a first-onset alcohol use disorder (OR = 3.12) and for a first-onset illicit drug use disorder (OR = 3.11). Preexisting SUDs failed to predict increased risk for PTSD development, however. This study provides further evidence that SUDs tend to follow PTSD development in comorbid women, in terms of relative order of onset.

These studies suggest that the temporality criterion of causality is indeed met in the case of comorbid PTSD–SUDs, at least among women. Specifically, PTSD tends to develop before the SUD in the large majority of comorbid women. The findings also converge in suggesting that women may be more susceptible than men to a form of comorbid PTSD–SUD in which the PTSD develops first. The temporality criterion is less clear as it pertains to men, with some findings suggesting that the PTSD develops first (Kessler et al., 1995), and others that the SUD develops first (Deykin & Buka, 1997). These temporal data are consistent with self-medication explanations for the comorbidity of PTSD and SUDs in women. Specifically, women with PTSD may come to abuse substances in an attempt to self-medicate their aversive PTSD symptoms. However, as noted by Chilcoat and Breslau (1998), although temporality is a necessary condition for causality, it cannot be used to confirm causal hypotheses. Moreover, the temporality criterion applies only to understanding the onset of comorbidity, not to potential reciprocal relations that may develop as the comorbidity becomes relatively more chronic. For example, even if self-medication for PTSD symptoms applies to the initiation of substance misuse among many female trauma victims, the possibility of a "vicious cycle" between these two forms of behavioral pathology developing over the longer term should be considered. Chronic substance abuse might lead to an intensification of PTSD symptoms over time. In turn, women with comorbidity may escalate their substance use in a further attempt to control these heightened PTSD symptoms.

One further caveat should be mentioned in interpreting these results of the investigations of temporality. All of the studies reviewed have relied on retrospective reports regarding the relative onset of symptoms of each disorder. Retrospective reports are subject to a number of biases that may limit their accuracy. Gender differences in the relative order of onset of PTSD and SUDs obtained using retrospective methods could be secondary to gender differences in memory or reporting biases. For example, it could be that women, more than men, perceive their current SUD as having been caused by their PTSD, and women may thus "misremember" the relative order of onset of symptoms of each disorder in a pattern consistent with these perceptions. To overcome these limitations, future research needs to use prospective, longitudinal methods to examine the relative order of onset of these two disorders in identified trauma victims (see Kilpatrick, Acierno, Resnick, Saunders, & Best, 1997, for sample methodology).

"Situational Specificity"

The self-medication hypothesis of PTSD–SUD comorbidity asserts that substances are used in an attempt to reduce or control the behavioral, affective, cognitive, and/or physiological symptoms of PTSD. In operant conditioning terminology, individuals with PTSD are said to learn to drink or to use drugs for their "negatively reinforcing" (e.g., tension-reducing, intrusive memory–dampening) effects (see Stewart, 1996, 1997). If, indeed, substance use serves a negative reinforcement function among traumatized individuals with PTSD, the heavy drinking/drug-taking behavior of those substance abusers with PTSD should be relatively "situation-specific." In other words, their substance use should be most frequent in contexts that have been associated in the past with a substance's tension-reducing effects (Stewart, Conrod, Samoluk, Pihl, & Dongier, 2000). In this section, we review studies that have been conducted to test this situational specificity hypothesis among male and female samples of patients with SUDs.

Sharkansky et al. (1999) administered measures of PTSD symptom severity and situation-specific drinking/drug taking to a sample of 86 veterans (84 men, 2 women) seeking treatment for a SUD at a VA medical center. DSM-IV (American Psychiatric Association, 1994) PTSD symptoms were assessed with the self-report PTSD Checklist (PCL; Blanchard, Jones-Alexander, Buckley, & Forneris, 1996). Situation-specific heavy drinking and drug taking were assessed with the 42-item Inventory of Drinking Situations (IDS-42; Annis, Graham, & Davis, 1987) and the Inventory of Drug Taking Situations (IDTS; Annis, Turner, & Sklar, 1996), respectively. The IDS-42 was administered to the 35% of the sample participants who identified alcohol as their primary drug of abuse. The IDTS was administered to the other 65% of the sample participants who reported a drug other than alcohol as their drug of choice (i.e., heroin, crack or cocaine, or marijuana). These instruments assess the frequency with which respondents drank heavily (IDS-42) or used drugs (IDTS) during the past year in eight types of situations: Unpleasant Emotions, Physical Discomfort, Pleasant Emotions, Testing Personal Control, Urges and Temptations, Conflict with Others, Social Pressure, and Pleasant Times with Others. These eight situations represent the situations in Marlatt and Gordon's (1985) taxonomy of typical situations for relapse to substance use among addicts. According to responses on the PCL, about 60% of the veteran substance abusers in the Sharkansky et al. (1999) study met DSM-IV (American Psychiatric Association, 1994) criteria for PTSD. Substance abusers with and without PTSD were compared on the eight subscales of the IDS-42 or IDTS. Consistent with the situational specificity hypothesis, a comorbid diagnosis of PTSD was associated with greater drinking/drug taking in situations involving Unpleasant Emotions, Physical Discomfort, and Conflict with Others. Comorbid PTSD was unrelated to frequency of drinking/drug taking in situations involving Pleasant Emotions, Testing Personal Control, Urges and Temptations, Social Pressure, or Pleasant Times with Others.

Because the Sharkansky et al. (1999) study was conducted with a sample of primarily male (i.e., 98% men) substance abusers, it remained unclear as to whether their findings might be generalizable to women. Thus, Stewart et al. (2000) attempted replication of the Sharkansky et al. (1999) study with women substance abusers. They administered a lifetime measure of trauma exposure and measures of PTSD symptom severity and situation-specific drinking to the same community-recruited sample of adult women substance abusers described previously for the Stewart, Conrod, Pihl, et al. (1999) study. DSM-IV (American Psychiatric Association, 1994) PTSD symptoms were assessed with the PSS-SR (Foa et al., 1993). Situation-specific heavy drinking was assessed with the IDS-42 (Annis et al., 1987). Self-reported rates of trauma exposure were high for several events (e.g., 42% reported histories of physical violence, and 47% reported histories of sexual victimization in childhood and/or adulthood). Forty-six percent of the sample met criteria for a DSM-IV (American Psychiatric Association, 1994) diagnosis of PTSD based on PSS-SR responses and the nature of the traumatic events reported. Consistent with the situational specificity hypothesis, and with the findings of Sharkansky et al. (1999), PTSD symptoms were significantly positively correlated with frequency of heavy drinking in situations involving Unpleasant Emotions, Physical Discomfort, and Conflict with Others. Also consistent with the Sharkansky et al. findings, PTSD symptoms were unrelated to frequency of heavy drinking in situations involving Testing Personal Control, Urges and Temptations, Social Pressure, or Pleasant Times with Others. Unexpectedly, and in contrast to the findings of Sharkansky et al., PTSD symptoms were also significantly negatively correlated with frequency of heavy drinking in situations involving Pleasant Emotions among the women substance abusers (see later for discussion of this negative correlation).

As later reported by Stewart, Conrod, Loughlin, Pihl, and Dongier (1999), all of those women in the Stewart et al. (2000) study who identified a drug other than alcohol as their primary drug of abuse were also administered the IDTS (Annis et al., 1996). Fifty-five percent of the original sample (N = 164 women) fell in this category, with reported drugs of choice ranging from heroin, cocaine or crack, and marijuana, to prescription anxiolytics and analgesics. Again consistent with the situational specificity hypothesis and with the findings of Sharkansky et al. (1999), PTSD symptoms were significantly positively correlated with frequency of drug taking in situations involving Conflict with Others, Unpleasant Emotions, and Physical Discomfort. And PTSD symptoms were again unrelated to frequency of drug taking in situations involving Testing Personal Control, Urges and Temptations, or Social Pressure. Unexpectedly, and in contrast to the findings of Sharkansky et al. (1999), PTSD symptoms were also significantly negatively correlated with frequency of drug taking in situations involving Pleasant Emotions and Pleasant Times with Others among this subsample of women substance abusers (Stewart, Conrod, Loughlin, et al., 1999). Because these additional data regarding correlations of PTSD symptoms with IDTS drug-taking situations have not been published elsewhere, they are presented in Table 9.1. Note that the IDTS subscales are grouped according to three, higher order, drug-taking situations (i.e., negatively reinforcing, positively reinforcing, and temptation) identified in a previous factor analysis of this inventory in substance abusers (Turner, Annis, & Sklar, 1997).

A direct comparison of the results of Sharkansky et al. (1999) with male substance abusers and those of Stewart, Conrod, Loughlin, et al. (1999) and Stewart et al. (2000) with female substance abusers indicates general support for the situational specificity hypothesis among trauma-

TABLE 9.1. Correlations between Frequency of Drug Taking in Specific Situations and Scores on a Self-Report Measure of PTSD Symptoms in 164 Women with SUDs Preferring Drugs Other Than Alcohol

IDS-42 drug-taking situation	PTSD symptoms
Negatively reinforcing situations	
Unpleasant emotions	$.13^*$
Physical discomfort	$.20^{***}$
Conflict with others	$.17^{**}$
Positively reinforcing situations	
Pleasant emotions	$-.21^{**}$
Pleasant times with others	$-.17^*$
Temptation situations	
Urges and temptations	$-.12$
Testing personal control	$.03$
Social pressure	$-.15$

Note. Significant correlations: $^*p < .05$; $^{**}p < .01$; $^{***}p < .005$. Subscales are grouped according to the three higher order drug-taking situation factors (Turner et al., 1997). PTSD symptoms assessed with the PTSD Symptom Scale—Self-Report (PSS-SR; Foa et al., 1993); drug-taking situations assessed with the Inventory of Drug Taking Situations (IDTS; Annis et al., 1996). Correlations between PTSD symptoms and negatively reinforcing IDTS drug-taking situations are evaluated with one-tailed tests given the hypothesized directional effects; all other correlations evaluated using two-tailed tests. Data from Stewart, Conrod, Loughlin, Pihl, and Dongier (1999).

tized men and women alike. Those with clinically significant levels of PTSD symptoms drink or take drugs more frequently, relative to other substance abusers, in potentially negatively reinforcing situations. This finding appears consistent across gender and trauma type (i.e., combat trauma, in the case of males; sexual/physical abuse/assault in the case of females). This suggests that relapse prevention efforts (Marlatt & Gordon, 1985) in males and females with comorbid PTSD–SUDs should focus on these types of situations as involving a high potential for relapse in this population.

However, a direct comparison of the results of the Sharkansky et al. (1999) and the Stewart, Conrod, Loughlin, et al. (1999) and Stewart et al. (2000) studies also suggests an important way in which men and women with comorbid PTSD may differ in terms of their context-specific drinking/drug use patterns. Male substance abusers with and without PTSD appear equally likely to consume alcohol or drugs in "positive" situations (i.e., those involving pleasant emotions and pleasant times with others). In contrast, female substance abusers with PTSD appear less likely than other female substance abusers to consume alcohol or drugs in such "positive" contexts (see Table 9.1). Recent research by Breslau, Chilcoat, Kessler, and Lucia (1999) suggests that the greater rates of PTSD in women compared to men (e.g., Breslau et al., 1991; Breslau, Davis, Andreski, Peterson, & Schultz, 1997; Kessler et al., 1995) are largely attributable to gender differences in the numbing/avoidance symptom cluster. Thus, the Stewart, Conrod, Loughlin, et al. (1999) and Stewart et al. (2000) gender-specific finding might be due to particular difficulties women with PTSD have experiencing pleasurable emotions (i.e., heightened emotional numbing). In other words, situations involving pleasurable emotions may be less likely to trigger substance abuse in women with PTSD, simply because such women rarely experience pleasurable emotions. This possibility has yet to be investigated empirically. It should be cautioned that such gender differences are merely suggestive, because a number of methodological differences between the Sharkansky et al. and Stewart et al. studies might account for the observed differences. We recommend that a future study be conducted in which male and female patients with SUDs, with and without comorbid PTSD, are directly compared on measures of situation-specific drinking and drug taking to investigate further the potential moderating effect of gender.

The Role of Anxiety Sensitivity and Anxiety/Depressive Symptoms

The study by Stewart et al. (2000) with community-recruited women with SUDs also provides information about the role of "anxiety sensitivity" (fear of anxiety-related sensations; Peterson & Reiss, 1992) in contributing to PTSD–SUD comorbidity among women. Anxiety sensitivity is a cognitive, individual-difference variable that has previously been shown to be a risk factor for substance abuse (see review by Stewart, Samoluk, & MacDonald, 1999) and to be elevated in PTSD (Taylor, Koch, & McNally, 1992). In fact, anxiety sensitivity levels are higher in PTSD than in all other anxiety disorders save panic disorder (Taylor et al., 1992). It has been suggested that anxiety sensitivity may represent a premorbid vulnerability factor for the development of PTSD following exposure to a traumatic event, because people with high anxiety sensitivity should be more likely to develop conditioned fear reactions (e.g., increased startle response) to trauma cues. In turn, the experience of anxiety-related PTSD symptoms may increase anxiety sensitivity levels (Taylor et al., 1992). Stewart et al. (2000) found in their sample of female substance abusers, that anxiety sensitivity mediated the observed associations between PTSD symptoms and situation-specific heavy drinking in negative contexts. In other words, female substance abusers with more frequent PTSD symptoms drink heavily in certain negative situations (e.g., contexts involving physical discomfort) at least partly because they are highly fearful of anxiety symptoms. No study to date has investigated potential differences in the role of anxiety sensitivity in explaining the comorbidity of PTSD and SUDs in women versus men. However, women consistently score higher relative to men on measures of anxiety sensitivity (see reviews by Stewart, Taylor, & Baker, 1997; Stewart & Baker, 1999). Thus, it might be speculated that fear of anxiety symptoms would play a greater role in motivating coping-related drinking/drug use among female substance abusers with PTSD than among their male counterparts. This suggestion requires empirical scrutiny in future research.

A study by Bonin, Norton, Asmundson, DiCurzio, and Pidlubny (2000) with 61 male and 30 female patients with SUDs, provides further information on the role of anxiety- and depression-related individual-difference variables in contributing to PTSD–SUD comorbidity among men versus women. These researchers conducted stepwise discriminant function analyses to determine which of a set of individual-difference factors pertaining to anxiety and depression could account for the most variance in PTSD diagnoses. These analyses were conducted separately within each gender group. The Beck Anxiety Inventory (BAI; Beck, Epstein, Brown, & Steer, 1988) alone accounted for about 69% of the variance for men, whereas the Beck Depression Inventory (BDI; Beck & Steer, 1987) alone accounted for about 75% of the variance for women. Consistent with suggestions that PTSD may present differently in men and women (Wolfe & Kimerling, 1997), Bonin et al.'s (2000) findings suggest that the emotional correlates of comorbid PTSD among those with a SUD may differ across gender. Their findings are consistent with clinical descriptions of ways in which men and women with comorbid PTSD–SUDs appear to vary (see review by Najavits et al., 1997). Bonin et al. found that a relation between depression and PTSD was particularly important for women patients with SUD. Similarly, comorbid women have been described in the clinical literature as being more self-blaming, more suicidal, and demonstrating more sexual dysfunction (i.e., all characteristics of depression; see DSM-IV [American Psychiatric Association, 1994]) relative to comorbid men (e.g., Bollerud, 1990; Herman, 1992; O'Donohue & Elliott, 1992).

The Role of PTSD Symptoms

The self-medication explanation of the relationship between PTSD and SUDs implies a mediating role for PTSD symptoms in the trauma–SUD relation. In other words, trauma exposure is related to increased rates of SUDs, because trauma results in PTSD symptoms, which patients attempt to control through drinking/drug misuse. In this section, we review two studies that have empirically investigated this potential mediating role of PTSD symptoms in women-only or mixed-gender samples.

Epstein, Saunders, Kilpatrick, and Resnick (1998) examined the potential mediating role of PTSD symptoms in explaining relations between childhood sexual abuse and alcohol problems in adult women. Participants were a random, nonclinical sample of 2,994 adult women interviewed about childhood sexual abuse history, and lifetime PTSD and alcohol abuse symptoms. The definition of childhood sexual abuse was conservative, including only instances involving penetration that occurred prior to age 18 years. PTSD was assessed using the National Women's Study Posttraumatic Stress Disorder Module (NWS PTSD; Resnick, Kilpatrick, Dansky, Saunders, & Best, 1993). Alcohol abuse was assessed by seven questions pertaining to the DSM-IV (American Psychiatric Association, 1994) criteria. A history of childhood sexual abuse was associated with a doubling of the number of alcohol abuse symptoms experienced in adulthood. Alcohol abuse was greater in sexual abuse victims who developed PTSD than among those who did not. Path analysis demonstrated significant pathways connecting childhood sexual abuse to PTSD symptoms, and PTSD symptoms to alcohol abuse. The association between childhood sexual abuse and adult alcohol abuse was completely mediated by PTSD symptoms. The authors suggested that PTSD may be an important variable affecting alcohol abuse patterns in women who were victims of sexual abuse in childhood (Epstein et al., 1998).

Bissonnette et al. (1997), using a mixed-gender sample, examined the potential mediating role of PTSD symptoms in explaining hypothesized relations between childhood familial abuse histories and excessive drinking in young adulthood. An undergraduate university sample of 379 students (144 males, 235 females) completed self-report questionnaires about childhood exposure to familial violence, and current PTSD symptoms and alcohol use patterns (i.e., weekly consumption, drinking to cope). Childhood maltreatment (defined as occurrence prior to age 18 years) was assessed using a 40-item instrument that encompassed witnessing violence between parents or stepparents, emotional/physical abuse by an adult, and/or sexual abuse experiences. Current PTSD symptoms were assessed using the 40-item version of the Trauma Symptom Checklist (TSC-40; Elliott & Briere, 1992). Drinking to cope was assessed with a single item from a measure of maladaptive coping strategies (Carver, Scheier, & Weintraub, 1989). Results revealed that childhood physical/emotional abuse predicts increased PTSD symptoms on the TSC-40 among both males and females, and that childhood sexual abuse contributed to increased PTSD symptoms in women only. Witnessing familial violence predicted increased weekly alcohol use among the males. However, alcohol consumption patterns of those experiencing greater versus lesser levels of PTSD symptoms failed to differ significantly, providing no support for the hypothesis that PTSD symptoms mediate the relation between childhood familial violence exposure and increased drinking behavior in young adulthood.

Students in the Bissonnette et al. (1997) study who reported greater levels of PTSD symptoms also indicated more coping-related drinking (collapsed across genders), which predicted increased weekly alcohol use among both males and females. In fact, other research suggests that alcohol consumption motivated by desires to cope with (i.e., avoid or reduce) negative emotional states is a strong predictor of alcohol-related problems over and above consumption levels alone (e.g., Cooper, Russell, Skinner, & Windle, 1992). Consistent with a self-medication model (Khantzian, 1985) of substance abuse in trauma victims, several studies indicate more self-reports of drinking or drug use to cope among victims sexually abused as children relative to controls with no sexual abuse histories (e.g., Harrison, Hoffmann, & Edwall, 1989; Hussey & Singer, 1993). Other research suggests that coping-motivated drinking is more common among young women than young men (Cooper, 1994), and that coping motives are a stronger predictor of heavy drinking among women than men (Cooper et al., 1992). Future research could employ validated measures of substance use motives (e.g., Stewart, Zeitlin, & Samoluk, 1996) to address the degree to which coping-motivated drinking or drug use explains the relation between PTSD symptoms and SUDs in women versus men.

Summary

Studies of the functional relations between PTSD and SUDs suggest some important gender differences. First, although a gradient of effect between symptoms of PTSD and SUDs appears to be evident among both men and women, this association may be more specific to PTSD arousal symptoms in women, at least in the case of alcohol use disorders. This finding remains to be explored further, through studies involving direct comparisons of men and women, and gender comparisons of comorbid patients' perceptions of relations between symptoms of their two disorders. Second, temporality studies suggest that women may be more susceptible than men to a form of comorbidity in which the PTSD develops first. However, this trend should be investigated further in longitudinal research. Third, studies of situation-specific substance use suggest that, consistent with a self-medication model, both men and women with comorbidity evidence a pattern of drinking/drug taking that is relatively specific to "negative" situations. However, only women show decreased drinking/drug taking in "positive" situations. Studies of the relevance of individual-difference factors indicate that anxiety sensitivity (fear of anxiety symptoms) is an important component of comorbidity in women. The relevance of anxiety sensitivity to comorbidity in males remains to be explored. Additionally, individual differences in depression appear important in comorbidity for women, whereas individual differences in anxiety appear important in comorbidity for men. Finally, studies of the potential mediating role of PTSD have established the status of PTSD symptoms as a mediator of the relationship between childhood sexual abuse and drinking problems in adult women. The mediating role of PTSD symptoms in explaining trauma exposure–SUD relations in men remains to be explored.

GENDER AS MODERATOR OF PTSD EFFECTS ON ADDITIONAL COMORBIDITY, SERVICE UTILIZATION, AND TREATMENT OUTCOME

Previous research suggests that persons with comorbid PTSD–SUDs present with more psychiatric and medical comorbidity relative to those with only one of these disorders (e.g., Brady et al., 1994; Najavits, Gastfriend, et al., 1998; Ouimette et al., 1996). They also appear to make more use of costly addiction treatment services (e.g., Brown, Recupero, & Stout, 1995; Brown, Stout, & Mueller, 1999; Druley & Pashko, 1988). Particularly worrisome are previous research results suggesting that patients with comorbid PTSD–SUDs display relatively poorer shorter and longer term treatment outcome (e.g., Brown et al., 1996; Druley & Pashko, 1988; Ouimette, Ahrens, Moos, & Finney, 1997, 1998a; Ouimette, Brown, & Najavits, 1998; Ouimette, Finney, & Moos, 1999). No previous studies have examined whether such effects vary by patient gender, however. Thus, Ouimette and Brown (1999) recently explored whether the expected associations between PTSD and higher rates of additional comorbidity, greater service utilization, and/or poorer treatment outcome vary by patient gender among patients with SUDs.

The Ouimette and Brown (1999) study involved two separate mixed-gender samples of adult patients with SUDs. The first sample was obtained from the Veterans Affairs (VA) Outcomes Monitoring Project (Moos, Finney, Federman, & Suchinsky, 2000; Ouimette, Kimerling, et al., 2000) and is hereafter referred to as the "VA sample." The subsample focused on here is the 106 women and 5,149 men with alcohol use disorders. These participants had sought inpatient or outpatient treatment at one of 150 VA facilities across the United States. Three-fourths of the patients were Caucasian, 28% were married or cohabiting, and 37% were employed. The average VA sample participant had achieved a high school education and was approximately 50 years old. In the VA sample, PTSD clinical diagnoses were obtained from VA databases. The second sample, obtained from a private hospital setting, is hereafter referred to as the "private hospital sample": 61 women and 52 men seeking treatment for an SUD. On average, private hospital sample participants were 37 years of age, 41% were married or cohabiting; and 50% were employed full-time. The average participant had achieved a high school education. The largest proportion of patients in the private hospital sample (i.e., 41%) had an alcohol use disorder only, and 28% had a drug use disorder only. The remaining 31% had both alcohol and drug use disorders. PTSD diagnoses were established using the Clinician-Administered PTSD Scale (CAPS; Blake et al., 1990).

Additional Psychiatric and Medical Comorbidity

In order to determine whether the expected relation between PTSD and greater additional psychiatric and medical comorbidity was moderated by gender, participants were assessed for the presence of a variety of forms of psychiatric disorders (VA and private hospital samples) and medical diagnoses (VA sample only). In the VA sample, chart diagnoses based on the ninth edition of the *International Classification of Diseases* (ICD-9; World Health Organization, 1978) were culled from VA nationwide databases. Specifically, each patient was coded for the presence or absence of any depressive disorder, any anxiety disorder (other than PTSD), and any medical diagnosis, respectively. In the private hospital sample, additional psychiatric comorbidity was assessed using the Structured Clinical Interview for DSM-III-R (SCID; Spitzer, Williams, & Gibbon, 1986). Focus was on rates of affective disorders (i.e., major depressive disorder, dysthymia, and bipolar disorder) and anxiety disorders other than PTSD (i.e., panic disorder, social phobia, simple phobia, obsessive–compulsive disorder, and generalized anxiety disorder). Patients with SUDs in each sample were grouped by gender and by the presence or absence of comorbid PTSD. Additional comorbid psychiatric and medical disorders were then examined as a function of gender, PTSD status, and their interaction, through moderated multiple regression analyses (cf. Baron & Kenny, 1986).

As hypothesized, patients with SUDs and PTSD exhibited higher rates of additional comorbid diagnoses than patients with SUD without PTSD (see Table 9.2). In the VA sample, PTSD-positive patients exhibited higher rates of depressive disorders, other anxiety disorders, and medical diagnoses than PTSD-negative patients (see Table 9.2). In the private hospital sample, PTSD-positive patients exhibited higher rates of major depressive disorder, bipolar disorder, and panic disorder relative to PTSD-negative patients (see Table 9.2). However, no significant interactions involving gender were observed in either sample, indicating that gender failed to moderate the relations between PTSD and comorbid disorders among patients with SUDs.

It should be cautioned that the lack of gender-moderating effects on psychiatric comorbidity is limited to those psychiatric disorders (i.e., anxiety and mood disorders) examined by Ouimette and Brown (1999). However, findings of Ouimette et al. (1996) suggest that comorbid borderline personality disorder and/or dissociative disorders may be particularly elevated in women with PTSD–SUDs. In addition, previous research has shown sexual dysfunction to be a common problem in females with SUD and sexual victimization histories (e.g., Covington & Kohen, 1984; see also reviews by Stewart & Israeli, 2002; Wilsnack, 1984). Relations between sexual victimization histories, sexual problems, and substance abuse have been observed even in community samples of women (Wilsnack, Vogeltanz, Klassen, & Harris, 1997). Moreover, female sexual dysfunctions involving pain and avoidance have been linked to sexual trauma histories (see re-

TABLE 9.2. Differences in Rates of Comorbid Psychiatric and Medical Diagnoses among PTSD-Positive versus PTSD-Negative Patients with SUDs from Two Settings

	PTSD status	
Setting	PTSD	No PTSD
VA sample	(N = 793)	(N = 4,462)
Psychiatric disorders		
Depressive disorders	49%	25%
Other anxiety disorders	21%	9%
Medical diagnosis	85%	74%
Private hospital sample	(N = 51)	(N = 62)
Psychiatric disorders		
Depressive disorders		
Major depressive disorder	79%	51%
Bipolar disorder	15%	0%
Other anxiety disorders		
Panic disorder	48%	19%

Note. PTSD diagnoses established with ICD-9 (World Health Organization, 1978) criteria and obtained from the VA database for the VA sample and with the CAPS (Blake et al., 1990) interview for the private hospital sample. Psychiatric and medical diagnoses established with ICD-9 criteria and obtained from the VA database for the VA sample. Private hospital sample's psychiatric diagnoses established with the SCID (Spitzer et al., 1986). No significant interactions with gender were obtained, so the data are collapsed across gender group. Data from Ouimette and Brown (1999).

views by Briere & Runtz, 1993; Sultan & Chambless, 1988). The degree to which gender might moderate the relation between PTSD–SUD and comorbid borderline personality disorder, dissociative disorders, and/or sexual dysfunctions remains to be explored in future research.

Service Utilization

In order to determine whether the expected relation between PTSD and higher service utilization was moderated by gender, VA patients' total number of visits for substance use services, psychiatric services, and medical services were culled from VA databases. Service utilization measures were examined through moderated multiple regression analyses as a function of gender, PTSD status, and their interaction. For all three service-utilization variables, significant main effects of PTSD status were obtained. Compared to PTSD-negative patients with alcohol use disorders, PTSD-positive patients with alcohol use disorders made significantly more psychiatric visits (means = 18.1 vs. 4.8), visits for treatment of substance abuse (means = 16.9 vs. 11.6), and medical visits (see Figure 9.1). However, this latter relation was qualified by a significant gender × PTSD status interaction: The effect of PTSD status on medical visits was much stronger among women than among men (see Figure 9.1).

The finding that PTSD status was associated with greater utilization of substance abuse services is consistent with previous findings in patients with SUDs (e.g., Brown et al., 1995, 1999; Druley & Pashko, 1988). However, Brown et al. (1999) also found that comorbid versus SUD-only patients did not differ in rates of use of psychiatric services, and that PTSD services, in particular, were rarely used by comorbid patients. Their results stand in contrast to the finding of Ouimette and Brown (1999) that use of psychiatric services was significantly elevated in patients with comorbidity relative to those with SUDs only. A number of factors may account for the discrepancy. First, the findings may reflect differing referral practices for patients with comorbidity across different treatment settings (VA setting in Ouimette & Brown, 1999 versus private hospital setting in Brown et al., 1999). Second, the VA study did not examine the type of problem for which psychiatric services were being accessed by patients with comorbidity. The discrepancy could be reconciled if comorbid patients in the VA study were overusing psychiatric services for mental health problems other than PTSD (e.g., for treatment of their elevated rates of mood or other anxiety disorders; see Table 9.2).

Ouimette and Brown's (1999) finding that the effect of comorbid PTSD on number of medical visits was greater among women substance abusers than among their male counterparts (see Figure 9.1) is consistent with previous research suggesting that trauma exposure is associated with somatic outcomes and long-term increases in medical care among women

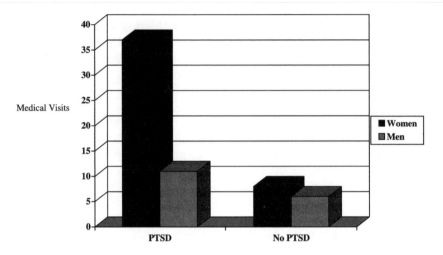

FIGURE 9.1. Moderating effect of gender on the relationship between PTSD status and service utilization in the VA sample of patients with SUDs (Ouimette & Brown, 1999). Bars represent mean number of medical visits.

(e.g., Koss & Heslet, 1992). This finding also converges with previous findings that PTSD is associated with poorer perceptions of physical health among women (Wolfe, Schnurr, Brown, & Furey, 1994). However, Ouimette and Brown's (1999) moderating effect of gender on medical visits was not accompanied by a similar moderating effect of gender on medical comorbidity in the VA sample. Although PTSD-positive patients with SUDs in the VA sample had significantly more comorbid medical disorders relative to PTSD-negative patients with SUDs (see Table 9.2), this effect of PTSD status was no stronger in the women than in the men with SUDs. Two possible explanations exist for this pattern of findings. First, women with comorbidity may be somatizing their psychological symptoms to a greater degree than do men with comorbidity. Thus, women with comorbidity may seek out medical services to a greater degree than their male counterparts. Second, health care providers may be funneling comorbid women into medical care more frequently than comorbid men, despite an absence of a true gender difference in medical comorbidity. Factors contributing to such possible gender biases in health care providers' referral practices require further investigation.

Treatment Course

In order to determine whether the expected relation between PTSD and poorer treatment outcome was moderated by gender, 6- to 12-month outcome data were collected for the VA sample, and 6-month outcome data were collected for participants in the private hospital sample. Sixty-three percent of the original VA sample and 86% of the original private hospital sample completed the treatment follow-up. Treatment outcome in the VA sample was assessed with the seven subscales of the ASI (McLellan et al., 1992). Treatment outcome in the private hospital sample was assessed with a Timeline Follow-Back (TLFB) interview (Sobell & Sobell, 1992) focusing on percentage of days abstinent and number of days to relapse (cf. Brown, Stout, & Meuller, 1996). For those with an alcohol use disorder at pretreatment, drinks per drinking day, and percentage of days heavy drinking were additional outcome measures covered in the TLFB interview (cf. Brown et al., 1996). Statistical analyses revealed that, for participants in the private hospital setting, PTSD status was associated with poorer treatment outcome on three of the four TLFB variables. Compared to patients with SUDs without comorbid PTSD, those with comorbid PTSD relapsed more quickly (35 days vs. 67 days from end of treatment to first relapse). Patients with comorbidity also drank more heavily on drinking days (means = 10 vs. 6 drinks per drinking day), and had a larger percentage of days during follow-up that were heavy drinking days (means = 58% vs. 40% heavy drinking days). Gender failed to moderate any of these effects of PTSD status on treatment outcome in the private hospital sample. For participants in the VA sample, PTSD status was associated with poorer treatment outcome on three of the seven ASI composite scores. Compared to patients with alcohol use disorder without comorbid PTSD, those with comorbid PTSD had higher treatment scores on the ASI psychiatric composite (means = .47 vs. .23), medical composite (means = .50 vs. .39), and family/social composite (means = .18 vs. .12). These findings are consistent with the results of previous research suggesting that PTSD–SUD comorbidity is associated with poorer treatment outcome (e.g., Brown et al., 1996; Druley & Pashko, 1988; Ouimette et al., 1997; Ouimette, Ahrens, Moos, & Finney, 1998; Ouimette, Brown, et al., 1998; Ouimette, Finney, et al., 1999).

One significant gender × PTSD status interaction was observed for the VA sample: For the ASI subscale tapping drug use problems, women with PTSD scored higher than women without PTSD at treatment follow-up; males with and without comorbid PTSD did not differ on this latter ASI subscale (see Figure 9.2). This gender-moderating effect occurred even with pretreatment drug use problems controlled. This suggests that women with comorbid PTSD–alcohol use disorders may be particularly vulnerable to problematic drug use outcomes. The degree to which these findings may be attributable to quality of care and/or patient noncompliance remains to be determined. For example, it is possible that coexisting drug use problems in women with PTSD–alcoholism are not attended to sufficiently in treatment, such that they remain a problem. Alternatively, alcoholic women with comorbid PTSD may be less compliant with treatment aftercare recommendations pertaining to their drug misuse (cf. Brady et al., 1994).

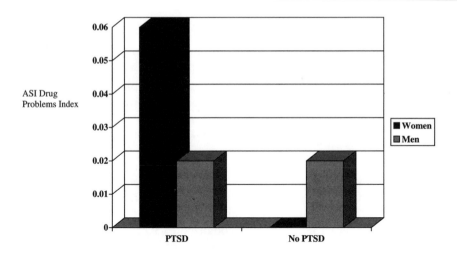

FIGURE 9.2. Moderating effect of gender on the relationship between PTSD and 6-month posttreatment outcome in the VA sample of patients with SUDs (Ouimette & Brown, 1999). Bars represent mean composite scores on the Drug Problems subscale of the Addiction Severity Index (McLellan et al., 1992).

Summary

The research reviewed in this section confirms that comorbid PTSD in patients with SUDs is associated with greater medical and other psychiatric comorbidity, greater service utilization, and poorer treatment outcome. Gender appears to be an important moderator of PTSD-status effects on certain aspects of service utilization and treatment outcome. Specifically, the effect of comorbid PTSD on patients' use of medical services appears stronger among women relative to men. The absence of similar gender-moderating effects with respect to medical comorbidity suggests that women with comorbidity in particular, make excessive use of medical services. Reasons for this overuse remain to be identified. Additionally, relative to pure alcohol use disorder patients, only women with comorbid PTSD–alcohol use disorder (but not comorbid men), show poorer treatment outcome with respect to problem drug use. This suggests that problematic drug use outcomes are a particular area of difficulty for such women.

ISSUES IN THE TREATMENT OF MEN AND WOMEN WITH COMORBID PTSD–SUDs

In this section, we review the findings on gender differences with respect to comorbid PTSD–SUDs in terms of their implications for the treatment of men and women. We review the controversies about whether treatment for comorbid patients should be sequential or simultaneous, and whether integrated treatments should be conducted in a mixed-gender or single-gender format.

Sequential versus Simultaneous Treatment for Comorbid Men and Women

Although most experts agree that both disorders need to be a focus of treatment, there has been controversy about which problem should be dealt with first, or whether both disorders should be treated simultaneously (see review by Brown & Wolfe, 1994). The most recent consensus appears to be that simultaneous treatment approaches, in which both disorders are a focus of treatment from the outset, are likely the best course of action. Given likely reciprocal relations between PTSD and SUDs, in which one disorder serves to maintain the other, attention to both disorders from the outset may enhance longer term outcome. If the PTSD symptoms are not treated, the patient may experience a reemergence or intensification of anxiety-related symptoms following sobriety, or during detoxification, that may precipitate relapse to alcohol/drug use (cf. Root, 1989). Conversely, the efficacy of psychological treatments for the PTSD may be compromised if patients are actively abusing substances during treatment (cf. Barlow, 2002). Presumably, these factors contribute to the poorer shorter and longer term treatment outcome of patients with SUDs and comorbid PTSD, reviewed earlier in this chapter. In fact, integrated, simultaneous treatments have been advocated for both comorbid male veterans (e.g., Boudewyns, Woods, Hyer, & Albrecht, 1991) and comorbid women with histories of victimization (e.g., Bollerud, 1990; Skorina & Kovach, 1986; Turner & Colao, 1985). Despite these recommendations, relatively little is known about the effective components of treatment for comorbid men or women.

Recent evidence suggests that although comorbid patients show poorer treatment outcome, more counseling sessions devoted to substance abuse and increased involvement in addiction self-help groups partially counteract the negative effects of comorbid PTSD on short-term treatment outcome among male veterans with SUDs (Ouimette, Ahrens, et al., 1998). This study also showed that comorbid males reported fewer psychological symptoms at discharge if they received treatment services high in support and structure. Recent evidence suggests that male veteran comorbid patients who utilized more outpatient substance abuse, psychiatric, and PTSD services in the first year following treatment were more likely to maintain a stable course of remission from substance use over a 2-year follow-up (Ouimette, Moos, & Finney, 2000). When these three types of services were examined in multiple regression analyses, PTSD-specific sessions emerged as the most significant predictor of longer term remission. These data are consistent with the notion that both PTSD- and SUD-focused treatment services are essential components of effective treatment for male patients with SUDs and comorbid PTSD (Ouimette, Ahrens, et al., 1998; Ouimette, Moos, & Finney, 2000). Less is known about the essential components of treatment for comorbid women. However, data from a mixed-gender sample of patients with comorbid PTSD–SUDs indicated that they have a clear preference for a simultaneous treatment approach (Brown et al., 1998).

Mixed-Gender versus Single-Gender Treatments

Just as controversy existed in the past regarding whether simultaneous or sequential treatment is most indicated for comorbid patients, there is current controversy about whether simultaneous treatment approaches should be gender-specific. For example, Triffleman, Carroll, and Kellog (1999) have developed a simultaneous treatment approach labeled "substance dependence PTSD therapy" (SDPT) designed for use among mixed-gendered civilian patients with varied sources of trauma. SDPT is conducted as an individual therapy and employs cognitive-behavioral techniques, including relapse prevention and coping skills training to tackle the SUD symptoms, and psychoeducation, stress inoculation training, and *in vivo* exposure to tackle the PTSD symptoms. This therapy approach has been manualized, and data from an open-trial pilot study suggest its efficacy (see Triffleman et al., 1999).

Others argue that the unique characteristics of men and women with comorbid PTSD–SUDs necessitate gender-specific treatment approaches. Najavits et al. (1997) argue that clinicians should not assume that simultaneous treatment approaches developed for combat-exposed, comorbid men can be transferred to women with comorbid PTSD–SUDs. Several differences between comorbid men and women have been outlined in this chapter (e.g., more self-blame, more suicide attempts, greater history of sexual victimization, more comorbid sexual dysfunctions, greater specificity of PTSD arousal symptoms to SUD symptoms among women). These differences suggest that treatments developed for combat-exposed, comorbid men likely need to be modified to treat comorbid women most appropriately. Ouimette, Kimerling, et al. (2000) have further suggested that mixed-gender therapy groups may be particularly difficult for females with comorbid PTSD–SUDs given the substantial sexual and physical victimization histories characteristic of these women and the fact that such mixed-gender groups might include male perpetrators of violence.

The differences between comorbid men and women outlined in the current chapter suggest several characteristics that may be useful in integrated therapy approaches for comorbid women. For example, the "gradient of effect" findings reviewed earlier (McFall et al., 1992; Stewart,

Conrod, Pihl, et al., 1999) suggest that arousal management training (e.g., Stockwell & Towne, 1989) may be a fruitful component of therapy for patients with comorbid PTSD–SUDs—particularly comorbid women (cf., Brown & Ouimette, 1999). Additionally, Ouimette and Brown (1999) further suggest that comorbid PTSD–alcoholic women, in particular, need to have any associated drug problems specifically addressed in treatment to enhance longer term outcome.

Although gender-specific integrated treatment approaches have long been advocated in the treatment of women with comorbid PTSD–SUDs who report histories of victimization (e.g., Bollerud, 1990; Skorina & Kovach, 1986; Turner & Colao, 1985), few of these therapies have been manualized or evaluated empirically for their efficacy. One exception is the integrated, simultaneous treatment approach developed by Najavits, Weiss, and Liese (1996). Their approach—"Seeking Safety"—involves cognitive-behavioral group psychotherapy that is specifically designed for women with this form of dual diagnosis. The results of an open-trial pilot study indicate positive treatment outcome effects on both PTSD and SUD symptoms, high attendance rates, strong patient–therapist alliance, and good patient satisfaction with this approach (Najavits, Weiss, Shaw, & Muenz, 1998).

Summary

Clearly, more research is needed to examine the role of gender in treatment outcome for clients with comorbid PTSD–SUDs, and whether gender-specific treatments are necessary and/or superior. However, some data suggest that single-gender treatment programs can confer substantial benefits for women with SUDs (see review by Hodgins, El-Guebaly, & Addington, 1997). Ouimette, Kimerling, et al. (2000) have recommended that when single-gender therapy groups are not available, comorbid women with abuse histories should be seen individually until symptoms are stabilized and linkages with appropriate adjunctive services have been established.

OVERALL SUMMARY AND CONCLUSION

Comorbid PTSD–SUDs is a problem for both women and men; however, women may be somewhat more likely than men to develop this dual diagnosis. Severity of trauma exposure increases the likelihood of developing this dual diagnosis in both women and men. Women's comorbidity may be more strongly linked to a history of physical and sexual victimization than that of men.

When functional relations between PTSD and SUDs are examined, women's pattern of comorbidity supports a model of PTSD developing first, then substance use. Possibly, men are more likely to develop PTSD secondary to a SUD, due to risky lifestyles associated with illicit substance abuse. Women's substance use appears to be more influenced by PTSD hyperarousal symptoms, and women are more fearful of anxiety sensations which perhaps fuels substance use. Both comorbid women and men appear to self-medicate in negative situations. Finally, women with this dual diagnosis may use medical services more often because of somatizing symptoms or improper referrals, and may have more problems with drug use.

We recommend that all individuals who experience trauma, especially women who have experienced sexual assault or have PTSD symptoms, should be educated about the risk for the development of substance use problems. Individuals with PTSD related to particularly severe trauma histories appear to be at greatest risk for SUDs; a thorough assessment of substance use is warranted through multiple means (self-report, interview, collateral informant). In turn, all patients with SUDs should be screened for trauma and PTSD, and male patients may be targeted for education about the potential consequences of the lifestyle associated with drug use. Providers should be aware that women with this dual diagnosis might somatize symptoms and overuse medical services, and that women with comorbid PTSD–alcoholism may have particular problems with recovery from concomitant drug abuse.

We recommend simultaneous treatment of PTSD and SUDs. Individual treatment or single-gender groups are recommended, with recognition of special issues associated with this dual diagnosis for women (e.g., sexual victimization, comorbid depression, hyperarousal, and anxiety sensitivity) and for men (e.g., combat). Women may benefit from treatments that focus on arousal management, such as relaxation training. Men may benefit from participation in self-help groups, along with formal treatment.

The evidence supports the examination of gender as an important individual difference variable for PTSD–SUD comorbidity. We hope that this chapter stimulates more theory and clinical research, as well as careful consideration of gender in clinical practice.

ACKNOWLEDGMENTS

This work was supported in part by a grant from the National Health Research Development Program, Health Canada (Dr. Stewart), and in part by the Department of Veterans Affairs Mental Health Strategic Health Group and the Health Services Research and Development Service (Dr. Ouimette). The views expressed in this chapter are those of the authors and do not necessarily represent the views of the Department of Veterans Affairs. We thank Rudolf H. Moos for his comments on this chapter.

REFERENCES

American Psychiatric Association. (1987). *Diagnostic and statistical manual of mental disorders* (3rd ed., rev.). Washington, DC: Author.

American Psychiatric Association. (1994). *Diagnostic and statistical manual of mental disorders* (4th ed.). Washington, DC: Author.

Annis, H. M., Graham, J. M., & Davis, C. S. (1987). *Inventory of Drinking Situations (IDS) user's guide*. Toronto: Addiction Research Foundation.

Annis, H. M., Turner, N. E., & Sklar, S. M. (1996). *Inventory of Drug-Taking Situations (IDTS) user's guide*. Toronto: Addiction Research Foundation.

Barlow, D. H. (2002). *Anxiety and its disorders: The nature and treatment of anxiety and panic* (2nd ed.). New York: Guilford Press.

Baron, R. M., & Kenny, D. A. (1986). The moderator–mediator distinction in social psychological research: Conceptual, strategic, and statistical considerations. *Journal of Personality and Social Psychology, 51,* 1173–1182.

Beck, A. T., Epstein, N., Brown, G., & Steer, R. A. (1988). An inventory for measuring clinical anxiety: Psychometric properties. *Journal of Counseling and Clinical Psychology, 56,* 893–897.

Beck, A. T., & Steer, R. A. (1987). *The Beck Depression Inventory manual*. Toronto: Psychological Corporation.

Bissonnette, M., Wall, A.-M., Wekerle, C., McKee, S. A., Hinson, R. E., & Tsianos, D. (1997). Is a post-traumatic stress disorder (PTSD) mediational model a valid framework for understanding undergraduate drinking behavior? [Summary]. *Alcoholism: Clinical and Experimental Research, 21,* 54A.

Blake, D. D., Weathers, F. W., Nagy, L. M., Kaloupek, D. G., Gusman, F. D., Charney, D., & Keane, T. M. (1990). Development of a clinician administered PTSD scale. *Journal of Traumatic Stress, 8,* 75–90.

Blanchard, E. B., Jones-Alexander, J., Buckley, T. C., & Forneris, C. A. (1996). Psychometric properties of the PTSD Checklist (PCL). *Behaviour Research and Therapy, 34,* 669–673.

Bollerud, K. (1990). A model for the treatment of trauma-related syndromes among chemically dependent inpatient women. *Journal of Substance Abuse Treatment, 7,* 83–87.

Bonin, M. F., Norton, G. R., Asmundson, G. J. G., DiCurzio, S., & Pidlubny, S. (2000). Drinking away the hurt: The nature and prevalence of PTSD in substance abuse patients attending a community-based treatment program. *Journal of Behavior Therapy and Experimental Psychiatry, 31,* 55–66.

Boudewyns, P. A., Woods, M. G., Hyer, L., & Albrecht, J. W. (1991). Chronic combat-related PTSD and concurrent substance abuse: Implications for treatment of this frequent "dual diagnosis." *Journal of Traumatic Stress, 4,* 549–560.

Brady, K. T., Dansky, B. S., Sonne, S. C., & Saladin, M. E. (1998). Posttraumatic stress disorder and cocaine dependence: Order of onset. *American Journal on Addictions, 7,* 128–135.

Brady, K. T., Killeen, T., Saladin, M., Dansky, B. S., & Becker, S. (1994). Comorbid substance abuse and PTSD: Characteristics of women in treatment. *American Journal on Addictions, 3,* 160–164.

Branchey, L., Davis, W., & Lieber, C. S. (1984). Alcoholism in Vietnam and Korean veterans: A long-term follow-up. *Alcoholism: Clinical and Experimental Research, 8,* 572–575.

Breslau, N., Chilcoat, H., Kessler, R., & Lucia, V. (1999). Vulnerability to assaultive violence: Sex differences in PTSD [Summary]. Presented as part of a symposium, Gender Issues in Posttraumatic Stress Disorder, R. Kimerling (Chair), *Final Program and Proceedings of the 15th Annual Meeting of the International Society for Traumatic Stress Studies,* pp. 87–88.

Breslau, N., Davis, G. C., Andreski, P., & Peterson, E. L. (1991). Traumatic events and posttraumatic stress disorder in an urban population of young adults. *Archives of General Psychiatry, 48,* 216–222.

Breslau, N., Davis, G. C., Andreski, P., Peterson, E. L., & Schultz, L. R. (1997). Sex differences in posttraumatic stress disorder. *Archives of General Psychiatry, 54,* 1044–1048.

Breslau, N., Davis, G. C., Peterson, E. L., & Schultz, L. R. (1997). Psychiatric sequelae of posttraumatic stress disorder in women. *Archives of General Psychiatry, 54,* 81–87.

Briere, J., & Runtz, M. (1993). Childhood sexual abuse: Long-term sequelae and implications for psychological assessment. *Journal of Interpersonal Violence, 8,* 312–333.

Brown, P. J., & Ouimette, P. C. (1999). Introduction to the special section on substance use disorder and posttraumatic stress disorder comorbidity. *Psychology of Addictive Behaviors, 13,* 75–77.

Brown, P. J., Recupero, P. R., & Stout, R. L. (1995). PTSD substance abuse comorbidity and treatment utilization. *Addictive Behaviors, 20,* 251–254.

Brown, P. J., Stout, R. L., & Gannon-Rowley, J. (1998). Substance use disorder–PTSD comorbidity: Patients' perceptions of symptom interplay and treatment issues. *Journal of Substance Abuse Treatment, 14,* 1–4.

Brown, P. J., Stout, R. L., & Mueller, T. (1996). Posttraumatic stress disorder and substance abuse relapse among women: A pilot study. *Psychology of Addictive Behaviors, 10,* 124–128.

Brown, P. J., Stout, R. L., & Mueller, T. (1999). Substance use disorder and posttraumatic stress disorder comorbidity: Addiction and psychiatric treatment rates. *Psychology of Addictive Behaviors, 13,* 115–122.

Brown, P. J., & Wolfe, J. (1994). Substance abuse and posttraumatic stress disorder comorbidity. *Drug and Alcohol Dependence, 35,* 51–59.

Carson, M., & Orr, S. (1999). Psychophysiologic responses in posttraumatic stress disorder: A comparison of male and female trauma populations [Summary]. Presented as part of a symposium, Gender Issues in Posttraumatic Stress Disorder, R. Kimerling (Chair), *Final Program and Proceedings of the 15th Annual Meeting of the International Society for Traumatic Stress Studies,* p. 88.

Carver, C. S., Scheier, M. F., & Weintraub, J. K. (1989). Assessing coping strategies: A theoretically based approach. *Journal of Personality and Social Psychology, 56,* 267–283.

C-DIS Management Group. (1991). *Computerized Diagnostic Interview Schedule (revised) for DSM-III-R [Computer software].* Ottawa: Author.

Chilcoat, H. D., & Breslau, N. (1998). Investigations of causal pathways between PSD and drug use disorders. *Addictive Behaviors, 23,* 827–840.

Cooper, M. L. (1994). Motivations for alcohol use among adolescents: Development and validation of a four-factor model. *Psychological Assessment, 6,* 117–128.

Cooper, M. L., Russell, M., Skinner, J. B., & Windle, M. (1992). Development and validation of a three-dimensional measure of drinking motives. *Psychological Assessment, 4*, 123–132.

Covington, S. S., & Kohen, J. (1984). Women, alcohol, and sexuality. *Advances in Alcohol and Substance Abuse, 4*, 41–56.

Dansky, B. S., Saladin, M. E., Brady, K. T., Kilpatrick, D. G., & Resnick, H. S. (1995). Prevalence of victimization and posttraumatic stress disorder among women with substance use disorders: Comparison of telephone and in-person assessment samples. *International Journal of the Addictions, 30*, 1079–1099.

Deykin, E. Y., & Buka, S. L. (1997). Prevalence and risk factors for posttraumatic stress disorder among chemically dependent adolescents. *American Journal of Psychiatry, 154*, 752–757.

Druley, K. A., & Pashko, S. (1988). Posttraumatic stress disorder in World War II and Korean combat veterans with alcohol dependency. In M. Galanter (Ed.), *Recent developments in alcoholism* (Vol. 6, pp. 89–101). New York: Plenum Press.

Elliott, D. M., & Briere, J. (1992). Sexual abuse trauma among professional women: Validating the Trauma Symptom Checklist–40 (TSC-40). *Child Abuse and Neglect, 16*, 391–398.

Epstein, J. N., Saunders, B. E., Kilpatrick, D. G., & Resnick, H. S. (1998). PTSD as a mediator between childhood rape and alcohol use in adult women. *Child Abuse and Neglect, 22*, 223–234.

Foa, E. B., Riggs, D. S., Dancu, C. B., & Rothbaum, B. O. (1993). Reliability and validity of a brief instrument for assessing posttraumatic stress disorder. *Journal of Traumatic Stress, 6*, 459–473.

Fullilove, M. R., Fullilove, R. E. III, Smith, M., Winkler, K., Michael, C., Panzer, P. G., & Wallace, R. (1993). Violence, trauma, and posttraumatic stress disorder among women drug users. *Journal of Traumatic Stress, 6*, 533–543.

Gallops, M., Laufer, R. S., & Yager, T. (1981). The Combat Scale, Revised. In R. S. Laufer, T. Yager, E. Frey-Wouters, & J. Donnelan (Eds.), *Legacies of Vietnam: Comparative adjustment of veterans and their peers* (Vol. 3, p. 444–448). Washington, DC: U.S. Government Printing Office.

Green, B. L., Lindy, J. D., Grace, M. C., & Gleser, G. C. (1989). Multiple diagnosis in posttraumatic stress disorder: The role of war stressors. *Journal of Nervous and Mental Disease, 177*, 329–335.

Harrison, P. A., Hoffmann, N. G., & Edwall, G. E. (1989). Differential drug use patterns among sexually abused adolescent girls in treatment for chemical dependency. *International Journal of the Addictions, 24*, 499–514.

Helzer, J. E., Robins, L. N., & McEvoy, L. (1987). Post-traumatic stress disorder in the general population: Findings of the Epidemiologic Catchment Area survey. *New England Journal of Medicine, 317*, 1630–1634.

Herman, J. L. (1992). *Trauma and recovery.* New York: Basic Books.

Hodgins, D. C., El-Guebaly, N., & Addington, J. (1997). Treatment of substance abusers: Single or mixed-gender programs? *Addiction, 92*, 805–812.

Hussey, D. L., & Singer, M. (1993). Psychological distress, problem behaviors, and family functioning of sexually abused adolescent inpatients. *Journal of the American Academy of Child and Adolescent Psychiatry, 32*, 954–961.

Keane, T. M., Caddell, J. M., Martin, B. W., Zimering, R. T., & Fairbank, J. A. (1983). Substance abuse among Vietnam veterans with posttraumatic stress disorders. *Bulletin of the Society of Psychologists in Addictive Behaviors, 2,* 117–122.

Keane, T. M., Caddell, J. M., & Taylor, K. L. (1988). Mississippi Scale for Combat-Related PTSD: Three studies in reliability and validity. *Journal of Consulting and Clinical Psychology, 56,* 85–90.

Keane, T. M., Gerardi, R. J., Lyons, J. A., & Wolfe, J. (1988). The interrelationship of substance abuse and posttraumatic stress disorder. In M. Galanter (Ed.), *Recent developments in alcoholism* (Vol. 6, pp. 27–48). New York: Plenum Press.

Keane, T. M., & Kaloupek, D. G. (1997). Comorbid psychiatric disorders in PTSD: Implications for research. In R. Yehuda & A. C. McFarlane (Eds.), *Psychobiology of posttraumatic stress disorder: Annals of the New York Academy of Sciences* (Vol. 821, pp. 24–34). New York: New York Academy of Sciences.

Keane, T. M., & Wolfe, J. (1990). Comorbidity in posttraumatic stress disorder: An analysis of community and clinical studies. *Journal of Applied Social Psychology, 20,* 1776–1788.

Kendall-Tackett, K. A., Meyer Williams, L., & Finkelhor, D. (1993). Impact of sexual abuse on children: A review and synthesis of recent empirical studies. *Psychological Bulletin, 113,* 164–180.

Kessler, R. C., Crum, R. M., Warner, L. A., Nelson, C. B., Schulenberg, J., & Anthony, J. C. (1997). Lifetime co-occurrence of DSM-III-R alcohol abuse and dependence with other psychiatric disorders in the National Comorbidity Survey. *Archives of General Psychiatry, 54,* 313–321.

Kessler, R. C., Sonnega, A., Bromet, E., Hughes, M., & Nelson, C. B. (1995). Posttraumatic stress disorder in the National Comorbidity Survey. *Archives of General Psychiatry, 52,* 1048–1060.

Khantzian, E. J. (1985). The self-medication hypothesis of addictive disorders: Focus on heroin and cocaine dependence. *American Journal of Psychiatry, 142,* 1259–1264.

Kilpatrick, D. G., Acierno, R. E., Resnick, H. S., Saunders, B. E., & Best, C. L. (1997). A 2–year longitudinal analysis of the relationships between violent assault and substance use in women. *Journal of Consulting and Clinical Psychology, 65,* 834–847.

Kimerling, R., Ouimette, P. C., & Cronkite, R. (1998). Women's Health Needs [Letter]. *Psychiatric Services, 49,* 1493.

Kofoed, L., Friedman, M. J., & Peck, R. (1993). Alcoholism and drug abuse in patients with PTSD. *Psychiatric Quarterly, 64,* 151–171.

Koss, M. P., & Heslet, L. (1992). Somatic consequences of violence against women. *Archives of Family Medicine, 1,* 53–59.

Kovach, J. A. (1986). Incest as a treatment issue for alcoholic women. *Alcoholism Treatment Quarterly, 3,* 1–15.

Kulka, R. A., Schlenger, W. E., Fairbank, J. A., Hough, R. L., Jordan, B. K., Marmar, C. R., & Weiss, D. S. (1990). *Trauma and the Vietnam War generation: Report of findings from the National Vietnam Veterans Readjustment Study.* New York: Brunner/Mazel.

LaCoursiere, R. B., Godfrey, K. E., & Ruby, L. M. (1980). Traumatic neurosis in the etiology of alcoholism: Vietnam and other trauma. *American Journal of Psychiatry, 137,* 966–968.

Malinosky-Rummell, R., & Hansen, D. J. (1993). Long-term consequences of childhood physical abuse. *Psychological Bulletin, 114*, 68–79.

Marlatt, G. A., & Gordon, J. R. (Eds.). (1985). *Relapse prevention.* New York: Guilford Press.

McFall, M. E., Mackay, P. W., & Donovan, D. M. (1991). Combat-related PTSD and psychological adjustment problems among substance abusing veterans. *Journal of Nervous and Mental Disease, 179*, 33–38.

McFall, M. E., Mackay, P. W., & Donovan, D. M. (1992). Combat-related posttraumatic stress disorder and severity of substance abuse in Vietnam veterans. *Journal of Studies on Alcohol, 53*, 357–363.

McLellan, A. T., Kushner, H., Metzger, D., Peters, R., Smith, I., Grison, G., Pettinati, H., & Argeriou, M. (1992). The fifth edition of the Addiction Severity Index. *Journal of Substance Abuse Treatment, 9*, 199–213.

Miller, W. R., & Marlatt, G. A. (1984). *Manual for the Comprehensive Drinker Profile.* Odessa, FL: Psychological Assessment Resources.

Moos, R. H., Finney, J. W., Federman, E. B., & Suchinsky, R. (2000). Specialty mental health care improves patients' outcomes: Findings from a nationwide program to monitor the quality of substance abuse care. *Journal of Studies on Alcohol, 61*, 704–713.

Najavits, L. M., Gastfriend, D. R., Barber, J. P., Reif, S., Muenz, L. R., Blaine, J., Frank, A., Crits-Christoph, P., Thase, M., & Weiss, R. D. (1998). Cocaine dependence with and without PTSD among subjects in the National Institute on Drug Abuse Collaborative Cocaine Treatment Study. *American Journal of Psychiatry, 155*, 214–219.

Najavits, L. M., Weiss, R. D., & Liese, B. S. (1996). Group cognitive-behavioral therapy for women with PTSD and substance use disorder. *Journal of Substance Abuse Treatment, 13*, 13–22.

Najavits, L. M., Weiss, R. D., & Shaw, S. R. (1997). The link between substance abuse and posttraumatic stress disorder in women: A research review. *American Journal on Addictions, 6*, 273–283.

Najavits, L. M., Weiss, R. D., & Shaw, S. R. (1999). A clinical profile of women with posttraumatic stress disorder and substance dependence. *Psychology of Addictive Behaviors, 13*, 98–104.

Najavits, L. M., Weiss, R. D., Shaw, S. R., & Muenz, L. R. (1998). "Seeking Safety": Outcome of a new cognitive-behavioral psychotherapy for women with posttraumatic stress disorder and substance abuse. *Journal of Traumatic Stress, 11*, 437–456.

O'Donohue, W., & Elliott, A. (1992). The current status of posttraumatic stress disorder as a diagnostic category: Problems and proposals. *Journal of Traumatic Stress, 5*, 421–439.

Ouimette, P. C., Ahrens, C., Moos, R. H., & Finney, J. W. (1997). Posttraumatic stress disorder in substance abuse patients: Relationship to one-year posttreatment outcomes. *Psychology of Addictive Behaviors, 11*, 34–47.

Ouimette, P. C., Ahrens, C., Moos, R. H., & Finney, J. W. (1998). During treatment changes in substance abuse patients with posttraumatic stress disorder: The influence of specific interventions and program environments. *Journal of Substance Abuse Treatment, 15*, 555–564.

Ouimette, P. C., & Brown, P. J. (1999). PTSD among female and male patients with substance use disorders [Summary]. Presented as part of a symposium, Gender Issues in Posttraumatic Stress Disorder, R. Kimerling (Chair), *Final Program and Proceedings of the 15th Annual Meeting of the International Society for Traumatic Stress Studies*, p. 87.

Ouimette, P. C., Brown, P. J., & Najavits, L. M. (1998). Course and treatment of patients with substance use and posttraumatic stress disorder comorbidity. *Addictive Behaviors, 23*, 785–795.

Ouimette, P. C., Finney, J. W., & Moos, R. H. (1999). Two-year post-treatment functioning and coping of substance abuse patients with posttraumatic stress disorder. *Psychology of Addictive Behaviors, 13*, 105–114.

Ouimette, P. C., Kimerling, R., Shaw, J., & Moos, R. H. (2000). Physical and sexual abuse among women and men with substance use disorders. *Alcoholism Treatment Quarterly, 18*, 7–17.

Ouimette, P. C., Moos, R. H., & Finney, J. W. (2000). Two-year mental health service use and course of remission in patients with substance use and posttraumatic stress disorders. *Journal of Studies on Alcohol, 61,* 247–253.

Ouimette, P. C., Wolfe, J., & Chrestman, K. R. (1996). Characteristics of posttraumatic stress disorder–alcohol abuse comorbidity in women. *Journal of Substance Abuse, 8*, 335–346.

Peterson, R. A., & Reiss, S. (1992). *Anxiety Sensitivity Index manual* (2nd ed.). Worthington, OH: International Diagnostic Systems.

Polusny, M. A., & Follette, V. M. (1995). Long-term correlates of child sexual abuse: Theory and review of the empirical literature. *Applied and Preventive Psychology, 4*, 143–166.

Rachman, S. J. (1991). A psychological approach to the study of comorbidity. *Clinical Psychology Review, 11*, 461–464.

Resnick, H. S., Kilpatrick, D. G., Dansky, B. S., Saunders, B. E., & Best, C. L. (1993). Prevalence of civilian trauma and posttraumatic stress disorder in a representative national sample of women. *Journal of Consulting and Clinical Psychology, 61*, 984–991.

Robins, L. N., Helzer, J. H., Croughan, J., & Ratcliff, K. S. (1981). The National Institute of Mental Health Diagnostic Interview Schedule: Its history, characteristics, and validity. *Archives of General Psychiatry, 38*, 381–389.

Root, M. P. P. (1989). Treatment failures: The role of sexual victimization in women's addictive behavior. *American Journal of Orthopsychiatry, 43*, 542–549.

Saladin, M. E., Brady, K. T., Dansky, B. S., & Kilpatrick, D. G. (1995). Understanding comorbidity between PTSD and substance use disorder: Two preliminary investigations. *Addictive Behaviors, 20*, 643–655.

Selzer, M. (1971). The Michigan Alcoholism Screening Test: The quest for a new diagnostic instrument. *American Journal of Psychiatry, 127*, 1653–1658.

Sharkansky, E. J., Brief, D. J., Peirce, J. M., Meehan, J. C., & Mannix, L. M. (1999). Substance abuse patients with posttraumatic stress disorder (PTSD): Identifying specific triggers of substance use and their associations with PTSD symptoms. *Psychology of Addictive Behaviors, 13*, 89–97.

Skorina, J. K., & Kovach, J. A. (1986). Treatment techniques for incest-related issues in alcoholic women. *Alcoholism Treatment Quarterly, 3*, 17–30.

Sobell, L. C., & Sobell, M. B. (1992). Timeline Follow-Back: A technique for assessing self-reported alcohol consumption. In R. Z. Litten & J. P. Allen (Eds.), *Mea-*

suring alcohol consumption: Psychological and biochemical methods (pp. 41–72). Totowa, NJ: Humana Press.

Spitzer, R. L., Williams, J. B., & Gibbon, M. (1986). *Structured Clinical Interview for DSM-III-R.* New York: Biometrics Research Department, New York Sate Psychiatric Institute.

Stewart, S. H. (1996). Alcohol abuse in individuals exposed to trauma: A critical review. *Psychological Bulletin, 120,* 83–112.

Stewart, S. H. (1997). Trauma memory and alcohol abuse: Drinking to forget? In J. D. Read & D. S. Lindsay (Eds.), *Recollections of trauma: Scientific evidence and clinical practice* (pp. 461–467). New York: Plenum Press.

Stewart, S. H., & Baker, J. M. (1999). Gender differences in anxiety sensitivity. *Anxiety Disorders Association of America Reporter, 10,* 1, 17–20.

Stewart, S. H., Conrod, P. J., Loughlin, H. L., Pihl, R. O., & Dongier, M. (1999). PTSD symptoms and situation-specific drug taking in women drug abusers [Summary]. Presented as part of a symposium, PTSD and Substance Use Disorder Comorbidity, P. C. Ouimette (Chair), *Final Program and Proceedings of the 15th Annual Meeting of the International Society for Traumatic Stress Studies,* pp. 67–68.

Stewart, S. H., Conrod, P. J., Pihl, R. O., & Dongier, M. (1999). Relationships between posttraumatic stress symptom dimensions and substance dependence in a community-recruited sample of substance-abusing women. *Psychology of Addictive Behaviors, 13,* 78–88.

Stewart, S. H., Conrod, P. J., Samoluk, S. B., Pihl, R. O., & Dongier, M. (2000). Posttraumatic stress disorder symptoms and situation-specific drinking in women substance abusers. *Alcoholism Treatment Quarterly, 18,* 31–47.

Stewart, S. H., & Israeli, A. L. (2002). Substance abuse and co-occurring psychiatric disorders in victims of intimate violence. In C. Wekerle & A.-M. Wall (Eds.), *The violence and addiction equation: Theoretical and clinical issues in substance abuse and relationship violence* (pp. 98–122). New York: Brunner–Routledge.

Stewart, S. H., Pihl, R. O., Conrod, P. J., & Dongier, M. (1998). Functional relationships among trauma, PTSD, and substance-related disorders. *Addictive Behaviors, 23,* 797–812.

Stewart, S. H., Samoluk, S. B., & MacDonald, A. B. (1999). Anxiety sensitivity and substance use and abuse. In S. Taylor (Ed.), *Anxiety sensitivity: Theory, research, and treatment of the fear of anxiety* (pp. 287–319). Mahwah, NJ: Erlbaum.

Stewart, S. H., Taylor, S., & Baker, J. M. (1997). Gender differences in dimensions of anxiety sensitivity. *Journal of Anxiety Disorders, 11,* 179–200.

Stewart, S. H., Zeitlin, S. B., & Samoluk, S. B. (1996). Examination of a three-dimensional drinking motives questionnaire in a young adult university student sample. *Behaviour Research and Therapy, 34,* 61–71.

Stockwell, T., & Towne, C. (1989). Anxiety and stress management. In R. K. Hester & W. R. Miller (Eds.), *Handbook of alcoholism treatment approaches: Effective alternatives* (pp. 222–230). Elmsford, NY: Pergamon Press.

Sultan, F. E., & Chambless, D. L. (1988). Sexual functioning. In E. A. Blechman & K. D. Brownell (Eds.), *Handbook of behavioral medicine for women* (pp. 92–102). Elmsford, NY: Pergamon Press.

Taylor, S., Koch, W. J., & McNally, R. J. (1992). How does anxiety sensitivity vary across the anxiety disorders? *Journal of Anxiety Disorders, 6,* 249–259.

Triffleman, E. G., Carroll, K., & Kellogg, S. (1999). Substance dependence posttraumatic stress disorder therapy: An integrated cognitive-behavioral approach. *Journal of Substance Abuse Treatment, 17*, 3–14.

Triffleman, E. G., Marmar, C. R., Delucchi, K. L., & Ronfeld, H. (1995). Childhood trauma and posttraumatic stress disorder in substance abuse inpatients. *Journal of Nervous and Mental Disease, 183*, 172–176.

Turner, N. E., Annis, H. M., & Sklar, S. M. (1997). Measurement of antecedents to drug and alcohol use: Psychometric properties of the Inventory of Drug-Taking Situations (IDTS). *Behaviour Research and Therapy, 35*, 463–483.

Turner, S., & Colao, F. (1985). Alcoholism and sexual assault: A treatment approach for women exploring both issues. *Alcoholism Treatment Quarterly, 2*, 91–103.

Wilsnack, S. C. (1984). Drinking, sexuality, and sexual dysfunction in women. In S. C. Wilsnack & L. J. Beckman (Eds.), *Alcohol problems in women: Antecedents, consequences, and intervention* (pp. 189–227). New York: Guilford Press.

Wilsnack, S. C., Vogeltanz, N. D., Klassen, A. D., & Harris, T. R. (1997). Childhood sexual abuse and women's substance abuse: National survey findings. *Journal of Studies on Alcohol, 58*, 264–271.

Wolfe, J., & Kimerling, R. (1997). Gender issues in the assessment of posttraumatic stress disorder. In J. P. Wilson & T. M. Keane (Eds.), *Assessing psychological trauma and PTSD* (pp. 192–238). New York: Guilford Press.

Wolfe, J., Schnurr, P. P., Brown, P. J., & Furey, J. (1994). Posttraumatic stress disorder and war-zone exposure as correlates of perceived health in female Vietnam War veterans. *Journal of Consulting and Clinical Psychology, 62*, 1235–1240.

World Health Organization. (1990). *Composite International Diagnostic Interview (CIDI)*. Geneva: Author.

World Health Organization. (1978). *Mental disorders: Glossary and guide to their classification in accordance with the Ninth Revision of the International Classification of Diseases (ICD-9)*. Geneva: Author.

Yager, T., Laufer, R., & Gallops, M. (1984). Some problems associated with war experience in men of the Vietnam generation. *Archives of General Psychiatry, 41*, 327–333.

10 | PTSD and Medical Comorbidity

RACHEL KIMERLING
GRETCHEN CLUM
JOY McQUERY
PAULA P. SCHNURR

Much research has documented the subjective and objective impairments in health status among individuals exposed to trauma and those diagnosed with posttraumatic stress disorder (PTSD). Readers are referred to several excellent reviews for an overview of this literature (Friedman & Schnurr, 1995; Koss, Koss, & Woodruff, 1991; Resnick, Acierno, & Kilpatrick, 1997; Schnurr & Jankowski, 1999). The purpose of this chapter is to explore the extent to which gender moderates the observed relationship between traumatic stress and impaired health status. Previous chapters of the book document gender differences in exposure to trauma over multiple domains and in multiple contexts. We now investigate the extent to which the effects of exposure are experienced and embodied by men and women in different ways. We then provide a preliminary exploration of pathways that may account for any gender differences observed. Our goal is to use our understanding of these issues to inform prevention interventions and health services for both men and women with PTSD.

WHY EXAMINE GENDER AND HEALTH OUTCOMES?

The prevailing view of gender and health status has long been encapsulated as "women get sick and men die." This statement refers to consistent gender differences found for morbidity and mortality. Mortality statistics for the United States suggest that women have a longer lifespan than men, living, on average, 6 years longer (Centers for Disease Control and Prevention, 1999). This survival advantage for women is observed in nearly every country in the world (Kinsella & Gist, 1998). Conversely, women experience greater lifetime rates of medical morbidity than men (Nathanson, 1977). The specific nature of these health conditions and the mechanisms associated with excess morbidity in women depend on a variety of social factors and are only broadly understood. In general, this research suggests that gender differences in health status result from a complex interaction between biological and social conditions. This means that when considering the health status of men and women, either gender may appear to have a health advantage, depending on the social group examined in the research study or the health outcome used as an indicator of health status. Considering the complexities involved in interpreting research on health status among the general population of men and women, it seems almost impossible to understand truly the relationship between PTSD and health status without accounting for gender. To fully explore the role of gender in the health status correlates of PTSD, our hope is that future research will address the broad influences of the biological, behavioral, and social aspects of gender. As a preliminary step toward accounting for gender in an effort to increase the understanding of the relationships among trauma, PTSD, and health status, the current chapter aggregates the literature of PTSD and health by gender of the participants. The pattern of results that we observe address several questions regarding gender, PTSD, and health that can guide future clinical research studies and clinical interventions.

OVERVIEW

This chapter is structured to review systematically the literature concerning the relationship of both PTSD and trauma exposure with health outcomes. Attention to gender in this field is in the early stages, and to date, few studies of trauma and PTSD have compared women and men for health status. In order to form hypotheses regarding gender, we highlight the few studies that have compared women and men, and discuss these results in the context of the research literature that has investigated health outcomes among both men and women. Because few studies have directly assessed morbidity and mortality among men and women with PTSD, we highlight these data and draw conclusions regarding the results with reference to the considerable literature on self-reported physical symptoms and self-rated health status. We conclude with a focus on research conducted with individuals diagnosed with specific conditions: gastrointestinal disorders, chronic pain, and sexually transmitted diseases. Significant research into these specific conditions has addressed their relationship to trauma and PTSD; however, these results and the concomitant gender issues are rarely examined in the context of the broader literature concerning PTSD and health status.

PTSD AND MEDICAL MORBIDITY

Studies Comparing Men and Women

To our knowledge, no published studies to date have directly compared women and men for the extent or type of medical comorbidity attendant with a diagnosis of PTSD. Research is only beginning to document the medical comorbidity with PTSD; however, an analysis of existing data can illuminate populations and diagnoses in need of further investigation. Most of the research has been conducted with samples of men and has utilized veteran samples. Some researchers have noted that because veterans are screened for health problems before entering the military, military samples may be healthier than representative community samples. This greater homogeneity in health status has the potential to obscure some of the relationships between trauma and health (Schnurr, 1996). Thus, the associations between PTSD and increased rates of medical morbidity observed in these populations may be more pronounced in nonveteran samples.

The National Vietnam Veterans Readjustment Study (NVVRS), a large representative sample of 1,632 male and female Vietnam veterans, has yielded informative results regarding the association between PTSD and self-reported health outcomes. The analyses did not directly compare women to men, but identical analyses were conducted separately for women and men. Results can serve as preliminary estimates that the relationship between PTSD and health conditions is comparable for women and men. Both female and male Vietnam Theater veterans with a current diagnosis of PTSD reported a greater number of active chronic physical health conditions and poorer self-rated health than their counterparts without PTSD (Kulka, Schlenger, & Fairbank, 1990).

Studies of Men

Most of these studies have examined medical morbidity after controlling for other factors also associated with health outcomes, such as age, behavioral risk factors, and socioeconomic status. These well-controlled studies are important to this literature, because they provide inroads in examining the unique contribution of PTSD to health outcomes. The data suggest that PTSD may be associated with increased rates of medical morbidity. A study of 327 male combat veterans seeking trauma-related mental health treatment assessed participants using standardized questionnaires and medical chart review (Beckham et al., 1998). Veterans with PTSD suffered from more health conditions according to both physician and patient self-report than did veterans without PTSD. This association persisted after controlling for age, socioeconomic status, minority status, combat exposure, alcohol use, and cigarette pack-year history. In addition, more severe PTSD was associated with poorer health as assessed by both physician and patient self-report.

The observation of a greater number of health conditions may indicate an increased frequency of specific disease states related to PTSD. A longitudinal analysis of a community sample of 605 older male veterans of World War II and the Korean War examined health status via physical exam. In these data, even after accounting for factors predictive of health status, such as age, smoking, alcohol use, and body weight at study entry, PTSD symptoms were associated with an increased risk for onset of several categories of physician-diagnosed medical problems common to older males: arterial, lower gastrointestinal, dermatological, and musculoskeletal disorders (Schnurr, Spiro, & Paris, 2000).

Self-reported morbidity data are similar. One of the largest studies of the physical and mental health of male veterans is the Centers for Disease Control (CDC) Vietnam Experience Study, a telephone survey of over 7,000 male veterans who served during the Vietnam War era (1988). A follow-up study of these participants examined the medical histories of 1,399 men approximately 20 years following combat exposure (Boscarino, 1997). A lifetime diagnosis of PTSD was associated with increased risk for a variety of chronic medical disorders. Risk was specifically increased for heart/circulatory disorders, nonsexually transmitted infectious disease, musculoskeletal disorders, digestive conditions, respiratory disorders, endocrine/metabolic conditions, and nervous system disorders. These analyses controlled for a number of factors thought to affect reporting of the onset of illness, including intelligence, race, region of birth, enlistment status, army medical profile, hypochondriasis, age, smoking, substance abuse, education, and income. The investigators also examined the effects of depression and other anxiety disorders, and found that PTSD was more strongly associated with health outcomes than were other psychiatric disorders, although they did not account for comorbidity among disorders. Nonveteran samples have been studied with less frequency, but those studies that exist are consistent with the veteran literature. For example, a study of Australian firefighters found that subjects with PTSD suffered more cardiovascular, respiratory, musculoskeletal, and neurological symptoms than those without a history of PTSD (McFarlane, Atchison, Rafalowicz, & Papay, 1994). Similar results were observed among a random sample of 363 military veterans exposed to mustard gas during World War II, in which men with PTSD reported more chronic health problems than did men without PTSD (Schnurr, Ford, et al., 2000).

Researchers have further investigated the specific association of PTSD with cardiovascular health among male veterans. In the CDC Vietnam Experience Study, chronic PTSD was associated with electrocardiogram (EKG) abnormalities, atrioventricular defects, and infarctions (Boscarino & Chang, 1999). Although depression and anxiety were also associated with positive EKG findings in these data, the association between PTSD and EKG abnormalities remained after controlling for these comorbid conditions. The analyses also accounted for factors related to coronary heart disease, including age, ethnicity, education, location of service, medications, drug and alcohol use, body mass index, and cigarette smoking. Another study found that Israeli veterans with combat-related PTSD demonstrated poorer performance on laboratory stress tests when compared to noncombat veterans, although no differences were observed in heart rate, blood pressure, or physical exam findings (Shalev, Bleich, & Ursano, 1990a). This study also controlled for behavioral risk factors for cardiovascular disease, including smoking and substance abuse.

Studies of Women

To date, few published studies have examined the relationship between PTSD and medical comorbidity specifically among women. No studies have yet examined objectively documented medical morbidity. Self-report of morbidity was assessed in a study of 109 female Vietnam veterans (Wolfe, Schnurr, Brown, & Furey, 1994). Women with PTSD were more likely to report current health problems, specifically, cardiovascular, gastrointestinal, gynecological, dermatological, opthalmological, and pain problems. These self-reported health problems were associated with PTSD even when war-zone exposure was controlled.

Discussion

Clearly, more data are needed to describe the extent of medical comorbidity with PTSD and to examine associated gender issues. Studies of men suggest that PTSD may be associated with increased risk of morbidity, and that cardiovascular, musculoskeletal, and gastrointestinal disorders may merit specific investigation. Are women with PTSD at risk for similar medical problems? Cardiovascular disease, for example, is the leading cause of death among women in the United States (Centers for Disease Control and Prevention, 1999). Unfortunately, the misperception that this disease is not a serious concern for women has resulted in a less assertive approach to research and treatment (Welty, 2001). In the past decade, medical research that has begun to address gender-specific risk factors and diagnostic procedures for cardiovascular disease can inform the methodology and design of studies examining the comorbidity of cardiovascular disease with PTSD among women. Researchers and clinicians must not conclude that medical disorders such as cardiovascular disease, gastrointestinal disorders, or musculoskeletal conditions are commonly comorbid with PTSD among men but not women, based on a lack of available empirical data. Instead, it is important to recognize the lack of research into women's health. More research is needed to investigate the relationship between PTSD and health status among both civilian and veteran women. We now turn to a discussion of trauma exposure and medical morbidity in an effort to better inform the interpretation of the literature reviewed earlier.

TRAUMA EXPOSURE AND MEDICAL MORBIDITY

Studies Comparing Men and Women

Similar to the PTSD literature, the literature concerning trauma and medical morbidity has yet to examine gender differences in health outcomes comprehensively. One cross-sectional study using a convenience sample of 1,359 middle- to upper-middle-class older men and women assessed sexual assault history in relation to 10 chronic medical conditions that were objectively confirmed by physician diagnosis or medical chart review (Stein & Barrett-Connor, 2000). Sex-specific, age-adjusted odds ratios (ORs) for lifetime risk of disorder were calculated. For coronary heart disease, hypertension, diabetes, osteoporosis, obesity, asthma, migraine, arthritis, fractures, and breast or prostate cancer, sexual assault history was associated with increased risk of thyroid disease in men and breast cancer and arthritis in women. The authors note that these findings were unexpected and do not appear to stem from a common pathology. The absence of a representative sample and/or the potentially constrained statistical power to detect effects for specific diagnoses may have affected the results. Results should be interpreted in the context of similar studies conducted with single-sex samples, reviewed subsequently in this section.

One notably comprehensive study has examined medical morbidity following childhood trauma exposure and merits discussion, although men and women were not compared in the analyses. The Adverse Childhood Experiences Study examined 9,508 health maintenance organization (HMO) enrollees for experiences such as sexual, physical, or psychological abuse; exposure to interparental violence; or living in a household in which one member was a substance abuser, mentally ill, suicidal, or imprisoned. The conceptualization of exposure included stressors beyond those traditionally considered traumatic. Although severe adversity appeared to be overrepresented among women, health outcomes were not compared on the basis of gender. More severe adversity, as defined by the report of a greater number of adverse childhood conditions, was associated with increased risk for adult medical morbidity. More severe exposure was linked to an increased risk for heart disease, cancer, chronic lung disease, skeletal fractures, and liver disease. The authors concluded that the effects of childhood adversity are so pronounced that such experiences should be considered a major risk factor for the leading causes of death among adults.

Studies of Men

The CDC Vietnam Experience Study compared veterans who served in the Vietnam theater and those who served in other locations to assess effects of combat exposure on health status (1988). Theater veterans reported more chronic medical problems than did Vietnam era veterans. When medical exams were performed with a subset of participants, theater veterans were found to have more hearing loss, lower sperm counts, and more abnormal sperm morphologies than era veterans. A similar study of Navy Vietnam veterans compared former prisoners of war (POWs) to a demographically matched group of veterans who were not POWs to examine the occurrence of medical diagnoses in the 14 years following military service (Nice, Garland, Hilton, Baggett, & Mitchell, 1996). Diagnoses were based on annual medical exams from 1976 to 1993. Investigators found that the POW group had a higher likelihood of disorders of the peripheral nervous system, joint problems, back problems, and peptic ulcer than non-POW veterans. The authors suggest that these illnesses may in large part be due to the physical effects of torture sustained during captivity.

Studies of Women

Several large studies have investigated medical morbidity in relation to trauma exposure among women. One of the largest studies of this type was an investigation of 1,225 randomly selected women subscribers of a large HMO. Women who reported childhood maltreatment compared to those without abuse histories revealed significantly higher rates of physician-diagnosed morbidity, including infectious disease, pain disorders, and other illnesses such as hypertension, asthma, or skin disorders. Medical charts of women who experienced multiple types of childhood maltreatment revealed the most diagnoses (Walker et al., 1999).

Studies of Women's Reproductive Health

A number of studies have specifically investigated the impact of trauma exposure on women's reproductive health. Although these data can not be compared to those obtained from men, the evidence of deleterious effects on reproductive health is an important facet of women's health that requires discussion. In a study of 191 women seen at an outpatient obstetrical/gynecological clinic, those who reported sexual, physical, or emotional abuse during childhood were more likely to be diagnosed with a gynecological disorder than nonabused women (Letourneau, Holmes, & Chasedunn-Roark, 1999). The disorders identified at higher rates in abused women included sexually transmitted diseases (STDs), excessive bleeding, vaginitis, cervical dysplasia, dysmenorrhea, and infertility.

Recent data suggest that intimate partner violence during pregnancy may be one of the leading causes of morbidity and mortality among pregnant women (Fildes, Reed, Jones, Martin, & Barrett, 1992; Frye, 2001). A study of 1,203 racially diverse women participating in prenatal care assessed exposure to interpersonal violence and conducted a chart review for pregnancy complications and birth outcomes following delivery (Parker, McFarlane, & Soeken, 1994). Exposure to violence during pregnancy was associated with low maternal weight gain, infections, anemia, and a briefer interpregnancy interval. Another study of 384 low-income, pregnant women found that violence during pregnancy was associated with twice the risk for preterm labor and chorioamnionitis compared to nonexposed women (Berenson, Wiemann, Wilkinson, Jones, & Anderson, 1994). Analyses of a representative sample of 6,143 women demonstrated an association of violence during pregnancy with an increased risk for delivery by cesarean section and antenatal hospitalization for kidney infection, premature labor, or physical trauma (Cokkinides, Coker, Sanderson, Addy, & Bethea, 1999). It appears evident that a variety of adverse outcomes are associated with violence during pregnancy. Researchers suggest that research in this area investigate the specific role of partner violence in physical trauma-related outcomes, and that studies should also be designed to investigate the role of psychological reactions to violence and the association with health outcomes (Petersen et al., 1997).

Discussion

Similar to results found in the PTSD literature, more research is needed to draw conclusions about any gender differences in the relationship between trauma exposure and medical morbidity. However, data from the Adverse Childhood Experiences Study strongly suggest that increased risk for health problems following trauma exposure is a serious issue for both men and women. Similar to studies of PTSD and health problems, studies of both men and women suggest that risk is increased for a broad range of health conditions. Notable in this literature is that both men and women appear to be at increased risk for reproductive health problem following trauma exposure, although the issue has been more extensively researched with women. Research that investigates PTSD diagnoses in conjunction with trauma exposure and reproductive health is needed. Such research would help to delineate how these reproductive health conditions are associated with characteristics of the trauma exposure and the extent to which the stress reactions to the trauma, PTSD, are associated with these conditions.

TRAUMA, PTSD, AND MORTALITY

The following review of mortality studies suggests that both trauma and PTSD have a negative impact on health, and that some aspects of the way trauma impacts health status may differ in men and women. Studies of all-cause mortality can serve as gross measures of the extent of health impairment associated with PTSD, whereas data that include cause of death can serve as a context for interpreting the morbidity studies previously reviewed.

Studies Comparing Men and Women

One study has investigated the relationship between exposure to trauma and mortality outcomes in a sample including both males and females. Sibai, Fletcher, and Armenian (2001) conducted a 10-year follow-up of 1,567 men and women exposed to war-related stressors in Lebanon. Increased numbers of war-related stressors were associated with increased risk for both cardiovascular disease-specific deaths and all-cause mortality. Although the data could not attest to differential rates of premature mortality following traumatic exposure, gender differences were found in the relationship between type of exposure and mortality risk. Both men and women displaced by war-related events showed the greatest mortality risks. For women, the experience of loss-related trauma was also associated with heightened mortality risk. These data attest to a potentially profound impact of traumatic exposure on health outcomes.

Studies of Men

Several studies suggest that exposure to trauma and PTSD is linked to early mortality among men, although primarily due to accidents and suicide. One of the largest studies of this type is a study of 16,257 male Vietnam veterans whose names were obtained from the Agent Orange Registry. The investigators compared mortality data of veterans with and without PTSD, and those of both groups to standardized mortality ratios for U.S. males (Bullman & Kang, 1994). Veterans with PTSD were almost four times more likely to die from suicide, and approximately three times more likely to die from accidental poisoning compared to veterans without PTSD. Results were similar when data regarding veterans with PTSD were compared to standard data of men in the United States of similar age and ethnicity, except that mortality risk for digestive diseases were also elevated. The CDC Vietnam Experience Study (1987) also found that the risk for early mortality increased by 17% among Vietnam theater veterans compared to Vietnam era veterans. This effect occurred primarily in the first 5 years following discharge and could be largely attributed to accidental deaths. The expected increase in mortality from cardiovascular symptoms was not observed.

Studies of Women

A study of mortality risk among 4,600 female Vietnam veterans and 5,300 female veterans who did not serve in Vietnam suggests that this issue is complex (Thomas, Kang, & Dalager, 1991). All-cause mortality rates did not differ between the Vietnam and era veterans. Both Vietnam and non-Vietnam veterans were less at risk for all-cause mortality (standardized mortality ratio [SMR] = 0.82 and 0.88, respectively), when compared to rates for U.S. women. This effect was primarily accounted for by a lower likelihood of death from circulatory disease. However, the effect for external causes of death was similar to that for male veterans. There was a small effect for increased mortality from external causes among female Vietnam veterans compared with non-Vietnam veterans (risk ratio = 1.33), primarily due to an excess of motor vehicle accidents (risk ratio = 3.19), although suicide rates were similar in both groups. The most pronounced effect was for cancers. Although rates for Vietnam veterans were similar to those among non-Vietnam veterans for all cancers, Vietnam veterans had twice the risk for mortality from cancers of the pancreas and uterine corpus compared with non-Vietnam veterans. Vietnam veterans also had significantly elevated rates of mortality from cancers of the pancreas (5 deaths, SMR = 3.27) and uterine corpus (4 deaths, SMR = 4.05) compared to U.S. women.

Discussion

The premature all-cause mortality associated with trauma, and potentially with PTSD, among both men and women attests to the profound impact of trauma exposure on health status. The Sibai et al. (2000) study found different types of exposure related to mortality among men and women. In this study, women, who are thought to be more relationship-oriented than men, were affected by loss-related trauma in ways that men were not. These results suggest that one of the ways gender may moderate the exposure–health relationship is through the process of appraisal and the construction of meaning.

Only one study has addressed PTSD and mortality, and we know very little about this relationship in both men and women. However, the presence of a psychiatric diagnosis has been linked to premature death (Black, 1998). Although fewer studies have examined mortality related to a specific disorder, studies of major depression also suggest that there is a risk for early mortality, similar to results from the PTSD study, related to suicide, accidents, and cardiovascular disease (Wulsin, Vaillant, & Wells, 1999).

Though mortality research is difficult to conduct, additional data will be informative regarding any specific effects of PTSD in men and women.

The subsequent literature review concerning PTSD and self-reported health can inform our understanding of the unique role that PTSD may play in health problems following trauma exposure among women and men.

PTSD AND SELF-REPORTED PHYSICAL SYMPTOMS

Studies Comparing Men and Women

Two sets of archival analyses on the NVRSS data inform hypotheses regarding gender. Taft et al. (1999) conducted a reanalysis of the NVRSS data using path analysis. They demonstrated that PTSD is related to a greater number of self-reported health conditions for both men and women. PTSD was also related to poorer functional status in both men and women. For men, both PTSD and the number of reported health conditions exerted independent effects on functional status, but for women, the number of physical health conditions alone accounted for the relationship between PTSD and functional status. These results suggest that PTSD may have an independent effect on functional status for men but affects women primarily via effects on health status.

Zatzick et al. (1997a, 1997b) performed separate archival analyses on the male and female subgroups from the NVVRS. In analyses of a subsample of 1,200 men, they found that PTSD was associated with poor functional outcomes such as physical limitations, fair or poor physical health, diminished well-being, and unemployment. This relationship persisted even when psychiatric comorbidity and an indicator of the graded severity of chronic illness were included in the model (Zatzick et al., 1997b). Analyses of 432 women from the NVVRS revealed similar results (Zatzick et al., 1997a). PTSD was associated with poorer self-rated health, more physical limitations, increased days in bed, and unemployment, after controlling for psychiatric comorbidity and an indicator of the graded severity of chronic illness.

A recent prospective study of 2,302 Gulf War veterans examined self-reported health in men and women assessed 18–24 months after return. Women reported more health problems than men, specifically, headaches, aches and pains, upset stomach, and dizziness. PTSD was predictive of physical health problems after controlling for demographic variables, exposure, and the baseline measures of physical health problems. Notably, the interaction between gender and PTSD symptoms was nonsignificant in the prediction of physical health problems, indicating no gender differences in the impact of PTSD symptoms on health problems (Wagner, Wolfe, Rotnitsky, Proctor, & Erickson, 2000).

Studies of Men

Most studies of men focused on veteran samples. For example, the Normative Aging Study of 1,079 male veterans from World War II and the Korean War found that men who had experienced both combat- and non-combat-related trauma reported more physical symptoms than those who had no trauma or a single type of trauma (Schnurr, Spiro, Aldwin, & Stukel, 1998). Furthermore, the doubly exposed combat and noncombat trauma group suffered more PTSD than any of the other groups, which the authors suggest indicates a possible mediational role for PTSD in relation to physical symptoms reporting, although it was not possible to test this directly. Many studies of male veterans and civilians have found PTSD to be associated with increased reports of a wide variety of physical symptoms among populations exposed to multiple types of trauma. The association between a diagnosis of PTSD and increased reports of physical symptoms has also been demonstrated in smaller Veteran samples from the United States, Israel, New Zealand, and Canada (Beckham et al., 1998; Litz, Keane, Marx, & Monaco, 1992; Ohry et al., 1994; Shalev et al., 1990b; Stretch, 1991). Similarly, in a sample of German firefighters, those with PTSD report more physical symptoms and poorer functional status than firefighters without PTSD (Wagner, Heinrichs, & Ehlert, 1998).

Studies of Women

Although fewer studies of women have included measures of PTSD, the bulk of data concerning trauma exposure and self-reported health among civilian populations has been conducted with women. The self-reported health and PTSD research in women is focused on two groups: female veterans and sexual assault victims. The female veteran samples do not preclude sexual assault; in fact, sexual assault and harassment constitute a frequently reported traumatic stressor in this sample (Wolfe et al., 1998).

Studies of female veterans have found that a diagnosis of PTSD is linked to increased reporting of heterogeneous physical symptoms and poorer self-rated health (Kimerling, Clum, & Wolfe, 2000; Wolfe et al., 1994). The association appears to persist even when the effects of depression and health risk behaviors are controlled. In the study by Wolfe et al. (1994), the relationship between PTSD and self-reported health was examined in a sample of 109 non-treatment-seeking female veterans of the Vietnam War. The investigators found that PTSD appeared to mediate partially the relationship between trauma and worsened self-reported health.

The sexual assault literature is generally consistent with the veteran literature. Investigators examined the role of depressive symptoms in the association between PTSD and physical symptoms reporting among a sample of 57 college women who had experienced sexual assault (Clum, Calhoun,

& Kimerling, 2000). Depression, PTSD, victimization history, assault severity, and physical reactions during the assault were examined. When all other factors were controlled, both depression and PTSD symptoms independently predicted reports of physical symptoms and perceived health status. When reproductive health symptoms were specifically examined, only PTSD was a significant predictor above and beyond other variables. In a group of women with chronic sexual assault-related PTSD, investigators examined the effects of negative life events, anger, depression and PTSD severity on physical symptom reports. In these data, only PTSD severity independently predicted health symptoms when all other factors were controlled (Zoellner, Goodwin, & Foa, 2000).

Discussion

These data consistently support a relationship between self-reported health and PTSD across both genders and serve as a complement to research examining morbidity. In studies comparing men and women, there appear to be few gender-based differences in the relationship between PTSD and self-reported health indices. One limitation is that the available studies are limited to veteran samples and may not be representative. The differences observed in self-report of physical symptoms between men and women in the general population may not extend to veteran populations, even those without exposure to trauma. While there is some evidence that when compared to men, women may report some physical symptoms at increased rates, female gender does not appear to moderate the relationship between PTSD and self-reported physical symptoms. The link between PTSD and increased reports of a variety of physical symptoms appears to be similar for both men and women.

TRAUMA AND SELF-REPORTED HEALTH

Studies Comparing Men and Women

The interaction among gender, race, and sexual assault has been examined in relation to the self-report of headache (Golding, 1999). Data from the Los Angeles and North Carolina sites of the Epidemiologic Catchment Area survey (ECA), a five-site cooperative study of a representative sample of U.S. residents that included data on mental health diagnoses (excluding PTSD), traumatic events, and health status (Eaton & Kessler, 1985), the National Study of Health and Life Experiences of Women (NHLES), a representative sample of U.S. women age 21 and over (Wilsnack, Wilsnack, & Klassen, 1986), the Adolescent Health Risk Study (AHRS), a sample of 13- to 18-year-old individuals from the New York area (Cooper, Peirce, & Huselid, 1994), and the Puerto Rico Methodologic Catchment Area Study

(PR-MECA), a subset of the larger MECA investigation of psychiatric issues among children ages 9–18 years were combined for these analyses. When controlling for gender and ethnicity, a history of sexual assault was associated with a greater likelihood of reported headaches. However, when the effects of gender and ethnicity were examined, results suggested an interaction between gender and ethnicity. Although there was no difference in association between sexual assault and headache for Latino men versus Latina women, there was a difference among whites. White men were more likely to have an association between headache and sexual assault than white women. This study is important in that instead of controlling for demographic factors such as ethnicity, ethnicity was used to add specificity to the relationship between trauma and health. Although significant statistical power is required to conduct such analyses, the large body of literature suggesting racial/ethnic and socioeconomic disparities in health status in the United States suggests that these types of inquiries may lead to informative results.

Gender did not appear to be an important factor in a study of men and women interviewed before and after a severe flood. Results suggested that more severe disaster exposure was linked to an increase in a variety of self-reported symptoms 18 months after the flood. Investigators who assessed for an interaction between physical symptoms and gender found that flood-exposed women were no more likely to report an increase in symptoms than flood-exposed men (Phifer, 1990).

The relationship between childhood abuse, self-reported health, and self-reported physical symptoms was investigated in a sample of 275 undergraduates. Approximately equal percentages of men and women reported abuse histories, although the type of abuse was different based on gender. Women had a higher preponderance of sexual abuse, whereas men experienced more physical abuse. Students with an abuse history, regardless of type of abuse, reported more physical symptoms measured as abdominal and cold symptoms than nonabused students (Salmon & Calderbank, 1996). No gender differences emerged.

Studies of Men and Women

Several well-designed studies have included both men and women in their samples. Although researchers have not analyzed the data by gender, their results are similar to those found in samples comparing men and women. The ECA data indicate that among a community sample of men and women, exposure to trauma was associated with increased reports of physical symptoms and poorer self-rated health (Ullman & Siegel, 1996). A prospective study of community residents exposed to a natural disaster in Puerto Rico found that the extent of disaster exposure was correlated with the severity of reports of physical symptoms, most notably, gastrointestinal and pseudoneurological symptoms (Escobar, Canino, Rubio-Stipec, & Bravo, 1992). The association between trauma and health status appears to extend to individuals of low socioeconomic status. A community sample of 1,128 male and female veterans explored the association between lifetime trauma and physical symptoms. The results were consistent with those of studies showing a stronger relationship between multiple trauma experiences and health status. Data revealed that most traumatic events occurred prior to military service. Furthermore, it was the lifetime accumulated trauma, whether trauma to self, sexual assault, or both, that predicted the number of physical symptoms reported (Martin, Rosen, Durand, Knudson, & Stretch, 2000).

Studies of Men

Studies of male veterans have documented long-term increases in physical symptom reports in association with trauma exposure. A study of World War II veterans from the Stanford–Terman data archives revealed an association between combat exposure and long-term self-reported health. During the 15 years following the war, those men exposed to combat were more likely to experience death or a decline in self-reported physical health than men with no combat exposure. This association remained despite controls for self-reported health immediately following the war (1945), rank, and theater status (Elder, Shanahan, & Clipp, 1997).

Studies of Women

Many of the large-scale, well-controlled studies of trauma exposure and health outcomes in women have been driven by a priori notions of a relationship between sexual assault and reproductive health symptoms. Though the results support this relationship, the dearth of studies investigating both cumulative trauma exposure among women and a range of health outcomes has led many researchers to interpret these results as suggesting a specific relationship between sexual assault and reproductive health. In light of the findings discussed earlier, we urge caution in adopting this interpretation.

Epidemiological data from the general adult population of the United States suggests that individuals exposed to one or more traumatic events over the lifetime report more physical symptoms and a greater number of chronic health conditions than do individuals not exposed to traumatic events. These studies account for the role of age, ethnicity, and socioeconomic status in the relationship between trauma exposure and health, but can account for gender to a lesser extent, because the majority of data from community samples are obtained only from women.

Data from selected ECA study sites have been analyzed specifically to examine relationships between sexual assault history and self-reported health among women. Results suggest that compared to women with no assault history, women who had been sexually assaulted are more likely to report health symptoms across a variety of organ systems and report poorer self-rated health (Golding, 1994). Other reanalyses of these data have documented associations between sexual assault and reproductive health symptoms, indicating that women who have experienced sexual assault report more reproductive health symptoms, such as excessive pain, painful intercourse, lack of sexual pleasure, irregular menstruation, and excessive bleeding (Golding, 1996). These data were combined with NHLES data, and analyses suggested that women who report gynecological symptoms (e.g., pain during menstruation, excessive bleeding, or sexual dysfunction) in their reproductive years are more likely to report a history of sexual assault than women without these symptoms, and that this association is consistent across demographic characteristics (Golding, Wilsnack, & Learman, 1998). These studies of sexual assault did not account for other types of trauma exposure. Because it is such a frequent form of traumatic exposure for women, sexual assault serves as a proxy for trauma exposure in these studies.

Other studies that include broader assessments of trauma exposure and physical symptoms suggest a more general relationship between the two. Among a diverse group of women HMO subscribers, victims of interpersonal violence reported poorer self-rated health status than did nonvictims (Koss, Woodruff, & Koss, 1990). In a longitudinal study, sexual assault victims recruited from an urban rape treatment center reported more physical symptoms over a variety of domains than did a demographically matched comparison group of nonassaulted women in a 1-year period, even when injuries sustained in the assault were excluded from analyses (Kimerling & Calhoun, 1994). Studies of treatment-seeking samples reveal associations between different types of trauma exposure and increased reports of a variety of physical symptoms. A study of 1,931 women sampled from multiple primary care clinics found that lifetime exposure to interpersonal violence was associated with increased physical symptom reporting, and that greater severity of exposure was linked to a greater number of physical symptoms (McCauley, Kern, Kolodner, Derogatis, & Bass, 1998). These analyses controlled for the effects of socioeconomic status on health outcomes.

Discussion

Data on self-reported physical symptoms suggest that women and men may be more similar than different. In contrast to data from the general population, among trauma populations women do not appear to report a greater number or severity of physical symptoms. These results suggest that exposure to trauma may attenuate some gender differences. For example, the gender disparities in rates of depression observed in the general population are not observed among trauma populations (see Orsillo et al., Chapter 8, this volume). Both men and women report a heterogeneous group of physical symptoms following trauma exposure. Of note is the lack of evidence for a specific relationship between sexual assault and reproductive health symptoms. Although the data on women reviewed thus far clearly indicate that trauma and PTSD have a negative impact on reproductive health, the stressors that elicit these symptoms do not seem to be limited to sexual trauma. As noted in other reviews in this volume, sexual assault, more common in women than men, is associated with a greater risk for PTSD than many other traumatic events. Thus, findings related to sexual assault may be better interpreted by viewing sexual assault as a proxy for severe trauma or PTSD risk. Other studies cited in this section (Martin et al., 2000; Schnurr et al., 1998) suggest that cumulative exposure over the lifetime may best predict symptom reports.

The studies reviewed here provide compelling evidence for associations of trauma and PTSD with health impairment over a variety of domains. Individuals exposed to trauma or diagnosed with PTSD appear to suffer premature mortality and an excess of medical conditions common to adults, and to report more physical symptoms. In general, these studies suggest that gender issues pertain more to the manner in which these studies are conducted than to differences between men and women in health outcomes. In other words, current research yields much data regarding sexual trauma and interpersonal violence in relation to self-reported health in populations of women, yet little data concerning PTSD or medical morbidity. Although more data has addressed objective health indicators and PTSD among males, little research has focused specifically on civilian populations of males and on non-combat-related trauma and PTSD. However, existing data suggest that these areas of research are important to our understanding of health outcomes for both women and men. This review suggests that the relationship between gender and health status observed in the general population may manifest differently among trauma populations. Therefore, researchers and clinicians must not allow a priori notions regarding gender and health status to shape PTSD research and treatment without sufficient empirical support. The following section further examines gender issues in the construction of research questions and health outcomes associated with trauma and PTSD with respect to specific health conditions that have received much research attention. In contrast to the previous sections, which have investigated health status among trauma-exposed populations, these studies have investigated the prevalence of trauma or PTSD among individuals seeking treatment for, or diagnosed with, a specific medical condition.

SPECIFIC DISEASE STATES

Several investigations have examined the prevalence of trauma or PTSD among individuals diagnosed with specific disease states in an effort to better understand psychosocial or behavioral contributions to etiology and course of disease. Considerable data exist regarding pain disorders, gastrointestinal disorders, and sexually transmitted infectious diseases (STDs), including HIV. In the following sections, we review the literature pertaining to each of these disorders. Conducting research with individuals diagnosed with a particular medical disorder is a challenging task. Several methodological issues must be addressed to allow accurate interpretation of results, and special attention should be directed to sampling strategies and assessment methods. The majority of the studies cited in the following sections have sampled patients from specialty medical clinics. A high prevalence of traumatic events among individuals seeking treatment for a given medical disorder does not necessarily indicate that exposure is associated with the likelihood of the medical condition. When research participants are sampled from treatment-seeking populations in specialty medical clinics, high rates of trauma exposure may indicate that these individuals are simply more likely to come to medical attention or to seek specialty care. Many of these studies focus on childhood sexual and physical abuse. Although childhood trauma clearly is associated with a range of deleterious outcomes, the studies reviewed in early sections of this chapter suggest that other adverse childhood experiences, as well as trauma occurring later in life, are also important determinants of adult health status. If only specific trauma events such as childhood sexual abuse are queried, then associations with health outcomes might appear specific to sexual abuse. However, because childhood sexual abuse frequently occurs in the context of other stressful and traumatic life events, and is associated with an increased risk for interpersonal violence in adulthood, statistical associations of health outcomes with childhood sexual abuse may be a proxy for a more general relationship between trauma exposure and health outcomes. Finally, because many of these studies are conducted with samples of either women or men, where effects of gender are not tested, or with samples of women alone, associations between trauma and health outcomes primarily among women appear to be pathological manifestations of trauma occurring without sufficient substantiation. The available research is discussed through the lens of gender, both in terms of the interpretation of the data and in the resulting manner in which these disease states are conceptualized by practitioners.

Gastrointestinal Disorders

Researchers have categorized gastrointestinal (GI) disorders into two types of diagnoses: structural/organic and functional disorders (Drossman, Li,

Leserman, Toomey, & Hu, 1996). Structural, or organic, GI diseases are associated with an identifiable organic pathology. Some of the more common organic diagnoses include Crohn's disease, ulcerative colitis, liver disease, or acid peptic disease. Functional GI disorders are diseases without clearly identified structural or biochemical etiology, including irritable bowel syndrome (IBS), nonulcer dyspepsia, and chronic functional abdominal pain. These conditions are thought to be general dysfunctions of the GI tract; it is suggested that individuals may have a particularly reactive colon that is easily triggered by stress or diet. These conditions have received particular research attention in an effort to establish a psychological component for cases in which an organic basis for the disorder is not apparent.

Estimates of the prevalence of childhood sexual or physical abuse among GI patients range from 31 to 56% and suggest that physical and sexual abuse are highly correlated in this population (Drossman et al., 1990; Scarinci, McDonald-Haile, Bradley, & Richter, 1994). Patients with abuse histories are more likely to receive functional as opposed to organic diagnoses (Drossman et al., 1990). GI clinic patients with abuse histories appear to have poorer functional status, more severe symptoms, and greater pain severity than their nonabused counterparts (Drossman et al., 1996). These patients also report more physical symptoms over a number of domains, including those related to musculoskeletal and genitourinary disorders, skin disturbance, respiratory illness, and pain (Drossman et al., 1990; Leserman, Li, Drossman, & Hu, 1998).

These data, collected primarily from samples of women, suggest that childhood sexual and physical abuse is overrepresented among individuals with GI disorders. However, a careful reading of this literature—with attention to both research methodology and gender—suggests that traumatic exposure may not be related to the presence or absence of the disorders, but is associated with a greater frequency of unexplained symptoms, functional impairment, and an increased likelihood of seeking specialty care (Drossman, 1995).

A multicenter study of men and women sampled from several health care settings in France proposed that patients with IBS are more likely to have suffered abuse or assault than several other groups of medical patients (Delvaux, Denis, & Allemand, 1997). Patients seeking treatment in GI clinics and diagnosed with IBS were compared to (1) patients seeking follow-up treatment for structural GI disorders, (2) patients seeking specialty treatment in opthamology, and (3) healthy patients seen for routine primary care. The investigators used a wide definition of sexual abuse that included verbal aggression. The study cited high rates of sexual abuse: 36% among IBS patients, significantly more than patients any other group (14% of follow-up GI patients, 13% of opthamology clinic patients, and 8% of primary care patients). Similar to other studies, sexual abuse was more often found among women than men patients. The authors conclude that childhood abuse may be particularly prevalent among IBS patients; however, the nonequivalence of the comparison groups in this study, and the nontraditional definition for sexual abuse, suggest interpretating these data with caution.

In fact, research conducted with 1,264 male and female patients in conjunction with routine HMO physical exams, suggests that some of the unexplained and/or functional GI symptoms observed in patients with trauma histories may be an artifact of the more general increased reports of physical symptoms observed in trauma-exposed men and women (Longstreth & Wolde-Tsadik, 1993). Reports of sexual abuse were associated with both GI and non-GI physical symptoms. Individuals who reported GI symptoms consistent with a diagnosis of IBS were also more likely to report a greater number of non-GI physical symptoms, a history of sexual abuse, and substance use. This relationship between trauma exposure and GI symptoms does not appear to be specific: Although severity of trauma exposure is associated with poorer outcomes for GI patients, outcomes depend on type of exposure (e.g., physical vs. sexual abuse) and whether exposure occurred during childhood compared to adulthood (Leserman, Drossman, Li, & Toomey, 1996).

Talley, Sara, Zinsmeister, and Melton (1994) surveyed a representative community sample of 919 men and women ages 40–49 in Minnesota to examine the association between trauma exposure and functional GI disorders such as IBS, heartburn, and dyspepsia. The investigators assessed lifetime history of sexual, physical, and emotional abuse. Forty-one percent of women and 11% of men reported a lifetime history of any abuse. Women were more than four times more likely to have been sexually abused, and more than five times as likely to have been physically abused as men in the sample. Significant cross-sectional associations were found between exposure to abuse and IBS, dyspepsia, and heartburn. Gender comparisons indicated that women were more likely to suffer from both IBS and dyspepsia, whereas men were more likely to suffer from heartburn. Thus, investigations limited to IBS or specific types of GI disorders may bias results, so that trauma exposure appears more associated with health outcomes among either women or men, depending on the particular disorder identified.

Although few studies have investigated PTSD among individuals diagnosed with GI disorders, such studies are potentially informative. These studies shift the focus for disease risk from a priori notions regarding specific types of trauma exposure, such as sexual abuse, to traumatic stress reactions. In a study of men and women seeking treatment for IBS, approximately 36% of the sample met criteria for a PTSD diagnosis that preceded the onset of IBS (Irwin et al., 1996). This prevalence rate, considerably higher than that found in the general population, suggests that further research with PTSD may enhance our understanding of the role of trauma in GI disorders.

Pain

PTSD is a common diagnosis among chronic pain patients. Among a sample of men and women seeking treatment for fibromyalgia, 56% met criteria for PTSD (Sherman, Turk, & Okifuji, 2000). In a sample of male veterans in outpatient care for PTSD, 80% reported a chronic musculoskeletal pain condition (Beckham et al., 1997). Results such as these have prompted investigators to consider a relationship between traumatic stress and pain disorders. Well-controlled studies that investigate potential mechanisms of a trauma–pain relationship among both men and women are needed to understand this relationship. Traumatic events in childhood have been observed among both men and women with chronic pain disorders in a variety of locations (Goldberg, 1994); however, much of the literature in this area has focused on a specific relationship between child sexual abuse and chronic pelvic pain in women.

Pelvic pain is common among women seeking gynecological treatment and is considered by clinicians to have a considerable psychosocial component (Fry, Crisp, & Beard, 1997). Researchers have observed high rates of childhood sexual abuse among women undergoing diagnostic laparoscopy for chronic pelvic pain compared to women undergoing the same procedure for fertility-related issues (Harrop-Griffiths et al., 1988; Walker et al., 1988). Other researchers have used categories of organic and idiopathic chronic pelvic pain to distinguish cases for which a medical basis for the complaints is easily diagnosed. These studies have found higher rates of sexual abuse in women with undiagnosed pelvic pain (Reiter & Gambone, 1990; Reiter, Shakerin, Gambone, & Milburn, 1991) than in women with readily identified organic bases for pain. Conversely, another study found that physical abuse, but not sexual abuse, was overrepresented among women presenting with chronic pelvic pain (Rapkin, Kames, Darke, Stampler, & Naliboff, 1990). The sexual trauma studies, however, have been interpreted by some researchers as consistent with widespread a priori psychodynamic explanations for the link between early sexual trauma and nonorganic pelvic pain. This hypothesis is prevalent in the clinical literature (Rosenthal, 1993). However, it is our opinion that this interpretation of the data is imprecise and pathologizes women medical patients.

Research that includes assessment of other pain disorders, lifetime trauma histories, and samples of both men and women provides support for a more general relationship between trauma exposure and pain. Among women sampled from primary care facilities, sexual trauma occurring in both childhood and adulthood was correlated not only with pelvic pain but also with a variety of other pain complaints (Jamieson & Steege, 1997). When women with chronic pelvic pain are compared to women seeking treatment for headache, both groups are more likely to report lifetime histories of sexual trauma than pain-free women (Walling et al., 1994). In a study of 426 male and female college students, sexual and physical abuse were both associated with reports of more severe pain symptoms and with pain in a greater number of body sites when compared to nonabused respondents (Fillingim, Wilkinson, & Powell, 1999). One study examined lifetime trauma history and pain severity using validated questionnaires with men and women seeking outpatient treatment for chronic pain (Spertus, Burns, Glenn, Lofland, & McCracken, 1999). Men and women reported comparable levels of trauma over the lifetime, with the exception of sexual assault, which was more prevalent among women (21.6% vs. 2.8% for childhood, and 25% vs. 2.8% for adulthood). Trauma-exposed patients reported more pain-related affective distress than nonexposed patients. Gender comparisons revealed that this effect was more pronounced among men than women. Furthermore, post hoc analyses revealed that even when controlling for sexual and physical assault, the general relationship between exposure and poor emotional adjustment to pain remained significant. The authors note that a gender bias in research limited to female samples and specific types of trauma may result in a lack of clear clinical conceptualization for the relationship between trauma exposure and pain syndromes among both men and women.

Sexually Transmitted Diseases

Gender issues have been a central factor in the investigation of the relationship among trauma exposure, PTSD, and STDs. Several studies have established a history of interpersonal violence among men and women with STDs, with a focus on HIV infection. One study of HIV-infected women estimated the lifetime rate of sexual assault at 43% (Zierler, Witbeck, & Mayer, 1996). A study of inner-city, low-income women, 88 of whom were infected with HIV, and a comparison group of 148 noninfected women investigated rates of exposure to interpersonal violence that met DSM-IV Criterion A for PTSD (Kimerling, Armistead, & Forehand, 1999). Whereas 66% of the HIV group were exposed to violence, rates in the comparison group were 40%. Although the difference between groups was statistically significant, both groups of women reported considerable exposure to violence. A follow-up study of PTSD among the women infected with HIV revealed that 35% of trauma-exposed women met full criteria for the disorder (Kimerling, Calhoun, et al., 1999). A cohort study of 168 men and women with HIV, and at risk for HIV, found that approximately 50% of the women and 20% of men reported lifetime rape (Zierler et al., 1991). Both men and women who had been raped were more likely to be infected with HIV than nonassaulted men and women. Men who reported rape in childhood were twice as likely to be infected with HIV than nonassaulted men. In a large national survey of male veterans, men diagnosed with both PTSD and substance abuse were approximately 12 times more likely to be infected with HIV than veterans without either diagnosis (Hoff, Beam-Goulet, & Rosenheck, 1997). Preliminary data suggest that PTSD may impact course of disease as well as risk for infection. In the Kimerling, Calhoun, et al. study (1999), for women diagnosed with PTSD, the disease progressed more rapidly than in women without PTSD, as indicated by rate of CD4/CD8 cell decline and number of opportunistic infections.

Clearly, trauma and PTSD are important issues among individuals with HIV. Although exposure to violence often occurs following infection with HIV (Zierler, 2001), researchers have proposed plausible behavioral mechanisms where trauma exposure serves as a risk factor for infection with STD, specifically, HIV infection. Violence can be linked to HIV and other STDs though several pathways. Most directly, sexual assault can result in STD for both men and women if the perpetrator is infected (Gostin et al., 1994; Holmes, 1999; Kobernick, Seifert, & Sanders, 1985). Other researchers have noted that intimate partner violence may contribute to the likelihood of STDs and HIV. In a sample of 165 ethnic minority, low-income women, researchers found that partners in violent relationships were less likely to use condoms, and that reported physical and verbal abuse, and threats of abuse as a result of initiating discussions about condom use (Wingood & DiClemente, 1997). Similarly, among a group of women who met geographic and demographic risk criteria for HIV infection, 42% reported engaging in unprotected and unwanted sexual activity as a result of force or threats of force (Kalichman, Williams, Cherry, Belcher, & Nachimson, 1998). There were high rates of intimate partner violence among these women, who also reported fears of violence as a result of requesting condom use by their male partners. Recent qualitative data suggest that among men who have sex with men, childhood sexual abuse may also be similarly linked to unwanted and unprotected sexual activity and relationship violence (Paul, Catania, Pollack, & Stall, 2001).

Studies of men with PTSD, reviewed in earlier sections of this chapter, have found increased rates of non-STDs. Associations between trauma and PTSD with STDs have been primarily found among women and men who have sex with men, and appear to be particularly associated with lifetime exposure to interpersonal violence. For males, childhood abuse may be particularly relevant. These observations have led researchers to focus on shared causal pathways for both interpersonal violence and HIV infection influenced by social inequalities related to gender, minority ethnicity, economic position, and sexual orientation (Zierler & Krieger, 1997). Additional research that further elucidates the role of trauma and PTSD in relation to behavioral risk for STDs might dramatically inform outreach and prevention efforts. For example, attention to violence in the social context of HIV and STDs would expand intervention strategies to address the consequences of violence. Additional data regarding the impact of trauma and

PTSD on functional status and course of disease among HIV-infected individuals could enhance treatment efforts.

CLINICAL IMPLICATIONS

The studies reviewed in this chapter suggest, as a whole, that PTSD is associated with adverse changes in health status. Study samples that represent diverse populations across different points in the lifespan and types of trauma converge, suggesting that PTSD is an important factor in health outcomes. In terms of objective health decrements and PTSD, significantly more evidence is available regarding men than women. The studies documenting objective health changes in men are largely well-controlled studies of male veterans that yield evidence of alterations in multiple body systems, among them arterial, lower GI, dermatological, muskuloskeletal, and EKG abnormalities. These important studies have begun to take into account and control for not only extant factors associated with disease, such as age and poor health behaviors, but also co-occurrence of psychiatric comorbidity. These studies stand in marked contrast to the objective health data available for women and studies that specifically investigate gender differences in health status. To date, no published studies have examined objective indicators of health status among female PTSD populations or addressed the ways women may differ from men in the medical comorbidity with PTSD. Clearly, more studies are required to draw conclusions about sex-specific relationships.

Although more research is needed, existing data have the potential to inform clinical practice substantially. Several important conclusions drawn from this literature review are relevant to the treatment of both women and men:

1. *There is little evidence for a specific relationship between childhood sexual abuse and any medical condition among men or women.* Childhood sexual abuse, a prevalent form of exposure among female trauma populations, is associated with risk for revictimization as an adult and is more prevalent among women than men. As a result, this form of exposure is closely associated with PTSD, which in turn is linked to increased rates of medical morbidity over a variety of domains, poorer functional status, and increased reports of physical symptoms. These phenomena are not a unique pathology of female medical patients, although this may appear to be the case, because females are more likely to experience childhood trauma, to disclose childhood sexual abuse, and to use medical services. However, research indicates that trauma and PTSD are associated with functional impairment and increased physical symptom reports in both women and men, and to a similar extent. Nor is any medical condition pathognomic of child-

hood sexual abuse. A diagnosis of pelvic pain or IBS, for example, does not suggest a trauma history per se. However, trauma exposure should play an important role in the formulation of medical treatment plans, even without a direct etiological role in "functional" disorders.

2. *Men and women with trauma exposure or PTSD experience a greater degree of functional impairment from their illness and evidence a poorer course of disease for a variety of medical conditions.* PTSD, the most common unrecognized anxiety disorder in medical settings (Fifer et al., 1994), has the greatest functional impact on health status among such disorders (Schonfeld et al., 1997). As a result, these patients may appear to have symptoms and impairment beyond what medical practitioners expect for a given illness. The overrepresentation of trauma-exposed men and women in specialty medical settings may be less associated with a pathological somatization of psychological distress than with treatment plans that do not fully account for the range of patients' impairment. Both mental health and medical providers must carefully consider ways in which the pervasive emotional and behavioral effects of trauma may influence patients' ability to adhere with treatment.

3. *Gender differences in health status observed in the general population may not correspond to those observed in trauma populations.* Exposure to trauma or PTSD may attenuate gender disparities in morbidity, mortality, and physical symptom reporting by interfering with the protective factor of gender. Although more objective data are needed, existing data suggest that men and women with PTSD are equally likely to experience poor health in each of these domains. However, men and women may experience different types of morbidity and health conditions. Unfortunately, we currently lack the research to determine whether PTSD hastens the onset of health conditions commonly experienced or is associated with specific pathologies in both men and women. We caution researchers and clinicians to avoid the assumption that specific health problems deserve more or less attention with respect to PTSD without empirical support. For example, PTSD certainly deserves greater attention in the prevention and treatment of STDs and HIV. Conversely, although "functional" GI disorders are investigated with respect to trauma exposure, few data can inform practitioners as to how PTSD may increase risk or affect the course of GI disorders with organic etiology. Some disorders, such as cardiovascular disease, are researched in men but not women. Clinicians should not assume, however, that PTSD does not pose an increased risk for cardiovascular disease among women.

4. *Women's health is an important research and treatment specialty in settings where PTSD populations receive care.* As noted previously, our knowledge of PTSD as it relates to objective indicators of women's health and medical morbidity is greatly lacking. Given that women experience roughly twice the rates of PTSD as men, seek medical treatment at greater

rates than men, and, as discussed previously, appear likely to experience medical morbidity at least at the same rates as men with PTSD, these data are especially important. Large numbers of women with PTSD are treated in medical settings without sufficient research to inform interventions. Research pertaining to PTSD and health may be particularly important in VA and public sector settings, where high rates of PTSD can be expected.

REFERENCES

Beckham, J. C., Crawford, A. L., Feldman, M. E., Kirby, A. C., Hertzberg, M. A., Davidson, J. R., & Moore, S. D. (1997). Chronic posttraumatic stress disorder and chronic pain in Vietnam combat veterans. *Journal of Psychosomatic Research, 43*(4), 379–389.

Beckham, J. C., Moore, S. D., Feldman, M. E., Hertzberg, M. A., Kirby, A. C., & Fairbank, J. A. (1998). Health status, somatization, and severity of posttraumatic stress disorder in Vietnam combat veterans with posttraumatic stress disorder. *American Journal of Psychiatry, 155*(11), 1565–1569.

Berenson, A. B., Wiemann, C. M., Wilkinson, G. S., Jones, W. A., & Anderson, G. D. (1994). Perinatal morbidity associated with violence experienced by pregnant women. *American Journal of Obstetrics and Gynecology, 170*(6), 1760–1766; discussion 1766–1769.

Black, D. W. (1998). Iowa record-linkage study: Death rates in psychiatric patients. *Journal of Affective Disorders, 50*(2–3), 277–282.

Boscarino, J. A. (1997). Diseases among men 20 years after exposure to severe stress: Implications for clinical research and medical care. *Psychosomatic Medicine, 59*(6), 605–614.

Boscarino, J. A., & Chang, J. (1999). Electrocardiogram abnormalities among men with stress-related psychiatric disorders: Implications for coronary heart disease and clinical research. *Annals of Behavioral Medicine, 21*(3), 227–234.

Bullman, T. A., & Kang, H. K. (1994). Posttraumatic stress disorder and the risk of traumatic deaths among Vietnam veterans. *Journal of Nervous and Mental Disease, 182*(11), 604–610.

Centers for Disease Control and Prevention. (1999). Mortality patterns—United States, 1997. *Morbidity and Mortality Weekly Report, 48*(30), 664–668.

Centers for Disease Control Vietnam Experience Study. (1987). Postservice mortality among Vietnam veterans. *Journal of the American Medical Association, 257*(6), 790–795.

Centers for Disease Control Vietnam Experience Study. (1988). Health status of Vietnam veterans: II. Physical health. *Journal of the American Medical Association, 259*(18), 2708–2714.

Clum, G. A., Calhoun, K. S., & Kimerling, R. (2000). Associations among symptoms of depression and posttraumatic stress disorder and self-reported health in sexually assaulted women. *Journal of Nervous and Mental Disease, 188*(10), 671–678.

Cokkinides, V. E., Coker, A. L., Sanderson, M., Addy, C., & Bethea, L. (1999). Physical violence during pregnancy: Maternal complications and birth outcomes. *Obstetrics and Gynecology, 93*(5, Pt. 1), 661–666.

Cooper, M. L., Peirce, R. S., & Huselid, R. F. (1994). Substance use and sexual risk taking among black adolescents and white adolescents. *Health Psychology, 13*(3), 251–256.

Delvaux, M., Denis, P., & Allemand, H. (1997). Sexual abuse is more frequently reported by IBS patients than by patients with organic digestive diseases or controls: Results of a multicentre inquiry. *European Journal of Gastroenterology and Hepatology, 9*(4), 345–352.

Drossman, D. A. (1995). Sexual and physical abuse and gastrointestinal illness. *Scandinavian Journal of Gastroenterology, 208*(Suppl.), 90–96.

Drossman, D. A., Leserman, J., Nachman, G., Li, Z., Gluck, H., Toomey, T. C., & Mitchell, C. M. (1990). Sexual and physical abuse in women with functional or organic gastrointestinal disorders. *Annals of Internal Medicine, 113*(11), 828–833.

Drossman, D. A., Li, Z., Leserman, J., Toomey, T. C., & Hu, Y. J. B. (1996). Health status by gastrointestinal diagnosis and abuse history. *Gastroenterology, 110*(4), 999–1007.

Eaton, W. W., & Kessler, L. G. (1985). *Epidemiologic field methods in psychiatry: The NIMH Epidemiologic Catchment Area program.* Orlando, FL: Academic Press.

Elder, G. H., Shanahan, M. J., & Clipp, E. C. (1997). Linking combat and physical health: The legacy of World War II in men's lives. *American Journal of Psychiatry, 154*(3), 330–336.

Escobar, J. I., Canino, G. J., Rubio-Stipec, M., & Bravo, M. (1992). Somatic symptoms after a natural disaster: A prospective study. *American Journal of Psychiatry, 149*(7), 965–967.

Fifer, S. K., Mathias, S. D., Patrick, D. L., Mazonson, P. D., Lubeck, D. P., & Buesching, D. P. (1994). Untreated anxiety among adult primary care patients in a health maintenance organization. *Archives of General Psychiatry, 51*(9), 740–750.

Fildes, J., Reed, L., Jones, N., Martin, M., & Barrett, J. (1992). Trauma: The leading cause of maternal death. *Journal of Trauma, 32*(5), 643–645.

Fillingim, R. B., Wilkinson, C. S., & Powell, T. (1999). Self-reported abuse history and pain complaints among young adults. *Clinical Journal of Pain, 15*(2), 85–91.

Friedman, M. J., & Schnurr, P. P. (1995). The relationship between trauma, posttraumatic stress disorder, and physical health. In M. J. Friedman, D. S. Charney, & A. Y. Deutch (Eds.), *Neurobiological and clinical consequences of stress: From normal adaptation to post-traumatic stress disorder* (pp. 507–524). Philadelphia: Lippincott Williams & Wilkins.

Fry, R. P., Crisp, A. H., & Beard, R. W. (1997). Sociopsychological factors in chronic pelvic pain: A review. *Journal of Psychosomatic Research, 42*(1), 1–15.

Frye, V. (2001). Examining homicide's contribution to pregnancy-associated deaths. *Journal of the American Medical Association, 285*(11), 1510–1511.

Goldberg, R. T. (1994). Childhood abuse, depression, and chronic pain. *Clinical Journal of Pain, 10*(4), 277–281.

Golding, J. M. (1994). Sexual assault history and physical health in randomly selected Los Angeles women. *Health Psychology, 13*(2), 130–138.

Golding, J. M. (1996). Sexual assault history and women's reproductive and sexual health. *Psychology of Women Quarterly, 20*(1), 101–121.

Golding, J. M. (1999). Sexual assault history and headache: Five general population studies. *Journal of Nervous and Mental Disease, 187*(10), 624–629.

Golding, J. M., Wilsnack, S. C., & Learman, L. A. (1998). Prevalence of sexual assault history among women with common gynecologic symptoms. *American Journal of Obstetrics and Gynecology, 179*(4), 1013–1019.

Gostin, L. O., Lazzarini, Z., Alexander, D., Brandt, A. M., Mayer, K. H., & Silverman, D. C. (1994). HIV testing, counseling, and prophylaxis after sexual assault. *Journal of the American Medical Association, 271*(18), 1436–1444.

Harrop-Griffiths, J., Katon, W., Walker, E., Holm, L., Russo, J., & Hickok, L. (1988). The association between chronic pelvic pain, psychiatric diagnoses, and childhood sexual abuse. *Obstetrics and Gynecology, 71*(4), 589–594.

Hoff, R. A., Beam-Goulet, J., & Rosenheck, R. A. (1997). Mental disorder as a risk factor for human immunodeficiency virus infection in a sample of veterans. *Journal of Nervous and Mental Disease, 185*(9), 556–560.

Holmes, M. (1999). Sexually transmitted infections in female rape victims [see comments]. *AIDS Patient Care and STDs, 13*(12), 703–708.

Irwin, C., Falsetti, S. A., Lydiard, R. B., Ballenger, J. C., Brock, C. D., & Brener, W. (1996). Comorbidity of posttraumatic stress disorder and irritable bowel syndrome. *Journal of Clinical Psychiatry, 57*(12), 576–578.

Jamieson, D. J., & Steege, J. F. (1997). The association of sexual abuse with pelvic pain complaints in a primary care population. *American Journal of Obstetrics and Gynecology, 177*(6), 1408–1412.

Kalichman, S. C., Williams, E. A., Cherry, C., Belcher, L., & Nachimson, D. (1998). Sexual coercion, domestic violence, and negotiating condom use among low-income African American women. *Journal of Women's Health, 7*(3), 371–378.

Kimerling, R., Armistead, L., & Forehand, R. (1999). Victimization experiences and HIV infection in women: Associations with serostatus, psychological symptoms, and health status. *Journal of Traumatic Stress, 12*(1), 41–58.

Kimerling, R., & Calhoun, K. S. (1994). Somatic symptoms, social support, and treatment seeking among sexual assault victims. *Journal of Consulting and Clinical Psychology, 62*(2), 333–340.

Kimerling, R., Calhoun, K. S., Forehand, R., Armistead, L., Morse, E., Morse, P., Clark, R., & Clark, L. (1999). Traumatic stress in HIV-infected women. *AIDS Education and Prevention, 11*(4), 321–330.

Kimerling, R., Clum, G. A., & Wolfe, J. (2000). Relationships among trauma exposure, chronic posttraumatic stress disorder symptoms, and self-reported health in women: Replication and extension. *Journal of Traumatic Stress, 13*(1), 115–128.

Kinsella, K., & Gist, Y. K. (1998). *International brief: Mortality and health.* Washington, DC: U.S. Department of Commerce, Economics and Statistics Administration, Bureau of the Census.

Kobernick, M. E., Seifert, S., & Sanders, A. B. (1985). Emergency department management of the sexual assault victim. *Journal of Emergency Medicine, 2*(3), 205–214.

Koss, M. P., Koss, P. G., & Woodruff, W. J. (1991). Deleterious effects of criminal victimization on women's health and medical utilization. *Archives of Internal Medicine, 151*(2), 342–347.

Koss, M. P., Woodruff, W. J., & Koss, P. G. (1990). Relation of criminal victimization to health perceptions among women medical patients. *Journal of Consulting and Clinical Psychology, 58*(2), 147–152.

Kulka, R. A., Schlenger, W. E., & Fairbank, J. A. (1990). *Trauma and the Vietnam War generation: Report of findings from the National Vietnam Veterans Readjustment Study.* New York: Brunner/Mazel.

Leserman, J., Drossman, D. A., Li, Z., & Toomey, T. C. (1996). Sexual and physical abuse history in gastroenterology practice: How types of abuse impact health status. *Psychosomatic Medicine, 58*(1), 4–15.

Leserman, J., Li, Z., Drossman, D. A., & Hu, Y. J. B. (1998). Selected symptoms associated with sexual and physical abuse history among female patients with gastrointestinal disorders: The impact on subsequent health care visits. *Psychological Medicine, 28*(2), 417–425.

Letourneau, E. J., Holmes, M. M., & Chasedunn-Roark, J. (1999). Gynecologic health consequences to victims of interpersonal violence. *Women's Health Issues, 9*(2), 115–120.

Litz, B. T., Keane, T. M., Marx, B., & Monaco, V. (1992). Physical health complaints in combat-related post-traumatic stress disorder: A preliminary report. *Journal of Traumatic Stress, 5*(1), 131–141.

Longstreth, G. F., & Wolde-Tsadik, G. (1993). Irritable bowel-type symptoms in HMO examinees: Prevalence, demographics, and clinical correlates. *Digestive Diseases and Sciences, 38*(9), 1581–159.

Martin, L., Rosen, L. N., Durand, D. B., Knudson, K. H., & Stretch, R. H. (2000). Psychological and physical health effects of sexual assaults and nonsexual traumas among male and female United States Army soldiers. *Behavioral Medicine, 26*(1), 23–33.

McCauley, J., Kern, D. E., Kolodner, K., Derogatis, L. R., & Bass, E. B. (1998). Relation of low-severity violence to women's health. *Journal of General Internal Medicine, 13*(10), 687–691.

McFarlane, A. C., Atchison, M., Rafalowicz, E., & Papay, P. (1994). Physical symptoms in post-traumatic stress disorder. *Journal of Psychosomatic Research, 38*(7), 715–726.

Nathanson, C. A. (1977). Sex, illness, and medical care: A review of data, theory, and method. *Social Science and Medicine, 11*(1), 13–25.

Nice, D. S., Garland, C. F., Hilton, S. M., Baggett, J. C., & Mitchell, R. E. (1996). Long-term health outcomes and medical effects of torture among US Navy prisoners of war in Vietnam. *Journal of the American Medical Association, 276*(5), 375–381.

Ohry, A., Solomon, Z., Neria, Y., Waysman, M., Bar-On, Z., & Levy, A. (1994). The aftermath of captivity: An 18-year follow-up of Israeli ex-POWs. *Behavioral Medicine, 20*(1), 27–33.

Parker, B., McFarlane, J., & Soeken, K. (1994). Abuse during pregnancy: Effects on maternal complications and birth weight in adult and teenage women. *Obstetrics and Gynecology, 84*(3), 323–328.

Paul, J. P., Catania, J., Pollack, L., & Stall, R. (2001). Understanding childhood sexual abuse as a predictor of sexual risk-taking among men who have sex with men: The Urban Men's Health Study. *Child Abuse and Neglect, 25*(4), 557–584.

Petersen, R., Gazmararian, J. A., Spitz, A. M., Rowley, D. L., Goodwin, M. M., Saltzman, L. E., & Marks, J. S. (1997). Violence and adverse pregnancy outcomes: A review of the literature and directions for future research. *American Journal of Preventive Medicine, 13*(5), 366–373.

Phifer, J. F. (1990). Psychological distress and somatic symptoms after natural disaster: Differential vulnerability among older adults. *Psychology and Aging, 5*(3), 412–420.

Rapkin, A. J., Kames, L. D., Darke, L. L., Stampler, F. M., & Naliboff, B. D. (1990). History of physical and sexual abuse in women with chronic pelvic pain. *Obstetrics and Gynecology, 76*(1), 92–96.

Reiter, R. C., & Gambone, J. C. (1990). Demographic and historic variables in women with idiopathic chronic pelvic pain. *Obstetrics and Gynecology, 75*(3, Pt. 1), 428–432.

Reiter, R. C., Shakerin, L. R., Gambone, J. C., & Milburn, A. K. (1991). Correlation between sexual abuse and somatization in women with somatic and nonsomatic chronic pelvic pain. *American Journal of Obstetrics and Gynecology, 165*(1), 104–109.

Resnick, H. S., Acierno, R., & Kilpatrick, D. G. (1997). Health impact of interpersonal violence: II. Medical and mental health outcomes. *Behavioral Medicine, 23*(2), 65–78.

Rosenthal, R. H. (1993). Psychology of chronic pelvic pain. *Obstetrics and Gynecology, Clinics of North America, 20*(4), 627–642.

Salmon, P., & Calderbank, S. (1996). The relationship of childhood physical and sexual abuse to adult illness behavior. *Journal of Psychosomatic Research, 40*(3), 329–336.

Scarinci, I. C., McDonald-Haile, J., Bradley, L. A., & Richter, J. E. (1994). Altered pain perception and psychosocial features among women with gastrointestinal disorders and history of abuse: A preliminary model. *American Journal of Medicine, 97*(2), 108–118.

Schnurr, P. P. (1996). Trauma, PTSD, and physical health. *PTSD Research Quarterly, 7*(3), 1–6.

Schnurr, P. P., Ford, J. D., Friedman, M. J., Green, B. L., Dain, B. J., & Sengupta, A. (2000). Predictors and outcomes of posttraumatic stress disorder in World War II veterans exposed to mustard gas. *Journal of Consulting and Clinical Psychology, 68*(2), 258–268.

Schnurr, P. P., & Jankowski, M. K. (1999). Physical health and post-traumatic stress disorder: Review and synthesis. *Seminars in Clinical Neuropsychiatry, 4*(4), 295–304.

Schnurr, P. P., Spiro, A., Aldwin, C. M., & Stukel, T. A. (1998). Physical symptom trajectories following trauma exposure: Longitudinal findings from the Normative Aging Study. *Journal of Nervous and Mental Disease, 186*(9), 522–528.

Schnurr, P. P., Spiro, A., 3rd, & Paris, A. H. (2000). Physician-diagnosed medical disorders in relation to PTSD symptoms in older male military veterans. *Health Psychology, 19*(1), 91–97.

Schonfeld, W. H., Verboncoeur, C. J., Fifer, S. K., Lipschutz, R. C., Lubeck, D. P., & Buesching, D. P. (1997). The functioning and well-being of patients with unrecognized anxiety disorders and major depressive disorder. *Journal of Affective Disorders, 43*(2), 105–119.

Shalev, A., Bleich, A., & Ursano, R. J. (1990a). Posttraumatic stress disorder: Somatic comorbidity and effort tolerance. *Psychosomatics, 31*(2), 197–203.

Shalev, A. Y., Bleich, A., & Ursano, R. J. (1990b). Somatic comorbidity of the post-traumatic stress disorder. In J. E. Lundeberg, U. Otto, & B. Rybeck (Eds.), *Wartime Medical Services Second International Conference, Stockholm, Sweden*, pp. 25–29.

Sherman, J. J., Turk, D. C., & Okifuji, A. (2000). Prevalence and impact of posttraumatic stress disorder-like symptoms on patients with fibromyalgia syndrome. *Clinical Journal of Pain, 16*(2), 127–134.

Sibai, A. M., Fletcher, A., & Armenian, H. K. (2001). Variations in the impact of long-term wartime stressors on mortality among the middle-aged and older population in Beirut, Lebanon, 1983–1993. *American Journal of Epidemiology, 154*(2), 128–137.

Spertus, I. L., Burns, J., Glenn, B., Lofland, K., & McCracken, L. (1999). Gender differences in associations between trauma history and adjustment among chronic pain patients. *Pain, 82*(1), 97–102.

Stein, M. B., & Barrett-Connor, E. (2000). Sexual assault and physical health: Findings from a population-based study of older adults. *Psychosomatic Medicine, 62*(6), 838–843.

Stretch, R. H. (1991). Psychosocial readjustment of Canadian Vietnam veterans. *Journal of Consulting and Clinical Psychology, 59*(1), 188–189.

Taft, C. T., Stern, A. S., King, L. A., & King, D. W. (1999). Modeling physical health and functional health status: The role of combat exposure, posttraumatic stress disorder, and personal resource attributes. *Journal of Traumatic Stress, 12*(1), 3–23.

Talley, N. J. F., Sara, L., Zinsmeister, A. R., Melton, L. J. (1994). Gastrointestinal tract symptoms and self-reported abuse: A population-based study. *Gastroenterology, 107*(4), 1040–1049.

Thomas, T. L., Kang, H. K., & Dalager, N. A. (1991). Mortality among women Vietnam veterans, 1973–1987. *American Journal of Epidemiology, 134*(9), 973–980.

Ullman, S. E., & Siegel, J. M. (1996). Traumatic events and physical health in a community sample. *Journal of Traumatic Stress, 9*(4), 703–720.

Wagner, A. W., Wolfe, J., Rotnitsky, A., Proctor, S. P., & Erickson, D. J. (2000). An investigation of the impact of posttraumatic stress disorder on physical health. *Journal of Traumatic Stress, 13*(1), 41–55.

Wagner, D., Heinrichs, M., & Ehlert, U. (1998). Prevalence of symptoms of posttraumatic stress disorder in German professional firefighters. *American Journal of Psychiatry, 155*(12), 1727–1732.

Walker, E., Katon, W., Harrop-Griffiths, J., Holm, L., Russo, J., & Hickok, L. R. (1988). Relationship of chronic pelvic pain to psychiatric diagnoses and childhood sexual abuse [see comments]. *American Journal of Psychiatry, 145*(1), 75–80.

Walker, E. A., Gelfand, A. N., Katon, W. J., Koss, M. P., Von Korff, M., Bernstein, D. E., & Russo, J. (1999). Adult health status of women with histories of childhood abuse and neglect. *American Journal of Medicine, 107*(4), 332–339.

Walling, M. K., Reiter, R. C., O'Hara, M. W., Milburn, A. K., Lilly, G., & Vincent, S. D. (1994). Abuse history and chronic pain in women: I. Prevalences of sexual abuse and physical abuse. *Obstetrics and Gynecology, 84*(2), 193–199.

Welty, F. K. (2001). Cardiovascular disease and dyslipidemia in women. *Archives of Internal Medicine, 161*(4), 514–522.

Wilsnack, R. W., Wilsnack, S. C., & Klassen, A. D. (1986). Antecedents and consequences of drinking and drinking problems in women: Patterns from a U.S. National Survey. *Nebraska Symposium on Motivation, 34*, 85–158.

Wingood, G. M., & DiClemente, R. J. (1997). The effects of an abusive primary partner on the condom use and sexual negotiation practices of African-American women. *American Journal of Public Health, 87*(6), 1016–1018.

Wolfe, J., Schnurr, P. P., Brown, P. J., & Furey, J. A. (1994). Posttraumatic stress disorder and war-zone exposure as correlates of perceived health in female Vietnam War veterans. *Journal of Consulting and Clinical Psychology, 62*(6), 1235–1240.

Wolfe, J., Sharkansky, E. J., Read, J. P., Dawson, R., Martin, J. A., & Ouimette, P. C. (1998). Sexual harassment and assault as predictors of PTSD symptomatology among U.S. female Persian Gulf War military personnel. *Journal of Interpersonal Violence, 13*, 40–57.

Wulsin, L. R., Vaillant, G. E., & Wells, V. E. (1999). A systematic review of the mortality of depression. *Psychosomatic Medicine, 61*(1), 6–17.

Zatzick, D. F., Marmar, C. R., Weiss, D. S., Browner, W. S., Metzler, T. J., Golding, J. M., Stewart, A., Schlenger, W. E., & Wells, K. B. (1997b). Posttraumatic stress disorder and functioning and quality of life outcomes in a nationally representative sample of male Vietnam veterans. *American Journal of Psychiatry, 154*(12), 1690–1695.

Zatzick, D. F., Weiss, D. S., Marmar, C. R., Metzler, T. J., Wells, K., Golding, J. M., Stewart, A., Schlenger, W. E., & Browner, W. S. (1997a). Post-traumatic stress disorder and functioning and quality of life outcomes in female Vietnam veterans. *Military Medicine, 162*(10), 661–665.

Zierler, S. (2001). Violence and HIV: Strategies for primary and secondary prevention. *Focus, 16*(6), 1–4.

Zierler, S., Feingold, L., Laufer, D., Velentgas, P., Kantrowitz-Gordon, I., & Mayer, K. (1991). Adult survivors of childhood sexual abuse and subsequent risk of HIV infection. *American Journal of Public Health, 81*(5), 572–575.

Zierler, S., & Krieger, N. (1997). Reframing women's risk: Social inequalities and HIV infection. *Annual Review of Public Health, 18*, 401–436.

Zierler, S., Witbeck, B., & Mayer, K. (1996). Sexual violence against women living with or at risk for HIV infection. *American Journal of Preventive Medicine, 12*(5), 304–310.

Zoellner, L. A., Goodwin, M. L., & Foa, E. B. (2000). PTSD severity and health perceptions in female victims of sexual assault. *Journal of Traumatic Stress, 13*(4), 635–649.

Part IV | Treatment

11 | Gender and PTSD Treatment

Efficacy and Effectiveness

DANA CASON
ANOUK GRUBAUGH
PATRICIA RESICK

This chapter is concerned with gender and research on posttraumatic stress disorder (PTSD) treatment efficacy and effectiveness. By far, treatment efficacy has been studied more than has treatment effectiveness. The efficacy of a treatment is established when a therapy is found to be superior to some sort of control condition. Efficacy studies usually involve random assignment of research participants to a treatment condition, time-limited and structured treatment protocols, and specific target outcomes. Treatment effectiveness, on the other hand, more broadly refers to whether treatment is helpful to consumers who seek treatment outside of the controlled conditions of an efficacy study. Rather than focusing on specific treatment outcomes, effectiveness studies are concerned with improvement in general functioning. Additionally, therapists in the field are rarely bound to a treatment protocol, and treatment duration is rarely predetermined. Ideally, ample research studies of PTSD treatment efficacy and effectiveness for male and female clients would be available for review in this chapter, because both efficacy and effectiveness studies are relevant for understanding gender issues. However, the bulk of this chapter focuses on efficacy research, because it is far more prevalent in the field.

We made concerted efforts to include all controlled PTSD treatment efficacy studies satisfying certain methodological considerations. For the purposes of this chapter, controlled PTSD treatment studies include any studies in which an active treatment condition is compared to a wait-list group, a control group for nonspecific treatment effects, and/or another active treatment. Treatment studies that did not utilize control groups were not included (e.g., Pitman et al., 1996a, 1996b), nor were studies wherein researchers provided neither effect sizes nor enough information to calculate effect sizes (e.g., Boudewyns & Hyer, 1996). PTSD diagnoses were based on DSM-III, DSM-III-R, or DSM-IV criteria, as determined by structured or unstructured clinical interviews.

In order to facilitate comparisons of the study results, we examined effect sizes. Generally speaking, an effect size reflects how much impact an intervention has had. More specifically, it is a measure of the magnitude of difference between treatment and control conditions, with the magnitude expressed in standard deviation units. In the research reviewed for this chapter, efficacy study populations fell into three groups: (1) both men and women who experienced a variety of traumatic experiences, (2) male military veterans with combat-related PTSD, and (3) female survivors of sexual or nonsexual assault. We used comparisons of effect sizes across the three types of studies to explore treatment responsiveness along the lines of gender.

Although epidemiological data suggest that women are twice as likely to develop PTSD (Kessler, Sonnega, Bromat, Hughes, & Nelson, 1995), comparisons of effect sizes suggest that women respond to treatment as well or better than do men. Among the possible factors contributing to the relative superiority of treatment for women are gender role variables such as familiarity and comfort with a wider range of emotions, more experience with interpersonal intimacy, and the tendency to use a range of coping strategies. However, greater treatment efficacy and/or higher effect sizes may also reflect the influence of factors that are theoretically independent of gender (e.g., methodological differences in the studies). We explore the studies, effect sizes, and related factors in depth. In order to provide a context for understanding differences in treatment efficacy and effectiveness, common treatment approaches are first described. Following a description of the common treatment approaches to PTSD, the findings of efficacy studies, along with possible moderating variables, are discussed. The chapter ends with a brief description of treatment effectiveness findings.

DESCRIPTION OF TREATMENTS

Exposure-Based Therapies

Exposure therapies were developed to treat specific anxiety disorders, such as phobias or obsessive–compulsive disorder. Inasmuch as PTSD has been conceptualized as an anxiety disorder, a logical step has been to adapt exposure-based treatments to trauma reactions. The underlying rationale of exposure treatments is that avoidance behaviors associated with PTSD interfere with the client's ability to process the traumatic event emotionally, subsequently reinforcing the negative and fearful feelings experienced during the trauma. Exposure techniques prevent the client from avoiding trauma-related memories, thus facilitating the habituation of the anxiety surrounding the traumatic event, while modifying the cognitive appraisal of feared situations.

Systematic desensitization, developed by Wolpe (1958) for the treatment of phobias, has been used with trauma survivors. In this treatment, therapist and client generate a hierarchy of fear cues that result from the traumatic event or generalize from conditioned cues. The client is trained in using relaxation skills and is then confronted with imaginal fear cues, along a graded hierarchy, while in a relaxed state. Within each session, the exposures are brief, repetitive, and focus exclusively on one fear cue alone. Mastery of low-level fear cues is followed by exposure to the next higher cue within the hierarchy. This review includes only one study that utilized the systematic desensitization protocol (Brom, Kleber, & Defares, 1989).

Another exposure technique, called flooding or direct therapeutic exposure (DTE), was introduced for the treatment of PTSD in the early 1980s. Flooding differs from systematic desensitization in that sessions are based on extended exposure to moderate or strong fear-producing cues. In addition to confronting fear cues in imagination, flooding also involves confrontation with real-life fear cues in the environment.

Another application of exposure therapy, prolonged exposure (PE), was developed and refined by Foa for use specifically with trauma victims (Foa, Rothbaum, Riggs, & Murdock, 1991). The treatment protocol for PE usually consists of nine 90-minute sessions that include breathing training for relaxation, imaginal exposures to the entire traumatic memory, and real-life exposures to trauma-related cues.

Exposures involving real-life fear cues involve clients' gradual confrontation of safe situations that evoke moderate levels of anxiety, and then following up with confrontations of more fearful situations. Subjective units of distress are assessed within the exposures to monitor emotional processing and the subsequent habituation (decrease) of anxiety. Although the live exposures may be conducted alone, clients are encouraged to begin with a coach, a trusted person who will accompany clients through the experiences.

Several studies reviewed for this chapter utilized a PE protocol for treating female assault survivors (Foa et al., 1991, 1999; Resick, Nishith, Weaver, Astin, & Feuer, 2000). It is worth noting, however, that the implementation of the PE protocol varied across studies. For example, some authors shortened the therapy sessions from 90 to 60 minutes (Foa et al., 1999; Tarrier et al., 1999). This is important to note, because it has been argued that the length of the exposure session is critical for the facilitation of emotional processing (Rachman, 1980).

Cognitive Therapy/Cognitive Processing Therapy

Cognitive processing therapy (CPT) was developed in order to facilitate the expression of affect and the appropriate accommodation of the traumatic event with more general schemas regarding oneself and the world (Resick & Schnicke, 1992; 1993). Resick and Schnicke (1992) argued that PTSD is not exclusively focused on the emotion of fear. Other strong emotions, such as anger, humiliation, shame, and sadness, may well result from the trauma. Furthermore, they emphasized the content of the meaning elements as an important focus. Drawing on the work of cognitive and constructivist theories, Resick and Schnicke proposed that beliefs about the traumatic event might become distorted in the victims' attempts to assimilate, or maintain old beliefs and schemas about themselves and the world. However, although accommodation of the new event into the person's memory and beliefs is desirable, overaccommodation (overgeneralization) may lead to extreme distortions about the safety or trustability of others, or overly harsh judgments about oneself. Resick (1995) has proposed that normal and expected emotions that likely result from danger are the ones that will abate through exposure. However, emotions that are the products of distorted thinking (e.g., "I should have prevented the event") may not necessarily habituate but, rather, may be continually manufactured. Hence, Resick and Schnicke (1992) proposed that the meaning of the event must be directly addressed in therapy.

Developed originally for use with rape and crime victims, CPT was adapted from basic cognitive techniques explicated by Beck and Emery (1985). However, while Beckian cognitive therapy usually focuses on challenging current maladaptive beliefs, CPT begins with the traumatic memory and focuses on feelings, beliefs, and thoughts directly emanating from the traumatic event. The therapist helps the clients to examine whether the traumatic event appears to disrupt or confirm beliefs held prior to the experience and to assess how much they may have overgeneralized from the event to their beliefs about themselves and the world. Clients are then taught to challenge their own self-statements and to modify extreme beliefs to bring them into balance.

It should be noted that CPT requires that the client read and reread a written account of the assault, which serves as an exposure exercise. In this manner, CPT addresses both dysfunctional beliefs about the meaning of the traumatic event via cognitive restructuring, as well as the arousal and avoidance associated with painful reminders of the assault via imaginal exposure.

Comparisons of the effectiveness of exposure and cognitive techniques have not yielded significant differences (Marks, Lovell, Noshirvani, Livanou, & Thrasher, 1998; Tarrier et al., 1999). Unlike CPT, the aforementioned studies used cognitive conditions that excluded any exposure-based components. Similarly, Resick et al. (2000) found no significant differences in PTSD or depression when comparing CPT and PE. However, CPT was found to be more effective in diminishing feelings of guilt.

Eye Movement Desensitization and Reprocessing

Eye movement desensitization and reprocessing (EMDR) is a controversial therapy that evolved from a personal observation. Shapiro (2001) developed EMDR on the basis of this observation and argued that lateral eye movements facilitate cognitive processing of the trauma. In its early presentations, EMDR was touted as a one-session cure for a range of disorders. However, recent studies are typically of trauma-related symptoms, with a course more similar to other trauma therapies. EMDR is now described as an eight-phase treatment that includes history taking, client preparation, target assessment, desensitization, installation, body scan, closure, and re-evaluation of treatment effects. EMDR includes exposure and cognitive components, as well as the lateral eye movements.

In the EMDR protocol, a client is asked to identify and focus on a traumatic image or memory (target assessment phase). Next, the therapist elicits negative belief statements about the memory. The client is asked to assign a rating to the memory and negative beliefs on an 11-point scale of distress and to identify the physical location of the anxiety. The therapist helps the client generate positive thoughts that would be preferable to associate with the memory. These are rated on a 7-point scale of how much the client believes the statement. Once the therapist has instructed the client in the basic EMDR procedure, the client is asked to do four things simultaneously during the desensitization phase: (1) visualize the memory; (2) rehearse the negative thoughts; (3) concentrate on the physical sensations of the anxiety; and (4) visually track the therapist's index finger. While the client does this, the therapist moves his or her index finger back and forth (two back and forth movements per second) 30–35 centimeters from the client's face. The procedure is repeated 24 times. Then the client is asked to blank out the memory and take a deep breath. Subsequently, the client brings back the memory and thoughts, and rates the level of distress. Sets of eye movements are repeated until the distress rating equals 0 or 1. At this point, the client describes how he or she feels about the positive cognition and gives a rating for it (installation phase).

The necessity for lateral eye movements has been called into question in studies that demonstrated equivalent results for EMDR with and without eye movements (Devilly, Spence, & Rapee, 1998; Renfrey & Spates, 1994). Without the lateral eye movements, EMDR is quite similar to other forms of cognitive-behavioral therapy in that the client thinks about the trauma, identifies negative cognitions associated with the trauma, and works toward positive cognitions as the traumatic memory is processed.

Therefore, any efficacy demonstrated by EMDR may be more attributable to the engagement of the traumatic memory and the inclusion of corrective information. Several recent studies have utilized EMDR (Carlson, Chemtob, Rusnak, Hedlund, & Muraoka, 1998; Jensen, 1994; Vaughn et al., 1994; Wilson, Becker, & Tinker, 1995; 1997).

Skills-Building Therapies

Skills-building techniques such as relaxation, assertiveness, social skills, and stress inoculation training are other approaches that have been used to alleviate symptoms of PTSD. These techniques are aimed at reducing distress and fostering more positive social environments through the acquisition of skills. One such program, stress inoculation training (SIT; Kilpatrick, Veronen, & Resick, 1982; Resick & Jordan, 1988; Veronen & Kilpatrick, 1983), is a cognitive-behavioral treatment package originally developed by Meichenbaum (1974) for the management of anxiety. The goals of SIT are to help clients understand and manage their trauma-related fear reactions, resulting in decreased avoidance behavior. The reduction in avoidance of fear-producing stimuli was assumed to result in the extinction or habituation of strong fear and anxiety responses. The SIT protocol consists of three phases: education, skills building, and application. SIT protocols range from 8 to 20 sessions depending on the needs of the client and the research study, but all versions use essentially the same component techniques. SIT has been used in both group and individual formats (Foa et al., 1991; 1999; Resick, Jordan, Girelli, Hunter, & Marhoefer-Dvorak, 1988).

The first sessions are educational in nature. Clients are given an explanation for their trauma symptoms based on two-factor theory (classical conditioning of fears and escape or avoidance of fear cues). They are taught to identify their different modes (or channels) of response, including emotions, behaviors, physical reactions, and thoughts. During subsequent sessions, clients are taught skills such as progressive muscle relaxation and the use of relaxation imagery. The relaxation skills are introduced to assist in three channels of response: physical, emotional, and cognitive. Concomitantly, coping skills are introduced that address the cognitive mode of response, such as thought stopping, covert rehearsal, problem solving, and guided self-dialogue (Kilpatrick et al., 1982; Resick & Jordan, 1988; Resnick & Newton, 1992).

In the third phase of treatment, clients learn how to apply these coping skills step-by-step in daily situations that provoke anxiety. The steps of stress inoculation include (1) assessing the probability of the feared event (including the discrimination between dangerous and safe situations); (2) managing avoidance behavior and fear reactions with cognitive restructuring, guided self-dialogue, and brief relaxation; (3) engaging in the feared behavior with the use of problem-solving skills and skills learned via role playing and covert modeling; and (4) reinforcing oneself to use skills in the feared situation (Meichenbaum, 1974). Before ending treatment, the therapist helps clients generate a fear hierarchy of events not addressed directly in therapy, on which clients are assigned continued work with the use of their coping skills after treatment.

Psychodynamic Therapies

Early in his career, Freud proposed that mental neurosis often arose following a traumatic event. Specifically, Freud hypothesized that hysteria, a condition characterized by somatic symptoms without a physical cause, was caused by the sexual abuse of children. Presented in the late 19th century, this view was met with indifference bordering on hostility. Freud's original theory was subsequently replaced by the belief that memories of sexual abuse were fantasies that emerged due to intrapsychic conflict between one's sexual impulses and inhibitions. In order to protect the ego, Freud proposed that the traumatic memory and associated emotions were repressed and unavailable to the conscious mind. Thus, the goal of treatment was to identify the pathological thought or memory, so that it could be treated. Subsequent psychoanalytic thought continued to deemphasize the role of external events and stressed Freud's concept of intrapsychic conflict and repressed infantile sexuality. This view dominated the psychoanalytic field for many years.

Modern psychodynamic theories continue to assert the importance of early psychological conflicts. Additionally, modern psychodynamic therapists place a greater emphasis on the therapeutic relationship, transference and countertransference, and developmental issues in general than on the other treatment approaches discussed in this chapter. Although modern psychodynamic therapies for traumatized victims generally focus on internal conflicts produced by the trauma, they have gradually adapted a more social-cognitive model of understanding trauma reactions. There is a strong similarity between social-cognitive and psychodynamic approaches, in that both focus on the impact of the traumatic event on the client's belief system. Similar to social-cognitive approaches, the individual is encouraged to reconcile the traumatic event by exploring the meaning attached to it and related schemas. Thus, the goal of most psychodynamic approaches is to integrate the traumatic event by exploring the psychological meaning attached to the event.

Although there is no unified "psychodynamic approach," a number of studies appear to fall within the psychodynamic tradition. Few of these studies, however, have systematically explored the effectiveness of psychodynamic approaches for the treatment of PTSD (Horowitz et al., 1984; Lindy, Green, Grace, & Titchener, 1983). However, the aforementioned studies were not included in this review because they lacked random assignment and control groups, and included heterogeneous diagnostic categories. A more rigorous investigation of the effectiveness of psychodynamic therapy was conducted by Brom and colleagues (1989), using a tailored psychodynamic approach aimed at resolving the intrapsychic conflict that resulted from the trauma. The results of this study are reviewed later in this chapter.

It is worth noting that a number of the approaches outlined earlier tend to be differentially selected for use with male and female trauma victims. Use of prolonged exposure and CPT, originally designed for use with female assault victims, continues to be predominant for the treatment of this population. Samples based on Vietnam veterans, however, tend to utilize EMDR or flooding treatments. As mentioned previously, EMDR without the lateral eye movements is similar to other forms of cognitive-behavioral therapy. Likewise, flooding is based on the same exposure principles as PE. Although there is no theoretical reason to suspect that these approaches would be differentially effective for male and female trauma victims, the generalizability of specific treatments for both genders should be investigated.

EFFICACY STUDIES

The majority of treatments outlined here have been empirically validated. However, scant attention has been paid to whether they have been equally effective for both men and women. The remainder of this chapter focuses on these treatment studies in order to delineate PTSD treatment efficacy/effectiveness along the lines of gender.

Studies reviewed herein vary a great deal in terms of participant characteristics, methodological design, assessment instruments, and types of treatments. These differences severely curtail our analysis of the relative efficacy of treatment for men and women. In describing conditions necessary for making statements about the relative efficacy of types of treatment, Cahill and Frueh (1997, p. 301) stated, "It is a generally accepted principle of research that two conditions must be met to assert that one treatment is superior to another. First, the groups of interest must differ in some degree on the variable under investigation. Second, they must not differ in any systematic way on any other variable." In the current situation, our interest is in making statements about the efficacy of treatment for two distinct populations: men and women. Unfortunately, the collected studies differ in systematic ways on multiple variables. As a result, we simply cannot make definitive statements about the superiority of treatment for one gender over the other. However, in this chapter, we strive to make a careful inquiry into patterns of treatment efficacy and gender.

Effect Size Comparisons

In order to facilitate such an investigation, effect sizes were calculated. An effect size reflects the magnitude of the difference between two groups, which is expressed in standard deviation units. Effect sizes can be thought of as the degree of departure from the null hypothesis (Wolf, 1986). In most cases (Brom et al., 1989; Carlson et al., 1998; Cooper & Clum, 1989; Devilly et al., 1998; Foa et al., 1991, 1999; Jensen, 1994; Keane, Fairbank, Caddell, & Zimering, 1989; Resick et al., 1988; 2000; Resick & Schnicke, 1992; Vaughn et al., 1994), the null hypothesis would be that the treatment condition did not produce changes that differ from those produced by a control condition. For example, Resick and colleagues (2000) reported that the effect size of CPT on PTSD symptoms was 2.78. This very large effect size means that participants in the CPT treatment condition improved 2.78 *SD* units more than did participants in the control condition. On the other hand, an earlier publication (Keane et al., 1989) reported that the effect size of implosive (flooding) therapy on a PTSD measure was 0.22. This much smaller effect size means that those who participated in implosion therapy only improved 0.22 *SD* units over those who did not.

In a few cases (Boudewyns & Hyer, 1990; Cusak & Spates, 1999; Devilly & Spence, 1999; Marks et al., 1998; Tarrier et al., 1999; Wilson et al., 1995), researchers reported effect sizes based on change scores, in which an effect size reflects differences in pre- and posttreatment scores from the same group of participants. For instance, Marks and colleagues (1998) reported an effect size of 1.00 for exposure therapy. This means that at posttreatment, participants had improved 1.00 *SD* units over their pretreatment scores. It has been suggested that effect sizes based on difference scores tend to be higher than those obtained by comparing treatment and control groups (Abramowitz, 1997). Therefore, effect sizes calculated with change scores are identified as such.

There are many ways to compute effect sizes (Wolf, 1986), none of which have been chosen as a gold standard. When possible, the effect sizes in this chapter were calculated using control and treatment group means and standard deviations following Cohen's (1988) convention:

$$\text{Effect size} = \frac{M_{\text{post-ctrl}} - M_{\text{post-trt}}}{\sigma'}$$

$$\text{where } \sigma'^2 = \frac{SD^2_{\text{post-ctrl}} + SD^2_{\text{post-trt}}}{2}$$

To facilitate comparisons at follow-up evaluations, the follow-up means and standard deviations replaced posttreatment means and standard deviations for the control groups. For studies based on change scores, pretreatment rather than control group scores were used as the comparison.

Treatment Findings

The most direct look into the relative efficacy of treatment for men and women can be found by examining studies in the first group of collected studies, the one involving both male and female participants (see Tables 11.1 and 11.2). Gender-specific effect sizes revealed that women did better than men in a study comparing imaginal exposure to cognitive therapy (Tarrier et al., 1999). However, gender differences in efficacy were not found in a study comparing exposure, cognitive restructuring, a combination of the two, and relaxation (Marks et al., 1998). Nor were gender differences observed in a study comparing EMDR to a wait-list control condition (Wilson et al., 1995, 1997). Gender differences were not addressed at all in several studies involving both male and female participants. These studies included a comparison of desensitization, hypnotherapy, and psychodynamic therapy (Brom et al., 1989); a comparison of variations of EMDR (Cusak & Spates, 1999); a comparison of EMDR and a protocol comprised of SIT, PE, and cognitive therapy components (Devilly & Spence, 1999), and a comparison of EMDR, image habituation, and relaxation (Vaughn et al., 1994).

Effect sizes reported for studies with exclusively male participants tended to be lower than those for studies with exclusively female participants (see Table 11.1). Exclusively male studies compared EMDR to relaxation (Carlson et al., 1998), flooding to standard treatment (Cooper & Clum, 1989), variations of EMDR to each other or to a control condition (Devilly et al., 1998), EMDR to a wait list (Jensen, 1994), and implosion to standard treatment (Keane et al., 1989). The average posttreatment effect size for men is 0.40.

Exclusively female studies compared PE, SIT, and supportive counseling to a wait-list condition (Foa et al., 1991); PE and SIT to a combination of the two (Foa et al., 1999); SIT, assertiveness training, and supportive therapy to a wait-list condition (Resick et al., 1988); CPT to a wait-list condition (Resick & Schnicke, 1993); and CPT and PE to a wait-list condition (Resick et al., 2000). The average posttreatment effect size for studies of women is 1.39. The tendency for women to benefit more than men remained at follow-up (average effect sizes of 0.79 to 0.65, respectively) (see Table 11.2) and when improvements in depressive symptoms were examined (average effect sizes of 0.73 to 0.48, respectively) (see Table 11.3).

Based on the relative magnitude of effect sizes, it appears that women fare equally well or better than men in controlled efficacy studies of PTSD

TABLE 11.1. PTSD Treatment Effect Sizes

Researchers	Gender	Trauma	Treatment	Measure	ES
Brom et al. (1989)	Both	Mixed	Desensitization	IES-int	0.92
				IES-av	1.09
			Hypnotherapy	IES-int	0.60
				IES-av	0.78
			Psychodynamic	IES-int	0.53
				IES-av	0.98
Cusak & Spates (1999)[b]	Both	Mixed	EMD	IES-int	1.59[a]
				IES-av	2.68[a]
			EMDR	IES-int	1.24[a]
				IES-av	1.44[a]
Devilly & Spence (1999)	Both	Mixed	TTP[c]	PSS-SR	1.81[a]
			EMDR	PSS-SR	0.75[a]
Marks et al. (1998)	Both	Mixed	Exposure	CAPS-sev	1.00[a]
			Cognitive restructuring (CR)	CAPS-sev	1.00[a]
			Exposure + CR	CAPS-sev	1.00[a]
			Relaxation	CAPS-sev	1.00[a]
Tarrier et al. (1999)[f]	(Male)	Mixed	Imaginal exposure	CAPS-sev	0.67[a]
	(Female)			CAPS-sev	1.22[a]
	(Male)		Cognitive therapy	CAPS-sev	1.21[a]
	(Female)			CAPS-sev	1.65[a]
Vaughn et al. (1994)	Both	Mixed	EMDR	SI-tot	1.53
			Image habituation	SI-tot	0.57
			Relaxation	SI-tot	0.50
Wilson et al. (1995)	Both	Mixed	EMDR	IES-int	1.66[a]
				IES-av	1.20[a]
Carlson et al. (1998)	Male	Combat	EMDR	IES-int	0.42
				IES-av	−0.05
			Relaxation	Mississippi	0.95
				IES-int	−0.09
				IES-av	−0.50
				Mississippi	−0.07
Cooper & Clum (1989)	Male	Combat	Flooding	MVEQ-sd[d]	1.11
				MVEQ-hs	0.71
				MVEQ-ps	1.14
Devilly et al. (1998)	Male	Combat	EMDR	Mississippi	0.00
			REDDR[e]	Mississippi	−0.31
Jensen (1994)	Male	Combat	EMDR	SI-tot	1.04
				Mississippi	−0.37

(continued)

TABLE 11.1. (*continued*)

Researchers	Gender	Trauma	Treatment	Measure	ES
Keane et al. (1989)	Male	Combat	Implosion	MMPI-ptsd	0.22
Foa et al. (1991)	Female	Rape	Prolonged exposure (PE)	PSS-I	0.44
			Stress inoculation training (SIT)	PSS-I	1.45
			Supportive counseling	PSS-I	0.20
Foa et al. (1999)	Female	Assault	PE	PSS-I	1.92
			PE + SIT	PSS-I	1.50
			SIT	PSS-I	1.61
Resick et al. (1998)	Female	Rape	SIT	IES-int	0.62
				IES-av	0.10
			Assertion training	IES-int	0.59
				IES-av	0.34
			Supportive therapy	IES-av	0.52
				IES-int	0.20
Resick & Schnicke (1992)	Female	Rape	Cognitive processing therapy (CPT) group	SCL-ptsd	0.64
Resick et al. (2000)	Female	Rape	CPT	CAPS-comb	2.81
				PSS-I	2.73
			PE	CAPS-comb	2.08
				PSS-I	1.87

Note. int, intrusion; av, avoidance.

[a]Effect sizes calculated with change scores.

[b]One-third of participants did not meet full criteria for PTSD.

[c]TTP, trauma treatment protocol, utilizing components of SIT, PE, and cognitive therapy.

[d]MVEQ, Modified Vietnam Experiences Questionnaire; sd, sleep disturbances; ps, psychotic-like symptoms; hs, hypersensitivity to sound.

[e]REDDR, reactive eye dilation desensitization and reprocessing, a treatment identical to EMDR but without the eye movement component.

[f]Gender-specific effect sizes provided by Nick Tarrier. Calculated with change scores.

treatments. However, the reasons for the trend are far from clear. It is possible that gender characteristics such as gender role socialization and the utilization of different types of coping strategies may predispose women to benefit more from treatment. It is also possible that factors independent of gender, such as research participant characteristics and trauma histories, criteria for inclusion, stringency of controls in research design, outcome measures, research methodology, and assessment strategies, played a role in these differences observed in effect sizes for men and women. These factors are reviewed next.

TABLE 11.2. Follow-Up PTSD Treatment Effect Sizes

Researchers	Gender	Trauma	Treatment	Time	Measure	ES
Brom et al. (1989)	Both	Mixed	Desensitization	3 mo	IES-int	0.78
					IES-av	0.68
			Hypnotherapy		IES-int	0.74
					IES-av	0.83
			Psychodynamic		IES-int	0.84
					IES-av	1.32
Devilly & Spence (1999)	Both	Mixed	TTP	3 mo	PSS-SR	1.78[a]
			EMDR		PSS-SR	0.31[a]
Marks et al. (1998)	Both	Mixed	Exposure	3 mo	CAPS-sev	2.00[a]
			Cognitive restructuring (CR)	6 mo	CAPS-sev	2.00[a]
			Exposure + CR		CAPS-sev	2.00[a]
			Relaxation		CAPS-sev	1.00[a]
			Exposure		CAPS-sev	2.00[a]
			CR		CAPS-sev	2.00[a]
			Exposure + CR		CAPS-sev	2.00[a]
Tarrier et al. (1999)[d]	(Male)	Mixed	Imaginal exposure	6 mo	CAPS-sev	1.10[a]
	(Female)				CAPS-sev	1.24[a]
	(Male)		Cognitive therapy		CAPS-sev	1.14[a]
	(Female)				CAPS-sev	1.44[a]
	(Male)		Imaginal exposure	12 mo	CAPS-sev	0.85[a]
	(Female)				CAPS-sev	0.87[a]
	(Male)		Cognitive therapy		CAPS-sev	0.80[a]
	(Female)				CAPS-sev	1.50[a]
Vaughn et al. (1994)	Both	Mixed	EMDR	3 mo	SI-tot	1.58
			Image habituation training		SI-tot	0.67
			Relaxation		SI-tot	0.89
Wilson et al. (1995/1997)	Both	Mixed	EMDR	3 mo	IES-int	1.74[a]
				15 mo	IES-av	1.23[a]
					IES-int	1.92[a]
					IES-av	1.28[a]
Boudewyns & Hyer (1996)	Male	Combat	Exposure	3 mo	VETS[b]	.12[c]
Carlson et al. (1998)	Male	Combat	EMDR	3 mo	IES-int	0.58
			Relaxation	3 mo	IES-av	0.37
			EMDR		Mississippi	1.05
			Relaxation		CAPS-sev	2.61
					IES-int	−0.19
					IES-av	−0.60
					Mississippi	0.11
					CAPS-sev	0.91
					Mississippi	0.80
					Mississippi	−0.80
Cooper & Clum (1989)	Male	Combat	Flooding	3 mo	MVEQ-sd	1.3
					MVEQ-hs	0.10
					MVEQ-ps	0.83

(continued)

TABLE 11.2. (*continued*)

Researchers	Gender	Trauma	Treatment	Time	Measure	ES
Devilly et al. (1998)	Male	Combat	EMDR	6 mo	Mississippi	−0.13
			REDDR	6 mo	Mississippi	−0.49
Keane et al. (1989)	Male	Combat	Implosion	6 mo	MMPI-ptsd	0.22
Foa et al. (1991)	Female	Rape	PE	3.5 mo	PSS-I	1.17
			SIT		PSS-I	0.85
			Supportive counseling		PSS-I	0.40
Foa et al. (1999)	Female	Assault	PE	3 mo	PSS-I	1.73
			PE + SIT		PSS-I	1.77
			SIT		PSS-I	1.06
			PE	6 mo	PSS-I	1.99
			PE + SIT		PSS-I	1.40
			SIT		PSS-I	1.52
			PE	12 mo	PSS-I	1.86
			PE + SIT		PSS-I	1.36
			SIT		PSS-I	1.19
Resick et al. (1988)	Female	Rape	SIT	6 mo	IES-int	0.40
					IES-av	0.48
			Assertion training		IES-int	0.22
					IES-av	0.54
			Supportive therapy		IES-int	0.28
					IES-av	0.55
Resick & Schnicke (1992)	Female	Rape	CPT group	3 mo	SCL-ptsd	0.81
				6 mo	SCL-ptsd	0.78

Note. hs, hypersensitivity to sound; ps, psychotic-like symptoms; sd, sleep disturbances; int, intrusion; av, avoidance.

[a]Effect sizes calculated with change scores.

[b]VETS, Veterans Adjustment Scale.

[c]Effect size provided by Paula Schnurr. Calculated with change scores.

[d]Gender-specific effect sizes provided by Nick Tarrier. Calculated with change scores.

FACTORS TO CONSIDER REGARDING GENDER AND TREATMENT OUTCOME

Person Variables

Gender Role Socialization

Gender socialization may play a role in the slight superiority of PTSD treatment responses among women in the studies reviewed for this chapter. Specifically, gender role socialization can influence the manner in which men and women experience and express emotions. In exploring the relationship between gender and psychotherapy response, the following issues are con-

TABLE 11.3. Effect Sizes for Depression Measures

Researchers	Gender	Trauma	Treatment	Time	Measure	ES
Devilly & Spence (1999)	Both	Mixed	TTP	Post	BDI	1.34[a]
				3 mo	BDI	1.31[a]
			EMDR	Post	BDI	0.68[a]
				3 mo	BDI	0.35[a]
Marks et al. (1998)	Both	Mixed	Exposure	Post	BDI	1.20[a]
				3 mo	BDI	1.50[a]
				6 mo	BDI	1.60[a]
			CR	Post	BDI	1.70[a]
				3 mo	BDI	1.00[a]
				6 mo	BDI	1.30[a]
			Exposure + CR	Post	BDI	1.80[a]
				3 mo	BDI	1.30[a]
				6 mo	BDI	1.50[a]
			Relaxation	Post	BDI	0.07[a]
				3 mo	BDI	1.00[a]
Tarrier et al. (1999)[b]	(Male)	Mixed	Imaginal exposure	Post	BDI	0.26[a]
				6 mo	BDI	0.06[a]
				12 mo	BDI	0.02[a]
	(Female)		Imaginal exposure	Post	BDI	1.12[a]
				6 mo	BDI	0.90[a]
				12 mo	BDI	0.40[a]
	(Male)		Cognitive therapy	Post	BDI	0.58[a]
				6 mo	BDI	0.08[a]
				12 mo	BDI	0.10[a]
	(Female)		Cognitive therapy	Post	BDI	1.07[a]
				6 mo	BDI	0.84[a]
				12 mo	BDI	0.84[a]
Vaughn et al. (1994)	Both	Mixed	EMDR	Post	HRSD	1.75
				3 mo	HRSD	1.44
			Image habitation	Post	HRSD	0.49
				3 mo	HRSD	0.39
			Relaxation	Post	HRSD	0.58
				3 mo	HRSD	1.13
Carlson et al. (1998)	Male	Combat	EMDR	Post	BDI	1.67
				3 mo	BDI	1.33
				9 mo	BDI	1.70
			Relaxation	Post	BDI	0.61
				3 mo	BDI	0.42
				9 mo	BDI	0.10
Cooper & Clum (1989)	Male	Combat	Flooding	Post	BDI	0.48
				3 mo	BDI	0.30
Devilly et al. (1998)	Male	Combat	EMDR	Post	BDI	0.24[a]
				6 mo	BDI	−0.07[a]
			REDDR	Post	BDI	−0.16[a]
				6 mo	BDI	0.10[a]

(continued)

TABLE 11.3. (*continued*)

Researchers	Gender	Trauma	Treatment	Time	Measure	ES
Foa et al. (1991)	Female	Sexual assault	SIT	Post	BDI	0.66
				3.5 mo	BDI	0.47
			PE	Post	BDI	0.16
				3.5 mo	BDI	1.04
			Supportive counseling	Post	BDI	0.00
				3.5 mo	BDI	−0.05
Foa et al. (1999)	Female	Assault	PE	Post	BDI	1.47
				3 mo	BDI	1.21
				6 mo	BDI	1.35
				12 mo	BDI	1.34
			SIT	Post	BDI	1.00
				3 mo	BDI	0.55
				6 mo	BDI	0.62
				12 mo	BDI	0.69
			PE + SIT	Post	BDI	0.91
				3 mo	BDI	0.65
				6 mo	BDI	0.97
				12 mo	BDI	0.80
Resick et al. (1988)	Female	Sexual assault	SIT	Post	SCL-dep	−0.72
				3 mo	SCL-dep	0.21
				6 mo	SCL-dep	0.20
			Assertion training	Post	SCL-dep	0.10
				3 mo	SCL-dep	0.10
				6 mo	SCL-dep	0.37
			Supportive counseling	Post	SCL-dep	0.13
				3 mo	SCL-dep	0.14
				6 mo	SCL-dep	0.05
Resick & Schnicke (1992)	Female	Sexual assault	CPT group	Post	SCL-dep	0.37
				3 mo	SCL-dep	0.68
				6 mo	SCL-dep	0.72
Resick et al. (2000)	Female	Sexual assault	CPT	Post	BDI	2.11
			PE	Post	BDI	1.18

[a]Effect sizes calculated with change scores.
[b]Gender-specific effect sizes provided by Nick Tarrier. Calculated with change scores.

sidered: (1) emotional expressiveness, (2) comfort with intimacy, (3) expression of anger, and (4) choice of coping strategies.

Although women are usually socialized to be emotionally expressive, nurturing, and to direct their achievement through affiliation with others, men are usually socialized to be emotionally inhibited, assertive, and independent (Gilbert, 1987; Kaplan, 1976). Because most forms of treatment emphasize the experience and expression of emotions, it seems reasonable to suggest that differences in socialization impact the degree of comfort that men and women have in therapy. For women, emotional expressiveness and concern with their own and others' feeling states are consistent with gender role expectations (Broverman, Vogel, Broverman, Clarkson, & Rosencratz, 1972). In fact, research has shown that women endorse a wider range and greater intensity of emotional experiences than do their male counterparts (Allen & Haccoun, 1976; Allen & Hamsher, 1974; Balswick & Avertt, 1977; Diener, Sandvik, & Larson, 1985; Smith & Klengel, 1982). It is unclear whether women experience more emotional variability or are simply more aware of and willing to acknowledge their emotions.

It seems plausible that gender socialization enters the therapy room just as it enters every other human interaction. Not surprisingly, it has been reported that men express less affect and are more cognitively oriented in therapy than women (Maracek & Johnson, 1980; Shay, 1996; Werrbach & Gilbert, 1987). It has also been suggested that mild forms of alexithymia, difficulty labeling and acknowledging feelings, are predictable consequences of gender socialization for men (Levant, 1990). Accordingly, alexithymia has been linked with impaired progress in therapy for male Vietnam veterans (Kosten, Krystal, Giller, Frank, & Dan, 1992). However, this relationship warrants further investigation, because a recent study demonstrated that alexithymia was not predictive of treatment outcome among a sample of female sexual assault victims (Kimball & Resick, 1999).

Another gender-related difference lies in comfort with interpersonal intimacy. Research findings suggest that women tend to have fewer but more intimate friendships than do men (Burda & Vaux, 1987; Turk-Charles, Rose, & Gatz, 1996). Women's familiarity with emotionality and intimacy among friends may make the therapeutic relationship more comfortable for them. Conversely, men may find the therapeutic relationship to be outside their normal experience and, hence, threatening.

Anger seems to be the one emotion that is not discouraged through male gender role socialization (Werrbach & Gilbert, 1987). However, at least for female clients, anger has been associated with poorer PTSD treatment outcome (Foa, Riggs, Massie, & Yarczower, 1995). Foa et al. found evidence that participants with higher levels of anger were less likely to become emotionally engaged during sessions of prolonged exposure. Emotional arousal is thought to be a marker of the activation of the fear network, one of the conditions that Foa and Kozak (1986) deemed necessary for successful processing of the traumatic event. Indeed, the experience of fear during early sessions of prolonged exposure is associated with better treatment outcomes (Foa et al., 1995). It has been suggested that anger might prevent the survivor from experiencing the fear necessary for recovery. Thus, it is possible that gender role messages that encourage men's anger, but not sadness or fear, interfere with their recovery from PTSD.

Gender role socialization has been hypothesized to impact coping behaviors among men and women. It has been observed that women are more likely to seek social support and use emotionally focused coping behaviors in the face of stressors (Ptacek, Smith, & Dodge, 1994; Ptacek, Smith, & Zanas, 1992). In contrast, men report using relatively more problem-focused coping behaviors. Although women and men both report that problem-focused coping strategies are more effective in the face of difficulties, such as typical life stressors (Ptacek et al., 1992; Diehl, Coyle, & Labouvie-Vief, 1996) and when struggling against depressive symptoms (Nolen-Hoeksema, Larson, & Grayson, 1999), a traumatic experience may produce difficulties that require emotional and affiliative strategies as well as cognitive ones for resolution; that is, an overreliance on cognitive coping strategies may hamper men's recovery from PTSD.

Social Support

Surprisingly, studies examining the relationship between social support and trauma recovery have yielded mixed results. Some studies suggest that social support facilitates recovery (Burgess & Holstrom, 1978; Ruch & Hennessey, 1982), whereas another failed to find a significant relationship between social support and recovery (Popiel & Susskind, 1985).

The symptoms of PTSD are likely to strain relationships with family and friends. In a study of Vietnam veterans, Herndon and Law (1985) found that symptoms of emotional numbing, irritability, and uncontrolled anger had a significant and deleterious affect on marital stability, resulting in decreased partner support. Compounding the marital estrangement, the larger community can often react with distance and discomfort to trauma survivors, particularly in light of the ambivalent and often hostile feelings evoked by American involvement in the Vietnam War. Herndon and Law further pointed out that many Vietnam veterans may have been away from their families and friends for long intervals of time and likely found that their relationships experienced some strain as they attempted to reconnect with "old" social support networks. This strain was likely exacerbated as the veteran's personality was affected by PTSD and depressive symptoms.

The difficulty that female assault survivors may have with social support networks, however, should not be understated. Female sexual assault victims may find it difficult to rely on family and friends because of feelings of shame and societal stigma about rape. Kubany and Manke (1995) identified several potential sources of trauma-related guilt, such as "wearing certain kinds of clothes" and "trusting the assailant" (p. 35). Indeed, a strong correlation was found between PTSD and trauma-related guilt severity in separate samples of Vietnam veterans and battered women (Kubany et al., 1995). Clinical and research findings also typically suggest that female assault victims' high levels of self-blame and shame likely affect their comfort in seeking out support (Meyer & Taylor, 1986). This is particularly important in light of evidence suggesting that postrape attributions based on self-blame have negative repercussions on adjustment measures (Meyer & Taylor, 1986). It is likely that, to some extent, self-blame is derived from a larger societal context that often assists in stigmatizing rape victims. Compared to victims of other crimes, rape victims are more likely to be blamed for the crime. Furthermore, victims who do not physically resist are more likely to be blamed (Burt, 1991). Given this context, it is not surprising that many rape victims are hesitant to seek help.

Changing conceptualizations of what legitimately qualifies as social support complicate findings on social support and recovery. Traditionally, social support was measured by the amount or frequency of contact as opposed to the perceived quality of the contact. However, growing evidence has suggested that perhaps quality is the more salient aspect of social support. Corroborating this view, several studies have demonstrated that network size is less predictive of recovery than the quality of the social interaction (Kessler, Price, & Wortman, 1985; Shinn, Lehman, & Wong, 1984). The research findings that suggest women tend to have more emotionally intimate relationships than men (Burda & Vaux, 1987; Turk-Charles, Rose, & Gatz, 1996) may have implications for the slight superiority of women to men in response to treatment; that is, women's responses to treatment may reflect the impact of both social support and the impact of formalized PTSD treatment.

Although gender role socialization (and related differences in the quality of social interactions) may favor women in the response to PTSD treatment, other factors certainly need to be considered when interpreting the seeming disparity in effect sizes for men and women. Paramount among these factors are the ways that the treatment populations may differ on variables other than gender.

Treatment Variables

Characteristics of Traumatic Events

The type of trauma experienced appears to have a substantial bearing on treatment outcome. Studies reviewed in this chapter have included participants with a broad range of traumatic experiences (e.g.,, combat duty, sexual assault, and accidents) that vary in intensity and duration. For example, Boudewyns and Hyer (1990) reported that their veteran participants were on combat duty for an average of 10.4 months. In contrast, 79% of participants in the Marks et al. study (1998) reported a discrete episode as their index event. Although the majority of the studies of female assault victims typically focused on discrete events during treatment, participants generally reported extensive trauma histories (e.g., Resick & Schnicke, 1992; Resick et al., 2000). Hence, it is difficult to judge whether characteristics of the traumatic event contributed to differences in effect sizes for men and women.

Time since the traumatic event also varied across studies and may have implications for treatment outcome. In treatment studies on veterans, two (Cooper & Clum, 1989) or even three (Devilly et al., 1998) decades had passed between the traumatization and treatment. Civilians in the Marks et al. study (1998) experienced the trauma an average of 4 years prior to participation; Brom et al. (1989) excluded participants who had experienced the target event more than 5 years prior to the pretreatment assessment. Again, the gender-specific impact of elapsed time since the traumatic event is not clear.

Overall, it appears that studies based on assault survivors or mixed trauma samples tend to report more discrete episodes, with smaller intervals between exposure to the trauma and treatment, than do studies of military veterans. These differences may be reflected in the larger effect sizes found for assault and mixed-trauma samples than for military combat samples. Consequently, they may be partially responsible for the differences in magnitude observed between male and female samples. These sample differences complicate conclusions about treatment efficacy and gender. However, it is not possible at this point to separate out the effects of the specific type of trauma from other salient factors.

Types of Control Groups

The nature of control groups is also relevant when the efficacy of treatments across studies is compared. In studies of Vietnam veterans, researchers were more likely to use "standard care" as the control group. Standard care typically involved group treatment, one-on-one counseling, and/or psychiatric services (Boudewyns & Hyer, 1990; Carlson et al., 1998; Cooper & Clum, 1989; Devilly et al., 1998; Jensen, 1994; Keane et al., 1989). In contrast, studies of civilian trauma survivors often used wait-list control groups (e.g., Foa et al., 1999; Resick & Schnicke, 1992; Resick et al., 2000). It may be that a control condition consisting of "standard care" is more likely than a wait-list condition to include nonspecific yet therapeutic effects associated with symptom improvement resulting in smaller effect sizes. The difference in types of control groups may temper interpretations of relative inferiority of treatments for male combat survivors.

Calculation of Effect Sizes

It should be reiterated that the formula for calculating effect sizes varied across studies. Many of the researchers utilizing mixed-gender samples furnished effect sizes based on change scores, which tend to be higher than those based on control groups (Abramowitz, 1997); the former may capitalize on statistical regression to the mean rather than actual treatment gains. Thus, the higher effect sizes found for mixed-gender research may partially reflect the greater reliance on change scores (see Tables 11.1 and 11.2). In contrast, male-only and female-only groups tended to use effect sizes based on differences between treatment and control groups. As such, the pattern of female-only groups faring better than male-only groups cannot be attributed to different methods of calculating and presenting effect sizes.

Implementation of Treatments

Differences across rape and veteran samples in treatment implementation likely affected the outcome of treatment. Issues related to treatment implementation include the use of manuals, homework assignments, treatment integrity monitoring, and the level of training the therapists receive. A significantly greater proportion of the rape treatment studies utilized treatment manuals and/or included an evaluation of treatment adherence by independent raters (Foa et al., 1991, 1999; Resick et al., 1988, 2000; Resick & Schnicke, 1992, 2000). These treatments also required clients to complete daily homework between sessions. Treatment modalities were also driven by a great deal of theory and research in the assault-related PTSD samples (e.g., PE and CPT). Furthermore, recognized experts in the particular treatment modality supervised the implementation of these therapies. It is likely that all of these factors contributed to the efficacy of treatments for the female-only studies.

In comparison, many of the studies using Vietnam veteran samples lacked information on how the treatments were implemented (e.g., Cooper & Clum, 1989) or failed to utilize treatments supported by a sound theoretical model (e.g., EMDR). Furthermore, between-session homework assignments were not typically used. However, a few researchers did utilize treatment manuals (Jensen, 1994; Keane et al., 1989) and included treatment adherence monitoring (Carlson et al., 1998). Boudewyns and Hyer (1996) used a manual as the basis of training but imposed minimal structure regarding the timing or content of the sessions. Although at times clinically necessary, deviations from a treatment protocol always introduce an element of variability that confounds conclusions.

Many of these veteran studies also failed to provide information on the level of therapist training provided (Cooper & Clum, 1989; Keane et al., 1989). Jensen (1994) utilized psychology interns who received 2-day, basic EMDR training. The authors indicated that the interns practiced their techniques on other interns, who posed as clients. Therapists in one study had varying levels of experience in different areas, ranging from psychiatric nursing to biofeedback and psychodynamic therapy training (Carlson et al., 1998). In contrast to the studies with female assault survivors, only one veteran study clearly reported using doctoral-level psychologists (Boudewyns & Hyer, 1990).

In general, we can tentatively state that treatments were implemented in a more theoretically and procedurally sound manner in studies with female assault victims than in studies with male or mixed-sample groups. Implications are that the relatively lower effect sizes for male combat veterans might reflect differences in treatment implementation, as well as the other factors discussed in this chapter.

Exclusionary Criteria

Generally, studies across combat, assault, and mixed-trauma samples excluded participants with unstable psychological conditions (i.e., psychosis or suspected organic brain damage, suicidality or self-harming behavior) (e.g., Boudewyns & Hyer, 1990; Carlson et al., 1998; Cooper & Clum, 1989; Foa et al., 1999; Jensen, 1994; Resick & Schnicke, 1992). It should be noted that studies using inpatient Vietnam veterans reported high levels of recently diagnosed substance abuse and/or dependence (Boudewyns & Hyer, 1990; Jensen, 1994). Boudewyns and Hyer (1990) reported that 70% of veterans admitted to the special treatment unit from which their sample was drawn admitted to a recent history of substance abuse. These rates are consistent with the National Vietnam Veterans Readjustment Study (NVVRS) finding that male Vietnam Theater veterans with PTSD are four times more likely to abuse alcohol or drugs as those without the disorder (Kulka et al., 1990). Furthermore, a strong association was found between substance abuse and other psychological problems, such as depression or lifetime dysthymia. Although veterans were prohibited from using alcohol during treatment, it seems plausible that a recent history of substance abuse/dependence could affect the course of treatment, which might be reflected in lower effect sizes for the male-only studies.

However, it should be noted that substance abuse and/or dependence is frequently reported among female assault victims (Kessler et al., 1995). Although studies based on female-only or mixed-gender samples excluded participants with active substance abuse and/or dependence, most of these studies did not report on past substance-related problems (e.g., Foa et al., 1991; Resick et al., 1988; Wilson et al., 1995). Thus, it is difficult to ascertain whether these rates are as high as those for veteran samples. We cannot conclude that civilian samples have less substance abuse and/or dependence. What we can conclude, however, is that a high proportion of Vietnam veterans have a chronic history of substance abuse that may complicate treatment responsiveness.

Compensation-Seeking Status

The role of compensation seeking among Vietnam veteran samples has been a frequently cited area of concern. Freuh, Gold, and De Arello (1997) found that compensation-seeking veterans were more likely to endorse psychopathology items and to produce "fake-bad" profiles on the Minnesota Multiphasic Personality Inventory (MMPI) than non-compensation-seeking veterans. Among the veteran samples reviewed in this chapter, a notable percentage of participants received some form of compensation from the federal government (e.g., Boudewyns & Hyer, 1996; Jensen, 1994). For example, Boudewyns and Hyer (1996) reported that 77% of their sample was either receiving or seeking disability pensions. Although not specifically mentioned in these articles, it is likely that many of the treatment-seeking veterans experienced difficulty obtaining or maintaining employment. Given the opportunity to receive, or continue to receive, benefits from the government based on a PTSD diagnosis and the potentially anxious experience of being employed, many Vietnam veterans stood to benefit from remaining symptom-positive. This influence may have occurred at a level beyond the veterans' conscious awareness; however, its existence should be recognized when examining treatment response. The possibility of a secondary gain might have affected the amount of improvement observed in veteran samples reviewed in this chapter.

In summary, compensation-seeking research participants were overrepresented in the male-only samples based in the United States. The influence wielded by the possibility of secondary gains for symptomatic participants in these samples may have contributed to the lower treatment efficacy found in these studies.

PTSD TREATMENT EFFECTIVENESS

The research reviewed and critiqued thus far has concerned treatment efficacy. Also of interest is treatment effectiveness. At this point, one published study of PTSD treatment effectiveness took place within the context of VA treatment centers (Rosenheck et al., 1996). Rosenheck et al. examined treatment effectiveness over a 2-year time span (1990–1991) across six VA sites with 525 veterans. The veterans were assessed at the initiation of treatment and at 4, 8, and 12 months posttreatment. As described earlier in this chapter, veterans presenting for PTSD treatment at VA centers represent a population with pervasive and chronic posttraumatic difficulties, high rates of psychiatric and substance abuse comorbidity, limited sociocultural resources (income, employment, social support), and a tendency to benefit less from treatment than do other PTSD populations.

Treatment gains reported by Rosenheck and colleagues (1996) are relatively modest or nonexistent. For example, mean scores on the Mississippi Scale for Caucasian veterans pre- and posttreatment were 122.14 and 120.16, respectively. Symptom severity changed minimally for African American veterans, from 126.28 at pretreatment to 126.33 at posttreatment. Gains on other psychological measures in this study were similarly modest or nonexistent. Furthermore, the effectiveness of PTSD treatment programs as measured by community adjustment variables, such as indices of employment, daily activities, and frequency and quality of close relationships, appears to be limited. For example, African Americans veterans worked an average of 4.93 days in the month preceding their entry into treatment. Twelve months after treatment, they averaged 6.5 days at work. The number of days worked for Caucasians at pretreatment and 12 months posttreatment was similar (6.91 and 7.07, respectively). The small gains suggest that the impressive results of efficacy studies have not yet filtered down into the general treatment community. It should be noted, however, that the effectiveness study predates many of the most efficacious clinical trials. Perhaps current advances among researchers are in the process of being disseminated to community clinicians.

No such effectiveness study has been done on predominately female or civilian populations. The vast number of military veterans returning from combat duty have made for a very special and easily identified at-risk population. In contrast, civilian victims of trauma are not easily identified; many keep their traumatic experiences a secret. Even when civilian traumas are acknowledged and treatment is sought, there is no centralized treatment delivery system (analogous to VA centers) through which civilians are served. Although the literature on treatment effectiveness is growing, little is known about differential responses to treatment among men and women.

CONCLUDING REMARKS

The relationships between gender and PTSD treatment efficacy and effectiveness are complex and multifaceted. We reviewed common treatment approaches in this chapter to help place the treatment studies within a theoretical context. Effect sizes were presented for PTSD treatment efficacy studies using male, female, and mixed-gender samples. Of the 18 studies reviewed and included in comparisons for this chapter, only seven involved both male and female participants. Of the seven studies, only three addressed gender differences in treatment effectiveness. Of those three, only one provided gender-specific effect sizes (Tarrier et al., 1999). Therefore, interpretations of differences in effect size may be regarded as potentially useful but still speculative.

Although epidemiological data suggest that women are twice as likely to develop PTSD as men (Breslau, Davis, Andreski, & Peterson, 1991; Breslau, Davis, Andreski, Peterson, & Schultz, 1997; Kessler et al., 1995), women appear to respond as well or better to treatment than men. Among the possible factors contributing to the relative superiority of treatment for women are gender role variables, such as familiarity and comfort with a wider range of emotions, more experience with interpersonal intimacy, and the tendency to use a range of coping strategies. However, methodological differences in the reviewed treatment studies also may have contributed to the appearance of relative superiority of treatment for women. Greater treatment efficacy and/or higher effect sizes may reflect the influence of factors that are theoretically independent of gender. Such factors include (1) more highly experienced therapists delivering more theoretically sound and protocol-driven treatments, (2) control groups in a wait list versus a standard care treatment condition, and (3) participant populations that are less likely to be seeking compensation and more likely to be employed and functioning at a higher level in the community. An important factor to consider when assessing the overall functioning of the samples included in this review is the issue of substance abuse. Epidemiological data clearly reveal that substance abuse often accompanies PTSD, and that greater proportions of males than females suffer from comorbid alcohol abuse and PTSD (Kessler et al., 1995). Although we cannot definitively state that substance abuse problems were more prominent among male or female samples included in this review, there is little reason to doubt that these samples would deviate from national prevalence rates. Clearly, higher rates of substance abuse in veteran studies would impact the efficacy of treatment.

Other methodological factors reviewed and deemed unlikely to be related to the relatively higher effect sizes found for studies with women include (1) the types of dependent variables used to assess improvement in the studies, and (2) the method of effect size calculation. It was not possible to determine whether influential variables, such as a greater severity or longer duration of the traumatic experiences, were disproportionately represented in male or female samples.

At this point, it is not possible to identify gender-specific, state-of-the-art interventions for PTSD. It does seem clear that, for both genders, interventions have become increasingly effective over time, and that interventions incorporating exposure and/or cognitive therapy are superior to interventions relying on relaxation and no treatment (Tables 11.1–11.3). It is our hope that future researchers will begin to routinely incorporate gender-specific effect sizes in their work, so that the current trend for women to benefit more than or as much as men can be further explored.

REFERENCES

Abramowitz, J. S. (1997). Effectiveness of psychological and pharmacological treatments for obsessive–compulsive disorder: A quantitative review. *Journal of Consulting and Clinical Psychology, 65,* 44–52.

Allen, J. G., & Haccoun, D. M. (1976). Sex differences in emotionality: A meta-dimensional approach. *Human Relations, 29,* 711–722.

Allen, J. G., & Hamsher, J. H. (1974). The development and validation of a test of emotional styles. *Journal of Consulting and Clinical Psychology, 42*, 663–668.

Balswick, J., & Avertt, C. P. (1977). Differences in expressiveness: Gender, interpersonal orientation and perceived parental expressiveness as contributing factors. *Journal of Marriage and the Family, 39*, 121–127.

Beck, A. T., & Emery, G. (1985). *Anxiety disorders and phobias: A cognitive perspective.* New York: Basic Books.

Boudewyns, P. A., & Hyer, L. (1990). Physiological response to combat memories and preliminary treatment outcome in Vietnam veteran PTSD patients treated with direct therapeutic exposure. *Behavior Therapy, 21*, 63–87.

Boudewyns, P. A., & Hyer, L. (1996). Eye movement desensitization and reprocessing (EMDR) as treatment for post-traumatic stress disorder (PTSD). *Clinical Psychology and Psychotherapy, 3*(3), 185–195.

Breslau, N., Davis, G. C., Andreski, P., & Peterson, E. (1991). Traumatic events and posttraumatic stress disorder in an urban population of young adults. *Archives of General Psychiatry, 48*, 216–222.

Breslau, N., Davis, G. C., Andreski, P., Peterson, E. L., & Schultz, L. R. (1997). Sex differences in posttraumatic stress disorder. *Archives of General Psychiatry, 54*, 1044–1048.

Brom, D., Kleber, R. J., & Defares, P. B. (1989). Brief psychotherapy for posttraumatic stress disorders. *Journal of Consulting and Clinical Psychology, 57*, 607–612.

Broverman, I. K., Vogel, S. R., Broverman, D. M., Clarkson, F. E., & Rosencratz, P. S. (1972). Sex-role stereotypes: A current appraisal. *Journal of Social Issues, 28*, 59–78.

Burda, P. C., & Vaux, A. C. (1987). The social support process in men: Overcoming sex-role obstacles. *Human Relations, 40*(1), 31–43.

Burgess, A. W., & Holmstrom, L. L. (1978). Recovery from rape and prior life stress. *Research in Nursing and Health, 1*, 165–174.

Burt, M. R. (1991). Rape myths and acquaintance rape. In A. Parrot & L. Bechhofer (Eds.), *Acquaintance rape: The hidden crime* (pp. 26–40). New York: Wiley.

Cahill, S. P., & Frueh, B. C. (1997). Flooding versus eye movement desensitization and reprocessing therapy: Relative efficacy has yet to be investigated—comment on Pitman et al. (1996). *Comprehensive Psychiatry, 38*(5), 300–303.

Carlson, J. G., Chemtob, C. M., Rusnak, K., Hedlund, N. L., & Muraoka, M. Y. (1998). Eye movement desensitization and reprocessing (EMDR) treatment for combat-related posttraumatic stress disorder. *Journal of Traumatic Stress, 11*, 3–25.

Cohen, J. (1988). *Statistical power analysis for the behavioral sciences* (2nd ed.). Hillsdale, NJ: Erlbaum.

Cooper, N. A., & Clum, G. A. (1989). Imaginal flooding as a supplementary treatment for PTSD in combat veterans: A controlled study. *Behavior Therapy, 20*, 381–391.

Cusak, K., & Spates, R. (1999). The cognitive dismantling of eye movement desensitization and reprocessing (EMDR) treatment of posttraumatic stress disorder (PTSD). *Journal of Anxiety Disorders, 13*(1–2), 87–99.

Devilly, G. J., & Spence, S. H. (1999). The relative efficacy and treatment distress of EMDR and a cognitive-behavior trauma treatment protocol in the amelioration of posttraumatic stress disorder. *Journal of Anxiety Disorders, 13*, 131–157.

Devilly, G. J., Spence, S. H., & Rapee, R. M. (1998). Statistical and reliable change with eye movement desensitization and reprocessing: Treating trauma within a veteran population. *Behavior Therapy, 29*, 435–455.

Diehl, M., Coyle, N., & Labouvie-Vief, G. (1996). Age and sex differences in strategies of coping and defense across the lifespan. *Psychology and Aging, 11*, 127–139.

Diener, E., Sandvik, E., & Larsen, R. J. (1985). Age and sex effects for emotional intensity. *Developmental Psychology, 21*(3), 542–546.

Foa, E. B., Dancu, C. V., Hembree, E. A., Jaycox, L. H., Meadows, E. A., & Street, G. P. (1999). A comparison of exposure therapy, stress inoculation training, and their combination for reducing posttraumatic stress disorder in female assault victims. *Journal of Consulting and Clinical Psychology, 67*, 194–200.

Foa, E. B., & Kozak, M. J. (1986). Emotional processing of fear: Exposure to corrective information. *Psychological Bulletin, 99*, 20–35.

Foa, E. B., Riggs, D. S., Massie, E. D., & Yarczower, M. (1995). The impact of fear activation and anger on the efficacy of exposure treatment for posttraumatic stress disorder. *Behavior Therapy, 26*, 487–499.

Foa, E. B., Rothbaum, B. O., Riggs, D. S., & Murdock, T. B. (1991). Treatment of posttraumatic stress disorder in rape victims: A comparison between cognitive behavioral procedures and counseling. *Journal of Consulting and Clinical Psychology, 59*, 715–723.

Freuh, B. C., Gold, P. B., & DeArello, M. A. (1997). Symptom overreporting in combat veterans evaluated for PTSD: Differentiation on the basis of compensation seeking status. *Journal of Personality Assessment, 68*, 369–384.

Gilbert, L. A. (1987). Gender issues in psychotherapy. In J. R. McNamara & M. A. Appel (Eds.), *Critical issues, developments, and trends in professional psychology* (Vol. 3, pp. 30–54). New York: Praeger.

Herndon, A. D., & Law, Jr., J. G. (1985). Post-traumatic stress and the family: A multimethod approach to counseling. In C. R. Figley (Ed.), *Trauma and its wake: Vol. II. The study and treatment of post-traumtic stress disorder* (pp. 264–280). New York: Brunner/Mazel.

Horowitz, M. J., Marmar, C., Weiss, D. S., Dewitt, K. N., & Rosenbaum, R. (1984). Brief psychotherapy of bereavement reactions: The relationship of process to outcome. *Archives of General Psychiatry, 41*, 438–448.

Jensen, J. (1994). An investigation of eye movement desensitization and reprocessing as a treatment for posttraumatic stress disorder symptoms of Vietnam combat veterans. *Behavior Therapy, 25*, 311–325.

Kaplan, A. G. (1976). Toward an analysis of sex-role related issues in the therapeutic relationship. *Psychiatry, 43*, 112–120.

Keane, T. M., Fairbank, J. A., Caddell, J. M., & Zimering, R. T. (1989). Implosive (flooding) therapy reduces symptoms of PTSD in Vietnam combat veterans. *Behavior Therapy, 20*, 245–260.

Kessler, R. C., Price, R. H., & Wortman, C. B. (1985). Social factors in psychopathology: Stress, social support, and coping processes. *Annual Review of Psychology, 36* 531–572.

Kessler, R. C., Sonnega, A., Bromet, E., Hughes, M., & Nelson, C. B. (1995). Posttraumatic stress disorder in the National Comorbidity Survey. *Archives of General Psychiatry, 52*, 1048–1060.

Kilpatrick, D. G., Veronen, L. J., & Resick, P. A. (1982). Psychological sequelae to rape: Assesssment and treatment strategies. In D. M. Dolays, R. L. Meredith, & A. R. Ciminero (Eds.), *Behavioral medicine: Assessment and treatment strategies* (pp. 473–497). New York: Plenum Press.

Kimball, L. A., & Resick, P. A. (1999). *Alexithymia in survivors of sexual assault: Predicting treatment outcome.* Unpublished manuscript, University of Missouri, St. Louis.

Kosten, T. R., Krystal, J. H., Giller, E. L., Frank, J., & Dan, E. (1992). Alexithymia as a predictor of treatment response in post-traumatic stress disorder. *Journal of Traumatic Stress, 5,* 563–573.

Kubany, E. S., Abueg, F. R., Owens, J. A., Brennan, J. M., Kaplan, A. S., & Watson, S. B. (1995). Initial examination of a multidimensional model of trauma-related guild: Applications to combat veterans and battered women. *Journal of Psychopathology and Behavioral Assessment, 17,* 353–376.

Kubany, E. S., & Manke, F. P. (1995). Cognitive therapy for trauma-related guilt: Conceptual bases and treatment outlines. *Cognitive and Behavioral Practice, 2,* 27–61.

Kulka, R. A., Schlenger, W. E., Fairbank, J. A., Hough, R. L., Jordan, B. K., Marmar, C. R., & Weiss, D. S. (1990). *Trauma and the Vietnam war generation.* New York: Brunner/Mazel.

Levant, R. F. (1990). Psychological services designed for men: A psychoeducational approach. *Psychotherapy, 27,* 309–315.

Lindy, J. D., Green, B. L., Grace, M., & Titchener, J. (1983). Psychotherapy with survivors of the Beverly Hills Supper Club fire. *American Journal of Psychotherapy, 37,* 593–610.

Maracek, J., & Johnson, M. (1980). Gender and the process of therapy. In A. M. Brodsky & R. Hare-Mustin (Eds.), *Women and psychotherapy: An assessment of research and practice* (pp. 67–93). New York: Guilford Press.

Marks, I., Lovell, K., Noshirvani, H., Livanou, M., & Thrasher, S. (1998). Treatment of posttraumatic stress disorder by exposure and/or cognitive restructuring: A controlled study. *Archives of General Psychiatry, 55,* 317–325.

Meichenbaum, D. (1974). *Cognitive behavior modification.* Morristown, NJ: General Learning Press.

Meyer, C. B., & Taylor, S. D. (1986). Adjustment to rape. *Journal of Personality and Social Psychology, 50,* 1226–1234.

Nolen-Hoeksema, S., Larson, J., & Grayson, C. (1999). Explaining gender differences in depressive symptoms. *Journal of Personality and Social Psychology, 77,* 1061–1072.

Pitman, R. K., Orr, S. P., Altman, B., Longpre, R. E., Poire, R. E., & Macklin, M. C. (1996a). Emotional processing and outcome of imaginal flooding therapy in Vietnam veterans with chronic posttraumatic stress disorder. *Comprehensive Psychiatry, 37,* 409–418.

Pitman, R. K., Orr, S. P., Altman, B., Longpre, R. E., Poire, R. E., & Macklin, M. C. (1996b). Emotional processing during eye movement desensitization and reprocessing therapy of Vietnam veterans with chronic posttraumatic stress disorder. *Comprehensive Psychiatry, 37,* 419–429.

Popiel, D. A., & Susskind, E. C. (1985). The impact of rape: Social support as a moderator of stress. *American Journal of Community Psychology, 13,* 645–676.

Ptacek, J. T., Smith, R. E., & Dodge, K. L. (1994). Gender differences in coping with stress when stressor and appraisals do not differ. *Personality and Social Psychology Bulletin, 20,* 421–430.

Ptacek, J. T., Smith, R. E., & Zanas, J. (1992). Gender, appraisal and coping: A longitudinal analysis. *Journal of Personality, 60*(4), 747–770.

Rachman, S. (1980). Emotional processing. *Behaviour Research and Therapy, 14,* 51–60.

Renfrey, G., & Spates, C. R. (1994). Eye movement desensitization: A partial dismantling study. *Journal of Behavior Therapy and Experimental Psychiatry, 25,* 231–239.

Resick, P. A. (1995, May). *Cognitive processing therapy for rape victims.* Workshop conducted at conference on PTSD sponsored by Manchester University, in conjunction with the British Association for Behavioural and Cognitive Psychotherapies, Manchester, UK.

Resick, P. A., & Jordan, C. G. (1988). Group stress inoculation training for victims of sexual assault: A therapists manual. In P. A. Keller & S. R. Heyman (Eds.), *Innovations in clinical practice: A source book* (pp. 99–111). Sarasota, FL: Professional Resource Exchange.

Resick, P. A., Jordan, C. G., Girelli, S. A., Hunter, C. K., & Marhoefer-Dvorak, S. (1988). A comparative outcome study of behavioral group therapy for sexual assault victims. *Behavior Therapy, 19,* 385–401.

Resick, P. A., Nishith, P., Weaver, T. L., Astin, M. C., & Feuer, C. A. (2000). *A comparison of cognitive processing therapy, prolonged exposure, and a waiting condition for the treatment of posttraumatic stress disorder in female rape victims.* Unpublished manuscript, University of Missouri, St. Louis.

Resick, P. A., & Schnicke, M. K. (1992). Cognitive processing therapy for sexual assault victims. *Journal of Consulting and Clinical Psychology, 60,* 748–756.

Resick, P. A., & Schnicke, M. K. (1993). *Cognitive processing therapy for rape victims: A treatment manual.* Newbury Park, CA: Sage.

Resnick, H. S., & Newton, T. (1992). Assessment and treatment of post-traumatic stress disorder in adult survivors of sexual assault. In D. W. Foy (Ed.), *Treating PTSD: Cognitive-behavioral strategies.* New York: Guilford Press.

Rosenheck, R., & Fontana, A. (1996). Race and outcome of treatment for veterans suffering from PTSD. *Journal of Traumatic Stress, 9,* 343–351.

Ruch, L. O., & Hennessey, M. (1982). Sexual assault: Victim and attack dimensions. *Victimology International Journal, 7,* 94–105.

Shapiro, F. (2001). *Eye movement desensitization and reprocessing: Basic principles, protocols, and procedures* (2nd ed.). New York: Guilford Press.

Shay, J. J. (1996). "Okay, I'm here but I'm not talking!": Psychotherapy with the reluctant male. *Psychotherapy, 33,* 503–513.

Shinn, M., Lehman, S., & Wong, N. W. (1984). Social interaction and support. *Journal of Social Issues, 40,* 55–76.

Smith, E. R., & Klengal, J. R. (1982). Cognitive and social bases of emotional expression: Outcome, attribution and affect. *Journal of Personality and Social Psychology, 43,* 1129–1141.

Tarrier, N., Pilgrim, H., Sommerfield, C., Faragher, B., Reynolds, M., Graham, E., & Barrowclough, C. (1999). Cognitive and exposure therapy in the treatment of PTSD: A randomized trial of cognitive therapy and imaginal exposure in the treatment of chronic posttraumatic stress disorder. *Journal of Consulting and Clinical Psychology, 67,* 13–18.

Turk-Charles, S., Rose, T., & Gatz, M. (1996). The significance of gender in the treatment of older adults. In L. L. Carstensen, B. A. Edelstein, & L. Dornbrand (Eds.), *The practical handbook of clinical gerontology* (pp. 107–128). Thousand Oaks, CA: Sage.

Vaughan, K., Armstrong, M. S., Gold, R., O'Connor, N., Jenneke, W., & Tarrier, N. (1994). A trial of eye movement desensitization compared to image habituation training and applied muscle relaxation in posttraumatic stress disorder. *Journal of Behavior Therapy and Experimental Psychiatry, 25,* 283–291.

Veronen, L. J., & Kilpatrick, D. G. (1983). Stress management for rape victims. In D. Meichenbaum & M. E. Jaremko (Eds.), *Stress reduction and prevention* (pp. 341–374). New York: Plenum Press.

Werrbach, J., & Gilbert, L. A. (1987). Men, gender stereotyping, and psychotherapy: Therapists' perceptions of male clients. *Professional Psychology: Research and Practice, 18,* 562–566.

Wilson, S. A., Becker, L. A., & Tinker, R. H. (1995). Eye movement desensitization and reprocessing (EMDR) treatment for psychologically traumatized individuals. *Journal of Consulting and Clinical Psychology, 63,* 928–937.

Wilson, S. A., Becker, L. A., & Tinker, R. H. (1997). Fifteen-month follow-up of eye movement desensitization and reprocessing (EMDR) treatment for posttraumatic stress disorder and psychological trauma. *Journal of Consulting and Clinical Psychology, 65,* 1047–1056.

Wolf, F. M. (1986). *Meta-analysis: Quantitative methods for research synthesis.* Beverly Hills, CA: Sage.

Wolpe, J. (1958). *Psychotherapy by reciprocal inhibition.* Stanford, CA: Stanford University Press.

12 | Gender and the Psychopharmacological Treatment of PTSD

KATHLEEN T. BRADY
SUDIE E. BACK

In recent years, the study of the pharmacotherapeutic management of posttraumatic stress disorder (PTSD) has received increasing attention. Eight years subsequent to the introduction of PTSD to DSM nosology, data from the first randomized medication trial showing efficacy for tricyclic antidepressants (TCAs; imipramine) and monoamine oxidase inhibitors (MAOIs; phenelzine) were published (Davidson et al., 1988; Frank, Kosten, Giller, & Dan, 1988; Kosten et al., 1991). Twenty years subsequent to that introduction, systematic evaluation of optimal treatment agents for PTSD is still at an early stage. Although a number of medications have shown potential and one medication (sertraline) has been approved by the FDA (in December 1999) for the treatment of PTSD, information related to gender differences that might inform pharmacological selection and application is notably absent. In this chapter, the role of gender in the psychopharmacological treatment of PTSD is explored. Following a brief overview of gender differences in PTSD that might impact pharmacological treatment, gender differences in pharmacokinetics and data concerning gender differences in medication response are reviewed.

GENDER DIFFERENCES IN PTSD

Chronicity

For many individuals, PTSD is a chronic condition. A substantial proportion of persons with PTSD report symptom duration of greater than 1 year

(Breslau, Davis, Andreski, & Peterson, 1991; Breslau & Davis, 1992; Zlotnick et al., 1999). As detailed in Chapter 1, this volume, by Norris et al., women are more likely than men to be diagnosed with PTSD. In addition, women are also more likely to suffer from PTSD symptoms for a longer period of time than men (Davis & Breslau, 1998). In the 1996 Detroit Area Survey, the overall median time to remission of PTSD was 24.9 months (Breslau et al., 1998). The rate of remission of PTSD among women was estimated to be four times longer than that for men (12.0 months in men vs. 48.1 months in women).

PTSD Symptom Constellations

Men and women differ in their response to traumatic events. On balance, men more often exhibit symptoms of aggression or violent impulses, whereas women usually exhibit symptoms of withdrawal or dysthymia (Janoff-Bulman & Frieze, 1987). Even among traumatized children, significant gender differences can be found, with boys demonstrating higher rates of externalizing disorders (e.g., oppositional defiant disorder, conduct disorder) in comparison to girls (Ackerman, Newton, McPherson, Jones, & Dykman, 1998). Women are more likely than men to withdraw from social contacts, relationships, close friendships, and sexual contact (Letourneau, Resnick, Kilpatrick, Saunders, & Best, 1996).

From the limited data available, it is reasonable to expect that men might be more likely than women to display symptoms from the Cluster D PTSD constellation (e.g., irritability, outbursts of anger). Davis and Breslau (1998) report that among people women with PTSD, women more frequently experience exaggerated startle response than men. It is unclear whether significant gender differences exist between rates of Cluster B (reexperiencing) and Cluster C (avoidance/numbing) PTSD symptoms. Available data suggest that women with PTSD experience intense physiological reactions to trauma-related stimuli and restricted affect more frequently then men with PTSD (Davis & Breslau, 1998). Research is needed to clarify further gender-specific differences in the presentation of PTSD that may be important in tailoring treatment interventions.

Comorbidity

A substantial proportion of individuals with PTSD meet lifetime criteria for at least one other psychiatric disorder. In the National Comorbidity Survey (NCS; Kessler, Sonnega, Bromet, Hughes, & Nelson, 1995), 88% of men and 79% of women with PTSD had a history of at least one other psychiatric disorder. Of these participants, 59% of men and 44% of women had more than three comorbid diagnoses. Frequently co-occurring disorders include major depression, other anxiety (e.g., social phobia, panic disorder, generalized anxiety disorder), substance use, and dissociative disorders (Brady, 1997; Breslau et al., 1991; Breslau, Davis, Peterson, & Schultz, 1997; Davidson, Hughes, Blazer, & George, 1991; Helzer, Robins, & McEvoy, 1987; Keane & Kaloupek, 1998; Shalev et al., 1998; Sierles, Chen, McFarland, & Taylor, 1983; Solomon & Davidson, 1997; Zlotnick et al., 1999). These patterns of comorbidity are important to assess and consider in selecting the most optimal pharmacological treatment adjunct.

Conclusions

There are substantial gender-related differences in the prevalence, chronicity, and presentation of PTSD. Some of these factors, particularly chronicity, comorbidity, symptom constellation, and associated features, may have important implications for pharmacological treatment.

GENDER DIFFERENCES IN PHARMACOKINETICS AND PHARMACODYNAMICS OF PSYCHOTROPIC MEDICATIONS

General Issues

In general, women are prescribed more psychotropic medications compared to men, yet little is known about the specific effects of gender on tolerability, safety, or efficacy of commonly used agents. There are significant gender differences in pharmacokinetic properties of psychotropic medications (Jensvold, Halbreich, & Hamilton, 1996; Pollock, 1997; Yonkers et al., 1995), including differences in absorption, drug distribution, bioavailability, and metabolism, which are reviewed below.

Absorption

The percentage of an agent that is absorbed from the gastrointestinal (GI) tract depends on properties of the drug (e.g., pH, lipophilicity, or fat solubility) and the physiology of the individual. Fat-soluble drugs are more readily absorbed. Women have a reduced rate of gastric emptying (Frezza et al., 1990; Hamilton & Yonkers, 1996) and more rapid internal transit time (Rao et al., 1987) that may lead to less absorption of orally administered medications. However, women have reduced gastric acidity compared to men (Hamilton & Yonkers, 1996; Grossman, Kirsner, & Gillespie, 1963), leading to more rapid absorption of agents that are weak bases (high pH), such as TCAs and benzodiazepines. Less gastric acid also causes less enzymatic breakdown in the GI tract, potentially leading to higher blood levels. To further complicate matters, gonadal hormones may play a role in changing GI transit time and absorption rates (Datz, Christian, & Moore, 1987; Horowitz, Maddern, & Chatterton, 1985). Although significant gender differences in gastric motility, gastric pH, and enzyme activity have been found, these effects are complex and may counterbalance each other. As such, the clinical utility of these differences remains undetermined.

Distribution

The biodistribution of an agent can be predicted by a number of factors, including individual variables such as body weight and adipose tissue mass, and characteristics of the drug, such as pH, lipid solubility (i.e., fat solubility), and protein binding. Women generally have lower body weight, reduced blood volume and a lower ratio of lean body mass to adipose tissue compared to men (Mayersohn, 1982). Although women's lower body weight and blood volume lead to higher plasma concentrations of an agent, the higher plasma percentage of body fat is associated with an initial greater volume of distribution and lower plasma concentrations for lipophilic drugs (i.e., fat-soluble drugs), such as the benzodiazepines. Lipophilic drugs, however, may accumulate in adipose tissue such that the half-life becomes prolonged in individuals with less lean body mass. Because elderly women, in general, have the greatest distribution of adipose tissue, they are the subgroup most prone to developing extensive accumulation of lipophilic medications.

Bioavailability

Many medications are bound to plasma proteins. This can have a profound effect on biodistribution because, generally, only the unbound portion of the drug crosses the blood–brain barrier and is bioactive. When two protein-bound drugs are administered at the same time, competitive displacement from protein binding can increase the bioavailability and potential toxicity of one of the drugs. Women have lower plasma protein binding than men. Most anxiolytic drugs are highly protein-bound. Benzodiazepines (99%) and the antidepressants fluoxetine, sertraline, paroxetine, and nefazodone (95%) are highly protein-bound (Preskorn, 1997). The TCAs (75–95%) and fluvoxamine (77%) are moderately protein-bound (Hamilton & Yonkers, 1996; Palmer & Benfield, 1994). Citalopram (50%) and venlafaxine (35%) have relatively low protein binding (Fredericson, 1978). As with the differences in absorption, the clinical relevance of gender differences in biodistribution have not been adequately explored.

Metabolism

Most psychotropic drugs, including the benzodiazepines and antidepressants, are metabolized by the liver. A substantial portion of the hepatic metabolism is mediated by the cytochrome P450 (CYP) enzyme system.

Certain isoenzymes (i.e., CYP2D6, CPP3A4, CYP1A1/2, CYP2C19) are responsible for the metabolism of most psychotropic medications. The most important, and complex, gender difference involves the CYP3A4 isoenzyme system, which metabolizes benzodiazepines. CPP3A4 activity is influenced by both gender and age such that premenopausal women have higher activity compared to men or to postmenopausal women (Pollack, 1997). This higher activity is likely to be associated with lower plasma concentrations, which can decrease the efficacy of benzodiazepines and increase vulnerability for developing withdrawal phenomena in premenopausal women treated with benzodiazepines.

SPECIAL ISSUES FOR WOMEN

Hormone Replacement Therapy

Female gonadal hormones, particularly estrogen and progesterone, have a regulatory role in the function of neurotransmitter systems involved in the pathophysiology of PTSD (Shear, 1997). Estrogen appears to facilitate serotonin function (Janowsky, Halbreich, & Rausch, 1996; Stahl, 1997). In addition, the locus ceruleus–norepinephrine-mediated stress response is attenuated by estrogen (Kirschbaum, Pirke, & Hellhammer, 1995; Lindheim et al., 1992). Progesterone is associated with biological effects that oppose the action of estrogen and has been linked to dysphoria and mood destabilization (Janowsky et al., 1996; Jensvold et al., 1996; Sherwin, 1996). Because these hormones play a critical role in the regulation of neurotransmitter systems involved in PTSD, they may be important in both enhancing susceptibility and influencing the clinical course and treatment of PTSD and other anxiety disorders. Although more than one-third of older women in the United States receives hormone replacement therapy (HRT), few data are available concerning its impact on pharmacokinetics or pharmacodynamics of psychotropic medications. The estrogen formulations used in HRT are metabolized through the CYP system; therefore, metabolism may be slowed and blood concentrations increased when they are coadministered with many antidepressant drugs. As will be discussed, other studies have demonstrated a more robust response to selective serotonin reuptake inhibitors (SSRIs) in premenopausal women compared to postmenopausal women or to men.

Menstrual Cycle

Plasma concentrations of medications may fluctuate during the menstrual cycle because of hormonal effects on drug metabolism. During the follicular phase, in general, there is a decrease in metabolism, leading to increased drug concentration. Metabolism peaks at midcycle (ovulation) and remains relatively high during the second half of the cycle, leading to decreased serum concentrations (Pollack, 1997; Hamilton & Yonkers, 1996; Kellermann & Luyten-Kellermann, 1978; Wilson et al., 1982). Although the clinical impact of these changes has not been studied, theoretically, these changes could be associated with an increased risk for adverse effects during the follicular phase, and increased risk for relapse during the luteal phase of the menstrual cycle.

Pregnancy

The risk–benefit ratio is certainly the most important issue in the decision to use medications during pregnancy. Risks associated with psychotropic medications include potential teratogenic effects (i.e., birth defects) as well as direct neonatal toxicity (Cohen & Rosenbaum, 1998). SSRIs are the agents that have demonstrated most efficacy in the treatment of PTSD (Brady et al., 2000). Fortunately, there is little evidence for teratogenicity or neonatal toxicity with these agents, although discontinuation of any medications that are not absolutely essential during pregnancy should always be considered.

There are substantial changes in a number of physiological parameters that determine the pharmacokinetic properties of drugs during pregnancy (Altshuler et al., 1996; Pollack, 1997). Gastric motility is decreased, whereas volume of distribution and cardiac output are increased. These changes all lead to reduced plasma drug concentrations as pregnancy progresses.

Lactation

Although there are remarkably few data on the issue of psychotropic medications during lactation, available data suggest that many medications are excreted into breast milk (Llewellyn & Stone, 1998). Generally, only a small percentage (0.1–6.2%) of the maternal dose is present in the infant. Nevertheless, because of reports of adverse events in infants exposed to psychotropic medications in breast milk, this should always be carefully monitored.

GENDER DIFFERENCES IN TREATMENT RESPONSE

Gender Differences in Efficacy

There are few data available on the issue of gender differences in response to psychotropic medications in the treatment of PTSD. Earlier studies of pharmacotherapeutic treatments for PTSD involving the TCAs and MAOIs (Davidson et al., 1990; Kosten et al., 1991) involved male veteran populations. In the more recent study of the MAOI brofaromine (Katz et al., 1995), no gender differences were reported.

Estrogen appears to have a critical role in the process of antidepressant-induced down-regulation of serotonin receptors. Data from animal studies suggest that the serotonin receptor adaptations necessary for the onset of antidepressant effects may be estrogen-dependent in women (Kendall, Stancel, & Enna, 1982). Antidepressant action may be substantially impaired in the absence of estrogen. Preliminary evidence indicates that estrogen is an important facilitator of serotonin response in humans. Postmenopausal women without estrogen replacement therapy (ERT) evidence a reduced serotonin response that can be effectively "normalized" with ERT (Halbreich et al., 1995). Moreover, depressed elderly women appear more likely to respond to SSRI antidepressant treatment when also receiving ERT (Schneider et al., 1997).

Although little is known about gender differences in the pharmacological treatment of PTSD, several studies indicate that there are gender-based differential responses to antidepressant treatments. In an analysis by gender, with pooled data from clinical trials of paroxetine, imipramine, and placebo in outpatients with major depression, women responded significantly better to paroxetine than to imipramine (Steiner et al., 1993). It is noteworthy that in the men, because of high placebo response rates, there were no significant differences among the three treatments, whereas women responded better to both active treatments compared with placebo.

Kornstein (1999) evaluated gender differences in treatment response to sertraline versus imipramine in chronic or "double" depression. A significant gender-by-treatment interaction was found for treatment response and dropout rates, with women having a more robust response to sertraline than to imipramine (57% vs. 46%, $p = .02$). Premenopausal women had a more robust response to sertraline than to imipramine (57% vs. 43%, $p = .01$), whereas response rates in postmenopausal women were similar (57% vs. 56%). The authors emphasize the importance of considering both gender and menopausal status in the selection of an antidepressant agent for a depressed patient.

The preferential response of women to SSRIs also was noted by Yonkers et al. (1995), who evaluated gender differences in response rates during a 12-week study of sertraline, imipramine, and placebo in the treatment of dysthymia. Significantly more women than men responded to sertraline (64% vs. 42%, $p = .02$). Women responded better to sertraline than to either imipramine or placebo, whereas for men there were no significant differences between any active treatment and placebo. The SSRIs in a number of different studies (Brady et al., 2000; Conner et al., 1999; van der Kolk et al., 1994) have demonstrated effectiveness in the treatment of PTSD. In the first published, placebo-controlled study of fluoxetine in the treatment of PTSD (van der Kolk et al., 1994), the study population was subdivided into those with combat- (N = 31) and non-combat-related (N = 33) PTSD. As would be expected, a much higher percentage of women were found in the non-combat-related group. Significant improvement in all symptom clusters of PTSD were found for the non-combat-related patients. It is not clear whether the differing between-group efficacy of fluoxetine treatment was related to gender, but it was certainly one variable that clearly differentiated the two groups. The nature of traumatic stressor, length of prior treatment, chronicity of symptoms, and the confounding effect of receiving disability benefits also differed between groups and may have contributed to differential treatment effects.

A gender-specific analysis of data from a recently published study of sertraline in PTSD treatment (Brady et al., 2000) indicated a more robust response in women compared to men (Brady & Farfel, 1999). Although the study was not designed to explore gender differences, women showed a more robust effect compared to men for all of the primary outcome measures (e.g., Clinician-Administered PTSD Scale, Clinical Global Impressions) and in the improvement in depressive symptoms. This difference may, in part, be explained by the higher number of women in the study compared to men, hence, more power to detect changes in women. Because the majority of women in the study were premenopausal, comparison of pre- versus postmenopausal response, in order to tease out potential contributions of estrogen to this preferential response, was not possible.

Comorbidity and Associated Features

As mentioned earlier, some of the psychiatric comorbidities and associated features seen in men and women with PTSD differ. In particular, women are more likely to have eating, dissociation, and somatization disorders. Men are more likely to have comorbid substance use disorders. Development of pharmacotherapies for comorbid conditions may provide another rational basis for gender differentiation in pharmacological treatment choice.

Dissociative symptoms, for example, may respond best to neuroleptic treatment (Friedman, 1988). For this reason, neuroleptics may be more useful in the treatment of PTSD in women compared to men. On the other hand, men with PTSD may experience more irritability, aggressivity, and difficulty with impulse control. In some studies (Ford, 1996; Lipper et al., 1986) these symptoms have been particularly responsive to treatment with mood-stabilizing anticonvulsant medications, such as carbamazepine. The gender differences in the incidence of these associated symptoms of PTSD suggest a preferential role for these agents in the treatment of PTSD in men.

PTSD Symptom Clusters and Treatment

PTSD is an extremely heterogeneous disorder, and its presentation may be markedly different from one individual to the next. It is possible that in addition to differences in comorbidity and associated symptoms in PTSD, gender-specific differences in symptom clusters may be important determinants of pharmacological specificity. As previously mentioned, women with PTSD experience more physiologic reactivity to trauma-related stimuli (intrusive symptoms), more restricted affect (avoidance symptoms), and more startle response (hyperarousal symptoms) than men (Davis & Breslau, 1998). As Friedman suggests (1997a), there is likely to be no "magic bullet" for the treatment of PTSD, but rather medications, or a combination of medications, targeting specific symptom constellations are likely to provide optimal pharmacological management. Both the TCAs (Davidson, Malik, & Sutherland, 1997; Kosten et al., 1991) and the MAOIs (Davidson et al., 1988; Kosten et al., 1991) have demonstrated efficacy in the treatment of intrusive symptoms. Although the SSRIs appear to be effective in the treatment of all symptom clusters in PTSD, the effect size for decreasing intrusive symptoms is smaller than that for arousal and avoidant symptoms (Brady et al., 2000). In women with prominent intrusive symptoms that do not respond fully to an SSRI, these other agents should be considered.

Avoidant symptoms, also prominent in women, have a robust response to both sertraline and fluoxetine (Brady et al., 2000; Conner et al., 1999). In contrast, there have been conflicting results concerning the effects of the TCAs on avoidant symptoms (Davidson et al., 1990; Friedman, 1997b). Arousal symptoms appear to be equally responsive to the SSRIs, TCAs, and MAOIs. Additionally, both clonidine and propranolol (Kolb, 1984) have been reported to be effective in decreasing arousal symptoms and should be considered as adjunctive therapies in resistant cases.

CONCLUSIONS

A number of gender differences are likely to effect blood levels, toxicity, side effects, and efficacy of the therapeutic agents used in the treatment of PTSD. To further complicate matters, gonadal hormones can also have an impact on a number of variables that affect therapeutic agents, such that efficacy and side-effect profiles may vary throughout the month in some individuals. Because of these issues, care must be taken to tailor individual, pharmacological treatment for women, with particular attention to variations in hormone levels as a result of HRT or menstrual cycle. Other issues specific to the use of medications in women concern the use of medications during pregnancy and breast feeding. Because of the lack of information about many of the agents commonly used, the risk–benefit of their use for pregnant or breast-feeding women must be carefully weighed. Regarding SSRIs, the agents most commonly used in the treatment of PTSD, there is not much evidence of teratogenicity or adverse impact on breast-feeding infants, but the data are limited and caution must be urged.

Systematic evaluation of the role of gender in the pharmacological management of PTSD has just begun. Gender-specific considerations in treatment selection will be guided by both the gender-specific features of PTSD (e.g., course of illness, comorbidity, presentation) and the gender differences in the pharmacokinetic and pharmacodynamic properties of psychotropic medications. As our knowledge base in both of these areas grows, recommendations concerning the most appropriate pharmacological treatment for men and women with PTSD can be refined.

REFERENCES

Ackerman, P. T., Newton, J. E. O., McPherson, W. B., Jones, J. G., & Dykman, R. A. (1998). Prevalence of post traumatic stress disorder and other psychiatric diagnoses in three groups of abused children (sexual, physical, and both). *Child Abuse and Neglect, 22*, 759–774.

Altshuler, L. L., Cohen, L., Szuba, M. P., Burt, V. K., Gitlin, M., & Mintz, J. (1996). Pharmacologic management of psychiatric illness during pregnancy: Dilemmas and guidelines. *American Journal of Psychiatry, 153*, 592–606.

Brady, K. T. (1997). Posttraumatic stress disorder and comorbidity: Recognizing the many faces of PTSD. *Journal of Clinical Psychiatry, 58*(Suppl. 9), 12–15.

Brady, K. T., & Farfel, G. (1999, November). *Effects of sertraline and placebo in women with PTSD.* Paper presented at the meeting of the International Society for Traumatic Stress Studies, Miami, FL.

Brady, K., Pearlstein, T., Asnis, G. M., Baker, D., Rothbaum, B., Sikes, C. R., & Farfel, G. M. (2000). Efficacy and safety of sertraline treatment of posttraumatic stress disorder. *Journal of the American Medical Association, 283*(14), 1837–1844.

Breslau, N., & Davis, G. C. (1992). Posttraumatic stress disorder in an urban population of young adults. *American Journal of Psychiatry, 149*, 671–675.

Breslau, N., Davis, G. C., Andreski, P., & Peterson, E. (1991). Traumatic events and posttraumatic stress disorder in an urban population of young adults. *Archives of General Psychiatry, 48*, 216–222.

Breslau, N., Davis, G. C., Peterson, E., & Schultz, L. R. (1997b). Psychiatric sequelae of posttraumatic stress disorder in women. *Archives of General Psychiatry, 54*, 81–87.

Breslau, N., Kessler, R. C., Chilcoat, H. D., Schultz, L. R., Davis, G. C., & Andreski, P. (1998). Trauma and posttraumatic stress disorder in the community. *Archives of General Psychiatry, 55*, 626–632.

Cohen, L. S., Rosenbaum, J. F. (1998). Psychotropic drug use during pregnancy: Weighing the risks. *Journal of Clinical Psychiatry, 59*(Suppl. 2), 18–28.

Conner, K. M., Sutherland, S. M., Tupler, L. A., Malik, M. L., & Davidson, J. R. T. (1999). Fluoxetine in post-traumatic stress disorder. *British Journal of Psychiatry, 175*, 17–22.

Datz, F. L., Christian, P. E., & Moore, J. (1987). Gender-related differences in gastric emptying. *Nuclear Medicine, 28*, 1204–1207.

Davidson, J. R. T., Hughes, D., Blazer, D. G., & George, L. K. (1991). Post-traumatic stress disorder in the community: An epidemiological study. *Psychological Medicine, 21*, 713–721.

Davidson, J., Kudler, H., Smith, R., Mahorney, S. L., Lipper, S., Hammett, E., Saunders, W. B., & Cavenar, J. O., Jr. (1990). Treatment of posttraumatic stress disorder with amitriptyline and placebo. *Archives of General Psychiatry, 47*(3), 259–266.

Davidson, J. R. T., Malik, M. L., & Sutherland, S. N. (1997). Response characteristics to antidepressants and placebo in post-traumatic stress disorder. *International Clinical Psychopharmacology, 12*, 291–296.

Davis, G. C., & Breslau, N. (1998, July). Are women at greater risk for PTSD than men? *Psychiatric Times,* pp. 65–66.

Ford, N. (1996). The use of anticonvulsants in posttraumatic stress disorder: Case study and overview. *Journal of Traumatic Stress, 9*, 857–863.

Frank, J. B., Kosten, T. R., Giller, E. L., & Dan, E. (1988). A randomized clinical trial of phenelzine and imipramine for posttraumatic stress disorder. *American Journal of Psychiatry, 145*, 1289–1291.

Fredericson, O. (1978). Preliminary studies of the kinetics of citalopram in man. *European Journal of Clinical Pharmacology, 14*, 69–73.

Frezza, M., di Padova, C., Pozzato, G., Terpin, M., Baraona, E., & Lieber, C. S. (1990). High blood alcohol levels in women. The role of decreased gastric alcohol dehydrogenase activity and first-pass metabolism [published errata appear in *New England Journal of Medicine*, 1990, May 24, *322*(21), 1540, and 1990, August 23, *323*(8), 553] [see comments]. *New England Journal of Medicine, 322*(2), 95–99.

Friedman, M. J. (1988). Toward rational pharmacotherapy for posttraumatic stress disorder: An interim report. *American Journal of Psychiatry, 145*, 281–285.

Friedman, M. J. (1997a). Drug treatment for PTSD: Answers and questions. In R. Yehuda & A. C. McFarlane (Eds.), Psychobiology of posttraumatic stress disorder. *Annals of the New York Academy of Sciences, 821*, 359–371.

Friedman, M. J. (1997b). Posttraumatic stress disorder. *Journal of Clinical Psychiatry, 58*(Suppl. 9), 33–36.

Grossman, M., Kirsner, J., & Gillespie, I. (1963). Basal and Histalog-stimulated gastric secretion in control subjects and in patients with peptic ulcer or gastric cancer. *Gastroenterology, 45*, 14–26.

Halbreich, U., Rojansky, N., Palter, S., Tworek, H., Hissin, P., & Wang, K. (1995). Estrogen augments serotonergic activity in postmenopausal women. *Biological Psychiatry, 37*(7), 434–441.

Hamilton, J., & Yonkers, K. (1996). Sex differences in pharmacokinetics of psychotropic medication: Part I. Physiological basis for effects. In M. Jensvold, U. Halbriech, & J. Hamilton (Eds.), *Psychopharmacology and women: Sex, gender, and hormones* (pp. 11–42). Washington, DC: American Psychiatric Association.

Helzer, J. E., Robins, L. N., & McEvoy, L. (1987). Post-traumatic stress disorder in the general population: Findings from the Epidemiologic Catchment Area Survey. *New England Journal of Medicine, 317*, 1630–1634.

Horowitz, M., Maddern, G. J., & Chatterton, B. E. (1985). The normal menstrual cycle has no effect on gastric emptying. *British Journal of Obstetrics and Gynecology, 92*, 743–746.

Janoff-Bulman, R., & Frieze, I. H. (1987). The role of gender in reactions to criminal victimization. In R. C. Barnett & L. Biener (Eds.), *Gender and stress* (pp. 159–184). New York: Free Press.

Janowsky, D., Halbreich, U., & Rausch, J. (1996). Association between ovarian hormones, other hormones, emotional disorders and neurotransmitters. In M. Jensvold, U. Halbreich, & J. Hamilton (Eds.), *Psychopharmacology and women: Sex, gender, and hormones* (pp. 85–106). Washington, DC: American Psychiatric Association.

Jensvold, M., Halbreich, U., & Hamilton, J. (Eds.). (1996). *Psychopharmacology and women: Sex, gender, and hormones.* Washington, DC: American Psychiatric Association.

Katz, R. J., Lott, M. H., Arbus, P., Crocq, L., Herlobsen, P., Lingjaerde, O., Lopez, G., Loughrey, G. C., MacFarlane, D. J., McIvor, R., et al. (1994). Pharmacotherapy of post-traumatic stress disorder with a novel psychotropic. *Anxiety, 1*(4), 169–174.

Keane, T. M., & Kaloupek, D. G. (1998). Comorbid psychiatric disorders in PTSD: Implications for research. *Annals of New York Academy of Sciences*, 24–34.

Kellermann, G., & Luyten-Kellermann, M. (1978). Antipyrine metabolism in man. *Life Sciences, 23*, 2485–2490.

Kendall, D., Stancel, G., & Enna, S. (1982). The influence of sex hormones on antidepressant-induced alterations in neurotransmitter receptor binding. *Journal of Neuroscience, 2*, 354–360.

Kessler, R. C., Sonnega, A., Bromet, E., Hughes, M., & Nelson, C. B. (1995). Posttraumatic stress disorder in the National Comorbidity Survey. *Archives of General Psychiatry, 52*, 1048–1060.

Kirschbaum, C., Pirke, K. M., & Hellhammer, D. H. (1995). Preliminary evidence for reduced cortisol responsivity to psychological stress in women using oral contraceptive medication. *Psychoneuroendocrinology, 20*, 509–514.

Kolb, L. C. (1984). Propranolol and clonidine in the treatment of the chronic posttraumatic stress disorders of war. In B. A. van der Kolk (Ed.), *Post-traumatic stress disorder: Psychological and biological sequelae* (pp. 97–107). Washington, DC: American Psychiatric Press.

Kornstein, S. G., Schatzberg, A. F., Thase, M. E., Yonkers, K. A., McCullough, J. P., Keitner, G. I., Gelenberg, A. J., Davis, S. M., Harrison, W. M., & Keller, M. B. (2000). Gender differences in treatment response to sertraline versus imipramine in chronic depression. *American Journal of Psychiatry, 157*(9), 1445–1452.

Kosten, T., Frank, J., Dan, E., McDougle, C. J., & Giller, E. L., Jr. (1991). Pharmacotherapy for posttraumatic stress disorder using phenelzine or imipramine. *Journal of Nervous and Mental Disease, 179*, 366–370.

Letourneau, E. J., Resnick, H. S., Kilpatrick, D. G., Saunders, B. E., & Best, C. L. (1996). Comorbidity of sexual problems and posttraumatic stress disorder in female crime victims. *Behavior Therapy, 27*, 321–336.

Lindheim, S. R., Legro, R. S., Bernstein, L., Stanczyk, F. Z., Vijod, M. A., Presser, S. C.. & Lobo, R. A. (1992). Behavioral stress responses in premenopausal women and the effects of estrogen. *American Journal of Obstetrics and Gynecology, 167*(6), 1831–1836.

Lipper, S., Davidson, J. R., Grady, T. A., Edinger, J. D., Hammett, E. B., Mahorney, S. L., & Cavenar, J. O., Jr. (1986). Preliminary study of carbamazepine in posttraumatic stress disorder. *Psychosomatics, 27*(12), 849–854.

Llewellyn, A., & Stone, Z. N. (1998). Psychotropic medications in lactation. *Journal of Clinical Psychiatry, 59*(Suppl. 2), 41–52.

Mayersohn, M. (1982). Drug disposition. In K. Conrad & R. Bressler (Eds.), *Drug therapy for the elderly* (pp. 31–63). St. Louis, MO: Mosby.

Palmer, K., & Benfield, P. (1994). Fluvoxamine: An overview of its pharmacological properties and review of its therapeutic potential in nondepressive disorders. *CNS Drugs, 1,* 57–87.

Pollock, B. G. (1997). Gender differences in psychotropic drug metabolism. *Psychopharmacology Bulletin, 33,* 235–241.

Preskorn, S. H. (1997). Clinically relevant pharmacology of selective serotonin reuptake inhibitors: An overview with emphasis on pharmacokinetics and effects on oxidative drug metabolism. *Clinical Pharmacokinetics, 1,* 1–21.

Rao, S. S., Read, N. W., Brown, C., Bruce, C., & Holdsworth, C. D. (1987). Studies on the mechanism of bowel disturbance in ulcerative colitis. *Gastroenterology, 93*(5), 934–940.

Schneider, L. S., Small, G. W., Hamilton, S. H., Bystritsky, A., Nemeroff, C. B., & Meyers, B. S. (1997). Estrogen replacement and response to fluoxetine in a multi-center geriatric depression trial. *American Journal of Geriatric Psychiatry, 5,* 97–106.

Shalev, A. Y., Freedman, S., Peri, T., Brandes, D., Sahar, T., Orr, S. P., & Pitman, R. K. (1998). Prospective study of posttraumatic stress disorder and depression following trauma. *American Journal of Psychiatry, 155*(5), 630–637.

Shear, M. K. (1997). Anxiety disorders in women: Gender-related modulation of neurobiology and behavior. *Seminars in Reproductive Endocrinology, 15,* 69–76.

Sherwin, B. (1996). Menopause, early aging and elderly women. In M. Jensvold, U. Halbreich, & J. Hamilton (Eds.), *Psychopharmacology and women: Sex, gender, and hormones* (pp. 225–240). Washington, DC: American Psychiatric Press.

Sierles, F. S., Chen, J., McFarland, R. E., & Taylor, M. A. (1983). Post-traumatic stress disorder and concurrent psychiatric illness. *American Journal of Psychiatry, 140,* 1177–1179.

Solomon, S. D., & Davidson, J. R. T. (1997). Trauma: Prevalence, impairment, service use, and cost. *Journal of Clinical Psychiatry, 58*(Suppl. 9), 5–11.

Stahl, S. (1997). Reproductive hormones as adjuncts to psychotropic medications in women. *Essential Psychopharmacology, 2,* 147–164.

Steiner, M., Wheadon, D. E., Kreider, M. S., et al. (1993). *Antidepressant response to paroxetine by gender.* Paper presented at the 146th annual meeting of the American Psychiatric Association, San Francisco, CA.

van der Kolk, B. A., Dreyfuss, D., Michaels, M., Shera, D., Berkowitz, R., Fisler, R., & Saxe, G. (1994). Fluoxetine in posttraumatic stress disorder. *Journal of Clinical Psychiatry, 55,* 517–522.

Wilson, K., Oram, M., Horth, C. E., & Burnett, D. (1982). The influence of the menstrual cycle on the metabolism and clearance of metaqualone. *British Journal of Clinical Pharmacology, 14,* 333–339.

Yonkers, K., & Hamilton, J. (1996). Sex differences in pharmacokinetics of psychotropic medication: Part II. Effects on selected psychotropics. In M. Jensvold, U. Halbreich, & J. Hamilton (Eds.), *Psychopharmacology and women: Sex, gender, and hormones* (pp. 43–72). Washington, DC: American Psychiatric Press.

Yonkers, K. A., Rush, A. J., Kornstein, S. G. et al. (1995). *Gender differences in the response to pharmacotherapy among early onset dysthymics.* Paper presented at the annual meeting of the American College of Neuropsychopharmacology.

Zlotnick, C., Warshaw, M., Shea, M. T., Allsworth, J., Pearlstein, T., & Keller, M. B. (1999). Chronicity in posttraumatic stress disorder (PTSD) and predictors of course of comorbid PTSD in patients with anxiety disorders. *Journal of Traumatic Stress, 12*(1), 89–100.

13 | Gender, Trauma Themes, and PTSD

Narratives of Male and Female Survivors

ELIZABETH D. KRAUSE
RUTH R. DeROSA
SUSAN ROTH

Traumatic events often create emotions and expectations that inform or challenge individuals' core beliefs about themselves, their relationships, and their life experiences. In addition, the impact of trauma may overwhelm routine coping processes and lead survivors to experience emotions and impulses that contradict their previous way of relating in the world and/or establish maladaptive patterns of behavior. One of the most central forces influencing how we view ourselves and the world, as well as how we function socially, is our gender socialization. In our culture, gender often forms one foundation of an individual's identity. How survivors respond to their traumas is likely shaped by their gender role socialization, and likewise, their gender identity may be influenced by the experience of trauma. This chapter explores how gender influences the processing of abuse-related traumatic events by focusing on qualitative research and case studies. Specifically, it reviews how gender, trauma themes, and posttraumatic stress may be associated for adult survivors of physical and sexual abuse.

Gender may be viewed as a complex aspect of identity that is shaped by multiple factors, including cultural and environmental influences, internalized schemas (stereotypes and social scripts), and human physiology. Men and women vary in the degree to which they identify with and behave in accordance with the cultural attributes assigned to their biological sex. Because one's sex is usually assigned at birth, men and women are exposed to profoundly different socialization experiences that are likely to exaggerate and intensify actual sex differences (Saxe & Wolfe, 1999). An understanding of the interaction between gender and posttraumatic processing would be advanced by a consideration of the influence of both sex role socialization and gender role identity.

Narrative investigations and case studies of male and female survivors of abuse support the notion that gender role identity plays a significant part in a person's adaptation to trauma and may be associated with posttraumatic stress disorder (PTSD). For instance, several studies have found that male survivors suffering from PTSD symptoms often report a lack of identification with their own gender and/or hypermasculine behavior (e.g., Bruckner & Johnson, 1987; Gill & Tutty, 1997; Lisak, 1995). Female survivors seeking treatment for PTSD symptoms have described feeling disconnected from other women, having difficulty identifying as female, and/or overidentifying with many of the negative attributes associated with femininity (Herman & Hirschman, 1981; Lebowitz & Roth, 1994; Roth & Newman, 1995). For example, women with PTSD often report passivity, helplessness, and a preoccupation with caring for others, often at the expense of caring for themselves.

These findings highlight how adaptation to abuse may be complicated by the effects of gender role identity, stereotypes, and sex role socialization. They also generate additional questions, such as what aspects of being a man or a woman influence difficulties in gender identification in the aftermath of abuse? What are the more personal meanings of abuse that may differ for men and women and be influential in PTSD symptomatology? Answering such questions may be critical for the development of successful therapeutic interventions for both male and female survivors.

One way investigators have come to understand both the processing of trauma and the development of PTSD is to examine the meanings people attribute to their traumatic experience and to their posttraumatic self (i.e., Horowitz, 1986, 1997; Janoff-Bulman, 1985; McCann & Pearlman, 1990; Roth & Newman, 1993, 1995). Researchers of this tradition have begun to identify and measure specific trauma meanings or themes that seem to predict chronic PTSD and often become targets of therapeutic change. These themes include cognitive–affective categories, such as helplessness, loss, rage, and self-blame. Although a number of studies have explored gender differences in rates of PTSD, little attention has been devoted to gender identity issues in the trauma theme literature. The kind of narrative analysis that has been used to evaluate trauma themes provides a naturalistic and rich context in which to begin answering some of our questions regarding gender, trauma meanings, and posttraumatic stress.

Thus, the current chapter begins with a review of therapy case studies and narrative investigations of trauma themes for male and female survivors of physical and sexual abuse. Unfortunately, trauma theme studies have tended to examine only one sex exclusively (e.g., Lebowitz & Roth, 1994; Lisak, 1995), limiting our ability to make generalizations across gender in terms of theory and treatment approaches.

To address this limitation, the second half of the chapter compares more directly men's and women's gender role socialization experiences and trauma theme processing. First, we provide a brief overview of some key sex role socialization issues. Then, thematic narratives of male and female survivors are examined and contrasted. In these comparisons, subtle, but meaningful, gender differences emerge in how salient trauma themes are conceptualized and how the survivor chooses or is driven to attempt to resolve them. We argue that gender-relevant constructions about abuse may contribute to the development and chronicity of PTSD symptoms, especially when these constructions restrict gender-discrepant emotions and prevent survivors from reframing trauma themes in meaningful and self-protective ways. In conclusion, we make recommendations about how the association between gender, trauma themes, and PTSD may be studied in future research and incorporated into treatments with abuse survivors.

TRAUMA THEMES FOR MALE AND FEMALE ABUSE SURVIVORS

Overview of the Trauma Theme Literature

Theories of PTSD that address social, cognitive, and emotional components have emphasized the wider impact of trauma and its consequences by focusing on the meanings people attribute to their traumatic experience and to their posttraumatic self (Horowitz, 1986, 1997; Janoff-Bulman, 1985; McCann & Pearlman, 1990; Roth & Newman, 1993, 1995). These theorists view PTSD as more a "disorder of meaning" than a "disorder of anxiety" (Meichenbaum, 1995). Individuals routinely develop narratives of significant life events that include descriptions of behavioral and affective reactions, causal explanations, and evaluations of changes and losses in their lives. Constructing one's experience in this way provides some coherence and meaning that may be essential to psychological well-being (Harvey, Orbuch, Weber, Merback, & Alt, 1992; Roth, Lebowitz, & DeRosa, 1997). Exposure to traumatic events tends to challenge adaptive representational processes, and in the worst case, may lead to "psychic death," a failure to engage in meaningful symbolization of experience (Lifton, 1979).

Horowitz's (1986, 1997) formulation of stress response syndromes was the first to link interruptions in meaningful symbolization and cognitive assimilation to the development and maintenance of PTSD. He hypothesizes that individuals have a psychological need to integrate new information with existing cognitive schemas. He defines "schemas" as internal representations of the world and self that have both conscious and unconscious aspects. A traumatic event presents an individual with information that is discrepant with these schemas. The greater the discrepancy, the more the new information may be affectively charged and cognitively avoided.

However, avoidance only maintains storage of the event in "active memory." With active memory stimulated, the mind continues to attempt integration of the novel material, causing memories of the trauma to intrude into consciousness in the form of flashbacks, nightmares, and/or unwanted thoughts. Horowitz argues that for resolution to occur, survivors must comprehend the emotional and cognitive impact of the trauma. Thus, theoretically, nonresolution or nonintegration of the traumatic material leads to the development and maintenance of PTSD symptomatology.

Theorists who have focused on interpersonal abuse have observed that assault victims, especially sexual assault victims, often encounter such schema-discrepant information that they engage in a variety of reactions that prevent them from integrating the event(s). Clinicians and researchers have observed that some victims overaccommodate or alter their beliefs, attributions, and expectations about themselves, others, and the world, in an extreme or maladaptive way (e.g., "Since I was raped, I do not trust men, any of them!") (Resick & Schnicke, 1992). Thus, moderate, rather than extreme, accommodation of traumatic material into one's schemas has become a goal of many therapies for abuse-related distress.

Researchers of this tradition have begun to identify specific trauma meanings or themes that seem to be salient in the process of recovering from physical and/or sexual abuse. For recovery or resolution to occur, these themes may need to be narrated in a way that both enhances their expression and puts them in perspective. It is these themes that researchers have tried to measure in order to represent the broad effects of trauma and to identify targets of therapeutic change beyond basic symptoms (Roth et al., 1997).

Although research has examined the types of trauma themes that arise in narratives of male and female survivors, the studies have included either men or women, but not both. In addition, the male and female trauma theme literatures have never been reviewed together, thus limiting our ability to make distinctions about the ways in which men and women might approach and process trauma themes differently. Understanding abuse sequelae within a framework that combines gender identity issues and cognitive–affective processing may have important therapeutic implications. This section reviews the trauma theme literature for women survivors, and then for men survivors.

Female Survivors and Trauma Themes

Although theoretical accounts of trauma themes are based on the experiences of men (i.e., combat veterans) and women (i.e., sexual abuse), most theme research has focused on female samples. Several common or universal abuse-related themes have been identified in female adult survivors' narratives in therapy transcripts (Finkelhor & Browne, 1985; Janoff-Bulman,

1985; Krupnick & Horowitz, 1981; McCann & Pearlman, 1990; Roth & Batson, 1997), trauma interviews (Luo, 1998; Roth & Lebowitz, 1988; Roth & Newman, 1993, 1995; Roth & Batson, 1993), and projective tests (Liem, O'Toole, & James, 1996). These themes include clinically meaningful affective and cognitive categories that seem initially to have been avoided following the abuse but tend to be confronted over the course of recovery. Although various names and slightly different definitions have been applied to many of the themes, the most common ones can be consolidated into the following categories: helplessness, rage, fear, loss, shame, self-blame/guilt, benign/meaningful world, trust, reciprocity, alienation, and legitimacy (Roth & Lebowitz, 1988; Roth & Newman, 1993, 1995; Roth & Batson, 1993, 1997). Definitions for these themes are presented in Table 13.1.

Evidence of reliability and validity of the themes in abused women's posttraumatic process has come from empirical studies using questionnaires (Coffey, Leitenberg, Henning, Turner, & Bennet, 1996; Edwards & Donaldson, 1989; Dutton, Burghardt, Perrin, Chrestman, & Halle, 1994) or quantitative coding systems (Roth & Lebowitz, 1988; Roth & Newman, 1995) designed to measure the saliency or resolution of each theme (i.e., the extent to which the victim has come to understand the relationship between the theme and his or her trauma, so that he or she is no longer preoccupied with or driven by the experience). Further support for the themes has come

TABLE 13.1. Summary of Trauma Themes

Helplessness—for example, a feeling that someone else has absolute power over you

Rage—for example, a feeling that your rage will be emotionally overwhelming

Fear—for example, behavior that is phobic and protective

Loss—for example, a feeling that a traumatic experience stole something from you

Self-blame/guilt—for example, a belief or feeling that you are in some way responsible for abuse perpetrated against you

Legitimacy—for example, a feeling of being deviant in your reaction to abuse

Shame—for example, feelings of humiliation for having been exposed to abuse

Alienation—for example, a feeling of being different and set apart from other people

Benign/meaningful world—for example, a belief that the world is unsafe, unrewarding, and/or unjust

Trust—for example, an expectation of others being unhelpful, capable of deception, betrayal, and exploitation

Self-worth—for example, a sense of being flawed or damaged

Reciprocity—for example, a feeling of being unworthy of giving and receiving love

Note. Adapted from Roth and Batson (1997). Copyright 1997 by The Free Press, Simon & Schuster, Inc. Adapted by permission.

from psychotherapy studies with rape and incest survivors in which treatment explicitly addressed many of the themes (Chard, Weaver, & Resick, 1997; Morgan & Cummings, 1999; Resick & Schnicke, 1992, 1993; Roth & Batson, 1997). Each of these treatment studies found theme-focused interventions to be associated with pre- to posttreatment reductions in PTSD symptomatology. In addition, both Morgan and Cummings (1999) and Roth and Batson (1997) found significant improvements in trauma theme resolution over the course of therapy.

Although many of the trauma themes described might be expected to be affected by gender role issues, the discourse on themes for female survivors has mostly occurred within a gender-neutral framework. This may be because men were initially left out of trauma theme research and treatment studies for sexual abuse survivors. Without a comparison group, female gender identity issues may not have seemed salient enough to address explicitly. Though theme-focused therapies may implicitly refer to gender constraints for women survivors, the treatment protocols have not discussed explicitly how the themes may be influenced by feminine gender socialization, and why challenging gender norms may be an important component of the therapeutic process.

A few exceptions to this gender-neutral framework come from feminist research and therapy approaches. For instance, Lebowitz and Roth (1994) examined how cultural beliefs or constructions about women, sexuality, and rape influence women's responses to sexual trauma. During trauma interviews, survivors spontaneously incorporated culturally generated constructions of femaleness, sexuality, and the meaning of rape into their descriptions of how they experienced the episode. They described what it means to be socialized as a woman in this society, which was linked to their experience of being raped. In addition, some women described how rape may function as a form of social control. These findings illuminate the impact of gender identity on women's attempts to make sense of their traumatic experiences during the recovery process. Lebowitz and Roth's study however, does not discuss explicitly how gender may be associated with the variety of themes that have been identified as central to traumatic responses and recovery, such as rage, helplessness, loss, and self-blame.

One study has examined the impact of a gender-based intervention on the saliency of trauma themes for female survivors. Morgan and Cummings (1999) compared a feminist group therapy for sexual abuse and a no-treatment control in terms of pre- to posttreatment change in trauma themes and PTSD symptoms. The intervention was based largely on Herman's (1992) feminist empowerment model; thus, it incorporated a critique of gender into the topics covered (i.e., self-nurturance, personal boundaries, self-blame, anger, relationships with mothers, dissociation, intimate relationships, self-awareness). Common trauma themes (anger and betrayal, guilt and shame, powerlessness, sadness and loss, vulnerability and isolation) and PTSD symptoms were measured with a standardized assessment instrument developed by Edwards and Donaldson (1989). Morgan and Cummings (1999) found significant pre- to posttreatment decreases in both trauma themes and PTSD symptoms for participants in the feminist group but not for those in the control group. Their study provides initial empirical support for the usefulness of addressing gender issues in trauma-focused therapies for women. By evaluating change in themes, in addition to PTSD symptoms, their findings verify the important association between themes and symptoms, and depict a complex portrait of the ways in which trauma and therapy may challenge schemas of self, others, gender, and so on.

Male Survivors and Trauma Themes

To date, most empirical studies of trauma themes and PTSD, and all of the theme-related treatment research, have failed to include male survivors. This may be because of higher rates of trauma reported by women compared to men, women's tendency to seek treatment more often than men, and cultural assumptions about abuse involving male perpetrators and female victims (Ellerstein & Canavan, 1980). Neglecting male survivors limits our ability to examine important gender differences in the meaning, intensity, and pattern of emergence of the themes in the recovery process. Such variations might point to different psychosocial predictors of traumatic stress in men and women. Considering the lack of systematic research on trauma themes and PTSD symptoms with abused men, the following review necessarily relies on a small number of qualitative studies and case reports.

Recent literature on male sexual abuse survivors has identified some of the same themes highlighted in women survivors' narratives. In addition, it has begun to address issues that may be significant in men's adaptation to sexual trauma. For instance, Lisak (1994) conducted a comprehensive thematic analysis of interviews with adult males with a history of childhood sexual abuse. He found support for the importance of the trauma themes often described for female abuse survivors, including anger, betrayal, fear, helplessness, isolation/alienation, legitimacy, loss, self-blame/guilt, and shame/ humiliation. In addition, Lisak found evidence for the salience of several themes that were not identified in studies with female survivors, including masculinity issues (damage to one's subjective sense of maleness or masculinity), homosexuality issues (irrational dread and loathing of homosexuality and homosexual people), and problems with sexuality (conflicts about sexual orientation and sexual difficulties).

Identification of these gender-relevant themes provides validation for the clinically based observations of others who have worked with male survivors (e.g., Dimock, 1988; Friedman, 1994; Harker, 1997; Hunter, 1990; Myers, 1989; Scott, 1992; Zamanian & Adams, 1997). These clinician researchers speculate that masculine gender role socialization, including social stigma against vulnerability, weakness, and homosexuality, may induce an overwhelming sense of powerlessness, shame, and silence among male survivors, which may in turn limit cognitive and emotional processing of traumatic events. Based on their work with male survivors, Lisak (1995) and others (Dimock, 1988; Friedman, 1994; Harker, 1997; Hunter, 1990; Myers, 1989; Scott, 1992; Zamanian & Adams, 1997) delineate how trauma themes and masculine conflicts might be confronted in therapy.

The work with male survivors has contributed significantly to the trauma literature by introducing masculine gender socialization into the study of traumatic stress and recovery. Unfortunately, no outcome studies have evaluated the efficacy of treatments that incorporate the themes, nor examined quantitatively changes in the themes over the course of psychotherapy with men. In addition, the studies have primarily included samples of Caucasian men and have neglected to consider issues that may be more prevalent among culturally diverse groups of male survivors. These research gaps might be expected considering that it was not until the mid- to late 1980s that attention first turned to males with a history of sexual abuse (Urquiza & Keating, 1990).

Summary

Overall, literature on trauma themes in male and female survivors' post-traumatic adaptation suggests that studies have focused on one sex or the other, and until recently, little attention has been devoted to addressing gender socialization issues directly in treatment. Although some studies have identified themes that may be particular to men (Lisak, 1994) or women (Roth & Lebowitz, 1988), altogether, more similarities than differences have been found in terms of the *types* of themes that are salient, including rage, fear, helplessness, loss, shame, self-blame/guilt, legitimacy, alienation, and trust/betrayal.

In addition to identifying common, important themes for male and female survivors, the reviewed studies suggest that gender identity schemas may be challenged by abuse for both men and women. These findings indicate that the roles of feminine and masculine gender issues in posttraumatic adaptation are more than just individual trauma themes. Trauma-related challenges to gender identification may lead survivors to engage in stereotyped thoughts and behaviors that attempt to reinforce their gender identity (i.e., hypermasculinity) or justify their schema-discrepant experiences (i.e., "I must have wanted it."). Recent theories of traumatic stress (Horowitz, 1986, 1997) and PTSD (Resick & Schnicke, 1992) suggest that such overaccommodating responses are likely to interfere with traumatic processing. Thus, male and female socialization experiences and extent of gender identification might be expected to have an impact on all of the trauma themes, particularly how the themes are expressed, and how the survivor chooses or is driven to attempt to resolve them.

In the remainder of this chapter, men's and women's gender role socialization experiences and trauma theme processing are compared directly. First, we provide a brief overview of some key issues surrounding gender socialization. Then, men's and women's thematic narratives are examined and contrasted. This detailed analysis demonstrates that some themes, assumed to be the same for men and women, differ in important ways, mostly as a function of gender role socialization. In addition, we suggest that affective trauma themes (i.e., fear and rage) often arise differently over the course of therapy for male and female survivors, and that this differential process may result from stereotypes and social codes regarding gender and emotional expression.

GENDER SOCIALIZATION OF ROLES, EMOTIONAL EXPRESSIVENESS, AND SEXUALITY

Gender role socialization refers to the process by which men and women are conditioned to feel, think, and behave in ways that are consistent with their culture's established norms of masculinity and femininity. Although gender development and the learning of sex role attributes are a lifelong process (Kagan, 1976), one's gender identity is firmly established as early as the age of 3 (Money & Wiedeking, 1980). Expectations about the ways in which males and females function in almost every personal and social domain are influenced by learned gender roles (Maccoby & Jacklin, 1974; Pleck, 1981).

Reviews of gender stereotypes regarding social roles and emotional expressiveness suggest that women are expected to have lower status and power positions (Miller, 1976); to do more family and child caretaking; to invest in relationships to a greater extent (Jordan, Kaplan, Miller, Stiver, & Surrey, 1991); to express more affiliative emotions, such as warmth and gratitude; and to demonstrate less physical aggression and anger (Brody, 1993) than men. Men, on the other hand, are expected to attain higher status and power; to maintain greater personal independence; to be providers, protectors, and warriors to a greater extent (Gilmore, 1990); to have stronger moral authority (Gilligan, 1982); and to express fewer emotions associated with vulnerability (Brody, 1993) than women.

Gender stereotypes have also pervaded the area of sexuality and sexual behavior. Reviews suggest that men are expected to have a greater sexual drive, to be more experienced with sex, to be more active sexually at a younger age, and to initiate sex more than do women (Bolton & MacEachron, 1988; Hoyenga & Hoyenga, 1979). Women's sexuality on the other hand tends to be conceptualized by the doctrine of feminine passivity or by the poles of "virgin" and "whore" (Lebowitz & Roth, 1994); that is, cultural messages abound that dichotomize women into sexual categories: A woman is considered either virginal, pure, and nonsexual, or dirty and promiscuous, if she is sexually active, whether she has sex by choice or against her will. In addition, women have traditionally been taught that it is their role not only to restrict their own sexual activity but also to set limits for male sexual behavior (Waites, 1993).

Research has demonstrated considerable cultural agreement regarding these stereotypes, especially the agentic–expressive distinction between men and women (Basow, 1992). Nevertheless, individual and cultural differences exist in terms of the extent to which men and women are exposed to and identify with these stereotypes. For example, African American men and women are stereotypically viewed as more similar to each other in terms of expressiveness and competence than are Anglo American men and women (Basow, 1992). Still, for most individuals in the United States, a number of these gender stereotypes are likely to be part of an identity schema that is active and conscious to different degrees and under difference circumstances. Stereotypes both mirror and construct the reality of gender differences (Brody, 1997). Over time, social codes are likely to become internalized, influencing men and women to express various emotions and behaviors while inhibiting others. Gender stereotypes are frequently used as a model against which individuals judge themselves. Consequently, whether or not individuals embody the positive characteristics associated with their gender may directly impact self-esteem.

In the face of trauma, when routine coping processes and core beliefs about oneself, one's relationships, and the social world are severely challenged, individuals may be especially unsure of how to respond. Traumatic events may introduce such novel circumstances that individuals may turn to external social cues, as well as internalized stereotypes and social scripts, to determine how to cope and make sense of their experiences. Thus, physical or sexual violence may be especially likely to activate gender role schemas regarding roles, emotionality, and sexuality.

COMPARING THEMATIC NARRATIVES
OF MALE AND FEMALE SURVIVORS

Considering this socialization framework, two conceptual questions are addressed in a comparison of themes identified in both male and female survivors' posttraumatic narratives: (1) How might gender issues influence men and women to struggle differently in resolving common trauma themes?, and (2) how might these gender-related struggles influence their own gender identity development? The examples chosen to compare men's and women's thematic responses come from published case studies and qualitative investigations of abuse survivors. We focus on studies that have identified groups of themes that seem central to PTSD and highlight the presence and/or absence of gender issues. Although there is no way to establish the representativeness of these samples, the consistency across investigators is compelling.

In terms of the characteristics of the individuals included, most studies of trauma themes have primarily sampled middle-class Caucasian Americans. However, some recent studies have examined trauma themes in the narratives of other groups, including African American and Chinese female survivors of sexual abuse. When available, narratives or findings from these studies are incorporated into the thematic comparisons. Although the data are currently too limited to consider the role of ethnic identity in regard to thematic adaptation or meaning making, the role of ethnic identity may be as central to an individual's traumatic experience as gender, and should be considered in future investigations.

Loss

Many male and female survivors associate their abuse with the destruction and loss of innocence. In addition, common coping responses, such as emotional numbing and dissociation, lead many individuals to have severe memory loss or selective memory for positive events. Recalling the abuse in therapy often leads individuals to sense that something has been stolen from them or that their whole sense of self has been disrupted. Men and women often similarly describe mourning for lost purity, naivete, and other psychological facets of childhood.

On closer examination, however, sex differences emerge in terms of the particular aspects of self that are perceived as lost following abuse. Many sexual abuse survivors describe feeling as if the trauma stripped them permanently of a positive gender identity. This overaccommodation to a "damaged" victim role tends to be related to feelings of loss and alienation from one's own sex. Although both men and women describe this experience, their narratives reflect differential gender stereotypes.

For women, loss of virginity or of what is socially considered a "perfect/pure" female body following assault causes survivors to feel that they have lost their right to womanhood or positive feminine sexuality:

> **Female S:** [After the rape I felt like] I am no longer a nice middle-class girl. . . . That was like proof that something irrevocable had happened and you can't get back. You've really lost something. . . . You've really changed. (Roth & Lebowitz, 1988, p. 93)

> **Female S:** If you want to know the truth, I feel angry about being a woman . . . and that bothers me a lot, feeling alienated from my own femaleness. I feel like I'm an inferior person because I'm female. In a way, I feel victimized by being female. And, the rape supports that . . . that's probably the thing

that interferes most with my happiness right now—not feeling happy about being a woman, not feeling good about myself as a human, who happens to be female. . . . Whenever I feel that alienated from myself, I feel bad about being a woman and unable to feel good about myself as a person, being female. That's the most painful thing. And the rape is so tied into that I can't sort it out. (Lebowitz & Roth, 1994, pp. 377–378)

Similarly, in a qualitative study of Chinese women with a history of childhood sexual abuse, survivors described feeling that they were different from and worse than other women: "stained," "worthless," and "incompetent" (Luo, 1998, p. 1017). If the rape coincided with the loss of their virginity, they often described no longer being "complete" (p. 1017). In addition, many worried about the consequences of their lost virginity on their self-value, sexual desirability, and future marriages (p. 1021): "In the future, how am I going to tell my husband that I have not been a virgin for so many years? . . . Will he believe my incest story, given that I have been withholding it for so long?"

These examples demonstrate the intricate ways in which a woman's identity may become intertwined with social constructions of female sexuality. As mentioned earlier, female sexuality tends to be culturally conceptualized by the poles of "virgin" and "whore." Indeed, in some Asian cultures, the loss of a woman's chastity is considered comparable to death (Luo, 1998). Considering this rigid bifurcation, women who are sexually abused may feel driven to overaccommodate to what they perceive as a negative feminine schema or, alternatively, to reject femininity following sexual traumatization. One of the factors maintaining female abuse survivors' low self-esteem is their lost virginity or the perception of their bodies as "dirtied." Being unable to "sort out" their own identity from social constructions of their female and sexual selves seems to prevent survivors from accommodating the experience in more positive, self-promoting ways. Consequently, they remain overwhelmed with PTSD symptoms and depression.

Many male survivors experience the powerlessness and vulnerability of abuse as a loss of their right to manhood:

Male S: Hell, I've got no manhood left. . . . He's made me into a woman. (Myers, 1989, p. 210)

Male S: When I got this job finally, for the first time I felt like one of them, you know, a guy. I felt very macho. I was one of the macho guys. I did it. I was a cowboy, I found a way to do it. But you know, inside really, it wasn't real. I was faking it and I knew it. (Lisak, 1995, p. 261)

Male S: You felt gay because you had been in bed with men. It's disgusting. . . . I've never been able to wipe that feeling away, you know. . . . It was terrible because . . . there aren't any gay he-men out there, are there? (Harker, 1997, p. 204)

These quotations resonate with other studies, which found that male survivors tend to equate threatened masculinity with loss of power, control, identity, selfhood, confidence, and independence (e.g., Myers, 1989). Indeed, in these narratives, male survivors emphasize the association they perceive between abuse and loss of masculinity and "acceptable sexuality" (e.g., heterosexuality). These constructions might be expected, considering our culture's strict bisection of masculinity and femininity–homosexuality. Masculinity is defined as much by the qualities it represents (e.g., control, independence, self-assertion, aggression, competitiveness, power, and strength) as by those qualities it rejects, namely, all that is considered feminine (e.g., vulnerability, passivity, dependence) (Chodorow, 1978; Lisak, 1995). Indeed, the lack of agency and the abject helplessness inherent in the experience of being sexually violated is especially threatening to masculine identity, because the abused male knows that these emotions breach cultural expectations of masculinity (Lisak, 1995). Thus, if a man cannot live up to these constructions of masculinity, then he may be deemed the alternative: feminine or gay. For traditional men, the extreme fear and disgust initiated by these threats prevent them from confronting their sexual concerns and exploring related meanings. As a result, they continue to be plagued with fears of inadequacy and to be denied positive identification with their maleness. In turn, their inability to reframe the experience in more tolerable ways most likely maintains PTSD symptomatology.

Although both male and female survivors describe cognitive shifts from positive to negative schemas of gender and sexuality, they may respond differently to the experience of loss. In some cases, feelings of having lost the alleged positive aspects of femininity lead female survivors not only to believe that they are "stained" or "worthless" but also to respond in ways that they feel confirm this negative self-schema:

> **Female S:** The marked thing I felt was that I had no choice but to be sexually active because this had happened to me. . . . I wasn't a virgin and I wasn't valued for that. . . . If the men I had semirelationships with wanted sex, what right did I have to deny them? Because I was a sleazy whore. (Roth & Lebowitz, 1988, p. 95)

In Luo's study (1998), Chinese survivors described similar responses to their abuse. One survivor changed her life completely: She slept during the day and had sex with strangers at night. Another survivor reported feeling guilty about her sexual desires since the abuse and considered herself an "evil" woman because of them. In addition, female survivors have been found to endorse rape-supportive attitudes to a greater extent than women without an abuse history (Briere, Smiljanich, & Henschel, 1994).

Many male survivors respond to feelings of lost masculinity by engaging in "hypermasculine compensation" (Lisak, 1995), exaggerated attempts to convince themselves and others that they embody all of the highly

stereotyped masculine characteristics, including interpersonal aggressiveness, inflated heterosexuality, and virulent homophobia:

> **Male S:** You had to portray a tough character . . . like smashing up, getting
> violent with things, furniture, cars, people. Like we were always beating
> something up. . . . We always had scruffy clothes, long hair—you had to
> portray this being tough. (Harker, 1997, pp. 202–203)

> **Male S:** By the time I was sixteen, I was having intercourse fairly often with
> a few different girls. By seventeen or eighteen, there were some occasional
> prostitutes and lots of masturbating. Overall, there have been many, many
> sex partners and frequent masturbation. I have basically done the things I
> always thought were masculine to do. (Dimock, 1988, pp. 207–208)

> **Male S:** When I'm not sexually active, I get down on myself, feel less confi-
> dent as a man, and also doubt my sexual orientation. (Myers, 1989, p. 210)

> **Male S:** I would have these fantasies all the time where I would beat up ho-
> mosexuals, pound on them with real violence. And I understand now where
> that was coming from—they threatened me. (Lisak, 1995, p. 262)

As seen in these examples, male survivors often rely on social constructions of masculinity to inform their efforts to compensate for lost gender
identification. Unfortunately, because these standards represent myths of
"he-man" masculinity and sexuality (Harker, 1997, p. 201), and are thus
unattainable, survivors are often left feeling inadequate and even "less con-
fident as a man." Still, these activities may be socially reinforced, because
they are consistent with cultural expectations, and internally reinforced, because they provide an immediate, albeit short-lived sense of control, confidence, and unemotionality.

Self-Blame/Guilt

Self-blame and feelings of guilt derive from the tendency of survivors to
hold themselves responsible in some way for the abuse perpetrated against
them. Such self-reproach may refer to a victim's feelings of culpability surrounding disclosure or lack of disclosure of the abuse (Lifton, 1996; Roth
& Newman, 1995). Additionally, it may refer to a victim's fear of initiating
the abuse (e.g., drinking too much, drawing attention to oneself) or of not
preventing it (e.g., avoiding the situation, fighting back). Self-blame tends
to be a common response of survivors, because it serves a number of seemingly self-protective functions, such as restoring a sense of control and
avoiding the experience of rage (Roth et al., 1997). However, it is not adaptive for victims to maintain the belief that they were to blame for the abuse
and its aftermath. Several studies have found significant relationships be-

tween self-blame and poor long-term adjustment (i.e., depression and PTSD) in women who have been sexually abused in childhood (Coffey et al., 1996; Wyatt & Newcomb, 1990).

Narrative studies and case examples have identified self-blame and guilt as salient themes in both men's and women's posttraumatic responses. However, when male and female survivors' descriptions of self-blame are compared side by side, subtle variations emerge that reflect how gender socialization may influence male and female survivors to conceptualize their self-reproach.

Women's narratives evidence their belief that they did something inappropriate, usually sexual, to initiate the abuse. Female survivors seem to blame themselves from the start as the instigator rather than as the victim, an interpretation that tends to be followed by characterological self-blame, such as "I must be a slut":

> Female S: I kept it inside and blamed myself for all that happened. I probably was a slut. (Calhoun & Resick, 1993, p. 71)

> Female S: He'd come into the room and I thought, I was making up the bed and I did something to entice him. I thought maybe my previous interest in sexual stuff had caused it. (Roth & Lebowitz, 1988, p. 93)

> Female S: I didn't even want my boobs to grow. I thought that would be temptation. I didn't want to look pretty, you know, that would be temptation. I always tempted him, ha. I felt really bad and I felt guilty. (Roth & Lebowitz, 1988, p. 93)

These narratives reveal the extent to which a woman's sexuality becomes intimately intertwined with her identity following sexual trauma and informs her understanding of her role in the event. Instead of blaming their perpetrators for objectifying their bodies and harming them, these survivors focus on how their bodies attracted abusive attention, and they reframe their sexuality, and therefore themselves, as deviant. These responses might be expected considering the sexual objectification of women's bodies in our culture (Fredrickson & Roberts, 1997). "Sexual objectification" refers to the socially sanctioned process by which a woman's sexual body is seen as an entity separate from her person, reduced to a mere instrument, or regarded as if it were capable of representing her (Bartky, 1990). When objectified, women are treated as bodies that exist for the use and pleasure of others, particularly men (Fredrickson & Roberts, 1997). When a survivor sees herself as a sexual object, not only does she feel responsible for the attention and abuse she receives, but also she believes she essentially deserves it (e.g., "I probably was a slut," and, from a quote presented earlier in the chapter, "If the men I had semirelationships with wanted sex, what right did I have to deny them? Because I was a sleazy whore").

In addition, the cognitive responses of female survivors ("I did something," "I tempted him") make sense considering cultural messages about women's role as sexual socializers. As described earlier, women have traditionally been taught that it is their role not only to restrict their own sexual activity but also to set limits for male sexual behavior. Beginning with biblical Eve, human anxieties and conflicts regarding sexuality have been blamed on women (Waites, 1993). The quotation, "I didn't even want my boobs to grow" highlights the extent to which survivors may feel they should suppress their own sexuality, even their body's development, in order to protect *men* from temptation.

Alternatively, male survivors seem to blame themselves, not for provoking the abuse, but for not being "man" enough or "smart" enough to prevent or stop it:

> **Male S:** I used to blame myself for it. I always thought I was a real smart two year old. So why didn't I get out of it. I blame myself. I don't blame him. I could have got out of it; I was plenty smart enough. (Lisak, 1994, p. 543)

> **Male S:** I do think I have some understanding of why I was a good candidate for abuse, but I think that deep down, if I were a real man, I should have been able to stop the abuse. It is hard for me as a male to tell people I was abused, because I am afraid they'll say I'm gay or that I'm a wimp for being stupid enough to let some fag abuse me. There is a part of me that keeps telling myself that I'm gay or a wimp because I let some asshole touch me. (Dimock, 1988, pp. 209–210)

These interpretations demonstrate the emphasis men place on the strength of their minds (intellect or suspicions) and how this power is supposed to protect them from vulnerability or victimization. Equally important seems to be their distress over not being physically strong enough to intervene and protect themselves. These attributions over time may lead to derogatory self-statements, such as "I am weak and vulnerable" or "I must be a wimp." In other words, not being smart enough or strong enough to protect oneself leads male survivors to fear that they are not a "real man." These responses might be expected considering cultural expectations about acceptable masculine behavior. In particular, two tenets of masculinity seem to be violated by the experience of sexual abuse: (1) societal beliefs that a man is expected to be able to defend himself against assault (Groth & Burgess, 1980), and (2) the male ethic of self-reliance (Finkelhor, 1984). The extent to which the male survivor's explanation of his abuse contradicts these cultural messages seems to be associated with self-blame, self-hatred, and PTSD symptomatology.

This comparison suggests that gender socialization may influence important differences in the issues that are salient to men and women surrounding the theme of self-blame. Considering that self-blame of any kind is associated with greater PTSD symptomatology and disruptions of beliefs (Edwards & Donaldson, 1989; Frazier & Schauben, 1994), confronting the relationships between gender socialization and these types of self-blame may assist men and women in contextualizing their attributions, redirecting blame to more appropriate sources, increasing self-esteem, and reducing PTSD symptomatology.

Helplessness/Powerlessness

Loss of control and having one's physical and psychological boundaries violated is an inherent aspect of sexual abuse for both men and women. Often, helpless feelings generalize beyond the actual assault or period of abuse and characterize other life circumstances. In addition, many survivors feel that the trauma opened their eyes to a world full of random and meaningless danger and evil. This sense of lost agency can be constant, or it can manifest only in response to perceived threat (Lifton, 1996; Roth & Newman, 1995).

Interestingly, the targets of male and female survivors' generalizations of helplessness may point to important gender socialization differences. Women's narratives suggest that the powerlessness they experience may become associated with definitions of femininity following assault, and may reinforce the belief that power is a privilege allocated to men, not to women. In addition, women may describe their powerlessness as pervading most relationships, including sexual, familial, and professional ones. The following examples from Roth and Newman (1992) are illustrative:

> **Female S:** I'm very afraid of men's power, and I mean in all sorts of ways— their physical power, their power in society, and their power interpersonally. They're real powerful and I feel powerless in a lot of ways in the face of that. I don't feel equal at all. I used to put that in an analogy of my feminism, of how men look down on women just generally. (p. 228)

> **Female S:** Or if I have to deal with people in a professional level, I'm afraid they're going to get me. But now I recognize that the reason I feel that way is because that's how I associate my perpetrators [as] these older authoritative men. And whenever I get in contact with older authoritative men, I feel their power. (p. 225)

In addition to these narrative examples, research on themes of power in survivors' projective stories and in studies of change in the experience of helplessness in sexually abused girls indicates that a sense of powerlessness pervades most aspects of female survivors' lives. Liem et al. (1996) found that women with a history of sexual abuse tend to be more sensitive, aware, and fearful of power in the world following their traumas than women without a history of abuse. Although there are no prospective studies of the development of a helplessness schema for women following their traumas, in-depth structured interviews with parents of sexually abused girls suggest that the girls had a more passive approach to life following abuse than previously (Pelcovitz, 1999).

These findings might be expected considering that, historically, women have had less access to power and less social support in positions of power than men in both personal and professional spheres. The powerlessness of abuse, coupled with reinforcing social cues about men's power and women's helplessness, may prevent female survivors from exploring their own agency and effectiveness, and may assist them in overaccommodating (as per Resick & Schnicke, 1992) to a feminine helplessness schema.

Like female survivors, abuse-related helplessness for men can generalize to other domains and sometimes result in exaggerated blaming of authorities (Friedman, 1994). However, a review of narratives and case examples (Lisak, 1994) suggests that male survivors often experience feelings of powerlessness in sexual encounters and relationships in particular:

> **Male S:** The defeat that I felt with my mother comes back often. I find it in my sexual relationships. A lot of times I'll allow people to be invasive because I'm used to it. And I've had a hard time setting up boundaries. I've had a hard time believing that my boundaries were worthwhile, that they were worth keeping. I guess I often felt like I was the property of somebody else. And that anybody could just do whatever they wanted. And that I didn't have a right to have feelings about it. (p. 534)

> **Male S:** All the scenes in college where the girls would seduce me, and I'd just kind of let them do whatever they want to do. Or I would do for them whatever they wanted me to do. And then just get out. (p. 534)

We hypothesize that male survivors' experiences of helplessness following their traumas may be more circumscribed than those of female survivors. For women, the experience of helplessness is consistent with female gender socialization; whereas for men, feeling helpless is discrepant with their masculine identity. Helplessness may be less globalized for men, because they may try to avoid reexperiencing helplessness in most domains of life. Unfortunately, such efforts often result in excessive behaviors that may be dangerous to themselves and harmful to others.

In addition to gender differences in responses to powerlessness, men and women also seem to use alternative means to regain control following abuse. These differences point to the fairly distinct spheres of power available to men and women in our society. For instance, narratives of female survivors suggest that one of the few avenues for power available to them is in manipulating their bodies through self-harm or sexual exploitation:

> **Female S:** Well, it's not okay to hurt, but in your mind, you tell yourself it is, rather than having other people hurting you. You can't deal with that, but you can deal with hurting yourself. (Calhoun & Resick, 1993, p. 78)

Similarly, a qualitative study of Chinese sexual abuse survivors found that, on the behavioral level, survivors felt driven to engage in risky sexual behaviors, including intercourse with multiple partners and prostitution, as a way to gain control in their lives. One college student survivor began a pattern of having sex with male strangers: "When she actually did it with a male stranger she felt that she was in control and in possession of that particular man" (Luo, 1998, p. 1017). Briere (1996) has also noted that many abused women come to use sex to achieve goals that are otherwise less available to them, such as limited control over powerful others, unmet needs for affection, and avoidance of loneliness. He hypothesizes that this option may seem appropriate to survivors, because, as women, they learn early in life that their sexuality is one of their most valued commodities.

Female survivors also describe finding other ways to gain control over the abuse dynamic, including verbal aggression and mental control:

> **Female S:** Men are raised with the obsession that sex and their ability to receive it and perform connotes their manhood and their self-worth. And so it's an obsession with men to conquer, and that's why they will go to the lengths that they do. Now, at the same time, I believe I can lay a man out; I don't need a gun. I can break men if I want to, just with my mind. I can take a man and have him on his knees, and I've done it. Physically on their knees, because I can take apart their mind and get to their little boy and make them vulnerable. Now, their games don't work with me, because I see through them. And it's because women know how to use their minds. I think men do too, but they haven't tried, because they're so busy trying to work on their sexual standpoint. (Roth & Newman, 1992, p. 224)

Likewise, in the words of an African American survivor:

> **Female S:** Gradually, my silence grew into a secret. I insisted that if someone were to be told about the rapes, *I* had to be the one to make the disclosure. If David [husband] told anyone, he had to tell me who the person was, so I would be prepared with a response when next I saw that person. Thus, I began to struggle to regain control of my life by trying to control the lives of others. (Pierce-Baker, 1998, p. 47)

Similar findings emerged from Chinese survivors' narratives. Probably in response to a sense of vulnerability to victimization, one 17-year-old survivor determined to become a "superwoman," so that she could control men ("order men around," in her own words) and protect herself from men's harm (Luo, 1998, p. 1020).

In contrast, the narratives of male survivors suggest that more stereotypically masculine methods, such as pursuing hypermasculine careers or physically dominating others, may be used by some men to gain control or power in the aftermath of abuse:

> Male S: Well, I decided to go in because the Marine Corps has a reputation as being the toughest. And, of course, I could never picture myself being in anything except the Marine Corps. (Lisak, 1994, p. 539)

> Male S: Sometimes when Thomas was doing that stuff to me, I said to myself: "When I get older, I want to be the one who does it, not the one who gets it." (Briere, 1996, p. 185)

> Male S: She was definitely raped. She definitely did that much of the thing against her will with my will. . . . I thought finally, wow, it wasn't that great, but at least I got that. I'm not a wimp. You can't tease me around like that. And I did what the man is supposed to do. And too bad she didn't love it. But she would next time, if we had another time. (Lisak, 1994, p. 539)

> Male S: So I always felt somewhat powerless in sex for awhile, except with the younger kids, where I felt in control. (Lisak, 1994, p. 534)

These narratives highlight some of the areas in which male survivors may pursue control and power in their lives when they endorse rigid gender stereotypes. The latter three survivors indicate that their abuse is in direct response to their own experiences of being "the one who gets it," "a wimp," or "powerless." Whereas verbal aggression, self-victimization, or sex with powerful men may seem like gender-appropriate avenues for women survivors to seek control, pursuing power through physical and sexual violence may be more likely to be perceived as "what the man is supposed to do."

Legitimacy

"Legitimacy" refers to whether or not survivors believe that their traumatic events can account for their subsequent emotional experiences. Both male and female victims often describe their reactions and emotions as deviant, invalid, or representing a deficit in functioning. For instance, some survivors think that they are "crazy," because they overreact to situations that seem unrelated to the abuse. Others doubt that the abuse actually occurred (Lifton, 1996; Roth & Newman, 1995).

Nevertheless, important differences abound between men's and women's descriptions of legitimacy that highlight their differential socialization experiences. For women, initial attempts to articulate or legitimize their experiences seem to be thwarted. Eventually, they come to rely on social cues to inform them about more "appropriate" ways to narrate their experience:

> Female S: A ten-year war had started in my mind. What he told me was true versus what I knew was true. He raped me. He manipulated me. He tortured and tormented me. He raped my mind and body. Back then, I didn't know what to believe or do, so I started lying about who I was, like in a fantasy. (Calhoun & Resick, 1993, p. 71)

> Female S: I told my college roommates. . . . Several of them didn't seem to understand the trauma of it. They looked at it not so much as a violation or a rape, but as, well, everyone has to lose their virginity. It was sort of downplayed. . . . I think that probably encouraged me to grasp for the "this is no big deal, let's cope" strategy, instead of focusing on the trauma. (Roth & Lebowitz, 1988, p. 97)

> Female S: Well I don't know if I call it a rape. I call it a sexual assault. I was orally raped so I don't know in the eyes of the law if I was raped, but somehow it is a protective device to say you were sexually assaulted. (Roth & Lebowitz, 1988, p. 97)

These examples demonstrate how female survivors come to internalize the interpretations of others and the law, even if these renditions contradict their own experiences. This response makes sense considering research that has identified some basic features of cultural invalidation and self-silencing of women, including women's often unsuccessful efforts to establish positions of agency in their professional lives and within relationships (Belenky, Clinchy, Goldberger, & Tarule, 1997). Belenky et al. (1997) observed that women in these contexts often have been ignored or unheard, which led them to become passively dependent on systems of authority rather than on their own sense of control and knowledge to make decisions or to articulate their experiences. Certainly, a woman's trauma and all of its underlying meanings cannot be worked through if her culturally constructed trauma narrative continues to be at odds with her authentic experience.

For men, one major obstacle to legitimizing their experiences seems to be that society at large, including the survivors themselves, fail to view men as victims (Lisak, 1994). Consequently, many male survivors ask how they can take their own traumas seriously:

> Male S: It's like, men aren't abused? You know, who ever heard of that? Who talks about that? If men aren't abused, how could I have been abused? (p. 536)

Male S: But as a man, in that same respect, I feel like this is typical of my life. There are all these women's organizations that are starting; they're becoming very conscious of not treating women as victims, not having violence toward women. But women have been victims and now they're reasserting themselves, and women are physically different from guys. So they can see themselves as victims. Maybe they themselves can see that victims are okay, they're good somehow; they martyred themselves. Some way, if you can have it black and white, good or evil, women were good and men were bad. Well, I'm the victim and I'm a guy, but guys are bad. So I can't even be a victim, right? (p. 536)

Indeed, several authors have highlighted the fact that in treatment literature and practice, as well as in media depictions of abuse, men tend to be portrayed as perpetrators and women as victims (Cermak & Molidor, 1996; Lisak, 1993). This social construction of gender roles can be detrimental to male survivors because of the likelihood that their abuse will be overlooked or downplayed by significant others and/or clinicians. One study found that even when presented with the same case information, clinicians were more likely to hypothesize that a client had a sexual abuse history if the client was female (Holmes & Offen, 1996). In light of such bias, male survivors tend to be denied protection, treatment, and the validation often needed to explore the impact of their traumas.

Although the issues described may be salient for Caucasian men and women, the absence of African American survivors' narratives in the trauma literature highlights the extent of this group's historical invalidation. In writing about the Clarence Thomas–Anita Hill senate hearings, Daniel (1995) points out that black women's experiences of sexual assault may be overlooked by professionals, the media, and others. She emphasizes that social constructions of black women tend to entail invisibility, devaluation, and lack of entitlement. One striking example of the silencing or delegitimization of black women's experiences of abuse is that they have had to rely on fiction as an outlet for publishing narratives about their sexual traumas, leaving the veracity of their experiences still under question (Daniel, 1995). To address this breach, Pierce-Baker (1998) collected and published black women's own narratives of their rape experiences, many of which illustrate this struggle with legitimacy:

Female S: One of my frustrations is knowing we black women accept being raped. And middle-class black women don't talk about rape. We sort of support society in viewing us as not being important as rape victims. Or we pretend it doesn't really happen. "She's just saying it." Or "You could have gotten out if you wanted to." Maybe it's a defense; we don't have control over our own sexuality historically—ever—with rape during slavery and all that. . . . A professor at the university said in class, in my presence, that "you can't get raped unless you go slinking through the ghetto." As if I'm not even a human being. I was sitting there! We're very disposable people, black women. (pp. 91–92)

Legitimacy may be an important theme for African American male survivors as well, because they may be one of the most neglected groups in the trauma field. Although one-fourth to one-third of all victims of sexual abuse are boys and one of every five sexually abused children is African American or Latino (American Humane Association, 1988), there have been far fewer empirical studies of sexually abused African American and Latino males than females, and no qualitative work on African American and Latino males' sexual trauma. Thus, the systematic study of themes particular to male and female survivors from these groups, and their differential patterns of coping, is still acutely needed for the development of gender and culturally sensitive interventions.

Anger and Fear

Anger and fear are important emotions associated with the experience of victimization for both men and women (Dimock, 1988; Lisak, 1993; Roth & Newman, 1995). Anger may be felt about the event itself, or it may be directed at one's attacker(s), at people who did not provide protection, at those who were not helpful in the aftermath, or at oneself in response to self-blaming cognitions (Roth & Newman, 1995). Fear associated with the trauma is often described as a continuous sense of dread that the abuse will be repeated or that further harm is imminent. Survivors often describe manifestation of their fear in avoidant, protective, and/or phobic behaviors.

Basic descriptions of anger and fear by survivors do not tend to differ by sex. Rather, gender differences in emotional expressiveness seem to play a role in how affective themes arise over the course of psychotherapy. Although most therapies for PTSD involve some type of "exposure" and initiate the experience of trauma-related emotions that clients have not previously confronted, it may be that certain affects are not as readily available or acceptable to clients based on the rigidity of their gender identity. A review of male and female narratives on anger and fear emphasizes the difficulty survivors experience when attempting to express gender-discrepant emotions.

For women, feelings of anger and the urge to hurt another individual (e.g., the perpetrator) in self-defense or out of rage may be experienced as extremely frightening because of their discrepancy with feminine gender socialization. The gender stereotype most documented and empirically supported is that females are the more emotionally expressive sex, and that they express more fear and sadness, and less direct anger, than do males (Brody & Hall, 1993; Timmers, Fischer, & Manstead, 1998). Consequently, following sexual trauma, experiences of anger may be suppressed or avoided, which may only lead to an intensification of helplessness and increase cognitive appraisals such as "I'm weak," "I'm no good," and "I'm to blame" (Lisak, 1995).

One study on the process of treatment for female sexual abuse survivors documented that the early sessions of therapy tend to be dominated by a discussion of gender-appropriate emotions, such as fear and helplessness (Roth & Batson, 1997). Anger, on the other hand, was the only affective theme that was not fully conscious (i.e., survivors did not describe awareness of the emotion, although there was evidence of its salience to them) at the beginning of treatment. However, 6 months into treatment, most survivors became aware that they were angry about the abuse and were attempting to address it.

In other case studies as well, female survivors' narratives emphasize that anger is acknowledged less early in therapy, because it threatens women's identity or sense of self-worth:

> Female S: I've turned some of this anger toward myself for letting the rape happen. This inward anger has created a war in my mind. This war took a lot of my self-confidence, esteem, and identity. (Calhoun & Resick, 1993, p. 67)

> Female S: I'm afraid of what I felt like. I'm afraid of experiencing the grief and anger. The anger more than the grief. That's the place that I'd say, if I've lost part of myself, it's in the ability to be angry, the ability to set limits and boundaries with other people. (Roth & Newman, 1992, p. 228)

Only after they have reframed the trauma in ways that emphasize their helplessness at the time of the trauma and deemphasize their self-blame do female survivors begin to express rage, feel it as overwhelming, and, over time, gain some control over it.

> Female S: When I started remembering, I knew it was rape, without a doubt. . . . Then I started to get angry. (Calhoun & Resick, 1993, p. 72)

> Female S: The other part that was hard for me once I acknowledged that I was an incest survivor was then working through and letting go of some of that anger once I even allowed myself to recognize that it was there. And then learning new kinds of behaviors . . . very hard. (Godbey & Hutchinson, 1996, p. 308)

Except for anger, most trauma-related emotions contradict masculine gender socialization. As described earlier, masculine gender identity demands strength, the denial of physical and emotional pain, and prohibits men from expressing and possibly even experiencing emotions that may lead to feelings of vulnerability (Lisak, 1995). Thus, inescapable pain, helplessness, and fear inherent in the experience of trauma are extremely schema-discrepant for men, especially those who have internalized rigid masculinity norms. Male survivors' narratives emphasize the saliency of cultural prescriptions of masculine expressiveness:

> **Male S:** As far as my masculine strengths are concerned, I'm not sure what are strengths and what are myths. What is it to be a man, and what is it to be a caring loving, intimate person? Shouldn't the two be connected? When fear or cowardice or tenderness enter my feelings, it seems to go against what I think I should be feeling. I would like to be able to feel those things without guilt. (Dimock, 1988, p. 210)

> **Male S:** It embarrasses me to see somebody sad. If I had to guess, it probably has to do with male programming. That you're not supposed to be sad and you're not supposed to cry. (Lisak, 1994, p. 538)

In an attempt to avoid the intense fear of lost manliness, male survivors may rely on anger as their sole emotional outlet, because it may be more easily accessed and more socially condoned (Briere, 1996; Dimock, 1988; Lisak, 1994). When asked early in therapy to write about his trauma, one survivor could only recollect his anger and aggressive impulses, even though he acknowledged to his therapist that he "should have been scared" (Neimeyer & Stewart, 1996):

> **Male S:** All these guys were kicking me in the head. But one in particular was running back and jumping on my face. I remember feeling intense rage mostly at the one jumping on me. I was thinking how I could hurt him easy if I could get up. I decided it would be worth getting shot just to get one good shot to his nose with the palm of my hand with an upward thrust. I decided I was going to do this no matter what, but every time I raised up, I would get knocked back to the ground. I tried many times to do this, I would guess 20 times. (p. 366)

This example highlights the way in which fear and vulnerability associated with traumatic events may be avoided or suppressed early in therapy by male survivors. Indeed, some have argued that men who abide strictly by gender stereotypes for emotional expressiveness often convert "nonmasculine" affects into anger (Mosher & Tomkins, 1988). Because traditional masculine socialization teaches men to avoid expression of vulnerable emotions, men may learn to rely on other ways of regulating their emotional pain, including cognitive avoidance strategies, such as dissociation, or behavioral distraction strategies, such as impulsive acts of aggression (Briere, 1996).

The embarrassment and guilt many male survivors experience when they feel or express vulnerability and fear, as well as their reliance on hypermasculine emotionality, may prevent them from disclosing their abuse to others, seeking treatment, and staying in therapy (Briere, 1996). As Blanchard (1986) noted: "Some young men will enter therapy and scrupulously avoid any discussion of their victimization, only to withdraw from counseling prematurely feeling confused and unfulfilled by the proceedings" (p. 20). Thus, it is imperative that therapists be cognizant of male survivors' ambivalence over expressing fear and helplessness, and find ways to normalize these affects while reassuring clients of their masculinity. These findings suggest that internalized gender codes may systematically interfere with the expression of emotion following traumatic experiences for both men and women, and be associated with gender-specific patterns of theme expression and resolution.

CONCLUSION: INTEGRATING GENDER INTO TRAUMA-FOCUSED RESEARCH AND THERAPY

The trauma theme literature and gender comparisons presented highlight how gender socialization regarding roles, sexuality, and emotional expressiveness influences the ways in which individuals make sense of their abuse and adapt in the aftermath. Men and women who abide by strict gender codes may be more susceptible to developing and maintaining posttraumatic stress if their response indeed limits them from experiencing and expressing gender-discrepant emotions, and prevents them from conceptualizing salient trauma themes in positive and self-protective ways. Addressing the interaction between trauma themes and gender in coping with abuse-related PTSD may be useful for both trauma researchers and clinicians.

Our review of the theme research emphasizes the need for studies that assess gender identity directly and/or include both male and female survivors. As demonstrated here, comparing men's and women's narratives unveils meaningful gender differences in cognitive and affective stress responses that may be overlooked by studies limited to forced-choice questionnaires. Research efforts that combine qualitative (i.e., coding of narratives or expressive behavior) and quantitative methods (i.e., standardized questionnaires or interviews) are recommended. A multimethod approach might elucidate further the relationships between sex, gender identity, trauma themes, and PTSD.

This review also underscores a need for trauma-focused treatment studies to evaluate therapies that address gender issues directly. Again, only one study that we are aware of (e.g., Morgan & Cummings, 1999) has examined the impact of a feminist intervention on change in trauma themes as well as PTSD symptomatology. This study represents a first step in addressing the importance of integrating gender issues in trauma-focused treatments.

Another important implication of the gender comparisons is that affective themes (i.e., anger and fear) over the course of therapy for men and women may arise differently. Psychotherapy process research that evaluates change in PTSD symptoms and trauma themes over the course of therapy is needed to test these preliminary hypotheses. Unfortunately, the study by Morgan and Cummings (1999) did not assess level of theme resolution and PTSD symptoms during the intervention. Thus, although they found pre- to posttreatment changes in these outcome measures, patterns of change in particular themes (i.e., anger and fear) and symptoms (i.e., emotional control and numbing) over the course of feminist psychotherapy could not be evaluated. We encourage future investigations that compare male and female survivors' expression of gender-consistent and -discrepant emotions at several time points during the intervention.

In terms of clinical applications, the gender comparisons and reports of gender-focused treatments for posttraumatic stress (Dimock, 1988; Lisak, 1995; Morgan & Cummings, 1999) suggest that incorporating techniques that assist clients in identifying and confronting rigid gender norms may be a key component of treatment. How might therapists incorporate a discussion of gender into trauma therapy? For both directive and nondirective interventions, therapists might consider incorporating psychoeducation, a method of sharing tools of analysis and interpretation with the client. By engaging in discussions or providing books and articles on gender, the therapist can introduce clients to controversies and debates about gender, and assist them in formulating a more flexible attitude toward their conceptualization of identity and sexuality (Brown, 1986; Lisak, 1995). Within such a framework, the clinician can then begin to incorporate gender issues into treatment as themes are addressed.

Although additional research is needed, the preliminary theme comparisons conducted here suggest that men and women may benefit from different therapeutic approaches to trauma-related emotions and schemas. Several clinicians have made recommendations about how therapists might approach emotional material with male survivors (Bolton, Morris, & MacEachron, 1989; Briere, 1996; Friedman, 1994; Scott, 1992; Zamanian & Adams, 1997). These interventions emphasize the importance of identifying and interpreting male survivors' ambivalence over expressing affects of vulnerability and their tendency to rely on defenses such as dissociation, intellectualization, and precipitous action. It seems imperative for therapists to normalize experiences of pain, fear, and helplessness, while reassuring male clients of their masculinity.

Dimock (1988) encourages clients to express their anger in order to gain access to other primary emotions, such as hurt and fear. One particular technique includes having the male survivor talk as if his abuser were present. The male group facilitates the survivor's expressiveness by giving him cues on what to say and asking him to raise his voice progressively. According to Dimock, "This process usually leads to other feelings. Often fear associated with the sexual abuse or painful feelings about what the abuse meant in a broader sense come to the surface and can be expressed at the same time" (p. 215). Within the safe and supportive environment of an all-male group, the client is more likely to experience vulnerable emotions as consistent rather than as discrepant with masculine gender identity.

The approach to emotional material with female survivors may require more focus on anger expression and assertiveness training than may be necessary for male clients. Therapists may need to facilitate labeling of rage and appropriate expression of angry feelings. Feminist therapists describe rehearsal of anger expression as an important component of the therapy process with women suffering from PTSD (Brown, 1986). Specific techniques include writing letters to the perpetrator(s) or others who did not protect or validate the survivor (either to send or solely to provide an emotional outlet), taking a course in martial arts, organizing a survivors' march, and so on (Bass & Davis, 1988). These techniques may assist the client in linking current rage conceptually with abuse experiences, and in confronting her perpetrator and/or those who did not protect her. They may also increase self-efficacy and a feeling of safety in the outside world, which may be especially important for clients who comply with strict codes of femininity (Briere, 1996).

In terms of exploring schematic trauma themes, the comparisons suggest that different material may need to be introduced or challenged with male versus female survivors. For instance, when helping to reframe self-blaming cognitions and associated guilt, therapists may need to focus on the interaction between societal norms and the survivor's personal history. With a female survivor, the clinician may need to spend more time exploring cultural messages that the client may have received that objectify women and teach them to feel responsible for male sexual aggressiveness. Alternatively, for male clients, the therapist may need to focus on socialization experiences that have led to an internalization of the male ethic of self-reliance and self-defense.

Whether implementing cognitive-behavioral approaches, such as cognitive restructuring, or using supportive–expressive therapy techniques, it is suggested that therapists carefully introduce alternative interpretations or perspectives when clients rely on detrimental gender stereotypes to explain their affective experiences and beliefs about self, others, and the world. Examining how cultural factors may have been reinforced or challenged in each client's unique life history is essential for understanding the significance of gender issues in the client's trauma resolution.

Despite the commonalities in men's and women's descriptions of trauma themes and the usefulness of methodologies that condense data across individuals, the importance of attending to the richness of individual experience both in treatment and psychological research needs to be emphasized

(Roth & Newman, 1992). In trauma-focused therapies, it is crucial for clinicians to maintain a broad lens that can incorporate the influence of gender and ethnic socialization, and a more narrowly focused lens that can attend to how the interaction of themes and gender may emerge for any particular individual.

Although this review points to the usefulness of addressing the interaction between trauma themes and gender in coping with abuse-related PSTD, we nevertheless recognize the limits of generalizing from case material. In addition, case studies and published narrative accounts that we did review are sparse, limiting our ability to take a closer look at all trauma themes discussed in the literature. As more qualitative and quantitative studies comparing male and female survivors' responses to abuse and therapeutic processes emerge, we hope that the findings will be added to the sketch of salient gender issues and trauma themes in PTSD. Such a delineation will provide a useful guideline for therapists conducting trauma focused therapies with men and women.

ACKNOWLEDGMENTS

We wish to express our appreciation to Dr. David Lisak for comments on an earlier draft of this chapter. Excerpted material from Roth and Lebowitz (1988), Lebowitz and Roth (1994), Myers (1989), Lisak (1994, 1995), Harker (1997), Dimock (1988), Calhoun and Resick (1993), Roth and Newman (1992), Pierce-Baker (1998), Briere (1996), Godbey and Hutchinson (1996), and Neimeyer and Stewart (1996) is reprinted with permission from the respective copyright holders.

REFERENCES

American Humane Association. (1988). *Highlights of official child neglect and abuse reporting, 1986.* Denver, CO: Author.

Bartky, S. L. (1990). *Femininity and domination: Studies in the phenomenology of oppression.* New York: Routledge.

Basow, S. A. (1992). *Gender stereotypes and roles* (3rd ed.). Pacific Grove, CA: Brooks/Cole.

Bass, E., & Davis, L. (1988). *The courage to heal: A guide for women survivors of child sexual abuse.* New York: Harper & Row.

Belenky, M. F., Clinchy, B. M., Goldberger, N. R., & Tarule, J. M. (1997). *Women's ways of knowing: The development of self, voice, and mind.* New York: Basic Books.

Blanchard, G. (1986). Male victims of child sexual abuse: A portent of things to come. *Journal of Independent Social Work, 1,* 19–27.

Bolton, F. G., Jr., & MacEachron, A. E. (1988). Adolescent male sexuality: A developmental perspective. *Journal of Adolescent Research, 3,* 259–273.

Bolton, F. G. Jr., Morris, L. A., & MacEachron, A. E. (1989). *Males at risk: The other side of child sexual abuse.* Newbury Park, CA: Sage.

Briere, J. (1996). Client gender issues. In *Therapy for adults molested as children: Beyond stereotypes* (pp. 182–201). New York: Springer.

Briere, J., Smiljanich, K., & Henschel, D. (1994). Sexual fantasies, gender, and molestation history. *Child Abuse and Neglect, 18,* 131–137.

Brody, L. R. (1993). On understanding gender differences in the expression of emotion: Gender roles, socialization and language. In S. Ablon, D. Brown, E. Khantzian, & J. Mack (Eds.), *Human feelings: Explorations in affect development and meaning* (pp. 87–121). Hillsdale, NJ: Analytic Press.

Brody, L. (1997). Gender and emotion: Beyond stereotypes. *Journal of Social Issues, 53,* 369–394.

Brody, L. R., & Hall, J. (1993). Gender and emotion. In M. Lewis & J. Haviland (Eds.), *Handbook of emotions* (pp. 447–460). New York: Guilford Press.

Brown, L. S. (1986). From alienation to connection: Feminist therapy with post-traumatic stress disorder. *Women and Therapy, 5,* 13–26.

Browne, A., & Finkelhor, D. (1986). Impact of child sexual abuse: A review of the research. *Psychological Bulletin, 99,* 66–77.

Bruckner, D., & Johnson, P. (1987, February). Treatment for adult male victims of childhood sexual abuse. *Social Casework,* pp. 81–87.

Calhoun, K. S., & Resick, P. A. (1993). Post-traumatic stress disorder. In D. H. Barlow (Ed.), *Clinical handbook of psychological disorders: A step-by-step treatment manual* (2nd ed., pp. 48–98) New York: Guilford Press.

Cermak, P., & Molidor, C. (1996). Male victims of child sexual abuse. *Child and Adolescent Social Work Journal, 13,* 385–400.

Chard, K. M., Weaver, T. L., & Resick, P. A. (1997). Adapting cognitive processing therapy for child sexual abuse survivors. *Cognitive and Behavioral Practice, 4,* 31–52.

Chodorow, N. (1978). *The reproduction of mothering.* Berkeley: University of California Press.

Coffey, P., Leitenberg, H., Henning, K., Turner, T., & Bennet, R. T. (1996). Mediators of the long-term impact of child sexual abuse: Perceived stigma, betrayal, powerlessness, and self-blame. *Child Abuse and Neglect, 20,* 447–455.

Daniel, J. H. (1995). The discourse on Thomas v. Hill: A resource for perspectives on the black woman and sexual trauma. In K. Weingarten (Ed.), *Cultural resistance: Challenging beliefs about men, women, and therapy* (pp. 103–122). New York: Harrington Park Press.

Dimock, P. T. (1988). Adult males sexually abused as children: Characteristics and implications for treatment. *Journal of Interpersonal Violence, 3,* 203–221.

Dutton, M. A., Burghardt, K. J., Perrin, S. G., Chrestman, K. R., & Halle, P. M. (1994). Battered women's cognitive schemata. *Journal of Traumatic Stress, 7,* 237–257.

Edwards, P. W., & Donaldson, M. A. (1989). Assessment of symptoms in adult survivors of incest: A factor analytic study of the responses to childhood incest questionnaire. *Child Abuse and Neglect, 13,* 101–110.

Ellerstein, N. S., & Canavan, J. W. (1980). Sexual abuse of boys. *American Journal of Diseases of Children, 134,* 255–257.

Finkelhor, D. (1984). *Child sexual abuse: Theory and research.* New York: Macmillan.

Finkelhor, D., & Browne, A. (1985). The traumatic impact of child sexual abuse: A conceptualization. *American Journal of Orthopsychiatry, 55,* 530–541.

Frazier, P., & Schauben, L. (1994). Causal attributions and recovery from rape and other stressful life events. *Journal of Social and Clinical Psychology, 31,* 1–14.

Fredrickson, B. L., & Roberts, T. (1997). Objectification theory: Toward understanding women's lived experiences and mental health risks. *Psychology of Women Quarterly, 21,* 173–206.

Friedman, R. M. (1994). Psychodynamic group therapy for male survivors of sexual abuse. *Group, 18,* 225–234.

Gill, M., & Tutty, L. M. (1997). Sexual identity issues for male survivors of childhood sexual abuse: A qualitative study. *Journal of Child Sexual Abuse, 6,* 31–47.

Gilligan, C. (1982). *In a different voice: Psychological theory and women's development.* Cambridge, MA: Harvard University Press.

Gilmore, D. D. (1990). *Manhood in the making: Cultural concepts of masculinity.* New Haven, CT: Yale University Press.

Godbey, J. K., & Hutchinson, S. A. (1996). Healing from incest: Resurrecting the buried self. *Archives of Psychiatric Nursing, 10,* 304–310.

Groth, A. N., & Burgess, A. W. (1980). Male rape: Offenders and victims. *American Journal of Psychiatry, 137,* 806–810.

Harker, T. (1997). Therapy with male sexual abuse survivors: Contesting oppressive life stories. In G. Monk, J. Winslade, K. Crocket, & D. Eston (Eds.), *Narrative therapy in practice: The archaeology of hope* (pp. 193–214). San Francisco: Jossey-Bass.

Harvey, J. H., Orbuch, T. L., Weber, A. L., Merback, N., Alt, R. (1992). House of pain and hope: Accounts of loss. *Death Studies, 16,* 99–124.

Herman, J. (1992). *Trauma and recovery.* New York: Basic Books.

Herman, J. L., & Hirschman, L. (1981). *Father–daughter incest.* Cambridge, MA: Harvard University Press.

Holmes, G., & Offen, L. (1996). Clinicians' hypotheses regarding clients' problems: Are they less likely to hypothesize sexual abuse in male compared to female clients? *Child Abuse and Neglect, 20,* 493–501.

Horowitz, M. J. (1986). *Stress response syndromes* (2nd ed.). Northvale, NJ: Jason Aronson.

Horowitz, M. J. (1997). *Stress Response Syndromes* (3rd ed.). Northvale, NJ: Jason Aronson.

Hoyenga, K. B., & Hoyenga, K. T. (1979). *The question of sex differences: Psychological, cultural, and biological issues.* Boston: Little, Brown.

Hunter, M. (1990). *Abused boys.* Lexington, MA: Lexington Books.

Janoff-Bulman, R. (1985). The aftermath of victimization: Rebuilding shattered assumptions. In C. R. Figley (Ed.), *Trauma and its wake: The study and treatment of post-traumatic stress disorder* (pp. 15–25). New York: Brunner/Mazel.

Jordan, J. V. Kaplan, A. G., Miller, J. B., Stiver, I. P., & Surrey, J. L. (1991). *Women's growth in connection: Writings from the Stone Center.* New York: Guilford Press.

Kagan, J. (1976). Psychology of sex differences. In F. Beach (Ed.), *Human sexuality in four perspectives* (pp. 87–114). Baltimore, MD: Johns Hopkins University Press.

Krupnick, J. L., & Horowitz, M. J. (1981). Stress response syndromes: Recurrent themes. *Archives of General Psychiatry, 38,* 428–435.

Lebowitz, L., & Roth, S. (1994). "I felt like a slut": The cultural context and women's response to being raped. *Journal of Traumatic Stress, 7,* 363–390.

Liem, J. H., O'Toole, J. G., & James, J. B. (1996). Themes of power and betrayal in sexual abuse survivors' characterizations of interpersonal relationships. *Journal of Traumatic Stress, 9,* 745–761.

Lifton, N. (1996). The thematic assessment measurement system: A measurement system for systematically tracking the process of recovery from sexual abuse. *Dissertation Abstracts International, 57*(4-B), 2937.

Lifton, R. J. (1979). *The broken connection: On death and the continuity of life.* New York: Simon & Schuster.

Lisak, D. (1993). Men as victims: Challenging cultural myths. *Journal of Traumatic Stress, 6,* 577–580.

Lisak, D. (1994). The psychological impact of sexual abuse: Content analysis of interviews with male survivors. *Journal of Traumatic Stress, 7,* 525–548.

Lisak, D. (1995). Integrating a critique of gender in the treatment of male survivors of childhood abuse. *Psychotherapy, 32,* 258–269.

Luo, T. (1998). Sexual abuse trauma among Chinese survivors. *Child Abuse and Neglect, 22,* 1013–1026.

Maccoby, E. E., & Jacklin, C. N. (1974). *The psychology of sex differences.* Stanford, CA: Stanford University Press.

McCann, I. L., & Pearlman, L. A. (1990). *Psychological trauma and the adult survivor: Theory, therapy, and transformation.* New York: Brunner/Mazel.

Meichenbaum, D. (1995). Disasters, stress and cognition. In S. E. Hobfoll & M. W. de Vries (Eds.), *Extreme stress and communities: Impact and intervention* (pp. 33–61). Norwell, MA: Kluwer Academic.

Miller, J. B. (1976). *Toward a new psychology of women.* Boston: Beacon Press.

Money, J., & Wiedeking, C. (1980). Gender identity/role: Normal differentiation and its transpositions. In B. B. Wolman & J. Money (Eds.), *Handbook of human sexuality* (pp. 269–284). Englewood Cliffs, NJ: Prentice-Hall.

Morgan, T., & Cummings, A. L. (1999). Change experienced during group therapy by female survivors of childhood sexual abuse. *Journal of Consulting and Clinical Psychology, 67,* 28–36.

Mosher, D. L., & Tomkins, S. S. (1988). Scripting the macho man: Hypermasculine socialization and enculturation. *Journal of Sex Research, 25,* 60–84.

Myers, M. F. (1989). Men sexually assaulted as adults and sexually abused as boys. *Archives of Sexual Behavior, 18,* 203–215.

Neimeyer, R. A., & Stewart, A. E. (1996). Trauma, healing, and the narrative emplotment of loss. *Families in Society, 77,* 360–375.

Pelcovitz, D. (1999). Betrayed by a trusted adult: Structured time-limited group therapy with elementary school children abused by a school employee. In N. B. Webb (Ed.), *Play therapy with children in crisis: Individual, group, and family treatment* (2nd ed., pp. 183–199). New York: Guilford Press.

Pierce-Baker, C. (1998). *Surviving the silence: Black women's stories of rape.* New York: Norton.

Pleck, J. H. (1981). *The myth of masculinity.* Cambridge, MA: MIT Press.

Resick, P. A., & Schnicke, M. K. (1992). Cognitive processing therapy for sexual assault victims. *Journal of Consulting and Clinical Psychology, 60,* 748–756.

Resick, P. A., & Schnicke, M. K. (1993). *Cognitive processing therapy for rape victims: A treatment manual.* Newbury Park, CA: Sage.

Roth, S., & Batson, R. (1993). The creative balance: The therapeutic relationship and thematic issues in trauma resolution. *Journal of Traumatic Stress, 6,* 159–179.

Roth, S., & Batson, R. (1997). *Naming the shadows: A new approach to individual and group psychotherapy for adult survivors of childhood incest.* New York: Free Press.

Roth, S., & Lebowitz, L. (1988). The experience of sexual trauma. *Journal of Traumatic Stress, 1,* 79–107.

Roth, S., Lebowitz, L., & DeRosa, R. (1997). Thematic assessment of posttraumatic stress reactions. In J. P. Wilson & T. M. Keane (Eds.), *Assessing psychological trauma and PTSD* (pp. 513–528). New York: Guilford Press.

Roth, S., & Newman, E. (1992). The role of helplessness in the recovery process for sexual trauma survivors. *Canadian Journal of Behavioral Science, 24,* 220–232.

Roth, S., & Newman, E. (1993). The process of coping with incest for adult survivors: Measurement and implications for treatment and research. *Journal of Interpersonal Violence, 8,* 363–377.

Roth, S., & Newman, E. (1995). The process of coping with sexual trauma. In G. S. Every, Jr. & J. M. Lating (Eds.), *Psychotraumatology: Key papers and core concepts in post-traumatic stress* (pp. 321–339). New York: Plenum Press.

Saxe, G., & Wolfe, J. (1999). Gender and posttraumatic stress disorder. In P. A. Saigh & J. D. Bremner (Eds.), *Posttraumatic stress disorder: A comprehensive text* (pp. 160–179). Boston: Allyn & Bacon.

Scott, W. (1992). Group therapy with sexually abused boys: Notes toward managing behavior. *Clinical Social Work Journal, 20,* 395–409.

Timmers, M., Fischer, A. H., & Manstead, A. S. R. (1998). Gender differences in motives for regulating emotions. *Personality and Social Psychology Bulletin, 24,* 974–986.

Urquiza, A. J., & Keating, L. M. (1990). The prevalence of sexual victimization of males. In M. Hunter (Ed.), *The sexually abused male: Vol. 1. Prevalence, impact, and treatment* (pp. 89–103). Lexington, MA: Lexington Books.

Waites, E. A. (1993). *Trauma and survival: Post-traumatic and dissociative disorders in women.* New York: Norton.

Wyatt, G. E., & Newcomb, M. (1990). Internal and external mediators of child sexual abuse in childhood. *Journal of Consulting and Clinical Psychology, 58,* 758–767.

Zamanian, K., & Adams, C. (1997). Group psychotherapy with sexually abused boys: Dynamics and interventions. *International Journal of Group Psychotherapy, 47,* 109–126.

14 | Gender Issues in Couple and Family Therapy Following Traumatic Stress

CHRISTINA A. BYRNE
DAVID S. RIGGS

The potential for psychological trauma to result in negative consequences for individuals who directly experience traumatic events is well documented. Traumatic events and their consequences may also affect family members, intimate partners, and others close to the traumatized individual (e.g., Jordan et al., 1992; Riggs, Byrne, Weathers, & Litz, 1998). Furthermore, supportive relationships with family members and intimate others may be important in an individual's recovery from traumatic experiences (e.g., Barrett & Mizes, 1988; Davidson, Hughs, Blazer, & George, 1991; Solomon, Waysman, & Mikulincer, 1990). For these reasons, clinicians and researchers have emphasized the potential value of incorporating couple and/or family therapy in treatment programs for individuals suffering from posttraumatic stress disorder (PTSD) and other difficulties following psychological trauma (e.g., Figley, 1988; Glynn et al., 1995; Reid, Wampler, & Taylor, 1996).

When utilizing family and couple approaches in the treatment of trauma survivors, it is important to consider how gender may influence the process. For example, gender role socialization may have a powerful effect on emotional expression, including the types of emotion considered appropriate to express, as well as when and how they are communicated. Gender may also be linked to individuals' perceptions of relationship dynamics, such as social support, that may impact the efficacy of family and couple-based interventions. Furthermore, there are gender differences in the types of traumas individuals are most likely to experience. Thus, in this chapter, as we review findings related to inclusion of intimate partners and family members in treatment for psychological sequelae of trauma, we draw attention to gender-related issues essential in understanding and applying these findings.

EFFECTS OF TRAUMA ON
COUPLE AND FAMILY RELATIONSHIPS

Psychological trauma has been associated with a variety of problems in couple relationships. Much of the research in this area is based on samples of male Vietnam veterans with and without combat-related PTSD symptomatology. Compared to veterans without PTSD, veterans with PTSD have reported greater relationship distress (Carroll, Rueger, Foy, & Donahoe, 1985; Caselli & Motta, 1995; Riggs et al., 1998), more relationship problems (Jordan et al., 1992; Riggs et al., 1998), higher levels of general hostility (Carroll et al., 1985), greater difficulties with intimacy (Roberts et al., 1982; Riggs et al., 1998), less verbal expressiveness and self-disclosure (Carroll et al., 1985), and more problems with sexual disinterest (Litz et al., 1992). PTSD symptomatology also places Vietnam veterans at risk for increased levels of aggression in their marital and cohabiting relationships. Veterans reporting higher levels of PTSD symptoms also report more frequent and severe levels of physical violence (Byrne & Riggs, 1996; Carroll et al., 1985; Jordan et al., 1992), and verbally and psychologically abusive behavior (Byrne & Riggs, 1996) toward their intimate partners.

The detrimental effects of trauma on relationships are evident in the reports of veterans' partners as well. For example, relative to reports by female partners of male Vietnam veterans without PTSD, partners of veterans with PTSD have reported more relationship problems (Jordan et al., 1992; Riggs et al., 1998), greater relationship distress (Riggs et al., 1998), and increased levels of physically (Jordan et al., 1992), psychologically, and verbally aggressive behavior (Byrne & Riggs, 1996) by their partners.

In addition to experiencing relationship difficulties, partners of traumatized individuals also appear to be at increased risk for psychological distress. This has been referred to as "secondary traumatization" (e.g., Figley & Kleber, 1995; Solomon, Waysman, et al., 1992), a process through which individuals close to the trauma survivor develop similar problems or symptoms. In a study of wives of Israeli combat veterans, those who reported PTSD symptoms in their husbands also reported higher levels of general distress compared to wives of veterans without noted PTSD symptomatology (Solomon, Waysman, et al., 1992). Similarly, among women married to or cohabiting with male Vietnam veterans, reports of overall psychological distress have been found to be significantly related to the veterans' PTSD severity (Beckham, Lytle, & Feldman, 1996).

Researchers have also examined intimate relationships of individuals abused as children. Women who experienced sexual abuse during childhood report greater dissatisfaction with their relationships (DiLillo & Long, 1999; Fleming, Mullen, Sibthorpe, & Bammer, 1999), more difficulties with trust (DiLillo & Long, 1999; Mullen, Martin, Anderson, Romans, & Herbison,, 1994), increased sexual problems or dissatisfaction (Finkelhor, Hotaling, Lewis, & Smith, 1989; Mullen et al., 1994), and poorer communication with their partners (DiLillo & Long, 1999) than women without a history of childhood sexual abuse. Like problems associated with combat trauma, negative correlates of childhood sexual abuse are apparent in partners' reports as well. Male partners of women sexually abused during childhood have reported lower relationship satisfaction and higher levels of general distress relative to male partners of women with no abuse history (Nelson & Wampler, 2000).

Similar findings have been noted in other traumatized populations. Compared to women without an assault history, female rape survivors have reported greater fears related to intimacy (Thelen, Sherman, & Borst, 1998) and higher rates of sexual dysfunction (Kilpatrick, Best, Saunders, & Veronen, 1988). Furthermore, in a sample of women with a history of criminal victimization, including sexual and nonsexual trauma, PTSD emerged as a strong predictor of sexual problems (Letourneau, Resnick, Kilpatrick, Saunders, & Best, 1996).

In addition to difficulties in their relationships with intimate partners, individuals who experience trauma also appear to be at increased risk for problems with other family members, specifically, their children. Compared to male Vietnam veterans without PTSD, veterans with PTSD have reported higher levels of parenting problems and poorer family adjustment (Jordan et al., 1992). Veterans' PTSD symptomatology is also associated with lower levels of overall family functioning (MacDonald, Chamberlain, Long, & Flett, 1999) and increased behavioral problems in their children (Caselli & Motta, 1995; Jordan et al., 1992).

As summarized earlier, findings from empirical studies provide clear evidence that the experience of trauma has the potential to disrupt interpersonal relationships and negatively affect intimate partners and family members of the traumatized individual. However, it is important to keep in mind the specific nature of this evidence and related limitations. For men, empirically based knowledge of the connection between trauma and interpersonal difficulties is based primarily on Vietnam combat veterans. For women, this knowledge stems largely from studies of child abuse survivors and from a small number of studies with sexual assault survivors. Little or no empirical data are currently available on interpersonal functioning in other populations, including men with histories of sexual abuse or sexual assault, female veterans, and survivors of other types of trauma.

INCLUDING INTIMATE PARTNERS AND FAMILY
MEMBERS IN TREATMENT OF TRAUMA SURVIVORS

Given the association between the experience of trauma and interpersonal difficulties, it follows that clinicians and researchers would consider including intimate partners and/or other family members in treatment for trauma survivors. Indeed, the clinical literature provides rich descriptions of the interpersonal problems faced by trauma survivors and their partners and family members, as well as suggestions about how to incorporate couple and/or family therapy into treatment programs. Specific populations that have received attention in this regard include heterosexual couples in which one or both partners has experienced childhood sexual abuse (Barnes, 1995; Buttenheim & Levendosky, 1994; Chauncey, 1994; Johnson, 1989; Maltas & Shay, 1995; Mennen & Pearlmutter, 1993; Nadelson & Polonsky, 1991; Reid et al., 1996; Wilson & James, 1992), homosexual couples in which one or both partners have as history of childhood trauma (Kerewksy & Miller, 1996; Klinger & Stein, 1996; Snyder, 1996), male Vietnam veterans and their partners/families (Brooks, 1991; Brown, 1984; Glynn et al., 1995; Hendrix, Jurich, & Schumm, 1995; Johnson, Feldman, & Lubin, 1995; Nelson & Wright, 1996; Lantz & Gregoire, 2000; Rosenheck & Thomson, 1986; Williams & Williams, 1980), male Israeli veterans (Rabin, 1995; Rabin & Nardi, 1991; Solomon, 1988; Solomon, Bleich, Shoham, Nardi, & Kotler, 1992; Waysman, Mikulincer, Solomon, & Weisenberg, 1993), female rape survivors (Barnes, 1995; Erickson, 1989; Hertz & Lerer, 1981; Mio & Foster, 1991; Silverman, 1978), and war refugee families (Arredondo, Orjuela, & Moore, 1989). Other authors have proposed treatment guidelines for trauma survivors and their partners and/or families more generally (e.g., Balcom, 1996; Compton & Follette, 1998; Figley, 1988, 1989; Harris, 1991; Johnson & Williams-Keeler, 1998).

In spite of the many descriptions of couple- and family-based interventions for PTSD, only one controlled treatment outcome study has been published to date. In this study, Glynn et al. (1999) randomly assigned 42 male Vietnam veterans with chronic, combat-related PTSD and one family member (typically a female intimate partner) to a wait-list control group, an exposure therapy group, or to a group receiving exposure therapy followed by behavioral family therapy. Consistent with the PTSD treatment literature, exposure therapy was effective in reducing veterans' reexperiencing and hyperarousal symptoms. However, behavioral family therapy did not add to the effectiveness of exposure therapy in reducing these symptoms, nor did it reduce avoidance and numbing symptoms as hypothesized. The authors offered several possible explanations for the failure to find that inclusion of family therapy led to greater improvement, including small sample size, difficulty of adapting the behavioral family therapy protocol (Mueser & Glynn, 1995) for couples, and insufficient course of intervention (Glynn et al., 1999). Limited generalizability of these results must also be kept in mind, because this study focused on a very specific group of trauma survivors.

Drawing largely from the clinical literature, there appear to be two primary approaches to including intimate partners and/or other family members in the treatment of trauma-related symptoms (Riggs, 2000). One approach, based on the idea that intimate partners or family members represent an important source of social support for the traumatized individual, focuses on utilizing these relationships in the recovery process for the traumatized individual. Another approach, based on the effects trauma may have on interpersonal relationships, partners, and family members, focuses on healing the systemic disruption believed to result from exposure to the trauma. These approaches share some techniques and goals, and are therefore not mutually exclusive (Riggs, 2000). For example, authors who recommend working with a partner or family members, so that they can provide beneficial support to the trauma survivor, also recognize that family members may be affected by the trauma themselves. Similarly, proponents of systemic approaches acknowledge the role of the family in providing support to the traumatized individual, as well as a safe recovery environment. Because so little empirical evidence exists to support directly or refute the effectiveness of these approaches and guide clinicians in their use, we review findings that highlight important issues to be aware of when considering the inclusion of intimate partners and family members in treating trauma survivors.

Role of Partners/Family Members in Treatment

According to the buffering model of social support, support protects individuals from potentially negative effects of stressful events (for review, see Cohen & Wills, 1985). Consistent with this model, social support has been found to be an important variable in understanding responses to trauma (Joseph, 1999; Kaniasty & Norris, 1992). Among female rape victims, higher levels of social support have been linked with reports of fewer somatic symptoms and enhanced perceptions of health (Kimerling & Calhoun, 1994). Retrospective studies of male Vietnam veterans have demonstrated a negative relationship between social support and PTSD, including social support soon after their return from Vietnam (Barrett & Mizes, 1988) as well as years later (Boscarino, 1995; Keane et al., 1985). Analysis of data from the National Vietnam Veteran Readjustment Study (NVVRS; Kulka et al., 1990) revealed social support as a mediator between war-zone stressors and PTSD both in female and male veterans (King, Fairbank, Keane, & Adams, 1998). In a prospective study of recent motor vehicle accident victims, individuals who developed delayed-onset PTSD in the year following the accident reported poorer social support during the first month after the accident compared to individuals who did not go on to develop PTSD (Buckley, Blanchard, & Hickling, 1996). Perceptions of social support shortly after the traumatic event have predicted development of PTSD in a prospective study of burn patients as well (Perry, Difede, Musngi, Frances, & Jacobsberg, 1992).

Whereas the presence of social support may be beneficial to individuals following trauma, perceived lack of support and existence of negative social relationships appear to have the opposite effect. Lack of support by a partner following sexual assault has been associated with increased levels of anxiety and depression, and decreased self-esteem in women (Moss, Frank, & Anderson, 1990). Problems with anxiety and low self-esteem were greatest among women who perceived their partners as supportive prior to the assault but not afterwards (Moss et al., 1990). Additionally, negative interpersonal interactions shortly after a sexual or nonsexual assault have been associated with women's PTSD symptom severity 3 months after the assault (Zoellner, Foa, & Brigidi, 1999). These findings demonstrate that involvement in interpersonal relationships is not necessarily beneficial to trauma survivors. Rather, it is the quality of these relationships that is important.

The relationship between social support and posttrauma symptomatology has led some authors to conclude that incorporating intimate partners and/or family members into treatment of traumatized individuals is important in recovery from PTSD (Figley, 1986; Fontana, Schwartz, & Rosenheck, 1997; Shehan, 1987). Research specific to social support by a partner enhances this conclusion: There is substantial evidence that intimate partners are often the primary source of social support for an individual (Beach, Martin, Blum, & Roman, 1993; McLeod, Kessler, & Landis, 1992; Syrotuik & D'Arcy, 1984).

As noted earlier, the idea that supportive family relationships are beneficial is not exclusive to interventions that propose support as a primary purpose of including intimate others in treatment for trauma survivors. A supportive environment is important in systemic interventions as well. In addition to providing support to the traumatized individual, couple and family interventions with trauma survivors may call on intimate partners and family members to participate in other ways. For example, they may be expected to learn more about the effects of trauma, to work on improving their relationship skills (e.g., communication skills), to increase their problem-solving abilities, and to examine and express their own emotional reactions to the trauma and/or the traumatized individual (Riggs, 2000).

Potential Difficulties

Although trauma interventions that involve intimate partners and family members appear compelling, clinicians must remain aware of possible difficulties that may arise.

There are several potential problems to consider with regard to the goal of facilitating increased support in a couple or family following trauma. First, some of the posttrauma sequelae that might be ameliorated through supportive relationships are associated with behaviors that could make it difficult for intimate others to be supportive. For example, PTSD is associated with increased interpersonal hostility in male Vietnam combat veterans (Beckham et al., 1996), and experiencing and displaying anger has been linked to decreased motivation in others to offer support (Lane & Hobfoll, 1992). Providing or receiving support from one's partner may also be difficult in the presence of relationship distress (Julien & Markman, 1991), which, as stated earlier, is associated with posttrauma symptomatology. Additionally, there is some evidence that the type of support considered beneficial by the recipient depends on the nature of the stressful event (Cutrona & Suhr, 1992). Behaviors intended as supportive may fall short of their goal or even have a negative effect on the individual with PTSD (Lehman, Ellard, & Wortman, 1986). Furthermore, providing support to a recently traumatized partner has been associated with significant distress in the supporting partner. For example, in a study of male disaster workers and their female partners following a plane crash, partners who provided social support to the disaster workers reported greater levels of intrusive symptomatology related to the crash than partners who did not provide support (Fullerton & Ursano, 1997).

Partners called on for support may also have their own trauma history. In order to fully understand relationship functioning, it is important to identify issues both partners bring to the dyadic system. Yet researchers studying the interpersonal effects of trauma have typically identified one partner as the traumatized individual. Taking the trauma history of both partners into consideration may provide a more complete and therefore more useful conceptualization of how posttrauma sequelae may disrupt the relationship. By doing so in a sample of male Vietnam veterans and their female partners, researchers found higher rates of PTSD among partners of veterans with PTSD than among partners of veterans without PTSD (Gallagher, Riggs, Byrne, & Weathers, 1998). In the absence of additional information, such findings could be conceptualized as the result of secondary traumatization, in which the partners' PTSD symptoms stem from the veterans' trauma and symptoms. However, higher rates of traumatic experiences were also found among partners of veterans with PTSD in this sample (Gallagher et al., 1998). Subsequent analyses demonstrated that PTSD symptoms experienced by each member of the couple influenced his or her own relationship satisfaction independently of the partner's PTSD symptoms (Riggs, Byrne, & Lam, 2001). In such dual-trauma couples, providing support may be particularly difficult (Balcom, 1996).

Gender differences related to social support and intimate relationships must also be considered in the context of involving intimate partners in treatment for posttrauma symptomatology. Researchers have found that women's reports of general well-being (Acitelli & Antonucci, 1994) and marital satisfaction (Julien & Markman, 1991) are more strongly related to perceptions of social support in marriage than are men's reports. Thus, the goal of increasing social support within an intimate relationship may be more beneficial for women than for men. As summarized by Barbee et al. (1993), researchers have also drawn attention to the role of gender in the ability of an individual to provide support to her or his partner. Women, who are traditionally socialized to be nurturing and emotionally expressive, may be better able to provide social support to their partners, particularly emotional support. Men, traditionally socialized toward autonomy and emotional control, may be more effective in providing instrumental support to their partners. If certain types of support are indeed more beneficial for some stressors than others (Cutrona & Suhr, 1992), considering these patterns of gender role socialization may be particularly important when involving intimate partners in the treatment of traumatized individuals. These patterns have implications for seeking out social support as well, with women having an easier time eliciting social support than men (Barbee et al., 1993).

As noted earlier, providing social support is not without costs, and these costs may differ for men and women. For example, in a study of disaster-related stress (Solomon, Smith, Robins, & Fischbach, 1987), men who were relied upon heavily for support by others reported increased alcohol use compared to men relied upon less heavily. Among women, being heavily relied upon by others was associated with increased somatic complaints. With regard to marital relationships, men highly satisfied with their relationships reported the lowest levels of symptomatology. For women, however, moderate satisfaction with their marital relationship was associated with the lowest levels of distress; women reporting high and low levels of satisfaction reported greater distress. Drawing on findings from another study of disaster-related stress in which women were more distressed than men by their partners' anxiety and/or depression (Gleser, Green, & Winget, 1981), Solomon et al. (1987) concluded that a similar dynamic might account for their own results; that is, women's distress may have been related to their spouses' problems and the level of support they provided to their spouses. Thus, women reporting the strongest marital relationships, and thus perhaps engaged in more nurturing behavior, were more distressed than those with moderately strong relationships characterized by lower demands for support. Consistent with this conceptualization, researchers studying Bosnian refugee couples found that women's reports of relationship distress were more strongly associated with their spouse's PTSD symptomatology than with their own PTSD symptoms (Spasojevic, Heffer, & Snyder, 2000).

Thus far in this section, we have focused primarily on issues related to increasing support in the relationships between trauma survivors and their partners and families. Trauma-related sequelae may pose challenges to other intervention strategies and goals as well. For instance, posttrauma symptoms, such as feelings of detachment from others and restricted range of emotion, may interfere with the desire and/or ability of trauma survivors to participate actively in family and couple-based interventions. Gender-related characteristics are also important to consider here. Compared to women, men have been found to be more reluctant to disclose negative emotions (Snell, Miller, Belk, Garcia-Falconi, & Hernandez-Sanchez, 1989). This reluctance may be especially pronounced in certain populations of trauma survivors. For example, Vietnam veterans, who were socialized into a very traditional masculine culture during their time in the military (Brooks, 1990) may find it particularly difficult to communicate openly with their families. Furthermore, maintaining relationships with important others appears central to women's self-esteem; in contrast, men's self-esteem has been associated with the ability to maintain their independence (Josephs, Markus, & Tafarodi, 1992). Thus, some of the goals of family and couple interventions may be more acceptable to women. Women are also likely to be more affected than men when others close to them experience negative life events (Kessler & McLeod, 1984). Thus, women may be more susceptible than men to secondary traumatization.

FURTHER CONSIDERATIONS AND RECOMMENDATIONS

As is clear from the previous discussion, there is much that we do not know about the use of couple- and family-based interventions for survivors of traumatic stress, particularly as characteristics of gender might influence these approaches. There is a shortage of empirical research on these treatments for trauma survivors, and discussion of gender issues is largely absent from the more extensive clinical literature. Therefore, we are left with many more questions than answers with regard to specific issues that might arise when conducting couple or family treatment with trauma survivors. We have identified four such issues that we think clinicians should consider when conducting couple or family therapy with trauma survivors.

First, although couple- and family-based interventions have been incorporated into treatment programs for both male and female trauma survivors, no comparisons of these treatments for men and women are available; that is, no data or clinical descriptions compare the efficacy or process of couple or family treatments across genders. As we described earlier, men and women are traditionally socialized such that they may seek and be able to provide different types of support to their partners. Similarly, traditional gender role socialization leads women, more than men, to derive their own self-worth from relationships with others. Thus, it seems likely that when incorporating couple or family therapy into treatments for trauma survivors, a therapist will encounter different issues with male compared to female survivors.

A second issue faced by clinicians working to incorporate couple or family therapy into their work with trauma survivors is the absence of information about how treatment might be affected by the type of trauma the survivor experienced. Although these therapies have been used with survivors of a range of traumatic events, including combat, rape, and child abuse, no information is available as to how these populations might differ in response to such treatment. It may be that the process and efficacy of family therapy will be substantially different for adult survivors of childhood sexual abuse than for someone recently injured in a car accident. In the present context, this is a particularly salient issue, because men and women are differentially at risk for different types of trauma. Therefore, clinicians must keep in mind that the use of couple or family therapy with trauma survivors may proceed differently for different clients both because of the client's gender, and because of the specific trauma that the client experienced.

A third consideration for therapists considering couple or family therapy for trauma survivors is whether the traumatic event preceded or followed the formation of the relationship. In cases in which the traumatic event occurred after the relationship (or family) was established (including cases in which a child was traumatized), the trauma represents an event that likely led to significant disruption of a functioning family. Therapy might focus on helping the family and survivor cope with this disruption, reestablishing the functional aspects of the "pretrauma" family, and improving family functioning in areas that were problematic prior to the trauma. In comparison, cases in which the traumatic event occurred prior to the formation of the relationship, it is likely that the survivor's trauma-related symptoms will have shaped the way in which the family developed. Treatment in these cases might need to focus on recognizing how the survivor's trauma affected the relationship, developing skills for functioning as a family, and managing the disruptions caused by the trauma-related symptoms. In dual-trauma couples in which both partners bring their own distinct trauma histories with them, these issues can be significantly more complicated.

Finally, clinicians working to incorporate couple or family therapy into their work with trauma survivors must consider which member or members of the family directly experienced the trauma. Family therapy in cases in which a single member of the family has experienced a trauma (by far the most prevalent situation described in the literature) may proceed in a relatively straightforward manner when focused on mutual support and improved communication. In contrast, when multiple family members, or even an entire family, are directly traumatized, the ability of the family to offer the necessary support or to invest the necessary energy in therapy may be substantially compromised.

SUMMARY

Although limited to specific populations, research provides evidence that trauma may have a deleterious effect on the interpersonal lives of trauma survivors and their partners and families. In spite of the perceived clinical utility of including intimate partners and family members in the treatment of posttrauma sequelae, empirical knowledge is extremely limited. Thus, in this chapter, we have reviewed related empirical findings that may be useful when deciding if and how to include intimate partners and family members in the treatment of posttrauma sequelae.

Descriptions of couple or family therapy for trauma survivors have tended to suggest that these approaches be used as an adjunct to other forms of treatment aimed more directly at alleviating posttraumatic symptoms (Riggs, 2000). Even when family therapy is recommended as the primary form of therapy (e.g., Erickson, 1989; Figley, 1995), individual treatment with the trauma survivor, either concurrently or prior to family therapy, is recommended. Only rarely, and almost exclusively in the case of traumatized children, does family therapy represent the exclusive, or even primary, mode of treatment for posttraumatic psychological symptoms. Indeed, in a review of the literature on the use of marital and family treatments for PTSD, Riggs (2000) concluded the following:

> Nothing is known about the efficacy of marital and family interventions alone as treatments for PTSD or other posttraumatic symptoms. Thus, pending further investigation, it is recommended at this time that, in the case of traumatized adults, marital and family therapy be conducted only in conjunction with (or following) treatment of the traumatized individual (or individuals) with interventions shown effective in reducing symptoms of PTSD. (p. 294)

Clearly, many clinicians have found it useful to incorporate couple and family therapy into their work with trauma survivors. Research focused on other disorders such as depression (e.g., Beach, Fincham, & Katz, 1996; Beach, Sandeen, & O'Leary, 1990; Jacobson, Dobson, Fruzzetti, Schmaling, & Salusky, 1991; O'Leary & Beach, 1990) and substance use (e.g.,

Fals-Stewart et al., 2000; O'Farrell & Fals-Stewart, 2000) also offer support for incorporating interventions aimed at couples or families for problems typically identified as individual issues. Because there is almost no empirical literature on the efficacy of couple and family therapy with trauma survivors at present, we can only speculate as to the utility of incorporating couple and family therapy into treatment programs for trauma-related problems. Research endeavors that focus on expanding the groups of trauma survivors studied, attending to gender and culture-related issues, and carrying out controlled treatment outcome studies would significantly enhance our understanding of the association between trauma and interpersonal functioning, and greatly facilitate intervention efforts.

REFERENCES

Acitelli, L. K., & Antonucci, T. C. (1994). Gender differences in the link between marital support and satisfaction in older couples. *Journal of Personality and Social Psychology, 4*, 688–698.

Arredondo, P., Orjuela, E., & Moore, L. (1989). Family therapy with Central American war refugee families. *Journal of Strategic and Systemic Therapies, 8*, 28–35.

Balcom, D. (1996). The interpersonal dynamics and treatment of dual trauma couples. *Journal of Marital and Family Therapy, 22*(4), 431–442.

Barbee, A. P., Cunningham, M. R., Winstead, B. A., Deriega, V. J., Gulley, M. R., Yankeelov, P. A., & Druen, P. B. (1993). Effects of gender role expectations on the social support process. *Journal of Social Issues, 49*, 175–190.

Barnes, M. F. (1995). Sex therapy in the couples context: Therapy issues of victims of sexual trauma. *American Journal of Family Therapy, 23*, 351–360.

Barrett, T. W., & Mizes, J. S. (1988). Combat level and social support in the development of posttraumatic stress disorder in Vietnam veterans. *Behavior Modification, 12*, 100–115.

Beach, S. R. H., Fincham, F. D., & Katz, J. (1998). Marital therapy in the treatment of depression: Toward a third generation of therapy and research. *Clinical Psychology Review, 18*, 635–661.

Beach, S. R. H., Martin, J. K., Blum, T. C., & Roman, P. M. (1993). Effects of marital and co-worker relationships on negative affect: Testing the central role of marriage. *American Journal of Family Therapy, 21*, 313–323.

Beach, S. R. H., Sandeen, R. R., & O'Leary, K. D. (1990). *Depression in marriage: A model for etiology and treatment.* New York: Guilford Press.

Beckham, J. C., Lytle, B. L., & Feldman, M. E. (1996). Caregiver burden in partners of Vietnam War veterans with posttraumatic stress disorder. *Journal of Consulting and Clinical Psychology, 64*, 1068–1072.

Beckham, J. C., Roodman, A. A., Barefoot, J. C., Haney, T. L., Helms, M. J., Fairbank, J. A., Hertzberg, M. A., & Kudler, H. S. (1996). Interpersonal and self-reported hostility among combat veterans with and without posttraumatic stress disorder. *Journal of Traumatic Stress, 9*, 335–342.

Boscarino, J. A. (1995). Post-traumatic stress and associated disorders among Vietnam veterans: The significance of combat exposure and social support. *Journal of Traumatic Stress, 8*, 317–336.

Brooks, G. R. (1990). Post-Vietnam gender-role strain: A needed concept? *Professional Psychology: Research and Practice, 21*, 18–25.

Brooks, G. R. (1991). Therapy pitfalls with Vietnam veteran families: Linearity, contextual naivete, and gender role blindness. *Journal of Family Psychology, 4*, 446–461.

Brown, P. C. (1984). Legacies of a war: Treatment and considerations with Vietnam veterans and their families. *Social Work, 29*, 372–379.

Buckley, T. C., Blanchard, E. B., & Hickling, E. J. (1996). A prospective examination of delayed onset PTSD secondary to motor vehicle accidents. *Journal of Abnormal Psychology, 105*, 617–625.

Buttenheim, M., & Levendosky, A. (1994). Couples treatment for incest survivors. *Psychotherapy, 31*, 407–414.

Byrne, C. A., & Riggs, D. S. (1996). The cycle of trauma: Relationship aggression in male Vietnam veterans with symptoms of posttraumatic stress disorder. *Violence and Victims, 11*, 213–225.

Carroll, E. M., Rueger, D. B., Foy, D. W., & Donohoe, C. P. (1985). Vietnam combat veterans with PTSD: Analysis of marital and cohabiting adjustment. *Journal of Abnormal Psychology, 94*, 329–337.

Caselli, L. T., & Motta, R. W. (1995). The effect of PTSD and combat level on Vietnam veterans' perceptions of child behavior and marital adjustment. *Journal of Clinical Psychology, 51*, 4–12.

Chauncey, S. (1994). Emotional concerns and treatment of male partners of female sexual abuse survivors. *Social Work, 39*, 669–676.

Cohen, S., & Wills, T. A. (1985). Stress, social support, and the buffering hypothesis. *Psychological Bulletin, 98*, 310–357.

Compton, J. S., & Follette, V. M. (1998). Couples surviving trauma: Issues and interventions. In V. M. Follette, J. I. Ruzek, & F. R. Abueg (Eds.), *Cognitive-behavioral therapies for trauma* (pp. 321–352). New York: Guilford Press.

Cutrona, C. E., & Suhr, J. A. (1992). Controllability of stressful events and satisfaction with spouse support behaviors. *Communication Research, 19*, 154–174.

Davidson, J. R., Hughes, D., Blazer, D. G., & George, L. K. (1991). Post-traumatic stress disorder in the community: An epidemiological study. *Psychological Medicine, 21*, 713–721.

DiLillo, D., & Long, P. J. (1999). Perceptions of couple functioning among female survivors of child sexual abuse. *Journal of Child Sexual Abuse, 7*, 59–76.

Erickson, C. A. (1989). Rape and the family. In C. R. Figley (Ed.), *Treating stress in families* (pp. 257–289). New York: Brunner/Mazel.

Fals-Stewart, W., O'Farrell, T. J., Feehan, M., Birchler, G. R., Tiller, S., & McFarlin, S. K. (2000). Behavioral couples therapy versus individual-based treatment for male substance-abusing patients: An evaluation of significant individual change and comparison of improvement rates. *Journal of Substance Abuse Treatment, 18*, 249–254.

Figley, C. R. (1986). Traumatic stress: The role of the family and social support system. In C. R. Figley (Ed.), *Trauma and its wake: Vol. II. Traumatic stress theory, research, and intervention* (pp. 39–52). New York: Brunner/Mazel.

Figley, C. R. (1988). A five-phase treatment of posttraumatic stress disorder in families. *Journal of Traumatic Stress, 1*(1), 127–141.

Figley, C. R. (1989). *Helping traumatized families.* San Francisco: Jossey-Bass.

Figley, C. R. (Ed.). (1995). *Compassion fatigue: Coping with secondary stress disorder in those who treat the traumatized.* New York: Brunner/Mazel.

Figley, C. R., & Kleber, R. J. (1995). Beyond the "victim": Secondary traumatic stress. In R. J. Kleber, C. R. Figley, & B. P. R. Gersons (Eds.), *Beyond trauma: Cultural and social dynamics* (pp. 75–98). New York: Plenum Press.

Finkelhor, D., Hotaling, G. T., Lewis, I. A., & Smith, C. (1989). Sexual abuse and its relationship to later sexual satisfaction, marital status, religion, and attitudes. *Journal of Interpersonal Violence, 4,* 379–399.

Fleming, J., Mullen, P. E., Sibthorpe, B., & Bammer, G. (1999). The long-term impact of childhood sexual abuse in Australian women. *Child Abuse and Neglect, 23,* 145–159.

Fontana, A., Schwartz, L. S., & Rosenheck, R. (1997). Posttraumatic stress disorder among female Vietnam veterans: A causal model of etiology. *American Journal of Public Health, 87,* 169–175.

Fullerton, C. S., & Ursano, R. J. (1997). Posttraumatic responses in spouse/significant others of disaster workers. In C. S. Fullerton & R. J. Ursano (Eds.), *Posttraumatic stress disorder: Acute and long-term responses to trauma and disaster* (pp. 59–75). Washington, DC: American Psychiatric Press.

Gallagher, J. G., Riggs, D. S., Byrne, C. A., & Weathers, F. W. (1998). Female partners' estimations of male veterans' combat-related PTSD severity. *Journal of Traumatic Stress, 11,* 367–374.

Gleser, G. C., Green, B. L., & Winget, C. (1981). *Prolonged psychosocial effects of disaster: A study of Buffalo Creek.* New York: Academic Press.

Glynn, S. M., Eth, S., Randolph, E. T., Foy, D. W., Leong, G. B., Paz, G. G., Salk, J. D., Firman, G., & Katzman, J. W. (1995). Behavioral family therapy for Vietnam combat veterans with posttraumatic stress disorder. *Journal of Psychotherapy Practice and Research, 4,* 214–223.

Glynn, S. M., Eth, S., Randolph, E. T., Foy, D. W., Urbaitis, M., Boxer, L., Paz, G. G., Leong, G. B., Firman, G., Salk, J. D., Katzman, J. W., & Crothers, J. (1999). A test of behavioral family therapy to augment exposure for combat-related posttraumatic stress disorder. *Journal of Consulting and Clinical Psychology, 67,* 243–251.

Harris, C. J. (1991). A family crisis-intervention model for the treatment of posttraumatic stress reaction. *Journal of Traumatic Stress, 4,* 195–207.

Hendrix, C. C., Jurich, A. P., & Schumm, W. R. (1995). Long-term impact of Vietnam War service on family environment and satisfaction. *Families in Society: The Journal of Contemporary Human Services, 16,* 498–506.

Hertz, D. G., & Lerer, B. (1981). The "rape family": Family reactions to the rape victims. *International Journal of Family Psychiatry, 2,* 301–315.

Jacobson, N. S., Dobson, K., Fruzzetti, A. E., Schmaling, D. B., & Salusky, S. (1991). Marital therapy as a treatment for depression. *Journal of Consulting and Clinical Psychology, 59,* 547–557.

Johnson, D. R., Feldman S. C., & Lubin, H. (1995). Critical interaction therapy: Couples therapy in combat-related posttraumatic stress disorder. *Family Process, 34,* 401–412.

Johnson, S. M. (1989). Integrating marital and individual therapy for incest survivors: A case study. *Psychotherapy, 21*(6), 96–103.

Johnson, S. M., & Williams-Keeler, L. (1998). Creating healing relationships for couples dealing with trauma: The use of emotionally focused marital therapy. *Journal of Marital and Family Therapy, 24,* 25–40.

Jordan, B. K., Marmar, C. R., Fairbank, J. A., Schlenger, W. E., Kulka, R. A., Hough, R. L., & Weiss, D. S. (1992). Problems in families of male Vietnam veterans with posttraumatic stress disorder. *Journal of Consulting and Clinical Psychology, 60*(6), 916–926.

Josephs, R. A., Markus, H. R., & Tafarodi, R. W. (1992). Gender and self-esteem. *Journal of Personality and Social Psychology, 63,* 391–402.

Joseph, S. (1999). Social support and mental health following trauma. In W. Yule (Ed.), *Post-traumatic stress disorders: Concepts and therapy* (pp. 71–91). West Sussex, UK: Wiley.

Julien, D., & Markman, H. J. (1991). Social support and social networks as determinants of individual and marital outcomes. *Journal of Social and Personal Relationships, 8,* 549–568.

Kaniasty, K., & Norris, F. H. (1992). Social support and victims of crime: Matching event, support, and outcome. *American Journal of Community Psychology, 20,* 211–241.

Keane, T. M., Scott, W. O., Chavoya, G. A., Lamparski, D. M., & Fairbank, J. A. (1985). Social support in Vietnam veterans with posttraumatic stress disorder: A comparative analysis. *Journal of Consulting and Clinical Psychology, 53,* 95–102.

Kerewksy, S. D., & Miller, D. (1996). Lesbian couples and childhood trauma: Guidelines for therapists. In J. Laird & R. Green (Eds.), *Lesbians and gays in couples and families* (pp. 298–315). San Francisco: Jossey-Bass.

Kessler, R. C., & McLeod, J. D. (1984). Sex differences in vulnerability to undesirable life events. *American Sociological Review, 49,* 620–631.

Kilpatrick, D. G., Best, C. L., Saunders, B. E., & Veronen, L. J. (1988). Rape in marriage and in dating relationships: How bad is it for mental health? *Annals of the New York Academy of Sciences, 528,* 335–344.

Kimerling, R., & Calhoun, K. S. (1994). Somatic symptoms, social support, and treatment seeking among sexual assault victims. *Journal of Consulting and Clinical Psychology, 62,* 333–340.

King, L. A., King, D. W., Fairbank, J. A., Keane, T. M., & Adams, G. A. (1998). Resilience–recovery factors in posttraumatic stress disorder among female and male Vietnam veterans: Hardiness, postwar social support, and additional stressful life events. *Journal of Personality and Social Psychology, 74,* 420–434.

Klinger, R. L., & Stein, T. S. (1996). Impact of violence, childhood sexual abuse, and domestic violence and abuse on lesbians, bisexuals, and gay men. In R. P. Cabaj & T. S. Stein (Eds.), *Textbook of homosexuality and mental health* (pp. 801–818). Washington, DC: American Psychiatric Press.

Kulka, R. A., Schlenger, W. E., Fairbank, J. A., Hough, R. L., Jordan, B. K., Marmar, C. R., & Weiss, D. S. (1990). *Trauma and the Vietnam War generation: Report of findings from the National Vietnam Veterans Readjustment Study.* New York: Brunner/Mazel.

Lane, C., & Hobfoll, S. E. (1992). How loss affects anger and alienates social support. *Journal of Consulting and Clinical Psychology, 60,* 935–942.

Lantz, J., & Gregoire, T. (2000). Existential psychotherapy with Vietnam veteran couples: A twenty-five year report. *Contemporary Family Therapy, 22,* 19–37.

Lehman, D. R., Ellard, J. H., & Wortman, C. B. (1986). Social support for the bereaved: Recipients' and providers' perspectives on what is helpful. *Journal of Consulting and Clinical Psychology, 54,* 438–446.

Letourneau, E. J., Resnick, H. S., Kilpatrick, D. G., Saunders, B. E., & Best, C. L. (1996). Comorbidity of sexual problems and posttraumatic stress disorder in female crime victims. *Behavior Therapy, 27,* 321–326.

Litz, B. T., Keane, T. M., Fisher, L., Marx, B., & Monaco, V. (1992). Physical health complaints in combat-related posttraumatic stress disorder: A preliminary report. *Journal of Traumatic Stress, 5,* 131–141.

MacDonald, C., Chamberlain, K., Long, N., & Flett, R. (1999). Posttraumatic stress disorder and interpersonal functioning in Vietnam War veterans: A mediational model. *Journal of Traumatic Stress, 12,* 701–707.

Maltas, C., & Shay, J. (1995). Trauma contagion in partners of survivors of childhood sexual abuse. *American Journal of Orthopsychiatry, 65,* 529–539.

McLeod, J. D., Kessler, R. C., & Landis, K. R. (1992). Speed of recovery from major depressive episodes in a community sample of married men and women. *Journal of Abnormal Psychology, 101,* 277–286.

Mennen, F. E., & Pearlmutter, L. (1993). Detecting childhood sexual abuse in couples therapy. *Families in Society: The Journal of Contemporary Human Services, 74,* 74–83.

Mio, J. S., & Foster, J. D. (1991). The effects of rape upon victims and families: Implications for a comprehensive family therapy. *American Journal of Family Therapy, 19* (2), 147–159.

Moss, M., Frank, E., & Anderson, B. (1990). The effects of marital status and partner support on rape trauma. *American Journal of Orthopsychiatry, 60,* 379–391.

Mullen, P. E., Martin, J. L., Anderson, J. C., Romans, S. E., & Herbison, G. P. (1994). The effect of child sexual abuse on social, interpersonal, and sexual function in adult life. *British Journal of Psychiatry, 165,* 35–47.

Mueser, K. T., & Glynn, S. M. (1995). *Behavioral family therapy for psychiatric disorders.* New York: Simon & Schuster.

Nadelson, C., & Polonsky, D. (1991). Childhood sexual abuse: The invisible ghost in couple therapy. *Psychiatric Annals, 21,* 479–484.

Nelson, B. S., & Wampler, K. S. (2000). Systemic effects of trauma in clinic couples: An exploratory study of secondary trauma resulting from childhood abuse. *Journal of Marital and Family Therapy, 26,* 171–184.

Nelson, B. S., & Wright, D. W. (1996). Understanding and treating posttraumatic stress disorder symptoms in female partners of veterans with PTSD. *Journal of Marital and Family Therapy, 22,* 455–467.

O'Farrell, T. J., & Fals-Stewart, W. (2000). Behavioral couples therapy for alcoholism and drug abuse. *Journal of Substance Abuse Treatment, 18,* 51–54.

O'Leary, K. D., & Beach, S. R. (1990). Marital therapy: A viable treatment for depression and marital discord. *American Journal of Psychiatry, 147,* 183–186.

Perry, S. W., Difede, J., Musngi, G., Frances, A. J., & Jacobsberg, L. (1992). Predictors of posttraumatic stress disorder after burn injury. *American Journal of Psychiatry, 149,* 931–935.

Rabin, C. (1995). The use of psychoeducational groups to improve marital functioning in high risk Israeli couples: A stage model. *Contemporary Family Therapy,* *17,* 503–515.

Rabin, C., & Nardi, C. (1991). Treating post traumatic stress disorder couples: A psychoeducational program. *Community Mental Health Journal, 27*(3), 209–224.

Reid, K. S., Wampler, R. S., & Taylor, D. K. (1996). The "alienated" partner: Responses to traditional therapies for adult sex abuse survivors. *Journal of Marital and Family Therapy, 22,* 443–453.

Riggs, D. S. (2000). Marital and family therapy. In E. B. Foa, T. M. Keane, & M. J. Friedman (Eds.), *Effective treatments for PTSD: Practice guidelines from the International Society for Traumatic Stress Studies* (pp. 280–301). New York: Guilford Press.

Riggs, D. S., Byrne, C. A., & Lam, L. M. (2001). *Traumatized relationships: Symptoms of posttraumatic stress disorder, intimacy, and marital adjustment in dual trauma couples.* Manuscript submitted for publication.

Riggs, D. S., Byrne, C. A., Weathers, F. W., & Litz, B. T. (1998). The quality of intimate relationships of male Vietnam veterans: Problems associated with posttraumatic stress disorder. *Journal of Traumatic Stress, 11,* 87–101.

Roberts, W. R., Penk, W. E., Gearing, M. L., Robinowitz, R., Dolan, M. P., & Patterson, E. T. (1982). Interpersonal problems of Vietnam combat veterans with symptoms of posttraumatic stress disorder. *Journal of Abnormal Psychology, 91,* 444–450.

Rosenheck, R., & Thompson J. (1986). "Detoxification" of Vietnam War trauma: A combined family–individual approach. *Family Process, 25,* 559–570.

Shehan, C. L. (1987). Spouse support and Vietnam veterans? adjustment to posttraumatic stress disorder. *Family Relations, 36,* 55–60.

Silverman, D. C. (1978). Sharing the crisis of rape: Counseling the mates and families of victims. *American Journal of Orthopsychiatry, 40,* 503–511.

Snell, W. E., Miller, R. S., Belk, S. S., Garcia-Falconi, R., & Hernandez-Sanchez, J. E. (1989). Men's and women's emotional disclosures: The impact of disclosure recipient, culture, and the masculine role. *Sex Roles, 21,* 467–486.

Snyder, M. (1996). Intimate partners: A context for the intensification and healing of emotional pain. *Women and Therapy, 19,* 79–92.

Solomon, S. D., Smith, E. M., Robins, L. N., & Fischbach, R. L. (1987). Social involvement as a mediator of disaster-induced stress. *Journal of Applied Social Psychology, 17,* 1092–1112.

Solomon, Z. (1988). The effect of combat-related posttraumatic stress disorder on the family. *Psychiatry, 51,* 323–329.

Solomon, Z., Bleich, A., Shoham, S., Nardi, C., & Kotler, M. (1992). The "Koach" project for treatment of combat-related PTSD: Rationale, aims, and methodology. *Journal of Traumatic Stress, 5*(2), 175–193.

Solomon, Z., Waysman, M., Levy, G., Fried, B., Mikulincer, M., Benbenishty, R., Florian, V., & Bleich, A. (1992). From front line to home front: A study of secondary traumatization. *Family Process, 31,* 289–302.

Solomon, Z., Waysman, M., & Mikulincer, M. (1990). Family functioning, perceived social support, and combat-related psychopathology: The moderating role of loneliness. *Journal of Social and Clinical Psychology, 9,* 456–472.

Spasojevic, J., Heffer, R. W., & Snyder, D. K. (2000). Effects of posttraumatic stress and acculturation on marital functioning in Bosnian refugee couples. *Journal of Traumatic Stress, 13,* 205–217.

Syrotuik, J., & D'Arcy, C. (1984). Social support and mental health: Direct, protective and compensatory effects. *Social Science and Medicine, 18,* 229–236.

Thelen, M. H., Sherman, M. D., & Borst, T. S. (1998). Fear of intimacy and attachment among rape survivors. *Behavior Modification, 22,* 108–116.

Waysman, M., Mikulincer, M., Solomon, Z., & Weisenberg, M. (1993). Secondary traumatization among wives of posttraumatic combat veterans: A family typology. *Journal of Family Psychology, 7,* 104–118.

Williams, C. M., & Williams, T. (1980). Family therapy for Vietnam veterans. In T. Williams (Ed.), *Post-traumatic stress disorder of the Vietnam veteran.* Cincinnati: Disabled American Veterans.

Wilson, K., & James, A. L. (1992). Child sexual abuse and couple therapy. *Sexual and Marital Therapy, 7,* 197–212.

Zoellner, L. A., Foa, E. B., & Brigidi, B. D. (1999). Interpersonal friction and PTSD in female victims of sexual and nonsexual assault. *Journal of Traumatic Stress, 12,* 689–700.

Part V | **Research and Policy**

15 | Gender Differences in Stress, Trauma, and PTSD Research

Application of Two Quantitative Methods

LYNDA A. KING
HOLLY K. ORCUTT
DANIEL W. KING

When one reads or hears the phrase "gender differences," the statistical situation that most readily comes to mind is the simple comparison of the scores of women and men on a particular variable. For example, we might ask the research question: "Following exposure to a common stressor, do women and men differ in posttraumatic stress disorder (PTSD) symptomatology as measured by their continuous symptom severity scores on the PTSD Checklist (PCL; Blanchard, Jones-Alexander, Buckley, & Forneris, 1996; Weathers, Litz, Herman, Huska, & Keane, 1993)?" This comparison is typically accomplished in one of two ways. Probably the most direct avenue is to evaluate the significance of the difference between independent group means (the PCL mean for men vs. that for women) using a t test or its equivalent F ratio. This strategy allows us to determine whether, on average, men score higher than women, or women score higher than men on the PCL. Similar information is available by relying on a bivariate regression analysis in which the dependent variable of interest, PCL score, is regressed on the independent variable of gender, and gender is coded in a dichotomous fashion (such as 1 = women and 0 = men). With this 1/0 coding scheme, the intercept in the regression equation is the mean for men, and the regression coefficient is the difference between the means of women and men. The significance of the regression coefficient—the gender difference—again may be evaluated by t or F, and the strength of the relationship—between gender and PCL score—can be captured in a correlation coefficient. Either approach may be used, and in both cases, the interpretation of a significant finding is the same.

Another simple comparison between genders can be made when the outcome of interest is a frequency count, a percentage of occurrence, or some documentation of proportion within levels of a categorical variable. In this regard, it may be of interest to determine whether women and men have different prevalence rates of PTSD; that is, do the data suggest a tendency for the diagnosis of PTSD to be more (or less) prevalent in women (or men)? We would count the number of PTSD-positive and PTSD-negative diagnoses for women and men separately, and then compute a chi-square test of the association between gender and diagnosis. A significant value for the chi-square statistic in this instance would lead to the conclusion that there is an association between gender and diagnosis and, hence, that there is a difference in prevalence rates for women and men. This particular examination of gender differences in frequency counts, percentages, or proportions could be extended to include research situations in which the comparison of women and men involves distributions across more than two categories: for example, full PTSD, partial PTSD, and no PTSD.

For any of these gender difference analyses, it is also possible to introduce "control variables" or covariates that statistically equate study participants before performing the gender-based comparison. Such a strategy is aimed at ruling out alternative influences for an observed gender difference on the outcome variable and possibly providing a more sensitive or powerful test of the difference between women and men. Consider the contrast between women and men who have experienced a common traumatic event, such as a natural or human-made disaster in their community. If one were interested in gender differences in PTSD symptom severity or prevalence rates, it might be appropriate to equate statistically all disaster victims on the intensity of the exposure. Removing the influence of exposure intensity in the comparison between women and men would more clearly answer the question: "Given an equal degree of exposure to the event, do women and men differ with regard to PTSD?" If PTSD is measured as a continuous variable (e.g., a symptom severity score on the PCL), then the gender difference question could be addressed with an analysis of covariance, a randomized block analysis of variance, or a multiple regression analysis. If PTSD is assessed as a categorical variable (e.g., frequencies, percentages, or proportions of persons classified as PTSD-positive or PTSD-negative, or as full PTSD, partial PTSD, or no PTSD), then log linear and logistic regression analyses are available.

Finally, though not as frequently used by researchers in the realm of gender differences, there are statistical tests for the difference between group variances. These procedures enable the researcher to decide whether there is evidence for a difference in the dispersion or spread of scores on a continuous variable. Lunneborg and Abbott (1983) demonstrated the logic for a likelihood ratio-based chi-square test for the difference between group variances, and the Statistical Package for the Social Sciences (SPSS) software package provides Levene's test of homogeneity of variance, a non-likelihood, ratio-based test recommended for non-normal data. To illustrate, in the National Vietnam Veterans Readjustment Study (Kulka et al., 1990), the dispersion of scores on the Mississippi Scale for Combat-Related PTSD (Keane, Caddell, & Taylor, 1988) was greater for male veterans who served in Vietnam than for female veterans who served in that war. The standard deviation for men was 22.35, whereas the standard deviation for women was 17.21, and the computed Levene statistic is significant, $F(1, 1617) = 47.07$, $p < .001$. Therefore, the spread or variance of scores for men is of higher magnitude than the spread or variance of scores for women. This finding is not surprising given that the subsample of women, mostly nurses, was quite homogeneous in education and other background characteristics, and their war-zone exposures were more uniform than those of the men who served in Vietnam (King, King, Foy, & Gudanowski, 1996; King, King, Gudanowski, & Vreven, 1995).

Thus, there is an entire collection of well-used methods that can identify differences between genders in their group mean scores, in their respective frequencies of occurrence of some event or condition, or in the dispersion of their scores. Regardless of the complexity of the analyses, the "bottom line" is to compare women and men on some aspect of the variable of interest.

Yet another type of research question is very important for a comprehensive understanding of gender differences. The question goes beyond the simple issue of differences in means, frequencies, or variances, and emphasizes female–male differences in the associations or relationships between or among variables. In this chapter, this notion of differential relationships as a function of gender provides an integrating theme to describe two seemingly unrelated methods. We begin with a presentation of moderated multiple regression analysis in which the interest is whether the relationship between a predictor and an outcome (say, intensity of trauma exposure and PTSD, or attitudes toward women and perpetration of domestic violence) is different for women than for men. We then discuss multiple group confirmatory factor analysis, the aim of which is to determine if the relationship between a latent variable or factor (e.g., PTSD) and a measured or observed variable (e.g., an item score, or perhaps a composite score on a handful of items measuring the same PTSD symptom cluster) is different for women than for men. Throughout our presentation, we attempt to provide a simple, not too mathematical conceptualization of the methods. We supplement, where possible, with illustrations and our own analyses with existing data sets.

MODERATED MULTIPLE REGRESSION

Perhaps the simpler of our two approaches to examining differential relationships as a function of gender is moderated multiple regression. In this section, we briefly introduce multiple regression. Then, we describe the concepts of interactions and moderator variables, followed by the special circumstance in which gender moderates the relationship between two continuous variables. We next demonstrate a moderated multiple regression analysis of the interaction between scores on a prominent measure of gender role ideology and gender in the prediction of intimate relationship violence. The section concludes with brief commentary on other issues and concerns, and recommendations for further reading on the topic.

Overview of Multiple Regression

Multiple regression is a class of statistical procedures intended to describe the association between an outcome, or dependent variable, and a weighted composite of two or more predictors, or independent variables. A very simple representation of a multiple regression equation would be

$$Y_i = B_0 + B_1 X_{1i} + B_2 X_{2i} + \ldots + B_k X_{ki} + e_i \qquad \text{(Eq. 1)}$$

Y_i is the dependent variable for person i; X_{1i}, X_{2i}, and as many as X_{ki} are independent variables for person i. The multiple regression equation has its roots in the algebra of a straight line, in that B_0 is the Y-intercept and the B_1 through B_k values are slopes. Each of these slopes indicates the change in the dependent variable (Y) per unit change in its associated independent variable (e.g., X_1) at constant or specified values of the other independent variables ($X_2 \ldots X_k$). The slopes also denote the unique contribution of an independent variable and are referred to as "regression coefficients." The e_i symbol recognizes the presence of a residual, or error, in the prediction of any single person's score on the dependent variable from the weighted composite of the various independent variables.

The weights in the composite (B_0 and B_1, $B_2 \ldots B_k$) are derived so as to satisfy optimally some specified function or criterion. One such criterion is the minimization of error, such that across all cases in the sample, the sum of the squared error terms (values of e) is as small as it can possibly be. Weights derived in this way are called "ordinary least squares estimates" and are the most typically used weights in multiple regression analysis. Under certain assumptions, these weights are maximum likelihood estimates, which allow for the implementation of parametric statistical theory. In other words, tests of statistical significance can be employed for both the intercept and regression coefficients, and for the model as a whole.

The independent variables may be either categorical (e.g., victim of prior violence vs. not a victim of prior violence; male vs. female gender) or continuous (e.g., a scaled measure of the severity of trauma exposure; age at time of exposure). The dependent variable likewise may be either categorical (as in the diagnosis of PTSD as present or absent) or continuous (as in symptom severity scores on the PCL or Mississippi Scale). We are particularly interested in the application of multiple regression to the case in which the dependent variable is continuous. (The case in which the dependent variable is categorical is beyond the scope of this chapter, and we refer the reader to major texts by Agresti, 1990, and Hosmer & Lemeshow, 1989.) Furthermore, in pursuit of our goal of describing differential relationships as a function of gender, our independent variables will be a mixture of categorical and continuous, with gender serving in the special role of moderator.

Introduction to Interactions and Moderator Variables

An understanding of differential relationships between a predictor and an outcome as a function of gender is most easily represented in a traditional 2 × 2 factorial design, in which the two levels of the gender categorical variable are crossed with two levels of another categorical variable. Let us assume that this second variable, denoted gender role ideology, classifies individuals with regard to their basic attitudes about the equality of women and men as either traditional or egalitarian. The dependent variable is a self-report of the number of incidents of physical violence directed toward an intimate partner. In other words, the researcher is asking whether the propensity to commit violent acts is a function of the individual's gender (constant over, or regardless of, gender role ideology) and/or a function of the individual's traditional–egalitarian attitudes about the equality of women and men (constant over, or regardless of, her or his gender). Each of these research questions defines a main effect. But a more interesting question may be the extent to which these variables *jointly* influence intimate relationship violence, such that some unique combination of the levels of gender and gender role ideology serves either to exacerbate or mitigate incidents of violence. This latter question reflects the notion of an interaction.

This research situation with two sets of contrived data is depicted in Table 15.1. Table 15.1a shows a pattern of cell means (for our dependent variable, intimate relationship violence) that might be obtained when we find main effects for both gender and ideology, but no interaction. Table 15.1b shows an alternative pattern of cell means that would indicate an interaction between gender and ideology (and also a main effect for ideology, but none for gender). The marginal values for the rows, rightmost on both tables, are the means for each level of ideology averaged over the levels of gender, and the marginal values for the columns, at the bottom of

TABLE 15.1. Illustration of Main Effects and Interaction: A Simple 2 × 2 Factorial Design

a. Main effects: No interaction

Ideology	Gender: F	Gender: M	
Traditional	1.50	2.50	2.00
Egalitarian	1.00	2.00	1.50
	1.25	2.25	

b. Gender × gender role ideology interaction

Ideology	Gender: F	Gender: M	
Traditional	1.00	2.50	1.75
Egalitarian	2.00	.50	1.25
	1.50	1.50	

Note. The dependent variable is the average number of incidents of intimate relationship violence. F, female; M, male.

each table, are the means for each level of gender averaged over the levels of ideology.

Concentrating first on Table 15.1a, the difference between the row marginal values (2.00 – 1.50 = .50) is the same as the difference between the traditional and egalitarian levels of ideology for both women (1.50 – 1.00 = .50) and men (2.50 – 2.00 = .50). Similarly, the difference between the column marginal values (1.25 – 2.25 = –1.00) is the same as the difference between women and men for both the traditional (1.50 – 2.50 = –1.00) and egalitarian (1.00 – 2.00 = –1.00) levels of ideology. This pattern of fictitious findings contrasts with that depicted in Table 15.1b. The column marginal values in Table 15.1b (both 1.50) suggest that there is no gender main effect; on average, women and men are reporting similar amounts of violence against their intimate partners. There is an apparent main effect for ideology; those holding traditional attitudes report more violence (1.75) than those holding egalitarian attitudes (1.25). Going further, beginning with the rows, the difference between the marginal values (1.75 – 1.25 = .50) is not equivalent to either the difference for women only (1.00 – 2.00 = –1.00) or the difference for men only (2.50 – .50 = 2.00). Likewise, the difference between the column marginal values (1.50 – 1.50 = 0) is not equal to the corresponding differences for individuals with a traditional ideology (1.00 – 2.50 = –1.50) or for individuals with an egalitarian ideology (2.00 – .50 = 1.50). In the instance in which there is no interaction (Table 15.1a), the effect of a given variable (e.g., ideology) is constant across the levels of the other variable (e.g., gender). When there is an interaction (Table 15.1b), the effect of a given variable is not constant across the levels of the other variable.

In our Table 15.1b example, women who are traditional in their ide-

ology report perpetrating fewer incidents of violence against their partners (mean of 1.00) than women who are egalitarian in their ideology
(mean of 2.00), whereas the opposite pattern is seen for men, with traditional men reporting perpetration of more violence (mean of 2.50) than
egalitarian men (mean of .50). Thus, the apparent influence of gender
role ideology on intimate relationship violence differs as a function of
gender; stated alternatively, the association between ideology and violence
is different for women and men. We conclude that there is a gender ×
gender role ideology interaction effect in accounting for intimate relationship violence.

Figure 15.1 is intended to clarify the results presented in Table 15.1,
especially the idea of an interaction in terms of differential relationships as
a function of gender. In both Figures 15.1a and 15.1b, the relationship between ideology and violence is graphed separately for women and men by
plotting values of the cell means (average violence scores) for each of the
two levels of ideology (traditional and egalitarian).

In Figure 15.1a, where there is no interaction, the main effect for gender is captured in the observation that the line for men is higher on the violence scale than the line for women. Similarly, the main effect for ideology
is captured in the observation that both lines are negatively inclined; hence,
persons with traditional attitudes are scoring higher on the violence scale
than persons with egalitarian attitudes. The parallelism, or uniform slopes,
of the two lines denote the lack of an interaction: The change in violence
scores, or difference in cell means, for women and men remains constant
across both levels of the ideology variable.

In Figure 15.1b, the interaction is obvious. Here, the relationship between ideology and violence clearly differs for women and men. Note the
slopes of the separate lines. For women, the change in violence scores, or
difference in cell means, is positive when moving from traditional to egalitarian ideology; for men, the corresponding change is negative. Thus, in
predicting the propensity to inflict intimate relationship violence from a
person's gender role ideology, it is extremely important to know the gender
of the person as well. Gender can be said to be a moderator of the relationship between ideology and violence. It might be noted that interactions can
be interpreted bidirectionally. For this illustration, we could have pursued
the relationship between gender and intimate relationship violence as a
function of gender role ideology. But because this chapter focuses on methods of detecting gender differences, gender is the appropriate moderator
variable.

Gender in Interaction with Continuous Independent Variables

Our example treated gender role ideology as a categorical variable having
two levels. The informed reader of gender research, however, is aware that

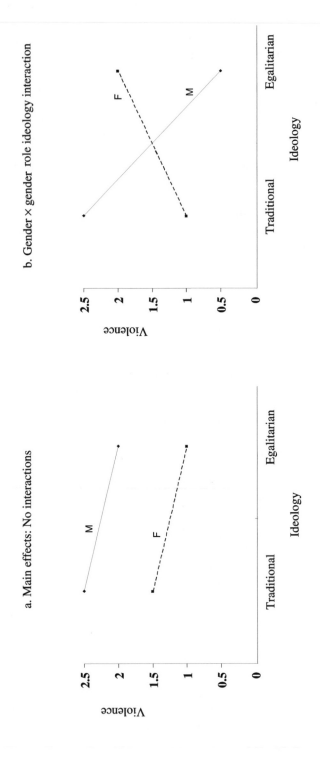

FIGURE 15.1. Graphical representation of the contrived data for the 2 × 2 factorial design. The dependent variable is the average number of incidents of intimate relationship violence. F, female; M, male.

this type of attitudinal variable is typically considered and measured as an ordered continuous dimension having multiple possible scores, ranging from low (traditional) to high (egalitarian); see, for example, the broadly used Attitudes Toward Women Scale (Spence & Helmreich, 1972), and the many assessment instruments catalogued by Beere (1990). Consequently, a more realistic representation of gender as a moderator of the ideology–violence relationship requires that the interaction represent the joint effect of the categorical gender variable and a continuous ideology variable. This generalizes to many questions in stress, trauma, and PTSD research, where the essential concern for female–male comparisons focuses on differential relationships between one or more continuous independent variables (e.g., intensity of trauma exposure, age at time of exposure, extent of social support network) and a continuous dependent variable (e.g., PTSD symptom severity). Thus, we extend our presentation to interactions in a multiple regression framework.

In multiple regression, an interaction between two predictor variables is represented by a third variable that is computed as the product of the two predictors. For example, a variable representing the interaction between X_1 and X_2 would be calculated as the product of scores on X_1 and X_2 for all cases; a variable representing the interaction of X_1 and X_3 would be calculated as the product of scores on X_1 and X_3 for all cases; and so on. With just two predictor variables and their interaction, the regression model would be

$$Y_i = B_0 + B_1X_{1i} + B_2X_{2i} + B_3X_{1i}X_{2i} + e_i \qquad \text{(Eq. 2)}$$

where all elements are as described previously (Eq. 1), the X_1X_2 product term carries the information of the interaction (Cohen & Cohen, 1983; Cohen, Cohen, Aiken, & West, 2002), and the B_3 regression coefficient delineates the unique contribution of the interaction term to the dependent variable. As noted by Jaccard, Turrisi, and Wan (1990), this coefficient is the change in relationship between one of the independent variables (say, X_2) and the dependent variable (Y) per unit change in the other independent variable (X_1), and vice versa. This interpretation can be seen by some minor manipulation of Eq. 2, most notably factoring X_2 from the third and fourth elements to the right of the equal sign:

$$Y_i = (B_0 + B_1X_{1i}) + (B_2 + B_3X_{1i})X_{2i} + e_i \qquad \text{(Eq. 3)}$$

Notice that this expression follows the general form for the equation of a straight line, documenting the relationship between two variables, X_2 and Y:

$$Y = \text{(intercept)} + \text{(slope)}X_2 + \text{error} \qquad \text{(Eq. 4)}$$

Here, the slope for the regression of Y on X_2 is $(B_2 + B_3X_1)$ and the intercept can be reconceptualized as $(B_0 + B_1X_1)$. Thus, the relationship between Y and X_2, as represented by the slope, changes as X_1 takes on different values. And, for each unit change in X_1, the slope for the regression of Y on X_2 changes by B_3 units, the value of the regression coefficient for the interaction term. By designating X_1 as gender, we now have a mechanism for representing differential relationships between the other independent variable (X_2) and the dependent variable (Y). The model can be expanded to accommodate more independent variables, either categorical or continuous, some possibly intended also to interact with gender, with each other, or not. The works by Cohen and Cohen (1983) and Cohen et al. (2002) provide excellent detailed elaboration on more complicated multiple regression analyses. What follows is a presentation of the analysis and interpretation of findings for a set of real data, incorporating additional basic concepts germane to the method.

Demonstration of Moderated Multiple Regression Analysis Using Existing Data

Description of the Data

For demonstration purposes, we draw from a portion of a study of intimate relationship violence among college students (Fitzpatrick, Salgado, Suvak, King, & King, 2002). The data set comprises the responses of 219 college students (155 women and 64 men) to three measures: (1) the physical violence subscale of the Conflict Tactics Scale (CTS; Straus, 1979), (2) the Dyadic Adjustment Scale (DAS, Spanier, 1976), and (3) the Sex-Role Egalitarianism Scale—Form KK (SRES; King & King, 1993, 1997). The CTS physical violence subscale is the measure of intimate relationship violence, with higher scores indicating more violent acts perpetrated by the study participant on her or his partner within a 1-year time frame. The DAS indexes the quality of the participant's relationship with her or his partner, again with higher scores representing more satisfaction and comfort with the relationship. The SRES assesses gender role ideology and provides continuous scores along a dimension bounded by traditional (lower end) to egalitarian (upper end). Lower scores reflect beliefs in line with more conventional role expectations for women and men, whereas higher scores indicate beliefs about the behaviors and characteristics of women and men that are more flexible and less tied to conventional role expectations. The primary research question of interest is as follows: Controlling for relationship quality, does the association between gender role ideology and intimate relationship violence differ as a function of participants' gender? Thus, this is a modest extension of the fictitious data previously used as a vehicle in this chapter.

Analyses

The gender variable was dummy coded, assigning a value of 1 to the female participants and a value of 0 to the male participants. In actuality, any two numbers could have been used, but this 1/0 coding scheme is recommended to simplify computations and afford direct interpretation of regression coefficients in terms of gender differences. Also recommended is the practice of centering any variable that is expected to interact with gender (e.g., Aiken & West, 1991; Jaccard et al., 1990; Cohen et al., 2002), in this case, gender role ideology as measured by the SRES. Centering is quite simple. It is transforming the distribution of original or observed scores, so that the mean of the transformed scores will be 0. This was easily accomplished by subtracting the original SRES mean from every original SRES score. The interaction term was next computed by multiplying the dummy coded gender score by the centered SRES score. The distribution of DAS scores was also centered to simplify later computations.

Using a standard statistical software package, a two-step hierarchical multiple regression procedure (Cohen & Cohen, 1983) was performed. At the first step, CTS scores were regressed on centered DAS scores, centered SRES scores, and gender. At the second step, CTS scores were regressed on centered DAS scores, centered SRES scores, gender, and the interaction between gender and SRES (ideology).

Results and Their Interpretation

Table 15.2 presents the results of the hierarchical multiple regression analysis predicting intimate relationship violence (CTS violence subscale scores). Note that this table provides only unstandardized regression coefficients (Bs); standardized coefficients (βs; betas) are omitted, because they are not as useful in interpreting interactions in moderated multiple regression. As shown in Table 15.2, at Step 1, relationship quality as measured by the DAS is the only significant variable. As one might predict, higher levels of relationship quality are associated with lower amounts of intimate relationship violence. The weighted composite of the three independent variables (DAS, SRES, gender) yielded a multiple correlation coefficient (R) of .201; 4% (the square of .201) of the variance in intimate relationship violence was accounted for by this composite.

When the interaction term (gender × SRES) was entered into the regression equation at Step 2, the value of R increased to .287, indicating that just over 8% (the square of .287) of the variance in intimate relationship violence was accounted for by the weighted composite (DAS, SRES, gender, gender × SRES). The significance of this increment (from 4% to 8%) is represented either in terms of a significant F statistic for the R^2 change, provided by many statistical software packages, or easily calculated (Cohen &

TABLE 15.2. Hierarchical Multiple Regression Results

Step	Variables in equation	Unstandardized coefficient (B)	Standard error	t	R
1	Intercept	1.837	.519	3.542***	
	DAS	−.049	.020	−2.395*	
	SRES	−.030	.021	−1.430	
	Gender	−.363	.621	−.585	.201
2	Intercept	1.415	.526	2.690***	
	DAS	−.046	.020	−2.306*	
	SRES	−.119	.035	−3.382**	
	Gender	−.030	.618	−.048	
	Gender × SRES	.135	.043	3.115**	.287

Note. DAS, Dyadic Adjustment Scale; SRES, Sex-Role Egalitarianism Scale.
*$p < .05$; **$p < .01$; ***$p < .001$.

Cohen, 1983; Cohen et al., 2002). The same information is carried in the significant t statistic (3.115) accompanying the regression coefficient for the interaction term, displayed in Table 15.2. Thus, there is support for the assertion of an interaction between gender and gender role ideology.

Note that, at Step 2, the unique contribution of SRES was significant, whereas at Step 1, it was not. An explanation for this shift can be found in the interpretation of the regression coefficients when interactions are not present versus when they are present. At Step 1, with no interaction being evaluated, the regression coefficient for SRES documents the effect of gender role ideology, holding constant gender and relationship quality. At Step 2, with the introduction of the interaction term, the SRES variable is evaluated for the condition in which the gender variable has a value of 0. In particular, its regression coefficient registers the association between gender role ideology and intimate relationship violence for male participants in the study, controlling for DAS. In this example, the regression coefficient is negative (−.119), indicating that as SRES scores increase toward the egalitarian end of the dimension, men tend to commit fewer acts of violence toward their partners. Conversely, the nonsignificant gender effect at Step 2 tells us that there is likely no difference between women and men in the amount of violence they perpetrate at an SRES value of 0, the mean SRES score following centering, again controlling for DAS. The intercept at Step 2 (1.415) denotes the score on the CTS violence subscale for men (coded 0) with an average score on the SRES (0) and on the DAS (0).

Using the regression coefficients from Step 2 of the multiple regression results, we can develop the equation for the regression of intimate relationship violence on relationship quality, gender role ideology, gender, and the interaction between gender and ideology. For simplicity, we drop the *i* sub-script but retain the e component in recognition of error in prediction.

$$Y = 1.415 - .046X_D - .119X_S - .030X_G + .135X_GX_S + e \qquad \text{(Eq. 5)}$$

where Y is the predicted CTS score for person i, X_D is the DAS score, X_S is the SRES score, X_G is gender, and X_GX_S is the interaction term for person i. We may use this equation to address further our key research question re-garding differential relationships between intimate relationship violence (Y) and gender role ideology (X_S) as a function of gender (X_G). Arranging terms in a manner similar to that depicted in Equations 3 and 4, we have

$$Y = (1.415 - .046X_D - .030X_G) + (-.119 + .135X_G)X_S + e \qquad \text{(Eq. 6)}$$

Substituting the mean DAS value (0), and alternative values for gender (1 and 0), we can develop two equations, one for the regression of violence on ideology for women, and one for men. For women, our equation becomes

$$Y = (1.415 - .046*0 - .030*1) + (-.119 + .135*1)X_S + e \qquad \text{(Eq. 7)}$$
$$Y = 1.385 + .016X_S + e \qquad \text{(Eq. 8)}$$

For men, the equation is

$$Y = (1.415 - .046*0 - .030*0) + (-.119 + .135*0)X_S + e \qquad \text{(Eq. 9)}$$
$$Y = 1.415 - .119X_S + e \qquad \text{(Eq. 10)}$$

Observe that the intercept and slope for men recapitulates the interpreta-tions stated previously.

   The two regression lines are graphed as Figure 15.2. It appears that the relationship between ideology and violence for women is only very slightly positive (regression coefficient of .016), whereas the relationship for men tends to be negative and stronger (regression coefficient of –.119). The sig-nificant regression coefficient for the gender × ideology interaction (Table 15.2) tells us that these relationships differ as a function of gender, and the value of this regression coefficient (.135) is the actual difference between the separate regression coefficients [.016 – (–.119) = .135]. But we can go further yet and determine the significance of the relationship within each gender, which is very likely of much interest to gender differences research-ers.

   Jaccard et al. (1990), among others, have provided a mechanism for evaluating the significance of the relationship between two continuous vari-ables within each group defining the levels of a moderator variable. This

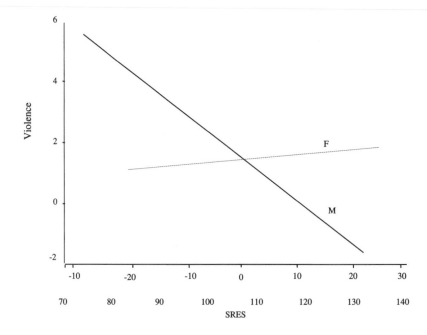

FIGURE 15.2. Association between gender role ideology and intimate relationship violence for women and men. Upper: centered scores; lower: raw scores.

procedure involves the computation of the standard error of the regression coefficient within a group, derived as a function of the variances and covariances among the components used to calculate that regression coefficient. To illustrate, in creating the regression equation for women in our sample (Eq. 7 and Eq. 8), two elements produced the final regression coefficient, −.119 and .135. These are the regression coefficients for SRES and gender × SRES taken from Table 15.2. Using the variances and covariance of these two elements—available as a part of multiple regression programs within most statistical software packages—standard errors can be calculated (see Jaccard et al., 1990, Appendix A), and tests of significance can be performed. For our data, the ideology–violence relationship was nonsignificant for women, $t(214) = .64$, NS, and significant for men, $t(214) = −3.38$, $p < .01$. An alternative method for directly computing and evaluating individual group simple slopes is provided by Cohen et al. (2002).

Additional Comments and Recommended Resources

Our presentation of moderated multiple regression necessarily is introductory and therefore limited and incomplete. Beyond the analyses already demonstrated, more questions can be answered about the nature of an interaction involving gender as a moderator variable. For example, as mentioned earlier, centering a predictor and dummy coding gender enables one to interpret the significance of the gender main effect at the mean of the predictor. But one can also go further and determine the significance of the difference between women and men on the outcome at any value of the predictor. In addition, in some circumstances, the researcher might wish to incorporate a curvilinear relationship between predictor and outcome, and propose that this relationship differs for women and men. The moderated multiple regression procedure allows for power polynomials and other strategies for assessing such curvilinearity. A three-way interaction between gender and two continuous predictors is possible, yielding information regarding differences in the interaction of the two continuous variables as a function of gender. Moreover, other categorical variables can be crossed with gender—race or ethnic identity and sexual orientation come to mind—and appropriately coded and included in the analysis to address more sophisticated questions about gender interactions. A set of multiple predictors also may be simultaneously incorporated in interaction with gender.

There are a few caveats in the search for gender differences in relationships using this methodology. Foremost is that interactions are often difficult to detect and replicate (Zedeck, 1971). What is more, when significant, the effect sizes are typically quite small, accounting for as little as 1–3% of the variance in the dependent variable (Champoux & Peters, 1987; McClelland & Judd, 1993). Interaction terms are known to be less reliable than their components and yield biased underestimates of their regression parameters. Nonetheless, moderated multiple regression, retaining the full range of scores on a predictor variable, is judged far superior to adopting a simple 2 × 2 factorial configuration, where scores on the predictor are dichotomized at some cutpoint (Cohen, 1983; West, Aiken, & Krull, 1996).

A few recommendations for further reading include the classic work by Cohen and Cohen (1983) and its successor (Cohen et al., 2002), and the texts by Darlington (1990), Draper and Smith (1998), and Pedhazur (1997), which provide comprehensive treatments of multiple regression and its applications, including interactions. The monographs by Jaccard et al. (1990) and Aiken and West (1991) focus exclusively on the analysis and interpretation of interactions and expand and supplement the issues presented here. There are many articles in the scientific literature on interactions and moderator variables. Among them are two of special note given the context of this section of the chapter: McClelland and Judd (1993) detailed reasons for failure to find or replicate interaction effects in field research, and Jaccard and Wan (1995) followed with an excellent assessment of problems with the reliability of interaction effects, closing with a suggestion for latent variable analysis (a topic to be introduced in the next section of this chapter). We also recommend the article by West et al. (1996), a demonstration of the analysis of interactions between categorical and continuous variables in the context of personality research; its content can easily be extrapolated to research on stress, trauma, and PTSD. Finally, O'Connor (1998) offers useful and free SAS and SPSS scripts to aid in the graphing of interactions. His programming was used to graph the interaction for this moderated multiple regression (Figure 15.2).

MULTIPLE-GROUP CONFIRMATORY FACTOR ANALYSIS

In our experience, PTSD theoreticians, researchers, and clinicians often pose the question of whether PTSD as a clinical entity or psychological variable is really the same for women as it is for men. This question of comparability of PTSD over genders addresses the issue of construct equivalence as represented in the literature on factorial invariance in confirmatory factor analysis (e.g., Byrne, Shavelson, & Muthen, 1989; Hancock, Stapleton, & Berkovits, 1999; Little, 1997; McArdle & Cattell, 1994; Meredith, 1993). In effect, the examination of factorial invariance can be couched in terms of the general theme of this chapter: here, the extent to which the relationship between a psychological construct, factor, or latent variable (PTSD) and scores on a manifest indicator of that variable (how an individual answers a PTSD item or set of items), differs for women compared to men. In this section, we concentrate on the confirmatory factor-analytic aspect of structural equation modeling. First, we provide a brief conceptual introduction to confirmatory factor analysis. Second, we discuss multiple-group modeling in confirmatory factor analysis and place the topic of factorial invariance in the context of gender differences. Third, we use an existing data set from a large-scale study of female and male Gulf War veterans to demonstrate a multiple-group confirmatory factor analysis. As before, we conclude with some commentary on issues and concerns, and recommendations for further reading.

Overview of Confirmatory Factor Analysis

Confirmatory factor analysis is a subset of the class of procedures known as structural equation modeling (e.g., Bollen, 1989; Bollen & Long, 1993; Hayduk, 1987, 1996; Hoyle, 1995; Kline, 1998; Loehlin, 1998; Marcoulides & Schumacker, 1996; Schumacker & Lomax, 1996; Schumacker & Marcoulides, 1998). It is the methodology associated with the specification and evaluation of the measurement component of a proposed structural equation model. This measurement component portrays hypothetical constructs or latent variables in terms of their observed scores or manifest indicators, typically, responses to items on some psychometric instrument.

Confirmatory factor analysis is used to test hypotheses about the underlying structure of the data; in other words, to what extent are there common entities or factors responsible for relationships or covariance patterns among the observed scores? The researcher must propose a priori a structure based on theory and/or previous factor analyses (exploratory or confirmatory), and then test how well the proposed structure fits the observed data.

To place confirmatory factor analysis in the context of multiple regression, as discussed in the previous section, we can express an individual's observed score on a particular PTSD item as follows:

$$Y_{ij} = B_{Y0} + B_{Y1}F_{i1} + B_{Y2}F_{i2} + \ldots + B_{Yk}F_{ik} + r_{ij} \qquad \text{(Eq. 11)}$$

In this equation, the dependent variable (Y_{ij}) represents a score for person i on item j. The independent variables (F_{i1}, F_{i2} ... F_{ik}) are scores on factors or latent variables for person i. These scores are not observed, and the number of factors is indeterminate and must be designated in advance by the researcher. As in the multiple regression equation described in the first section of this chapter, B_{Y0} is the Y-intercept, and B_{Y1}, B_{Y2} ... B_{Yk} are slopes or regression coefficients. In this case, they are called "factor loadings" and denote the contribution of each factor or latent variable to the prediction of the observed score. The more a factor is implicated in an observed score, the stronger will be the factor loading or regression coefficient. The residual, a composite of both error and specificity carried by the observed score or manifest indicator, is symbolized as r_{ij}. For a given confirmatory factor analysis, there are as many equations as there are items or manifest indicators (Weathers, Keane, King, & King, 1997).

In proposing a factor structure in a confirmatory factor analysis, the researcher stipulates whether the intercepts, regression coefficients (factor loadings), and residuals of these equations, as well as factor means and factor variances, are to be estimated, or whether they should take on a specified value, usually 0 or 1. Such decisions essentially define the hypothesized pattern of loadings, the number of factors, which factors are predictors of which manifest indicators, and characteristics of the latent variable(s). One or more of these elements also may be subject to equality constraints, wherein they are specified to be equivalent to other elements, or some function of other elements. Additional considerations in model specification include whether the factors will be allowed to associate with one another, and whether residuals will be free to covary. Under most conditions, each manifest indicator is specified to load on only one factor; its loading on the other factors are fixed at 0 to facilitate interpretation of the solution. Also, residuals are normally not free to covary in confirmatory factor analysis. As a consequence of these decisions, a conceptual "mapping" of the postulated factor structure results, including a factor loading matrix augmented by intercepts for the regression of manifest indicators on factor scores, a matrix of residual variances for the manifest indicators, a matrix of variances and covariances among the factors, and a vector of factor means.

A number of methods for estimating the parameters in the hypothesized factor structure are available. Each seeks to optimize the "fit" between relationships actually observed in the data (typically characteristics of the manifest indicators: their means, variances, and covariances) and those that can be reproduced from the parameter estimates (intercepts, loadings, variances, etc.) in the hypothesized factor structure. Under certain assumptions, and for designated estimation procedures, the resulting fit function, a weighted sum of squared deviations multiplied by the number of cases minus 1, yields a noncentral chi-square statistic. Its degrees of freedom are equal to the difference between the number of means, variances, and unique covariances among the manifest indicators, and the number of parameters estimated in the model. An estimate of the noncentrality parameter is equal to the value of the computed noncentral chi-square minus the number of degrees of freedom. (The noncentrality parameter and the degrees of freedom are required to define the noncentral chi-square distribution.)

Low values of chi-square, relative to the degrees of freedom, indicate good fit and thus support the hypothesized factor structure. High values of chi-square, relative to the degrees of freedom, cast doubt upon the researcher's a priori factor structure. Given inherent problems with the chi-square statistic as the sole index of model–data fit, several additional goodness-of-fit indices have been developed (for profiles of those available, see Hu & Bentler, 1995, 1998; Joreskog & Sorbom, 1993a; Marsh, Balla, & McDonald, 1988). The more prominent fit indices at this writing include the Tucker–Lewis index (TLI; Bentler & Bonett, 1980; Tucker & Lewis, 1973), the comparative fit index (CFI; Bentler, 1990), the LISREL goodness-of-fit index (GFI; Joreskog & Sorbom), the root mean square error of approximation (RMSEA; Steiger, 1990), and the standardized root mean square residual (SRMR; Hu & Bentler, 1998). As we demonstrate later, there are procedures for evaluating the best among a series of competing models.

Multiple-Group Modeling: The Search for Construct Equivalence

Within the realm of structural equation modeling—and particularly for confirmatory factor analysis—we have the capability to pose questions about the similarity or equivalence of networks of relationships across two or more mutually exclusive groups. When multiple-group modeling is applied to confirmatory factor analysis, we are asking the extent to which a postulated factor structure holds across groups. In the earlier section on moderated multiple regression, we emphasized differential relationships between predictors and outcomes as a function of gender. In multiple-group confirmatory factor analysis, the representation is parallel, with manifest indicators being outcomes or dependent variables, and the factors being predictors or independent variables. There are slopes and intercepts, and they may or may not differ across genders. For example, when women and men respond to items on the PCL in reference to a common traumatic event (e.g., a natural disaster within their community, exposure to political terror and violence in their homeland, service in a war zone), we may be interested in whether the 17 items, scored for severity, have the same meaning for women and men. Stated another way, to what degree do the same factors appear relevant across genders and seem to contribute equally to reports of symptom severity for women and men? Other questions are also possible, the important point being that multiple-group confirmatory factor analysis supplies a mechanism for assessing comparability of factor structures for women and men (or any other grouping typology of interest).

The process of determining group differences in factor structures involves evaluation of a sequence of nested factor models. One model is said to be nested within another model when the pattern of associations present in the former is the same as for the latter, but there are fewer parameter estimates in the former than in the latter. A factor-analytic model having a larger number of parameter estimates is said to be more saturated than a model with a smaller number of parameter estimates. Other conditions held constant, the larger the number of parameter estimates in a model, the smaller will be the value of the chi-square statistic, which, as noted earlier, is an index of the discrepancy between the means, variances, and unique covariances of the observed data, and those reproduced by the proposed model. Put another way, the more information in the proposed model—a larger number of parameters being estimated with fewer degrees of freedom—the closer will be the model–data fit. The goal of science, of course, is parsimony, the quest to explain observed behavior or any other phenomenon as simply as possible (Mulaik & James, 1995). Therefore, for any structural equation modeling endeavor, we desire to represent our observations with a model containing a minimum of superfluous, irrelevant, or unnecessary parameters. As we evaluate or compare a series of nested models, we are searching for the simplest, least parameterized model that also retains strong model–data fit.

With regard to differences between factor structures for women and men, the test of nested models primarily emphasizes the notion of equivalence: Are the parameters that describe the factor structure for women equivalent to the parameters that describe the factor structure for men? Which are equivalent, and which are not equivalent? If two parameters are set equal to one another in a structural equation model, only one parameter is actually being estimated, not two. A multigroup confirmatory factor-analytic model with equality constraints on, for example, the factor loadings across groups, has fewer parameter estimates than one with factor loadings estimated separately for each group. Hence, a model with equality constraints is nested within a model without such constraints. By systematically imposing equality constraints of parameters across genders, we are able to compare more constrained with more saturated models and evaluate equivalence, thereby appraising gender differences.

A number of statistical methods are available for comparisons among constrained models. A frequently used approach is the test of significance of the difference between the chi-square statistics for two nested models. Keeping in mind that the chi-square statistic for a more constrained model is likely greater than (and never less than) that for a more saturated model, and that the chi-square statistic is an indicator of "misfit," the concern is whether the imposition of an equality constraint damages (as evidenced by an increase in chi-square) the model–data fit sufficiently to declare that the parameter(s) should not be constrained to be equivalent. Alternatively, is the damage so minor that a more parsimonious model (with equivalent values for the parameters across groups) is a better representation of the data? Sequential chi-square difference testing (Anderson & Gerbing, 1988; Steiger, Shapiro, & Browne, 1985), with the difference between two chi-square statistics evaluated at the difference between their associated degrees of freedom, assists in making these judgments. It has been suggested (e.g., Little, 1997) that the chi-square difference test may be too sensitive. Other statistics are available, including the Akaiki information criterion (AIC; Akaiki, 1987), corrected Akaiki information criterion (Bozdogan, 1987), expected cross-validation index (ECVI; Browne & Cudeck, 1993), and Bayesian information criterion (BIC; Muthen & Muthen, 1998). The values of these indices carry no meaning in and of themselves; they are used to determine the best of a series of models, with preference given to models having values closer to 0. The researcher consults the chi-square difference test results in conjunction with these indices to reach conclusions about which model best fits the data.

What remains before we proceed to our example using real data is a brief discussion of exactly what constraints should be applied and in what order to examine gender differences in factor structures. Equality constraints can be applied to intercepts, factor loadings, residuals, factor variances, and factor covariances. Moreover, it is not necessary to constrain all intercepts, all factor loadings, all residuals, and so on, across genders; rather, particular pairs within each of these categories might be chosen, based on some rationale or theoretical basis. Joreskog and Sorbom (1993b) provide a guide to conducting tests of equivalence using the LISREL software, beginning with an evaluation of the equivalence of the observed variances and covariances across groups, then proceeding to evaluations of the equivalence of the number of factors and pattern of loadings (configural invariance), the values of the loadings (factorial or metric invariance), the values of the residuals, and, finally, the values of the factor variances and covariances. Marsh (1994) proposed a slightly different progression, beginning with the test of configural invariance, then factorial invariance, followed by equivalence of factor covariances, variances, and residuals. He commented that invariance of factor variances and invariance of measurement residuals are usually of lesser substantive importance to the equality of factor structures.

Meredith (1993) and Little (1997) argued that a demonstration of "strong factorial invariance" requires the equality of both intercepts and factor loadings. They specifically noted that the residuals should be free to vary across groups, reasoning that the imposition of equality constraints on the residuals would introduce bias into estimates of other model parameters. They also distinguished between a measurement level of invariance, concerned with intercepts and factor loadings, and a latent level of invariance, concerned with factor means, variances, and covariances. Byrne et al. (1989) introduced partial factorial invariance as a less stringent requirement in exploring the equivalence of factor structures. From their perspective, it might be sufficient to demonstrate that equality constraints on a single intercept and a single factor loading are all that are required. Hancock et al. (1999) supported this position. Obviously, consensus on what constitutes equivalence of factor structures is not yet achieved.

Demonstration of Multiple-Group Confirmatory Factor Analysis Using Existing Data

Description of the Data

For the purposes of example, we now introduce analyses on a portion of data from a longitudinal study of Gulf War veterans. The original data collection occurred within 5 days of the soldiers' return from the Gulf region in 1991 (for additional details, see Wolfe, Erickson, Sharkansky, King, & King, 1999). Follow-up data collections occurred in 1992–1993 and 1997–1998. Data presented here were obtained in the initial 1991 assessment. The sample consisted of 2,949 Army personnel deployed from and returning to Ft. Devens, Massachusetts: 240 women and 2,702 men, with 823 from regular active duty status, 587 from the Reserves, and 1,505 from the National Guard. The focal instrument was the Mississippi Scale for Combat-Related PTSD (Keane et al., 1988), modified for Gulf War personnel (Wolfe, Brown, & Kelley, 1993). To provide a reasonably straightforward demonstration of multiple-group confirmatory factor analysis, we created four composite, or subscale, scores from responses to the 35 items on this scale: a simple average item score across 11 items measuring reexperiencing and situational avoidance, 11 items measuring withdrawal and numbing, 8 items measuring arousal and lack of behavioral or emotional control, and 5 items measuring self-persecution (guilt and suicidality) (King & King, 1994). The primary research question of interest is: Does the structure of PTSD, as measured by the four subscales of the Mississippi Scale, differ as a function of gender? Placed in terms of the guiding theme of this chapter, does the relationship between the hypothetical construct of PTSD and its four manifest indicators differ for women and men?

Analyses

Analyses were accomplished using Arbuckle's (1997) AMOS software package. A series of nested, single-factor means and covariance structures, multiple-group confirmatory factor analyses was conducted using maximum likelihood estimation. The most saturated model, the one with the largest number of estimated parameters, was one in which both the intercepts and loadings, as well as the residuals, were estimated. For the next model in the series, we constrained the factor loadings to be equivalent for women and men. The third model constrained the intercepts to be equivalent. And the fourth model placed equality constraints on the factor variances. Because the model contained only one factor, there were no factor covariances to be considered. Various indices of fit and relative fit, available from the AMOS software, were used to evaluate the strengths of the several models.

Results and Their Interpretation

Table 15.3 presents the results of analyses of the nested, multiple-group models. The first row of Table 15.3 summarizes the findings for the most saturated model and supports an assertion for configural invariance across genders; that is, for both women and men, a single-factor model with four manifest indicators of the PTSD construct appears to provide a reasonably good representation of the observed data. Evidence for this assertion is best seen in the values for the two incremental fit indices, the TLI and the CFI. Both exceed the .95 criterion of good fit recently mandated by Hu and Bentler (1998). Moreover, the value for the RMSEA is less than .05, another standard of good fit set forth by Browne and Cudeck (1993).

The second row of Table 15.3 reports the findings for a model in which the factor loadings are equivalent across genders. When this model is compared to the most saturated model, the chi-square difference ($\Delta\chi^2$) is nonsignificant, indicating that constraining loadings to be equivalent and the attendant change in degrees of freedom (Δdf), do not significantly damage model–data fit. Furthermore, there is a drop in the values of the AIC and the ECVI, the two indices specifically intended to compare models. These decreases also suggest that the more parsimonious, equal-factor loadings model is a better representation of the data. The RMSEA likewise

TABLE 15.3. Results of Multiple-Group Confirmatory Factor Analysis

Model	χ^2	df	TLI	CFI	RMSEA	90% CI	AIC	ECVI	$\Delta\chi^2$	df
1. Saturated	31.501	4	.996	.999	.048	.034–.065	79.501	.027		
2. Equal factor loadings	35.673	7	.998	.999	.037	.036–.050	77.673	.026	4.172	3
3. Equal factor loadings and equal intercepts	151.561	10	.992	.996	.069	.060–.079	187.561	.064	115.888[*]	3
4. Equal factor loadings, equal intercepts, and equal factor variances	165.216	11	.992	.996	.069	.060–.079	199.216	.068	13.665[*]	1

Note. TLI, Tucker–Lewis Index; CFI, comparative fit index; RMSEA, root mean square error of approximation.
[*]$p < .001$.

decreases in value, a good sign that fit is enhanced with this model. TLI and CFI remain high.

On the other hand, adding the constraint that the intercepts be equivalent across genders is probably not advisable. As shown in the third row of Table 15.3, when this constraint is added, there is a significant increase in the chi-square, accompanied by large increases in the AIC, ECVI, and RMSEA. The RMSEA increases above the .05 recommended cutpoint. In fact, its 90% confidence interval (.060–.079) does not enclose the value .05. Thus, it is better to consider leaving the separate intercepts for women and men free to vary, and conclude that they differ from one another. Information in the fourth row of Table 15.3 indicates that it is also unwise to constrain the variance of the PTSD factor to be equivalent across genders. Consequently, the model that best fits the data is one in which the factor loadings for women and men are equivalent but the intercepts and factor variances are different.

The models of best fit are depicted in Figures 15.3 and 15.4. These displays incorporate what is known as reticular action model (RAM) theory (McArdle & Boker, 1990; McArdle & McDonald, 1984) conventions for presenting a structural equation model. Equations in the form of Equation 11 can be written directly from Figures 15.3 and 15.4. On each display, the large circle represents the PTSD latent variable; the squares represent the four manifest indicators, our observed subscale scores; the smaller circles represent residuals; the small horseshoe-shaped, double-headed arrow, a sling, associated with the PTSD latent variable, represents the factor variance; the same type of horseshoe-shaped, double-headed arrows attached to the residuals represent residual variance; and the triangle is a constant

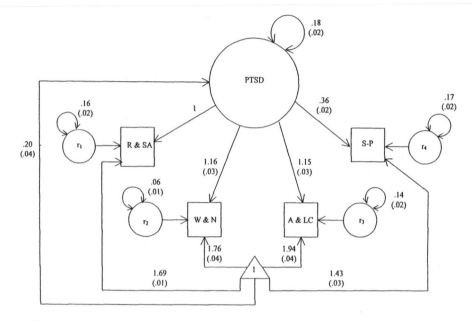

FIGURE 15.3. Graphical representation of the factor-analytic model for women. PTSD, posttraumatic stress disorder; R & SA, reexperiencing and situational avoidance; W & N, withdrawal and numbing; A & LC, arousal and lack of control; S-P, self-persecution (guilt and suicidality).

used to represent means and intercepts. Values are also shown for all parameter estimates, with their standard errors in parentheses. All parameter estimates for both women and men have critical ratios (the estimate divided by its standard error) that exceed 2.00. Although the sampling distribution of these critical ratios is not exactly known, Joreskog and Sorbom (1993b) noted that a value greater than 2.00 suggests statistical significance at $p <$ .05.

Note that the path from the PTSD latent variable to the reexperiencing and situational avoidance manifest indicator has a value of 1, with no standard error for either women or men. Note also that the value for the intercept of the regression of PTSD on this manifest indicator is the same for women as for men, and that the mean of the PTSD latent variable for men is equal to 0. These specific constraints set the origin and scale for the latent PTSD variable, a necessity for model identification. The issue of model identification is very complex; the reader is referred to some of the more comprehensive texts on structural equation modeling (e.g., Bollen, 1989; Kline, 1998; Loehlin, 1998; Schumacker & Lomax, 1996). Many of the commercially available software programs set these particular constraints by default.

Figures 15.3 and 15.4 also provide information about the difference between group means on the latent variable. The mean for the latent variable for men is equal to 0 (see preceding paragraph), and the corresponding mean for women is .20. Its associated critical ratio (.20/.04 = 5.00) represents a test of the significance of this estimate from 0. Therefore, for this example, women's PTSD scores exceeded those of men.

As pointed out by Horn and Meredith (1998), an interpretation of the intercepts in a factor-analytic model is that they are a function of the means of the component of the residual that is specific to the manifest variable itself (and not held in common with the latent factor, in our example, PTSD). For purposes of demonstration, we conducted only an overall test of the equivalence of the intercepts (third row, Table 15.3) and found that somewhere among the intercepts, there is at least one difference across genders. We could go further to evaluate the source of the overall difference: for example, if the single intercept for withdrawal and numbing for women (note the 1.76 value in Figure 15.3) is equivalent to that for men (note the 1.91 value in Figure 15.4), or if the intercept for arousal and lack of control for women (1.94) is equivalent to that for men (1.72). Gender differences in

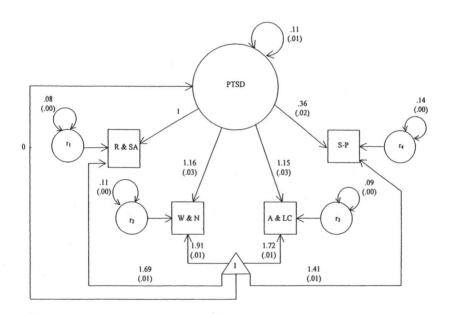

FIGURE 15.4. Graphical representation of the factor-analytic model for men. PTSD, posttraumatic stress disorder; R & SA, reexperiencing and situational avoidance; W & N, withdrawal and numbing; A & LC, arousal and lack of control; S-P, self-persecution (guilt and suicidality).

the intercepts for a particular symptom cluster would suggest that, above and beyond what the four symptom clusters hold in common with one another (presumably, PTSD), women and men differ on another component specific to that cluster, but outside what is PTSD.

Additional Comments and Recommended Resources

Our presentation of multiple-group confirmatory factor analysis might appear somewhat different from most of the published literature that includes this analytic procedure. Typically, confirmatory factor analysis represents what is formally called the analysis of covariance structures, the goal of which is to best reproduce the matrix of variances and covariances among observed scores. We have presented an augmented approach, the analysis of means and covariance structures, the goal of which is to best reproduce the vector of means of the observed scores as well. While slightly more complicated, advantages are obvious in the form of additional information about possible group differences on specific factors, as represented by differences in the intercepts, and group differences in the means of the latent variable(s). Moreover, as suggested by Yung and Bentler (1999), incorporating mean structures into a multiple-group confirmatory factor analysis may yield more stable estimates of the factor loadings.

We also might add that examining differences in relationships between women and men can go beyond confirmatory factor analysis, the measurement component of structural equation modeling, and be applied to the structural component of structural equation modeling. In the latter situation, the concern would be whether associations between latent variables in a theoretical network differ across genders. The basic strategy would be quite similar to that demonstrated in this chapter for the measurement component. Subsequent to establishing factorial invariance, the researcher could test for gender-based differences by means of equality constraints placed on path coefficients and intercepts in the structural model.

As with our discussion of moderated multiple regression, this presentation of multiple-group confirmatory factor analysis is rather cursory. We strongly encourage the interested reader attempting this type of procedure to seek out more extensive treatments of the topic. Among a growing list of very good texts on the larger subject of structural equation modeling are the works of Bollen (1989), Hayduk (1987, 1996), Kline (1998), Loehlin (1998), and Schumacker and Lomax (1996). Additionally, the books edited by Bollen and Long (1993), Hoyle (1995), and Marcoulides and Schumacker (1996) contain chapters that are excellent summaries of special issues in the field. A very approachable ("how to") text on multivariate statistics by Tabachnick and Fidell (1996) contains a chapter on structural equation modeling. McArdle (1996) provided a succinct overview of the confirmatory factor-analytic methodology, directed at the general community of scientists and academics. Finally, Keith (1997) describes an application of confirmatory factor analysis to the process of understanding the construct of intelligence; a similar approach could be taken to explore the structure underlying PTSD and to understand gender differences in PTSD. Journals directly devoted to new developments in structural equation modeling include *Structural Equation Modeling: A Multidisciplinary Journal, Multivariate Behavioral Research, Applied Psychological Measurement,* and the *Journal of Educational and Behavioral Statistics.* Software available for structural equation modeling includes AMOS (Arbuckle, 1997), EQS (Bentler, 1995), Mplus (Muthen & Muthen, 1998), Mx (Neale, 1993), and LISREL 8/SIMPLIS/PRELIS 2 (Joreskog & Sorbom, 1993a, 1993b, 1993c).

REFERENCES

Agresti, A. (1990). *Categorical data analysis.* New York: Wiley.

Aiken, L. S., & West, S. G. (1991). *Multiple regression: Testing and interpreting interactions.* Newbury Park, CA: Sage.

Akaiki, H. (1987). Factor analysis and AIC. *Psychometrika, 52,* 317–332.

Anderson, J. C., & Gerbing, D. W. (1988). Structural equation modeling in practice: A review and recommended two-step approach. *Psychological Bulletin, 103,* 411–423.

Arbuckle, J. L. (1997). *AMOS user's guide.* Chicago: SPSS.

Beere, C. A. (1990). *Gender roles: A handbook of tests and measures.* New York: Greenwood Press.

Bentler, P. M. (1990). Comparative fit indices in structural models. *Psychological Bulletin, 107,* 238–246.

Bentler, P. M. (1995). *EQS structural equations program manual.* Encino, CA: Multivariate Software.

Bentler, P. M., & Bonett, D. G. (1980). Significance tests and goodness of fit in the analysis of covariance structures. *Psychological Bulletin, 88,* 588–606.

Blanchard, E. B., Jones-Alexander, J., Buckley, T. C., & Forneris, C. A. (1996). Psychometric properties of the PTSD Checklist (PCL). *Behaviour Research and Therapy, 34,* 669–673.

Bollen, K. A. (1989). *Structural equations with latent variables.* New York: Wiley.

Bollen, K. A., & Long, J. S. (Eds.). (1993). *Testing structural equation models.* Newbury Park, CA: Sage.

Bozdogan, H. (1987). Model selection and Akaiki's information criteria (AIC). *Psychometrika, 52,* 345–370.

Browne, M. W., & Cudeck, R. (1993). Alternative ways of assessing model fit. In K. A. Bollen & J. S. Long (Eds.), *Testing structural equation models* (pp. 136–162). Newbury Park, CA: Sage.

Byrne, B. M., Shavelson, R. J., & Muthen, B. (1989). Testing for the equivalence of factor covariance and mean structures: The issue of partial measurement invariance. *Psychological Bulletin, 105,* 456–466.

Champoux, J. E., & Peters, W. S. (1987). Form, effect size, and power in moderated regression analysis. *Journal of Occupational Psychology, 60*, 243–255.

Cohen, J. (1983). The cost of dichotomization. *Applied Psychological Measurement, 7*, 249–253.

Cohen, J., & Cohen, P. (1983). *Applied multiple regression/correlation analysis for the behavioral sciences* (2nd ed.). Mahwah, NJ: Erlbaum.

Cohen, J., Cohen, P., Aiken, L. S., & West, S. G. (2002). *Applied multiple regression/correlation analysis for the behavioral sciences* (3rd ed.). Mahwah, NJ: Erlbaum.

Darlington, R. B. (1990). *Regression and linear models.* New York: McGraw-Hill.

Draper, N. R., & Smith, H. (1998). *Applied regression analysis* (3rd ed.) New York: Wiley.

Fitzpatrick, M. F., Salgado, D. M., Suvak, M. K., King, L. A., & King, D. W. (2002). *Associations of gender and gender-role ideology with behavioral and attitudinal features of intimate partner aggression.* Manuscript under review.

Hancock, G. R., Stapleton, L. M., & Berkovits, I. (1999, April). *Loading and intercept invariance within multisample covariance and mean structure models.* Paper presented at the meeting of the American Educational Research Association, Montreal, Canada.

Hayduk, L. A. (1987). *Structural equation modeling with LISREL: Essentials and advances.* Baltimore: Johns Hopkins University Press.

Hayduk, L. A. (1996). *LISREL: Issues, debates, and strategies.* Baltimore: Johns Hopkins University Press.

Horn, J., & Meredith, W. (1998, October). *Factorial invariance in longitudinal research.* Paper presented at the conference on New Methods for the Analysis of Change, State College, PA.

Hosmer, D. W., & Lemeshow, S. (1989). *Applied logistic regression.* New York: Wiley.

Hoyle, R. H. (Ed.). (1995). *Structural equation modeling: Concepts, issues, and applications.* Thousand Oaks, CA: Sage.

Hu, L., & Bentler, P.M. (1995). Evaluating model fit. In R. H. Hoyle (Ed.), *Structural equation modeling: Concepts, issues, and applications* (pp. 76–99). Thousand Oaks, CA: Sage.

Hu, L., & Bentler, P. M. (1998). Fit indices in covariance structure modeling: Sensitivity to underparameterized model specification. *Psychological Methods, 3*, 424–453.

Jaccard, J., Turrisi, R., & Wan, C. K. (1990). *Interaction effects in multiple regression.* Thousand Oaks, CA: Sage.

Jaccard, J., & Wan, C. K. (1995). Measurement error in the analysis of interaction effects between continuous predictors using multiple regression: Multiple indicator and structural equation approaches. *Psychological Bulletin, 117*, 348–357.

Joreskog, K. G., & Sorbom, D. (1993a). *LISREL 8: Structural equation modeling with the SIMPLIS command language.* Chicago: Scientific Software.

Joreskog, K. G., & Sorbom, D. (1993b). *LISREL 8 user's reference guide.* Chicago: Scientific Software.

Joreskog, K. G., & Sorbom, D. (1993c). *PRELIS 2 user's reference guide.* Chicago: Scientific Software.

Keane, T. M., Caddell, J. M., & Taylor, K. L. (1988). Mississippi Scale for Combat-Related Posttraumatic Stress Disorder: Three studies in reliability and validity. *Journal of Consulting and Clinical Psychology, 56*, 95–102.

Keith, T. Z. (1997). Using confirmatory factor analysis to aid in understanding the constructs measured by intelligence tests. In D. P. Flanagan, J. L. Genshaft, & P. L. Harrison (Eds.), *Contemporary intellectual assessment: Theories, tests, and issues* (pp. 373–402). New York: Guilford Press.

King, D. W., King, L. A., Foy, D. W., & Gudanowski, D. M. (1996). Prewar factors in combat-related posttraumatic stress disorder: Structural equation modeling with a national sample of female and male Vietnam veterans. *Journal of Consulting and Clinical Psychology, 64,* 520–531.

King, D. W., King, L. A., Gudanowski, D. M., & Vreven, D. L. (1995). Alternative representations of war zone stressors: Relationships to posttraumatic stress disorder in male and female Vietnam veterans. *Journal of Abnormal Psychology, 104,* 184–196.

King, L. A., & King, D. W. (1993). *Manual for the Sex-Role Egalitarianism Scale: An instrument to measure attitudes toward gender-role equality.* London, Ontario: Research Psychologists Press/Sigma Assessment Systems.

King, L. A., & King, D. W. (1994). Latent structure of the Mississippi Scale for Combat-Related Posttraumatic Stress Disorder: Exploratory and higher-order confirmatory factor analyses. *Assessment, 1,* 275–291.

King, L. A., & King, D. W. (1997). Sex-Role Egalitarianism Scale: Development, psychometric properties, and recommendations for future research. *Psychology of Women Quarterly, 21,* 71–87.

Kline, R. B. (1998). *Principles and practice of structural equation modeling.* New York: Guilford Press.

Kulka, R. A., Schlenger, W. F., Fairbank, J. A., Hough, R. L., Jordan, B. K., Marmar, C. S., & Weiss, D. S. (1990). *Trauma and the Vietnam War generation: Report on the findings from the National Vietnam Veterans Readjustment Study.* New York: Brunner/Mazel.

Little, T. D. (1997). Mean and covariance structures (MACS) analyses of cross-cultural data: Practical and theoretical issues. *Multivariate Behavioral Research, 32,* 53–76.

Loehlin, J. C. (1998). *Latent variable models: An introduction to factor, path, and structural analyses* (3rd ed.). Mahwah, NJ: Erlbaum.

Lunneborg, C. E., & Abbott, R. D. (1983). *Elementary multivariate analysis for the behavioral sciences: Applications of basic structure.* New York: Elsevier/North-Holland.

Marcoulides, G. A., & Schumacker, R. E. (Eds.). (1996). *Advanced structural equation modeling: Issues and techniques.* Mahwah, NJ: Erlbaum.

Marsh, H. W. (1994). Confirmatory factor analysis models of factorial invariance: A multifaceted approach. *Structural Equation Modeling: A Multidisciplinary Journal, 1,* 5–34.

Marsh, H. W., Balla, J. R., & McDonald, R. P. (1988). Goodness-of-fit indexes in confirmatory factor analysis: The effect of sample size. *Psychological Bulletin, 103,* 391–410.

McArdle, J. J. (1996). Current directions in structural factor analysis. *Current Directions in Psychological Science, 5,* 11–18.

McArdle, J. J., & Boker, S. M. (1990). *RAMpath: Path diagram software.* Denver: Data Transforms.

McArdle, J. J., & Cattell, R. B. (1994). Structural equation models of factorial invariance in parallel proportional profiles and oblique confactor problems. *Multivariate Behavioral Research, 29,* 63–113.

McArdle, J. J., & McDonald, R. P. (1984). Some algebraic properties of the reticular action model for moment structures. *British Journal of Mathematical and Statistical Psychology, 37,* 234–251.

McClelland, G. H., & Judd, C. M. (1993). Statistical difficulties of detecting interactions and moderator effects. *Psychological Bulletin, 114,* 376–390.

Meredith, W. (1993). Measurement invariance, factor analysis and factorial invariance. *Psychometrika, 58,* 525–543.

Mulaik, S. A., & James, L. R. (1995). Objectivity and reasoning in science and structural equation modeling. In R. H. Hoyle (Ed.), *Structural equation modeling: Concepts, issues, and applications* (pp. 76–99). Thousand Oaks, CA: Sage.

Muthen, L. K., & Muthen, B. O. (1998). *Mplus user's guide.* Los Angeles: Author.

Neale, M. C. (1993). *Mx: Statistical modeling.* Richmond: Medical College of Virginia.

O'Connor, B. P. (1998). SIMPLE: All-in-one programs for exploring interactions in moderated multiple regression. *Educational and Psychological Measurement, 58,* 836–840.

Pedhazur, E. J. (1997). *Multiple regression in behavioral research: Explanation and prediction* (3rd ed.). Fort Worth: Harcourt Brace.

Schumacker, R. E., & Lomax, R. G. (1996). *A beginner's guide to structural equation modeling.* Mahwah, NJ: Erlbaum.

Schumacker, R. E., & Marcoulides, G. A. (Eds.). (1998). *Interaction and nonlinear effects in structural equation modeling.* Mahwah, NJ: Erlbaum.

Spanier, G. B. (1976). Measuring dyadic adjustment: New scales for assessing the quality of marriage and similar dyads. *Journal of Marriage and the Family, 38,* 15–28.

Spence, J. T., & Helmreich, R. (1972). The Attitudes Toward Women Scale: An objective instrument to measure the attitudes toward the rights and roles of women in contemporary society [Ms. No. 153]. *JSAS: Catalog of Selected Documents in Psychology, 2,* 66–67.

Straus, M. A. (1979). Measuring intrafamily conflict and violence: The Conflict Tactics (CT) Scales. *Journal of Marriage and the Family, 41,* 75–88.

Steiger, J. H. (1990). Structural model evaluation and modification: An internal estimation approach. *Multivariate Behavioral Research, 25,* 173–180.

Steiger, J. H., Shapiro, A., & Browne, M. W. (1985). On the multivariate asymptotic distribution of sequential chi-square statistics. *Psychometrika, 50,* 253–264.

Tabachnick, B. G., & Fidell, L. S. (1996). *Using multivariate statistics* (3rd ed.). New York: HarperCollins.

Tucker, L. R., & Lewis, C. (1973). A reliability coefficient for maximum likelihood factor analysis. *Psychometrika, 38,* 1–10.

Weathers, F. W., Keane, T. M., King, L. A., & King, D. W. (1997). Psychometric theory in the development of posttraumatic stress disorder assessment tools. In J. Wilson & T. M. Keane (Eds.), *Assessing psychological trauma and PTSD* (pp. 98–135). New York: Guilford Press.

Weathers, F. W., Litz, B. T., Herman, D. S., Huska, J. A., & Keane, T. M. (1993, October). *The PTSD Checklist: Reliability, validity, and diagnostic utility.* Paper presented at the annual meeting of the International Society for Traumatic Stress Studies, San Antonio, TX.

West, S. G., Aiken, L. S., & Krull, J. L. (1996). Experimental personality designs: Analyzing categorical by continuous variable interactions. *Journal of Personality, 64,* 1–48.

Wolfe, J., Brown, P. J., & Kelley, J. M. (1993). Reassessing war stress: Exposure and the Persian Gulf War. *Journal of Social Issues, 49,* 15–31.

Wolfe, J., Erickson, D. J., Sharkansky, E. J., King, D. W., & King, L. A. (1999). Course and predictors of posttraumatic stress disorder among Gulf War veterans: A prospective analysis. *Journal of Consulting and Clinical Psychology, 67,* 520–528.

Yung, Y., & Bentler, P. M. (1999). On added information for ML factor analysis with mean and covariance structures. *Journal of Educational and Behavioral Statistics, 24,* 1–20.

Zedeck, A. (1971). Problems with the use of "moderator" variables. *Psychological Bulletin, 76,* 295–310.

16 | Mental Health Policy and Women with PTSD

MARY C. BLEHAR
BRUCE CUTHBERT
KATHRYN M. MAGRUDER

Community lifetime prevalence estimates of posttraumatic stress disorder (PTSD) range from 1.3% to 12.3% (e.g., Davidson, Hughes, Blazer, & George, 1991; Helzer, Robins, & McEvoy, 1987; Kessler, Sonnega, Bromet, Hughes, & Nelson, 1995; Resnick et al., 1993). Moreover, women are fully twice as likely to be affected as men (Hidalgo & Davidson, 2000). Despite this high prevalence and striking gender disparity, little attention has been paid to particular PTSD issues in women. The reason for this discrepancy has most likely been the fact that PTSD originally entered the psychiatric lexicon as a postcombat syndrome (Figley, 1978); therefore, the diagnosis has primarily been associated with male veterans. With the advent of community epidemiological surveys, the scope of PTSD in women has only recently come to be more fully appreciated. A range of traumas may trigger PTSD (Breslau, Chilcoat, Kessler, Peterson, & Lucia, 1999; Kessler et al., 1995), but in women, the diagnosis has been particularly associated with assaultive violence, such as rape. The extent of sexual and physical violence against women, however, and its full significance as a public health problem, remain to be precisely determined. Typically, clinical and intervention studies of PTSD in female victims of sexual assault have been conducted in specialized crisis intervention settings. The impact of PTSD in women not seeking treatment in relation to

The opinions expressed herein are solely those of the authors and do not represent the official policies or positions of the National Institute of Mental Health.

sexual trauma is largely unknown. Furthermore, the salience of assaultive violence overshadows the fact that it does not represent the primary cause of PTSD or the only source of its increased prevalence among women. In the National Comorbidity Survey, the sudden unexpected death of a loved one was a more commonly reported cause of PTSD in the community, accounting for nearly one-third of PTSD cases (Kessler et al., 1995). Thus, the full range of potential traumatic events must be considered for a comprehensive accounting.

In this chapter, we view PTSD in women from a public health perspective. From this perspective, we consider prevalence of PTSD in community and clinical settings, risk factors, sequelae, comorbidity, and associated disability. We note that despite the significance and seriousness of these problems, they receive little attention. Furthermore, we view interventions not only in terms of efficacy but also in terms of effectiveness in multiple settings and their potential to have a public health impact. From this perspective, it is important to view basic neurobiology and clinical research in terms of potential translation into interventions and services that may prevent the onset of symptoms and disorder, and have a beneficial impact on functional outcomes of women with PTSD. We then discuss applied research on screening and interventions, particularly in primary care and obstetrics–gynecology settings. Policy implications of this research will be explored in a final section.

CLINICAL CONSIDERATIONS IN WOMEN WITH PTSD

The vast majority of persons with PTSD meet criteria for at least one other mental disorder, and a substantial percentage have three or more other psychiatric diagnoses (Kessler et al., 1995). The most common co-occurring diagnoses with PTSD are depressive disorders, substance use disorders, and other anxiety disorders. There is a substantial amount of symptom overlap between PTSD and other psychiatric diagnoses, particularly major depressive disorder, and high rates of comorbidity may to some extent reflect this overlap. In any case, symptom overlap may contribute to diagnostic confusion and to underdiagnosis of PTSD, particularly because trauma histories are not specifically obtained in many clinical situations.

There are, however, reports of gender differences in comorbidities. Differences in risk for development of PTSD following exposure to a trauma have been linked to past history of depression and anxiety disorders, and these diagnoses are more common in women than in men. Men with PTSD are more likely to have histories of comorbid alcohol and other substance abuse and dependence. In a Detroit community sample, Breslau, Davis, Andreski, Peterson, and Schultz (1997a; Breslau et al., 1998) examined the relationship between exposure to trauma and rates of PTSD (Breslau,

Chilcoat, Kessler, & Davis, 1999). Preexisting anxiety disorders or major depressive disorders, higher in women than men, played a part in the observed gender difference in PTSD, but even controlling for these factors did not attenuate the difference in PTSD entirely. Lifetime prevalence rates of exposure to traumatic events and number of traumatic events did not vary by gender, but the prevalence of PTSD was higher for women than for men exposed to traumatic events (hazards ratio = 2.3). The gender difference in PTSD was markedly greater if trauma exposure occurred in childhood rather than later.

Other findings (Davidson et al., 1998) indicate that a history of depression is an independent predictor of chronic PTSD, along with specific trauma-related variables. Vulnerability to PTSD following rape has been associated with familial vulnerability to major depression. The authors suggest that some forms of PTSD and depression may share common vulnerability factors, with PTSD representing a type of depression in which neurobiological substrates and clinical phenomenology are modified by extreme stress.

In a clinical description of the sequelae of PTSD, Foa and associates, in a long-term program of research emphasizing female victims of PTSD, note that schemas of the self and the world can be altered on a long-term basis following a trauma such as rape or another crime. Thus, previous schemas of safety and security give way to a more anxiety-provoking view of the environment as a constant threat (Foa & Rothbaum, 1998). In a study of the psychiatric sequelae of PTSD in women, Breslau, Davis, Peterson, and Schultz (1997b) assessed the risk for first-onset major depression, anxiety, and substance use disorders associated with prior PTSD. PTSD signaled increased risk for first-onset major depression (hazards ratio = 2.1) and alcohol use disorder (hazards ratio = 3.0). Women with preexisting anxiety and PTSD had significantly increased risk for first-onset major depression. Additional analysis showed that preexisting major depression increased women's vulnerability to PTSD-inducing effects and risk for exposure to traumatic events.

A growing body of research indicates that the neurobiological consequences of trauma occurring early in development may be more pervasive and long-lasting than trauma occurring in adulthood (e.g., Heim et al., 2000; Weiss, Lonhhurst, & Mazure, 1999). Women with childhood histories of sexual abuse have different comorbidities and a less favorable course than women who have experienced traumas as adults. Women with histories of sexual abuse have higher lifetime rates of attempted suicide—particularly if the sexual trauma occurred before 16 years of age. Chronic PTSD is also associated with both higher rates of childhood risk factors and risk exposures, and more somatic symptoms and functional disability (Davidson, Hughes, George, & Blazer, 1996).

THE NEUROBIOLOGY OF PTSD:
TRANSLATIONAL IMPLICATIONS

The neurobiology of PTSD has received considerable attention in the past two decades, and a more focused picture is gradually coming into view (e.g., Charney, Deutsch, Krystal, Southwick, & Davis, 1993; Yehuda, 2000). Clinical findings in PTSD are also beginning to be integrated with basic research on relevant gender differences in stress and emotional responding.

A substantial body of evidence points to dysregulation of activity in the hypothalamic–pituitary–adrenal (HPA) axis in PTSD. Findings, however, have been somewhat unexpected in view of classic conceptions of the body's stress response. Cortisol levels, known to rise in response to acute stress situations, are diminished in chronic PTSD (e.g., Mason, Giller, Kosten, & Harkness, 1988; Yehuda et al., 1990). These findings, however, are consistent with primate models of extended stress, in which inescapable and unpredictable shocks delivered to rhesus monkeys over a number of weeks resulted initially in elevations of cortisol metabolites but then led to decreases in levels after approximately 4 weeks (e.g., Brady, 1975). An additional clinical finding is that administration of dexamethasone, a synthetic glucocorticoid that normally inhibits cortisol secretion due to negative feedback systems, produces even more exaggerated suppression in PTSD patients.

The "fight-or-flight" model of stress response has been assumed for the most part to apply to males and females equally, but this may not be the case. A small but growing body of work has demonstrated gender differences in animal models of stress (e.g., Shors, Lewczyk, Pacynski, Mathew, & Pickett, 1998). The literature on childhood anxiety disorders consistently indicates that females have higher rates of these disorders than males, particularly after early childhood, and there has been considerable theorizing about the ethological evolutionary bases of these behaviors (Bowlby, 1988). A recent analysis of event-related depression found that women are more likely than men to report an episode following a traumatic life event (e.g., Maciejewski, Prigerson, & Mazure, 2001). Therefore, it is important to integrate research on gender differences in biological vulnerability to stressors with the emergent clinical research findings in PTSD and other mental disorders that disproportionately affect women.

A considerable literature indicates that females are consistently more sensitive to painful stimuli (e.g., Berkley, 1997; Unruh, 1996). Although a variety of factors, including stimulus and social variables, affect pain responses, this overall tendency may contribute to development of PTSD following events that involve actual pain or the threat of aversive stimulation. Furthermore, basic studies of emotion have shown consistently that women are more sensitive to negative stimuli than men, whereas men react more strongly to appetitive stimuli. These effects may be due in part to socialization, but they can nevertheless be measured at all levels, including central nervous system patterns (e.g., Lang et al., 1998). Additionally, hormonal and neurotransmitter systems that regulate stress responses in the body have been studied for their involvement in PTSD, and these systems are modulated by the effects of endogenous sex steroids (McEwen, Alves, Bulloch, & Weiland, 1998).

Levels of catecholamines, such as epinephrine, have also been reported to be elevated in PTSD (Bremner et al., 1997). Among other functions, catecholamines affect the storage and consolidation of memory through actions on the hippocampus. Accordingly, it has been suggested that PTSD may be considered at least in part a disorder of memory, and the intrusive thoughts, dissociation, and other memory-related phenomena in PTSD support this view (e.g., see Pitman, 1989. Studies of memory effects in PTSD may be profitably integrated with the emerging clinical literature on the memory-enhancing impact of estrogen in females (e.g., Costa, Reus, Wolkowitz, Manfredi, & Lieberman, 1999).

Furthermore, the degree of dissociation manifested in the peritraumatic period has been identified as a risk factor for the development of PTSD. Although women are generally found to have higher rates of other dissociative disorders than men, there has been little study of gender differences in dissociation immediately following trauma. Gilboa and Foa (reported in Hembree & Foa, 2000) divided recent rape victims into groups with peak symptoms occurring either immediately after the trauma or 4–6 weeks after the rape. Consistent with the idea that rapid-onset symptoms reflect emotional engagement and processing of the trauma, patients in the first group showed less severe PTSD. In summary, a program of research has yet to elaborate the gender differences in the biology of PTSD, and such elaboration holds considerable promise for clinical applications.

RECOGNITION OF PTSD IN HEALTH CARE SETTINGS

This section focuses primarily on PTSD in primary care and obstetrics–gynecology settings, which have received little attention to date but are especially important when one views PTSD from a public health perspective. In addition to women in primary care settings, a large number of women of childbearing age use obstetrics–gynecology settings for their primary care. Interventions in these settings may benefit large numbers of women who are currently not provided with treatment services for PTSD. Space limitations preclude a thorough consideration of issues regarding services for women with PTSD in mental health and substance abuse treatment settings, but issues raised in this section bear similar relevance to these clinical sites.

Recent evidence indicates that PTSD is common in general medical or specialty mental health settings but largely unrecognized by health care providers. Two studies in general medical settings report prevalences ranging from 6% (Davidson et al., 1998) to 18% (J. Miranda et al., personal communication, 2000). Schonfeld, Verboncoeur, Lipschutz, Lubeck, and Buesching (1997) found PTSD—although largely undetected—to be the second most common mental disorder following major depression in primary care settings. In another study, 95% of women participating in a study of severe premenstrual syndrome reported at least one sexual abuse event, with PTSD present in nearly two-thirds of the abused women (Golding, Taylor, Menard, & King, 2000). A study of PTSD in a mental health clinic found that 25% of outpatients qualified for a PTSD diagnosis, but health care providers detected only one-third of cases (Zimmerman & Mattia, 1999). A study of the occurrence of traumatic events and PTSD symptoms in an inpatient affective disorders sample found that 84% of patients identified at least one traumatic event, and symptoms consistent with PTSD were highly prevalent. However, only 6 of the 343 patients had chart diagnoses of PTSD. More than twice as many women as men showed symptoms of PTSD despite equivalent reports of potentially traumatizing experiences (Escalona, Tupler, Saur, Krishnan, & Davidson, 1997). If PTSD is underrecognized in specialty mental health settings, it then seems probable that it will be even more underrecognized in general health care settings.

Even when other mental disorders (especially depression, panic disorder, and substance abuse disorders) are recognized and treated in primary care or specialty settings, few health care providers query patients about history of traumatic experiences, despite evidence that PTSD may complicate treatment and outcome of other presenting conditions. For instance, in a study conducted in a health maintenance organization, a history of PTSD was associated prospectively with elevated rates of somatic complaints (Andreski, Chilcoat, & Breslau, 1998).

Furthermore, the contribution of sexual trauma and PTSD to a variety of pain conditions is thought to be considerable. Chronic pelvic pain has been estimated to account for 10% of outpatient gynecology consultations, approximately 20% of laparoscopic procedures, and 12% of hysterectomies performed in the United States (Reiter, 1990). However, a significant number of women undergoing these procedures do not report symptomatic improvement. In general, there is evidence that a high proportion of women seeking gynecological treatment for pelvic pain have experienced sexual trauma, including childhood molestation, incest, and rape (Reiter & Gambone, 1990). Golding, in a recent review of the literature, noted that the rates of sexual assault ranged from 26 to 82% in patients with chonic pelvic pain (Golding, 1999). Walker et al. (1995) reported that in a sample of women scheduled for diagnostic laparoscopy, women with chronic pelvic pain reported significantly higher rates of childhood and adult sexual victimization.

Despite the association between chronic pain and abuse in obstetrics–gynecology settings, women are not routinely asked about such experiences. In one study (Robohm & Buttenheim, 1996), 82% of women who experienced sexual abuse as children were not asked about history of abuse, despite reporting more discomfort in a gynecological examination. Rapkin et al. (1990) examined the association between abuse and a variety of painful conditions, and did not find a significantly stronger association between abuse and chronic pelvic pain, and abuse and other kinds of chronic bodily pain. They suggested that abuse experiences many promote chronicity of many painful conditions. Consistent with this hypothesis, Jamieson and Steege (1997) found that all pain syndromes occur with higher frequency in women reporting sexual abuse in either childhood or adulthood. Similarly, fibromyalgia occurs with significantly higher frequency in victims of sexual abuse (Walker et al., 1997). Overall, the evidence indicates that women who have suffered sexual abuse are at risk for a wide variety of adverse health outcomes (Golding, 1999; Walker, Gelfand, et al., 1999), and incur significantly higher health costs (Walker, Unutzer, et al., 1999).

It is highly likely, then, that PTSD is common in both primary care and obstetrics–gynecology settings. Despite its association with high rates of other medical morbidity and cost of care, few studies have documented recognition rates by health care providers or tested the effectiveness of screening interventions for improving the rates of recognition and treatment of PTSD.

It is reasonable, therefore, to consider the benefit of screening for PTSD in such settings, but a number of barriers to recognition and treatment of PTSD pose a challenge to those who would propose screening. The first barrier, inherent in the PTSD syndrome, is that individuals may avoid discussion of the PTSD-precipitating traumatic experience and instead express symptoms somatically. Other barriers include both a lack of health care providers' recognition of the symptoms of PTSD and an appreciation of its potential impact on patient health care. Additionally, the field has been slow to develop screening instruments that can be adapted for use in fast-paced primary care settings. Yet other barriers are found in the service delivery system, including a dearth of effective treatments for PTSD that can be offered in a primary care setting and limited systems for referral of individuals with acute or complicated PTSD to specialty mental health settings. These barriers are considered from the perspective of their impact on women with PTSD.

BARRIERS TO RECOGNITION: PATIENT

Barriers to recognition of PTSD begin at the patient level. PTSD is often difficult to detect, particularly in those whose primary expression of the disorder involves avoidance of trauma-related issues, along with somatization of symptoms. Psychologically distressed primary care patients have a tendency to communicate their distress through somatic symptoms and general medical complaints. This emphasis on somatic symptoms not only limits the ability of the primary care provider to recognize the presence of a mental disorder but also often leads to expensive and unnecessary diagnostic tests and procedures. Moreover, many individuals with PTSD rarely reveal even the slightest hint of severe disorder directly, thus compromising the likelihood of detection in brief primary care visits.

For many women, sexual abuse and violence are experiences so traumatic and humiliating that they are reluctant to disclose them. Unless a woman has had the opportunity to form a confiding relationship with the care provider, there is no assurance that even face-valid screening questions for PTSD will be answered candidly. Hence, even targeted screening techniques may underestimate the impact of PTSD, if patients are not comfortable disclosing relevant experiences. In this regard, it may be useful to assess the potential acceptability to patients of self-screening scales for PTSD, such as those devised by Davidson and colleagues (Davidson et al., 1997; Meltzer-Brody, Churchill, & Davidson, 1999) for comparison with clinical interviews or screening.

BARRIERS TO RECOGNITION: PROVIDER/PRACTICE

At the provider level, lack of clinical competencies in dealing with an elusive disorder such as PTSD almost guarantees a low recognition rate. There is a need to train primary care physicians in initial detection, counseling, and referral procedures, which may help women with PTSD acknowledge symptoms and accept the need for interventions, as well as study the best methods for eliciting information needed to make a diagnosis.

Although significant progress has been achieved in professional primary care training in screening depressive, anxiety, and alcohol use disorders (Ewing, 1984; Eisenberg, 1992; Katon et al., 1995), little or no formal training has been directed toward the detection or education concerning the potential impact of PTSD on general health conditions. Failure to recognize PTSD may in fact contribute to the limited success in dealing with depressive, anxiety, and alcohol use disorders in primary care. Because PTSD symptoms overlap with symptoms of all these disorders, and PTSD is the second most common mental disorder (next to depression) in primary care settings (Schonfeld et al., 1997), it is likely that PTSD may be either the primary disorder (mistakenly identified and treated as depression, panic disorder, or an alcohol-related disorder) or a comorbid condition. In either case, not recognizing PTSD contributes to low treatment success.

At the practice level, the increasing demands on general health care systems to treat high volumes of patients and to operate primary care clinics with high patient–provider ratios necessitate brief and infrequent visits that make difficult the screening and treatment of a wide spectrum of psychiatric and substance use disorders.

The problem of violence against women has been recognized as an issue by obstetricians and gynecologists, who often function as primary care doctors for women of childbearing age. Few resources within this setting, however, are devoted to recognition of clinically significant symptoms of PTSD. The American College of Obstetricians and Gynecologists (ACOG) advocates screening for domestic violence in the clinical setting, but this is not consistently implemented, and many clinicians ask questions only when they suspect domestic violence (Horan, Chapin, Klein, Schmidt, & Shulkin, 1998). Such a procedure may fail to identify many women who might otherwise be identified using systematic screening procedures.

LACK OF SCREENING INSTRUMENTS

Even in primary care systems that feasibly and effectively screen for depressive disorders with brief, reliable, and valid screening tools, the lack of equally effective PTSD screening tools prevents accurate recognition of the disorder and handicaps providers' attempts to recognize the syndrome in their patients. The development of quick screens that are useful in the primary care setting and recognition of the costs of undiagnosed PTSD will likely set the stage for more screening research in this area in the coming years. There are a number of high-quality, psychometrically valid instruments for diagnosing and assessing the severity of PTSD: Mississippi Scale for Combat-Related PTSD (Keane, Caddell, & Taylor, 1988); Clinician-Administered PTSD Scale (Blake et al., 1995); PTSD Checklist (Blanchard, Jones-Alexander, Buckley, & Forneris, 1996; Weathers, Litz, Herman, Huska, & Keane, 1993); MMPI-2/Keane PTSD Subscale (Lyons & Keane, 1992). Nonetheless, there are currently no PTSD screening instruments validated for use in primary care settings. The ideal screening instrument must be brief—much like the CAGE questionnaire for identification of alcohol problems (Ewing, 1984)—in order to be feasibly utilized in a primary care environment. The briefest, validated tool to date (the Mississippi Scale—Short Form) is still 11 items long (Fontana & Rosenheck, 1994). In response to this lack, however, attempts are under way to develop appropriate screening measures. For instance, Read, Stern, Wolfe, and Ouimette

(1997) developed a brief screening measure for use in a primary care center, although no validation against DSM criteria was conducted. In a more extensive study, Breslau, Peterson, Kessler, and Schultz (1999) reported on the development of a seven-symptom screening scale that uses items from the NIMH Diagnostic Interview Schedule (DIS). The authors reported that a cutoff score of 4 on this scale yields sensitivity of 80% and specificity of 97%. To date, however, a limitation of most instruments has been lack of validation against a "gold standard" of clinical assessment for PTSD and the relatively limited age range of study participants.

INTERVENTION ISSUES

Implementation of an effective screening intervention procedure will likely increase recognition rates, with more women requiring treatment for PTSD. This in turn raises the issue of how the health care provider determines the appropriateness of managing these problems in a primary care clinic versus a specialty PTSD treatment setting. Although psychiatric treatment of mild to moderate depression and anxiety disorders in primary care settings has been found to be feasible and effective (Katon et al., 1995; Schulberg et al., 1996), the typical heterogeneity and severity of PTSD and its commonly associated psychiatric and substance-related comorbidities constitute a complexity that often requires specialist intervention. Efficacious treatment approaches for PTSD indicate high-intensity combination pharmacotherapies (Hamner, Horne & Ulmer, 1997; Friedman, Davidson, Mellman, & Southwick, 2000) and a broad spectrum of individual and group psychotherapies (Boudewyns & Hyer, 1990; Cooper & Clum, 1989; Foa & Meadows, 1997; Frueh, Turner, & Beidel, 1995; Frueh, Turner, Beidel, Mirabella, & Jones, 1996; Keane et. al., 1989) that require delivery by specialists outside of primary care.

Until recently there have been no specific approved indications for PTSD among psychotropic drugs commonly prescribed in primary care settings. With the advent of FDA-approved treatments for PTSD using compounds already familiar to general medical practitioners in the treatment of depression, there will likely be increased impetus to screen for PTSD in primary care. A number of selective serotonin reuptake inhibitors (SSRIs) have been found in efficacy studies to offer some benefits for PTSD (for a review, see Davidson, 1997). Sertraline received FDA approval recently for PTSD (Brady et al., 2000). Gender analysis of treatment data from the sample indicated that the compound was efficacious for PTSD in women but not men (K. T. Brady, personal communication, 2000). The reason for this gender difference may reflect greater overall clinical severity and more treatment-resistant comorbidity (e.g., chronic alcoholism) in men than in women in the sample. The

RESEARCH AND POLICY

possibility of biologically mediated gender differences in response to the SSRIs, however, cannot be ruled out (Kornstein et al., 2000). Findings of gender differences in treatment effectiveness highlight yet again the value of a focus on gender issues in treatment settings. On a practical level, a finding such as that reported for sertraline in PTSD treatment will provide renewed impetus for gender analysis of clinical trials.

Despite the likelihood of increased impetus for identification and treatment of PTSD in primary care settings, specialty care, however, will likely be required for many newly diagnosed or severe, chronic PTSD patients. Guidelines need to be developed to ensure appropriate referral to and engagement in the specialty clinics, and for treatment in primary care and mental health service delivery systems.

Given this complexity of PTSD etiologies, diagnoses, and treatments, appropriate referral becomes a critical issue for services research. However, a number of potential obstacles may interfere along the sequence of events: administration of the screening, communication of results to the primary care provider, action taken to refer patients formally from primary care to specialty clinics, and engagement in specialty treatment. Thus, it will be important to develop and test a variety of methods to involve front-line service managers and primary care team leaders, in order to prompt front-line providers to watch for the results of the PTSD screen and to take timely action.

SUMMARY

PTSD has been underrecognized in general health care and many specialty mental health settings. It is a highly prevalent, potentially disabling disorder, twice as common in women as in men. The emerging picture of gender differences and the scope of PTSD in women suggest a number of implications for health policy. First, there is a need to develop better studies of the clinical epidemiology of PTSD in women and its functional impact on clinical course, and to relate these findings to intervention development and services research. There may be practical utility for treatment planning in subtyping PTSD based on patterns of comorbidities.

Research is also needed to provide a basis for assessing the relative utility of screening and referral procedures in different medical settings. With better estimates, the policymaker would be in a better position to allocate the primary care and mental health resources necessary for recognizing and treating PTSD. Given the large number of women using general medical and obstetrics–gynecology settings for primary care, there would seem to be considerable potential to reach a substantial proportion of women with undiagnosed PTSD through screening in these settings.

PTSD differs from other mental disorders in that it is often associated with a clear triggering event. Because of this, there are significant and perhaps unique possibilities for preventive interventions in cases of identifiable traumatic experiences. For instance, it is possible that prophylactic pharmacotherapy in individuals who have experienced a traumatic event will become standard practice. Preventive interventions in turn may reduce the morbidity associated with traumatic events and provide renewed impetus for more screening. Because of the etiological heterogeneity of PTSD, there needs to be assessment of the utility of a variety of pharmacological and psychosocial–behavioral prophylactic approaches in women with a range of trauma experiences. For instance, women with long-standing chronic PTSD, or PTSD related to childhood events, may not be candidates for pharmacological prophylaxis for the primary disorder; but in cases of retraumatization, women may benefit greatly from prophylaxis. Likewise, women with serious mental illnesses may be at increased risk for the development of PTSD; this consideration (and its prevention) may need to become a more integral component of treatment and rehabilitative services.

Women who have no prior history of PTSD but have experienced a traumatic event may also derive considerable benefit from prophylaxis. There is growing appreciation of the range of events that may lead to PTSD or PTSD-like syndromes that cause functional impairment. For instance, the National Comorbidity Study (Kessler et al., 1995) identified sudden loss of a loved one as a common trauma source, but recently bereaved individuals have heretofore received little research attention from the perspective of prevention. Prigerson and colleagues (1997) have identified a syndrome of traumatic grief that has many features in common with full-blown PTSD. By virtue of demographic patterns, this syndrome is more common in older women than in older men or younger persons. With screening and assessment procedures, it may be possible to identify women at high risk for the development of a traumatic grief syndrome and to initiate preventive interventions in those at clinically high risk for traumatic stress syndrome manifestation.

It is also possible to foresee biological assessments for PTSD, such as measuring cortisol and catecholamine activity in mental health care specialty clinics, if not in general medical practice settings such as emergency rooms, where individuals may have experienced a potentially traumatizing event. Such practices would have been entirely impracticable even a few years ago. Within the past decade, however, relatively straightforward assays for salivary cortisol have been developed (e.g., Odber, Cawood, & Bancroft, 1998), with a simple cotton swab to gather the necessary sample. Similarly, assays for the catecholamine metabolites also have become available and can similarly be analyzed readily. These measures could be taken at repeated intervals of 3–6 months for some time after severe traumatic events, such as a rape or a motor vehicle accident, in order to provide a biological marker of subsequent risk for PTSD.

Even without such sophisticated measures, it would be highly important for staff at the care setting to collect a history of prior traumatic events. Such a history could then provide a guide for both prevention and near-term treatment, as well as for awareness of risk for subsequent development of PTSD. Such measures could provide guidelines for those patients who should receive extended treatment following a trauma, including preventive treatments designed to provide some inoculation, if possible, against PTSD onset or exacerbation. Such assessments may also identify patients in whom somatic complaints may indicate undetected PTSD. When women with a traumatic exposure have been identified, there may be considerable additional benefit to identifying those with a past history of depression and anxiety disorders as being at particularly high risk for development of PTSD. Likewise, as indicated previously, there may be value in assessing certain groups (e.g., women with chronic or recurrent affective disorders) for histories of trauma and comorbid PTSD symptoms, because such a history is associated with treatment resistance and poorer long-term outcome.

A substance use disorder comorbid with PTSD may also develop as patients attempt to self-medicate the painful symptoms of PTSD. Withdrawal from substance abuse may exacerbate PTSD symptoms (Brady, Killeen, Brewerton, & Lucerini, 2000). Appropriate treatment of PTSD in substance abusers is a controversial issue because of a widely held belief that addressing issues related to the trauma in early recovery can precipitate relapse. In particular, the issues of treatment of PTSD in women substance abusers have rarely been addressed. These women may benefit from different kinds of treatment approaches integrated into primary care (same-sex groups) than are typically offered for men with these disorders. The high prevalence of sexual abuse and PTSD in women with substance abuse is an additional reason to plan interventions and service settings that facilitate revelation of such experiences in a nonthreatening and supportive environment.

From a longer term, policy perspective, the literature on PTSD augurs the need to provide early and effective interventions for childhood trauma, particularly abuse, in order to provide primary prevention of adverse developmental risk not only for mood and anxiety disorders but also general medical complications that result from dysregulated HPA axis development (e.g., McEwen, 2000). This would require the development of new approaches to screening for trauma and preventive interventions in children, and a new focus on gender differences in childhood vulnerability to the anxiety disorders.

Finally, in order to best inform public policy for women with PTSD, the basic science translation must begin to attend closely to differences in gender-related biological factors that may mediate gender differences in prevalence and clinical course of PTSD. Behavioral differences in stress behaviors relative to gender differences in prevalence and the functional consequences of clinical PTSD in males and females remain an open question. The challenge to integrate behavioral and physiological research from a variety of basic and human studies is with what is known about gender differences in stress response relative to PTSD, the long term consequences of stress such as occurs in PTSD, and gender differences in response to interventions. The benefits to be derived from such translational endeavors seem particularly geared to provide better interventions in both men and women with PTSD and other stress related mental disorders.

REFERENCES

Andreski, P., Chilcoat, H., & Breslau, N. (1998). Post-traumatic stress disorder and somatization symptoms: A prospective study. *Psychiatry Research*, *79*(2), 131–138.

Berkley, K. J. (1997). Sex differences in pain. *Behavioral and Brain Sciences, 20*, 371–380.

Blake, D. D., Weathers, F. W., Nagy, L. M., Kaloupek, S. G., Gusman, F. D., Charney, D. S., & Keane, T. M. (1995). The development of a clinician-administered PTSD scale. *Journal of Traumatic Stress, 8*, 75–90.

Blanchard, E., Jones-Alexander, J., Buckley, T., & Forneris, C. (1996). Psychometric properties of the PTSD checklist. *Behaviour Research and Therapy, 34*, 669–673.

Boudewyns, P. A., & Hyer, L. (1990). Physiological response to combat memories and preliminary treatment outcome in Vietnam veteran PTSD patients treated with direct therapeutic exposure. *Behavior Therapy, 21*, 63–87.

Bowlby, J. (1988). *A secure base: Parent–child attachment and healthy human development*. New York: Basic Books.

Brady, J. V. (1975). Toward a behavioral biology of emotion. In L. Levi (Ed.), *Emotions: Their parameters and measurement* (pp. 17–45). New York: Raven Press.

Brady, K. T., Killeen, T. K., Brewerton, T., & Lucerini, S. (2000). Comorbidity of psychiatric disorders and posttraumatic stress disorder. *Journal of Clinical Psychiatry, 61*, 22–32.

Brady, K. T., Pearlstein, T., Asnis, G. M., Baker, D., Rothbaum, B., Sikes, C. R., & Farfel, G. M. (2000) Efficacy and safety of sertraline treatment of posttraumatic stress disorder: A randomized controlled trial. *Journal of the American Medical Association, 283*(14), 1837–1844.

Bremner, J. D., Randall, P., Veermetten, E., Staib, L., Bronen, R. A., Mazure, C., Capelli, S., McCarthy, G., Innis, R. B., & Charney, D. S. (1997). Magnetic resonance imaging-based measurement of hippocampal volume in posttraumatic stress disorder related to childhood physical and sexual abuse: A preliminary report. *Biological Psychiatry, 41*, 23–32.

Breslau, N., Chilcoat, H. D., Kessler, R. C., & Davis, G. C. (1999). Previous exposure to trauma and PTSD effects of subsequent trauma: Results from the Detroit Area Survey of trauma. *American Journal of Psychiatry, 156*(6), 902–907.

Breslau, N., Chilcoat, H. D., Kessler, R. C., Peterson E. L., & Lucia, V. C. (1999). Vulnerability to assaultive violence: Further specification of the sex difference in post-traumatic stress disorder. *Psychological Medicine, 29*(4), 813–821.

Breslau, N., Davis, G. C., Andreski, P., Peterson, E. L., & Schultz, L. (1997). Sex differences in posttraumatic stress disorder. *Archives of General Psychiatry, 54*(11), 1044–1048.

Breslau, N., Davis, G. C., Peterson, E. L., & Schultz, L. (1997). Psychiatric sequelae of posttraumatic stress disorder in women. *Archives of General Psychiatry, 54*(1), 81–87.

Breslau, N., Kessler, R. C., Chilcoat, H. D., Schultz, L. R., Davis, G. C., & Andreski, P. (1998). Trauma and posttraumatic stress disorder in the community: The 1996 Detroit Area Survey of trauma. *Archives of General Psychiatry, 55*(7), 626–632.

Breslau, N., Peterson, E. L., Kessler, R. C., & Schultz, L. R. (1999). Short screening scale for DSM-IV posttraumatic stress disorder. *American Journal of Psychiatry, 156*(6), 908–911.

Charney, D. S., Deutch, A. Y., Krystal, J. H., Southwick, S. M., & Davis, M. (1993). Psychobiologic mechanisms of posttraumatic stress disorder. *Archives of General Psychiatry, 50*, 294–305.

Cooper, N. A., & Clum, G. A. (1989). Imaginal flooding as a supplementary treatment for PTSD in combat veterans: A controlled study. *Behavior Therapy, 20*, 381–391.

Costa, M. M., Reus, V. I., Wolkowitz, O. M., Manfredi, F., & Lieberman, M. (1999). Estrogen replacement therapy and cognitive decline in memory-impaired postmenopausal women. *Biological Psychiatry, 46*, 182–188.

Davidson, J. R. T. (1997). Biological therapies for posttraumatic stress disorder: An overview. *Journal of Clinical Psychiatry, 58*(Suppl. 9), 29–32.

Davidson, J. R. T., Book, S. W., Colket, J. T., Tupler, L. A., Roth, S., David, P., Hertzberg, M., Mellman, T., et al. (1998). Psychiatric disorders in primary care patients receiving complementary medical treatments. *Comprehensive Psychiatry, 39*, 16–20.

Davidson, J. R. T., Book, S. W., Colket, J. T., Tupler, L. A., Roth, S., David, P., Hertzberg, M., Mellman, T., Beckham, J. C., Smith, R. D., Danson, R. M., Katz, R., & Feldman, M. E. (1998). Assessment of a new self-rating scale for post-traumatic stress disorder. *Psychological Medicine, 27*, 153–160.

Davidson, J. R. T., Hughes, D., Blazer, D. G., & George, L. K. (1991) Posttraumatic stress disorder in the community: An epidemiological study. *Psychological Medicine, 21*(3), 713–721.

Davidson, J. R. T., Hughes, D. C., George, L. K., & Blazer, D. G. (1996) The association of sexual assault and attempted suicide within the community. *Archives of General Psychiatry, 53*(6), 550–555.

Davidson, J. R. T., Rampes, H., Eisen, M., Fisher, P., Smith, R. D., & Malik, M. (1998). Psychiatric disorders in primary care patients receiving complimentary medical treatments. *Comprehensive Psychiatry, 39*, 16–20.

Eisenberg, L. (1992). Treating depression and anxiety in primary care: closing the gap between knowledge and practice. *New England Journal of Medicine 326*, 1080–1083.

Escalona, R., Tupler, L. A., Saur, C. D., Krishnan, K. R. R., & Davidson, J. R. (1997). Screening for trauma history on an inpatient affective-disorders unit: A pilot study. *Journal of Traumatic Stress, 10*(2), 299–305.

Ewing, J. A. (1984). Detecting alcoholism: The CAGE questionnaire. *Journal of the American Medical Association, 252,* 1905–1907.

Figley, C. R. (1978). *Stress disorders among Vietnam veterans: Theory, research and treatment.* New York: Brunner/Mazel.

Foa, E. B., & Meadows, E. A. (1997). Psychosocial treatments for posttraumatic stress disorder: A critical review. *Annual Review of Psychology, 48* 449–480.

Foa, E. B., & Rothbaum, B. O. (1998). Treating the trauma of rape: Cognitive behavioral therapy for PTSD. New York: Guilford Press.

Fontana, A., & Rosenheck, R. (1994). A short form of the Mississippi Scale for Measuring Change in Combat-Related PTSD. *Journal of Traumatic Stress, 7* 407–414.

Friedman, M. J., Davidson, J. R. T., Mellman, T. A., & Southwick, S. M. (2000). Pharmacotherapy. In E. B. Foa & T. M. Keane (Eds.), *Effective treatments for PTSD: Practice guidelines from the International Society for Traumatic Stress Studies* (pp. 326–329). New York: Guilford Press.

Frueh, B. C., Turner, S. M., & Beidel, D. C. (1995). Exposure therapy for combat-related PTSD: A critical review. *Clinical Psychology Review, 15,* 799–817.

Frueh, B. C., Turner, S. M., Beidel, D. C., Mirabella, R. F., & Jones, W. J. (1996). Trauma Management Therapy: A preliminary evaluation of a multicomponent behavioral treatment for chronic combat-related PTSD. *Behaviour Research and Therapy, 34,* 633–643.

Golding, J. M. (1999). Sexual-assault history and long-term physical health problems: Evidence from clinical and population epidemiology. *Current Directions in Psychological Science, 8*(6), 191–194.

Golding, J. M., Taylor, D. L., Menard, L., & King, M. J. (2000). Prevalence of sexual abuse history in a sample of women seeking treatment for premenstrual syndrome. *Journal of Psychosomatic Obstetrics and Gynecology, 21*(2), 69–80.

Hamner, M., Ulmer, H., & Horne, D. (1997). Buspirone potentiation of antidepressants in the treatment of PTSD. *Depression and Anxiety, 5,* 137–139.

Heim, C., Newport, J., Heit, S., Graham, Y. P., Wilcox, M., Bonsall, R., Miller, A. H., & Nemeroff, C. B. (2000). Pituitary—adrenal and autonomic responses to stress in women after sexual and physical abuse in childhood. *Journal of the American Medical Association, 284,* 592–597.

Helzer, J. E., Robins, L. N., & McEvoy, L. (1987). Posttraumatic stress disorder in the general population: Findings of the Epidemiologic Catchment Area survey. *New England Journal of Medicine, 317,* 1630–1634.

Hembree, E. A., & Foa, E. B. (2000). Posttraumatic stress disorder: Psychological factors and psychosocial interventions. *Journal of Clinical Psychiatry, 61,* 33–39.

Hidalgo, R. B., & Davidson, J. R. T. (2000). Selective serotonin reuptake inhibitors in posttraumatic stress disorder. *Journal of Psychopharmacology, 12*(1) 70–76.

Horan, D. L., Chapin, J., Klein, L., Schmidt, L. A., & Shulkin, J. (1998). Domestic violence screening practices of obstetrician–gynecologists. *Obstetrics and Gynecology, 92*(5), 785–789.

Jamieson, D. J., & Steege, J. F. (1997). The association of sexual abuse with pelvic pain complaints in a primary care population. *American Journal of Obstetrics and Gynecology, 177*(6), 1408–1412.

Katon, W., VonKorff, M., Lin, E., Walker, E., Simon, G. E., Bush, T., Robinson, P., & Russo, J. (1995). Collaborative management to achieve treatment guidelines: Impact on depression in primary care. *Journal of the American Medical Association, 273*(13), 1026–1031.

Keane, T. M., Caddell, J. M., & Taylor, K. L. (1988). Mississippi scale for Combat-Related Posttraumatic Stress Disorder: Three studies in reliability and validity. *Journal of Consulting and Clinical Psychology, 56*, 85–90.

Kessler, R. C., Sonnega, A., Bromet, E., Hughes, M., & Nelson, C. B. (1995). Posttraumatic stress disorder in the National Comorbidity Survey. *Archives of General Psychiatry, 52*(12), 1048–1060.

Kornstein, S. G., Schatzberg, A. F., Thase, M. E, Yonkers, K. A., McCullough, J. P., Keitner, G. I., Gelenberg, A. J., Davis, S. M., Harrison, W. M., & Keller, M. B. (2000). Gender differences in treatment response to sertraline versus imipramine in chronic depression. *American Journal of Psychiatry, 157*, 1445–1452.

Lang, P. J., Bradley, M. M., Fitszimmons, J. R., Cuthbert, B. M., Scott, J. D., Moulder, B., & Nangia, V. (1998). Emotional arousal and activation of the visual cortex: An fMRI analysis. *Psychophysiology, 35*,199–210.

Lyons, J. A., & Keane, T. M. (1992). Keane PTSD Scale: MMPI and MMPI-2 update. *Journal of Traumatic Stress, 5*, 111–117.

Maciejewski, P. R., Prigerson, H. G., & Mazure, C. M. (2001). Sex differences in event-related risk for major depression. *Psychological Medicine, 31*, 593–604.

Mason, J. W., Giller, E. L., Kosten, T. R., & Harkness, L. (1988). Elevation of urinary norepinephrine/cortisol ratio in posttraumatic stress disorder. *Journal of Nervous and Mental Disease, 176*, 498–502.

McEwen, B. S. (2000). The neurobiology of stress: From serendipity to clinical relevance. *Brain Research, 886*, 172–189.

McEwen, B. S., Alves, S. E., Bulloch, K., & Weiland, N. G. (1998). Clinically relevant basic science studies of gender differences and sex hormone effects. *Psychopharmacology Bulletin, 34*(3), 251–259.

Meltzer-Brody, S., Churchill, E., & Davidson, J. (1999). Derivation of the SPAN, a brief diagnostic screening test for post-traumatic stress disorder. *Psychiatry Research, 88*, 63–70.

Odber, J., Cawood, E. H., & Bancroft, J. (1998). Salivary cortisol in women with and without perimenstrual mood changes. *Journal of Psychosomatic Research, 45*, 557–568.

Pitman, R. K. (1989). Posttraumatic stress disorder, hormones, and memory. *Biological Psychiatry, 26*, 221–223.

Prigerson, H. G., Bierhals, A. J., Kasl, S. V., Reynolds, C. F., 3rd, Shear, J. K., Day, N., Beery, L. C., Newsom, J. T., & Jacobs, S. (1997). Traumatic grief as a risk factor for mental and physical morbidity. *American Journal of Psychiatry, 154*, 616–623.

Rapkin, A. J., Kames, L. D., Darke, L. L., Stampler, F. M., & Naliboff, B. D. (1990). History of physical and sexual abuse in women with chronic pelvic pain. *Obstetrics and Gynecology, 76*, 92–96.

Read, J. P., Stern, A. L., Wolfe, J., & Ouimette, P. C. (1997). Use of a screening instrument in women's health care: Detecting relationships among victimization history, psychological distress, and medical complaints. *Women and Health, 25*(3), 1–17.

Reiter, R. C. (1990). Chronic pelvic pain. *Clinical Obstetrics and Gynecology, 33,* 117–118.

Reiter, R. C., & Gambone, J. C. (1990). Demographic and historical variables in women with idiopathic chronic pelvic pain. *Obstetrics and Gynecology, 75,* 428–432.

Resnick, H. S., Kilpatrick, D. G., Dansky, B. S., Saunders, B. E., & Best, C. L. (1993). Prevalence of civilian trauma and posttraumatic stress disorder in a representative national sample of women. *Journal of Consulting and Clinical Psychology, 61,* 984991.

Robohm, J. S., & Buttenheim, M. (1996). The gynecological care experience of adult survivors of childhood sexual abuse: A preliminary investigation. *Women and Health, 24,* 59–75.

Schonfeld, W. H., Verboncoeur, C. J., Lipschutz, R. C., Lubeck, D. P., & Buesching, D. P. (1997). The functioning and well-being of patients with unrecognized anxiety disorders and major depressive disorder. *Journal of Affective Disorders, 43*(2), 105–119.

Schulberg, H. C., Madonia, M. J., Block, M. R., Coulehan, J. L., Scott, C. P., Rodriguez, B., & Black, A. (1996). Major depression in primary care practice: Clinical characteristics and treatment implications. *Psychosomatics, 36,* 129–137.

Shors, T. J., Lewczyk, C. L., Pacynski, M., Mathew, P. R., & Pickett, J. (1998). Stages of estrous mediate the stress-induced impairment of associative learning in the female rat. *Neuroreport: An International Journal for the Rapid Communication of Research in Neuroscience, 9,* 419–423.

Unruh, A. M. (1996). Gender variations in clinical pain experience. *Pain, 65,* 123–167.

Walker, E. A., Gelfand, A., Katon, W. J., Koss, M. P., Von Korff, M., Bernstein, D., & Russo, J. (1999). Adult health status of women with histories of childhood abuse and neglect. *American Journal of Medicine, 107,* 332–339.

Walker, E. A., Katon, W. J., Hansom, J., Harrop-Griffiths, J., Jones, M. L., Hickok, L. R., & Russo, J. (1995). Psychiatric diagnosis and sexual victimization in women with chronic pelvic pain. *Psychosomatics, 36*(6), 531–540.

Walker, E. A., Keegan, D., Gardner, G., Sullivan, M., Bernstein, D., & Katon, W. J. (1997). Psychosocial factors in fibromyalgia compared with rheumatoid arthritis: II. Sexual, physical, and emotional abuse and neglect. *Psychosomatic Medicine, 59,* 572–577.

Walker, E. A., Unutzer, J., Rutter, C., Gelfand, A., Saunders, K., VonKorff, M., Koss, M., & Katon, W. (1999). Costs of health care use by women HMO members with a history of childhood abuse and neglect. *Archives of General Psychiatry, 56,* 609–613.

Weathers, F. W., Litz, B. T., Herman, D. S., Huska, J. A., & Keane, T. M. (1993). *The PTSD Checklist (PCL): Reliability, validity, and diagnostic utility.* Paper presented at the Annual Meeting of the International Society for Traumatic Stress Studies, San Antonio, TX.

Weiss, E. L., Longhurst, J. G., & Mazure, C. M. (1999). Childhood sexual abuse as a risk factor for depression in women: Psychosocial and neurobiological correlates. *American Journal of Psychiatry, 156*(6), 816–828.

Yehuda, R. (2000). Cortisol alterations in PTSD. In A. Shalev (Ed.), *International handbook of human response to trauma* (pp. 265–283). New York: Kluwer Academic/Plenum.

Yehuda, R., Southwick, S. M., Nussbaum, G., Wahby, V., Giller, E. L., & Mason, J. W. (1990). Low urinary cortisol excretion in patients with posttraumatic stress disorder. *Journal of Nervous and Mental Disease, 178*, 366–369.

Zimmerman, M., & Mattia, J. L. (1999). Is posttraumatic stress disorder underdiagnosed in routine clinical settings? *Journal of Nervous and Mental Disease, 187*, 420–428.

Index